MANUAL OF OBSTETRIC ANESTHESIA

Second Edition

MANUAL of OBSTETRIC ANESTHESIA

Second Edition

EDITED BY
Gerard W. Ostheimer, M.D.

Professor of Anaesthesia
Harvard Medical School
Interim Chairman
Department of Anesthesia
Brigham and Women's Hospital
Boston, Massachusetts

Churchill Livingstone
New York, Edinburgh, London, Melbourne, Tokyo

Library of Congress Catologing-in-Publication Data
Manual of obstetric anesthesia / edited by Gerard W. Ostheimer. — 2nd ed.
p. cm.
Includes bibliographical references and index.
ISBN 0-443-08743-1
1. Anesthesia in obstetrics—Handbooks, manuals, etc.
I. Ostheimer, Gerard W.
[DNLM: 1. Anesthesia, Obstetrical—handbooks. WO 231 M294]
RG732.M36 1992
617.9'682—dc20
DNLM/DLC
©for Library of Congress 91-36281
CIP

Distributed in the United Kingdom by Churchill Livingstone, Robert Stevenson House, 1–3 Baxter's Place, Leith Walk, Edinburgh EH1 3AF, and by associated companies, branches, and representatives throughout the world.

Accurate indications, adverse reactions, and dosage schedules for drugs are provided in this book, but it is possible that they may change. The reader is urged to review the package information data of the manufacturers of the medications mentioned.

The Publishers have made every effort to trace the copyright holders for borrowed material. If they have inadvertently overlooked any, they will be pleased to make the necessary arrangements at the first opportunity.

Assistant Editor: *Ann Ruzycka*
Copy Editor: *Paul Bernstein*
Production Designer: *Angela Cirnigliaro*
Production Supervisor: *Sharon Tuder*

Printed in the United States of America

First published in 1992 7 6 5 4 3 2 1

To my mother, Margaret A. Ostheimer,
for her unfailing love and support,
and
to Benjamin G. Covino, Ph.D., M.D.,
teacher, researcher, chairman,
whose grand plan we carry on.

Contributors

Katherine Amundson, M.D.
Resident, Department of Anesthesiology, University of Maryland Medical Center, Baltimore, Maryland

John E. Arnold, M.D.
Anesthesiologist, Sharp Memorial Hospital, San Diego, California

Angela M. Bader, M.D.
Assistant Professor, Department of Anaesthesia, Harvard Medical School; Anesthesiologist, Department of Anesthesia, Brigham and Women's Hospital, Boston, Massachusetts

Lori Bannon, M.D.
Clinical Fellow, Department of Anaesthesia, Harvard Medical School; Resident, Department of Anesthesia, Brigham and Women's Hospital, Boston, Massachusetts

William H. Barth, Jr., M.D.
Assistant Chief of Obstetrics, Department of Obstetrics and Gynecology, Wilford Hall United States Air Force Medical Center, Lackland Air Force Base, Texas

David J. Birnbach, M.D.
Assistant Professor, Departments of Anesthesiology and Obstetrics and Gynecology, Columbia University College of Physicians and Surgeons; Director of Obstetric Anesthesia, St. Luke's/Roosevelt Hospital, New York, New York

Corey A. Burchman, M.D.
Chairman, Department of Anesthesiology, U.S. Naval Hospital, Ceiba, Puerto Rico; Clinical Associate, Department of Anesthesia, Massachusetts General Hospital, Harvard Medical School, Boston, Massachusetts

Gerald A. Burger, M.D.
Chairman and Program Director, Department of Anesthesiology, U.S. Naval Hospital, San Diego, California

Randall L. Busch, M.D.
Clinical Fellow, Department of Anaesthesia, Harvard Medical School; Resident, Department of Anesthesia, Brigham and Women's Hospital, Boston, Massachusetts

William R. Camann, M.D.
Assistant Professor, Department of Anaesthesia, Harvard Medical School; Anesthesiologist, Department of Anesthesia, Brigham and Women's Hospital, Boston, Massachusetts

Harvey Carp, Ph.D., M.D.
Assistant Professor, Department of Anesthesia, Oregon Health Sciences University School of Medicine; Director of Obstetric Anesthesia, Department of Anesthesia, University Hospital, Portland, Oregon

Paula D.M. Chantigian, M.D.
Obstetrician and Gynecologist, Olmsted Medical Group, Rochester, Minnesota

Robert C. Chantigian, M.D.
Assistant Professor, Department of Anesthesiology, Mayo Medical School; Director of Obstetric Anesthesia, Mayo Clinic, Rochester, Minnesota

Paul M. Chetham, M.D.
Instructor, Department of Anaesthesia, Harvard Medical School; Anesthesiologist, Department of Anesthesia, Brigham and Women's Hospital, Boston, Massachusetts

Stephen B. Corn, M.D.
Instructor, Department of Anaesthesia, Harvard Medical School; Anesthesiologist, Department of Anesthesia, Brigham and Women's Hospital, Boston, Massachusetts

Mary A. Courtney, M.D.
Instructor, Department of Anaesthesia, Harvard Medical School; Anesthesiologist, Department of Anesthesia, Brigham and Women's Hospital, Boston, Massachusetts

Benjamin G. Covino, Ph.D., M.D.*
Professor, Department of Anaesthesia, Harvard Medical School; Chairman, Department of Anesthesia, Brigham and Women's Hospital, Boston, Massachusetts

Paul Cramp, M.B., Ch.B.
Visiting Assistant Professor, Department of Anesthesiology, Oregon Health Sciences University School of Medicine, Portland, Oregon

Sanjay Datta, M.D.
Associate Professor, Department of Anaesthesia, Harvard Medical School; Director of Obstetric Anesthesia, Brigham and Women's Hospital, Boston, Massachusetts

Gilbert Fanciullo, M.D.
Instructor, Department of Anaesthesia, Harvard Medical School; Anesthesiologist, Department of Anesthesia, Brigham and Women's Hospital, Boston, Massachusetts

Michael J. Fasano, M.D.
Fellow, Obstetric Anesthesia, Department of Anesthesiology, University of Maryland School of Medicine; Resident, Department of Anesthesia, Hospital of the University of Maryland, Baltimore, Maryland

* Deceased.

F. Michael Ferrante, M.D.
Assistant Professor, Department of Anaesthesiology, Harvard Medical School; Director, Pain Treatment Service, Department of Anesthesia, Brigham and Women's Hospital, Boston, Massachusetts

Paul E. Forzley, M.D.
Instructor, Department of Anaesthesia, Harvard Medical School; Anesthesiologist, Department of Anesthesia, Brigham and Women's Hospital, Boston, Massachusetts

John A. Fox, M.D.
Instructor, Department of Anaesthesia, Harvard Medical School; Anesthesiologist, Department of Anesthesia, Brigham and Women's Hospital, Boston, Massachusetts

Philip Hartigan, M.D.
Instructor, Department of Anaesthesia, Harvard Medical School; Anesthesiologist, Department of Anesthesia, Brigham and Women's Hospital, Boston, Massachusetts

Barbara L. Hartwell, M.D.
Assistant Professor, Department of Anaesthesia, Harvard Medical School; Anesthesiologist, Department of Anesthesia, Brigham and Women's Hospital, Boston, Massachusetts

Martha A. Hauch, M.D.
Assistant Professor, Department of Anaesthesia, Harvard Medical School; Anesthesiologist, Department of Anesthesia, Brigham and Women's Hospital, Boston, Massachusetts

Laurel A. Hortvet, M.D.
Anesthesiologist, Department of Anesthesia, Hartford Hospital, Hartford, Connecticut

Timothy Huckaby, M.D.
Director of Anesthesia, Arnold Palmer Hospital for Children and Women, Orlando, Florida

Catherine O. Hunt, M.D.
Anesthesiologist, Department of Anesthesia, Brigham and Women's Hospital, Boston, Massachusetts

Ronald J. Hurley, M.D.
Assistant Professor, Department of Anaesthesia, Harvard Medical School; Associate Director of Obstetric Anesthesia, Department of Anesthesia, Brigham and Women's Hospital, Boston, Massachusetts

Calvin Johnson, M.D.
Assistant Professor, Department of Anesthesiology, Wayne State University School of Medicine; Vice-Chief, Department of Anesthesia, Chief, Section of Obstetric Anesthesia, Hutzel Hospital, Detroit, Michigan

Mark D. Johnson, M.D.
Assistant Professor, Department of Anaesthesia, Harvard Medical School; Anesthesiologist, Department of Anesthesia, Brigham and Women's Hospital, Boston, Massachusetts

Robert M. Knapp, D.O., J.D.
Anesthesiologist, Department of Anesthesiology, Women and Infants' Hospital, Providence, Rhode Island

Robert F. LaPorta, M.D., Ph.D.
Anesthesiologist, North Shore University Hospital, Manhasset, New York

Kathleen A. Leavitt, M.D.
Assistant Professor, Department of Anesthesiology, George Washington University Medical School; Assistant Director of Obstetrical Anesthesia, George Washington University Hospital, Washington, D.C.

Catherine K. Lineberger, M.D.
Associate, Department of Anesthesiology, Duke University School of Medicine; Faculty Anesthesiologist, Duke University Medical Center, Durham, North Carolina

Barbara L. Loferski, M.D.
Instructor, Department of Anaesthesia, Harvard Medical School; Anesthesiologist, Department of Anesthesia, Brigham and Women's Hospital, Boston, Massachusetts

Steven A. Lussos, M.D.
Clinical Fellow, Department of Anaesthesia, Harvard Medical School; Resident, Department of Anesthesia, Brigham and Women's Hospital, Boston, Massachusetts

Eileen P. Lynch, M.D.
Instructor, Department of Anaesthesia, Harvard Medical School; Anesthesiologist, Department of Anesthesia, Brigham and Women's Hospital, Boston, Massachusetts

T. Philip Malan, Jr., Ph.D., M.D.
Clinical Assistant Professor, Department of Anesthesiology, University of Arizona College of Medicine, Tucson, Arizona

Andrew M. Malinow, M.D.
Assistant Professor, Departments of Anaesthesiology and Obstetrics and Gynecology, University of Maryland School of Medicine; Director of Obstetric Anesthesia, Department of Anesthesia, University of Maryland Medical Center, Baltimore, Maryland

Virgil S. Manica, M.D.
Clinical Fellow, Obstetric Anesthesia, Department of Anaesthesia, Harvard Medical School; Resident, Department of Anesthesia, Brigham and Women's Hospital, Boston, Massachusetts

Ramon Martin, M.D.
Assistant Professor, Department of Anaesthesia, Harvard Medical School, Boston, Massachusetts; Postdoctoral Associate, School of Science, Massachusetts Institute of Technology, Cambridge, Massachusetts; Anesthesiologist, Department of Anesthesia, Brigham and Women's Hospital, Boston, Massachusetts

Elizabeth M. McGrady, M.B., Ch.B.
Visiting Assistant Professor, Section of Obstetric Anesthesia, Department of Anesthesiology, University of Maryland School of Medicine, Baltimore, Maryland

Kenneth J. Mintz, M.D.
Clinical Instructor, Department of Anesthesiology, State University of New York Health Science Center at Syracuse, Syracuse, New York; Anesthesiologist, Binghamton General Hospital, Binghamton, New York

Beth H. Minzter, M.D.
Clinical Fellow, Department of Anaesthesia, Harvard Medical School; Resident, Department of Anesthesia, Brigham and Women's Hospital, Boston, Massachusetts

BettyLou Koffel Mokriski, M.D.
Assistant Professor, Department of Anesthesiology, University of Maryland School of Medicine, Baltimore, Maryland

Deborah H. Moran, M.D.
Assistant Professor, Department of Anesthesia, Bowman Gray School of Medicine of Wake Forest University, Winston-Salem, North Carolina

Nancy E. Oriol, M.D.
Instructor, Department of Anaesthesia, Harvard Medical School; Director, Obstetric Anesthesia, Department of Anesthesia, Beth Israel Hospital, Boston, Massachusetts

Gerard W. Ostheimer, M.D.
Professor, Department of Anaesthesia, Harvard Medical School; Interim Chairman, Department of Anesthesia, Brigham and Women's Hospital, Boston, Massachusetts

Robert A. Peterfreund, M.D.
Assistant, Department of Anesthesia, Massachusetts General Hospital, Harvard Medical School, Boston, Massachusetts

Michael D. Popitz, M.D.
Instructor, Department of Anaesthesia, Harvard Medical School; Staff Anesthesiologist, Beth Israel Hospital, Boston, Massachusetts

Marcia A. Procopio, M.D.
Instructor, Department of Anaesthesia, Harvard Medical School; Anesthesiologist, Department of Anesthesia, Brigham and Women's Hospital, Boston, Massachusetts

Nancy L. Ray, M.D.
Director of Obstetric Anesthesia, Akron City Hospital and Saint Thomas Hospital, Summa Health System, Akron, Ohio

Jude Anne McMahon Rowe, R.N.
Former Clinical Research Associate, Department of Anesthesia, Brigham and Women's Hospital, Boston Massachusetts

Arthur Runyon-Hass, M.D.
Clinical Instructor, Department of Anesthesia, Brigham and Women's Hospital, Boston, Massachusetts

Gerald M. Sacks, M.D.
Assistant Professor, Department of Anesthesiology, University of Southern California School of Medicine, Los Angeles, California; Chairman, Department of Anesthesiology, Rancho Los Amigos Medical Center, Downey, California

William Schimpke, M.D.
Clinical Fellow, Department of Anaesthesia, Harvard Medical School; Fellow, Department of Anesthesia, Brigham and Women's Hospital, Boston, Massachusetts

Daniel N. Schneeweiss, M.D.
Anesthesiologist, Valley Anesthesiology, Yakima, Washington

Mark J. Segal, M.D.
Assistant Professor, Department of Anesthesiology, Tulane University School of Medicine; Anesthesiologist, Tulane Medical Center Clinic Hospital, New Orleans, Louisiana

Jonathan H. Skerman, B.D.Sc., M.Sc.D., D.Sc.
Professor, Departments of Anesthesiology and Obstetrics and Gynecology, School of Medicine, Louisiana State University School of Medicine; Director of Obstetric Anesthesia, Louisiana State University Medical Center, Shreveport, Louisiana

Julien Vaisman, M.D.
Attending Physician, Department of Medicine, Wise Appalachian Regional Healthcare, Wise, Virginia

Jasmine V. Vartikar, M.D.
Assistant Clinical Professor, Department of Anesthesiology, Tufts University School of Medicine; Chief, Department of Anesthesia, St. Margaret's Hospital for Women, Boston, Massachusetts

Pamela H. Vehring
Administrative Assistant, Department of Anesthesia, Brigham and Women's Hospital, Boston, Massachusetts

Dimitri Voulgaropoulos, M.D.
Clinical Assistant Professor, Department of Anesthesiology, University of Arizona College of Medicine, Tucson, Arizona

Marsha L. Wakefield, M.D.
Assistant Professor, Department of Anesthesiology, Medical College of Georgia School of Medicine, Augusta, Georgia

Elizabeth B. Walker, R.N.C.
Clinical Specialist in Inpatient Obstetrics, University Hospital, Louisiana State University Medical Center, Shreveport, Louisiana

Donald H. Wallace, M.D.
Assistant Professor, Department of Anesthesiology, Director of Obstetric Anesthesia, University of Texas Southwestern Medical School at Dallas, Dallas, Texas

Preface to the Second Edition

The Second Edition of the *Manual of Obstetric Anesthesia* is in many ways a completely new book. Chapters have been completely rewritten or updated to include our current practice. The chapters on understanding the mother and fetus have been rewritten. The chapter on perinatal pharmacology has been expanded, particularly in the area of intraspinal opioids. The former sections of this chapter dealing with nonpharmacologic pain relief and drug interactions have been enlarged, and are now full chapters in the Second Edition. The techniques of obstetric anesthesia have been revised and new areas of interest have been added.

The most frequently heard comment concerning the First Edition was that readers wanted to have additional information on the high-risk parturient. We have responded to that request in the Second Edition by devoting a chapter specifically to the high-risk parturient; in addition, increased coverage of areas of special consideration has been added. The chapter on the neonate has been updated to reflect current practice, and a chapter on education, organization, and standards has been added for completeness.

These revisions and expansions in the Second Edition include some duplication of information in the different sections of the *Manual.* This duplication has been done purposefully, so that the reader would have all the necessary information on any particular subject gathered together in one place. Our goal continues to be to provide the essential information on any particular subject along with the appropriate anesthetic considerations for the management of that particular problem.

I wish to inform the reader of several changes in vocabulary. I believe terminology should provide appropriate descriptions of what actually takes place, and should be updated when necessary to reflect practice in the 1990s. Thus, I have used terms such as "acute oxygenation" or "denitrogenation" to replace "preoxygenation." "Opioid" has replaced "narcotic," except where the term "narcotic" was more descriptive. "Intraspinal" defines the area within the spinal canal and includes both "epidural" and "subarachnoid." These terms are more definitive than "major conduction" or "regional anesthesia," which should be applied to the entire usage of local anesthetics for various procedures.

The purpose of the Second Edition of the *Manual of Obstetric Anesthesia* remains exactly the same as the First Edition. We are providing the most up-to-date clinical information on obstetric anesthesia that is possible. In fact, in this edition we have looked ahead to the utilization of developing agents to provide obstetric and surgical pain relief in the future. By necessity, more references have been added to each section because of the major expansion in basic and clinical research in obstetric anesthesia during the 1980s.

I am delighted that the Second Edition of the *Manual* has been entirely produced by long-standing colleagues in obstetric anesthesia at the Brigham and Women's Hospital, including former trainees who are now leaders in obstetric anesthesia, and a third generation that has been taught by former fellows and residents in obstetric anesthesia at both the Boston Hospital for Women and now the Brigham and Women's Hospital.

The Second Edition of the *Manual* is dedicated to my mother, who has been a constant source of support over my entire medical career, and to Benjamin G. Covino, Ph.D., M.D., who was my chairman, my mentor, and my friend. Dr. Covino had the foresight, character, and charisma to amalgamate the departments that made up the Department of Anesthesia at the Brigham and Women's Hospital into one of the leading departments of anesthesia in the world today. Finally, very special thanks are due to Marlene Major for her administrative assistance in bringing all the parts of the Second Edition together. Our thanks to our publisher, Churchill Livingstone, particularly Toni Tracy, and to Ann Ruzycka and Paul Bernstein, who provided the final touches.

Gerard W. Ostheimer, M.D.

Preface to the First Edition

The *Manual of Obstetric Anesthesia* is the outgrowth of the physiologic and pharmacologic approach to pain relief for the obstetric patient developed over the last 25 years at the Boston Lying-In Hospital, which became the Boston Hospital for Women, and finally, the Brigham and Women's Hospital. This manual is dedicated to Jess B. Weiss, M.D., who began and nurtured the practice of obstetric anesthesia as we know it today. Superb clinical care is the foundation on which our approach to obstetric anesthesia has been developed.

Dr. Weiss was instrumental in changing the practice of predelivery sedation and reliance on general anesthesia without airway protection to the utilization of spinal anesthesia for delivery, which eventually evolved to the employment of epidural anesthesia for labor and vaginal or cesarean delivery.

In the late 1960s, Dr. Weiss began the first clinical laboratory devoted solely to studies in obstetric anesthesia. The initial investigations on the pharmacologic effects of local anesthetics used for epidural anesthesia emanated from that laboratory.

In 1966, the Boston Lying-In Hospital and the Free Hospital for Women became the Boston Hospital for Women. In 1969, Milton H. Alper, M.D. became Chief of Anesthesia at the newly formed institution and was as instrumental in the academic development of the department as Dr. Weiss was in its clinical development.

At the beginning of the 1980s, the Boston Hospital for Women joined the Peter Bent Brigham and Robert Breck Brigham Hospitals to form the Brigham and Women's Hospital and your editor assumed the responsibility for obstetric anesthetic care in the new institution.

Residents in Anesthesia from throughout the United States, but particularly from the Harvard-affiliated hospitals, have been instructed in the concepts put forth in this manual. Our approach has always been conservative—but progressive—to preserve the well-being of the parturient and her fetus. Over 150,000 parturients have been delivered in our institution under this protective mantle of clinical care during the last 25 years.

The *Manual of Obstetric Anesthesia* is not to be considered a textbook. Its references are current and selective. Several texts currently available will help to provide additional background information. Our purpose is to provide the most up-to-date clinical information on obstetric anesthesia that is possible.

The approach to clinical care that is presented in the following pages could only be the result of an extraordinary effort by the current and past staff in obstetric anesthesia in this institution. Special thanks must be given to Dianne Visconti for her repeated typing of what seemed to be an endless manuscript; Donna Stampone, M.S.N., for her outstanding editorial assistance in making our thoughts understandable to all those interested in obstetric anesthesia, and to Churchill Livingstone, particularly Bill Schmitt, the editor who believed in this project, and Ann Ruzycka, who pulled all the loose ends together.

Gerard W. Ostheimer, M.D.

Contents

1

Understanding the Mother*

PHYSIOLOGIC ADAPTATIONS DURING PREGNANCY

Pregnancy involves major physiologic and anatomic adaptation by all the maternal organ systems. The anesthesiologist caring for the pregnant patient must understand these physiologic changes in order to provide safe analgesia and anesthesia to the mother and enable safe delivery of the fetus.

CARDIOVASCULAR SYSTEM

Cardiac Output

Oxygen consumption increases during pregnancy, and maternal cardiac output rises to meet these demands[1] (Table 1-1). The rise in cardiac output is a result of increased heart rate and decreased afterload, as stroke volume does not change appreciably during normal pregnancy.[2] Cardiac output rises most rapidly during the second trimester (Fig. 1-1) and then remains steady until term, when labor and uteroplacental transfusion of blood into the intravascular system cause further increases in cardiac output.

Blood Volume

Blood volume increases by 35 percent during pregnancy compared with during the nonpregnant state.[3] The stimulus for this change is controversial. Increased mineralocorticoid levels during pregnancy may predispose to progressive sodium and water retention with consequent enlargement of the intravascular space (the "overfill" hypothesis). Alternatively, primary enlargement of this space owing to hormonal (prostaglandin, progesterone) vasodilation and placental arteriovenous shunting may be the stimulus for secondary renal sodium and water retention (the "underfill" hypothesis).[4] Recent evidence seems to favor primary peripheral vasodilation early in the first trimester (underfill) as the cause of subsequent blood volume expansion.[5]

Uterine Size and Vascularity

The gravid uterine blood flow is 20 to 40 times above the nonpregnant level, accounting for 20 percent of maternal cardiac output at term. Uterine vascular resistance is markedly reduced during gestation, producing a low-pressure circuit in "parallel" with a maternal circulation characterized by reduced systemic vascular resistance.

The enlarged uterus produces mechanical compression of surrounding vascular structures, known as aortocaval compression or the "maternal supine hypotensive syndrome".[6] In the supine position, compression of the inferior vena cava decreases venous return, resulting in decreased stroke volume and hypotension; compression of the aorta further decreases uterine perfusion and may result in fetal distress. Normal maternal compensatory responses to aortocaval compression consist of tachycardia and lower-extremity vasoconstriction.

The Pericardium

Recent noninvasive studies have demonstrated a high incidence of asymptomatic pericardial effusion during normal pregnancy.[7] The stimulus is unknown, as plasma volume and protein fraction changes do not seem to correlate with the development of such effusion.[5]

Vascular Tone

Normal parturients are less responsive to vasopressor and chronotropic agonists.[8,9] Epinephrine, isoproterenol, and angiotensin II all show dose-related blunting of effect during pregnancy. Down-regulation of α- and β-adrenergic receptors has been postulated as the cause

* The text, Tables 1-1 and 1-3, and redrawing of Figures 1-1, 1-2, and 1-4 are from International Anesthesiology Clinics Vol. 27, No. 4, Winter 1989, with permission.

Table 1-1. Maternal Cardiovascular Alterations at Term

Variable	Change	Rate (%)
Cardiac output	↑ ↑ ↑ ↑	40
Stroke volume	± ↑	0–30
Heart rate	↑ ↑	15
Systolic blood pressure	↓	0–5 mmHg
Diastolic blood pressure	↓ ↓	10–20 mmHg
Total peripheral resistance	↓ ↓	15
Central venous pressure	+	0
Pulmonary wedge pressure	–	0
Ejection fraction	–	0

Adapted from Mashini et al.[2] and Skaredoff and Ostheimer,[56] with permission.)

of these phenomena. However, the presence of vasodilatory prostaglandins may play a role as well, since (1) inhibitors of prostaglandin synthesis have been shown to reverse vascular unresponsiveness to catecholamines, and (2) toxemic patients who have an abundance of vasoconstricting prostaglandins (e.g., thromboxane) are more sensitive to exogenous catecholamines.

Clinical Implications

Aortocaval compression should always be avoided. Parturients should not be allowed to rest in the supine position, but rather be encouraged to maintain uterine displacement by a right or (preferably) left lateral tilt of the pelvis (Fig. 1-2). Sympathetic blockade due to spinal or epidural anesthesia interferes with the mechanisms that compensate for aortocaval compression, sometimes causing profound hypotension in the absence of adequate uterine displacement and intravascular volume expansion. Conditions involving a particularly large uterus (e.g., multiple gestation, polyhydramnios, or diabetes mellitus) predispose to the risk and consequences of aortocaval compression.[6]

Engorgement of the epidural vasculature (Battson's plexus) makes puncture or cannulation of an epidural vein more likely than in the nonpregnant patient during initiation of epidural anesthesia. Likewise, negative pressure in the epidural space may not be consistently found in the parturient,[10] theoretically rendering the "hanging drop" technique for identification of the epidural space less successful in the pregnant patient than in nonpregnant patients.

Patients with cardiac disease may tolerate pregnancy poorly. The increased blood volume and decreased systemic resistance may cause decompensation in patients with stenotic valvular lesions and may worsen right-to-left shunting in the presence of uncorrected congenital heart defects. In contrast, parturients with regurgitant valvular lesions usually do quite well during pregnancy. Although coronary artery disease is rare among women of childbearing age, a gradual trend to older parturients may increase the incidence of myocar-

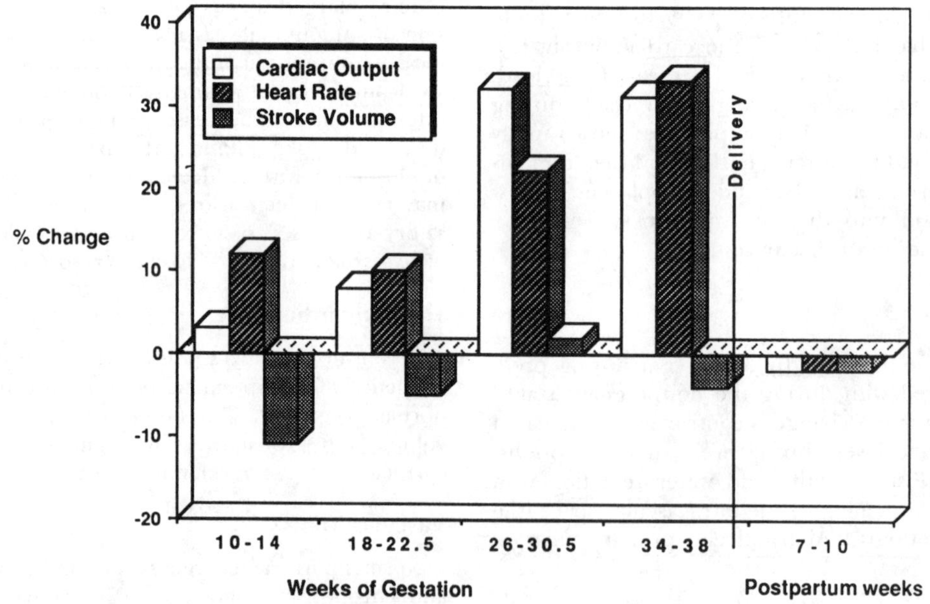

Fig. 1-1. Hemodynamic changes during pregnancy. (Adapted from Mashini et al.,[2] with permission.)

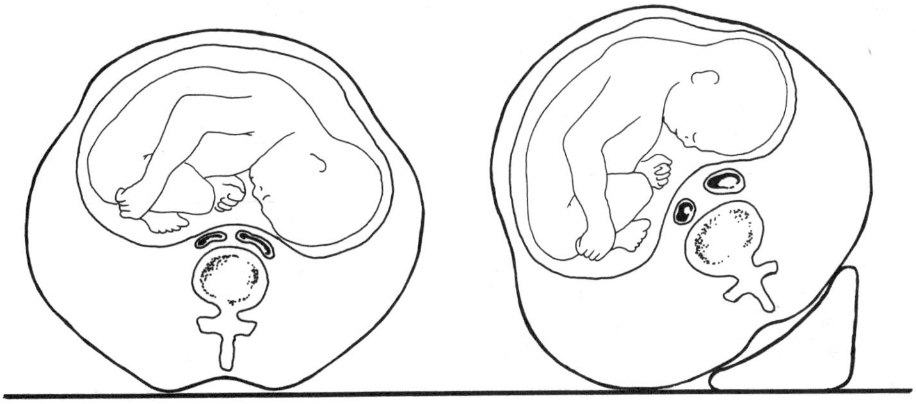

Fig. 1-2. Aortocaval decompression with left lateral tilt.

dial ischemia, infarction, or both during gestation.[11] The hypermetabolic demands of pregnancy suggest that invasive monitoring be considered in parturients with known or suspected atherosclerotic, spastic, or thrombotic coronary artery disease. In addition, the differential diagnosis of hemodynamic instability from any cardiac etiologic factor should include echocardiographic evaluation to rule out pericardial effusion.

RESPIRATORY SYSTEM

The Upper Airway

Whereas generalized peripheral edema is a common nuisance in pregnancy, edematous changes of the upper airway may be life threatening. Mucous membranes become extremely friable during the third trimester, and manipulation of the upper airway, such as may occur during insertion of nasal airways or nasogastric tubes, or during nasotracheal intubation, should be done with great care to avoid severe bleeding. Toxemic patients are particularly susceptible to airway and vocal cord edema.[12] The possibility of technically difficult intubation requiring small-diameter endotracheal tubes (i.e., 6.0 mm or less) should always be kept in mind when caring for such patients.

Respiratory Mechanics

The expanding uterus produces cephalad displacement of the diaphragm; thus, functional residual capacity (FRC) is decreased.[13] Total lung capacity, vital capacity, and inspiratory capacity all remain unchanged, however, because of compensatory subcostal widening and enlarging of the thoracic anteroposterior diameter.[14] The increased oxygen consumption of pregnancy is compensated by a 70 percent increase in alveolar ventilation at term.[15] This is accomplished by increases in both tidal volume (40 percent) and respiratory rate (15 percent). Enhancement of tidal volume is largely due to rib cage volume displacement, and less so to abdominal (diaphragmatic) movement.[14] The rise in alveolar ventilation exceeds the oxygen demands of the parturient and is probably a result of elevated progesterone levels, which increase the ventilatory response to carbon dioxide.[16] (Table 1-2).

Gas Exchange

Ventilatory augmentation produces a respiratory alkalosis with compensatory renal excretion of bicarbonate and, hence, partial pH correction.[15] Oxygenation is improved during normal pregnancy; arterial PO_2 values are typically slightly higher than in the nongravid state

Table 1-2. Maternal Respiratory Alterations at Term

Variable	Change	Rate (%)
Minute ventilation	↑ ↑ ↑ ↑	50
Alveolar ventilation	↑ ↑ ↑ ↑ ↑	70
Tidal volume	↑ ↑ ↑	40
Respiratory rate	↑	15
Closing volume	± ↓	0
Airway resistance	↓ ↓	36
Vital capacity	±	0
Inspiratory lung capacity	±	0
Functional residual capacity	↓ ↓	20
Total lung capacity	±	0
Expiratory reserve volume	↓ ↓	20
Residual volume	↓ ↓	20
Oxygen consumption	↑ ↑	20

(From Skaredoff and Ostheimer,[56] with permission.)

Table 1-3. Acid Base Values in Pregnancy versus the Nonpregnant State

Variable	Nonpregnant State	Pregnancy
pH	7.38–7.42	7.38–7.42
PaO_2 (mmHg)	90–100	100–110
$PaCO_2$ (mmHg)	35–45	28–32

(Table 1-3). Physiologic dead space at term is decreased.[17] It is likely that increased cardiac output with favorable ventilation-perfusion matching in upper lung zones accounts for both the increased PO_2 values and the decreased dead space.

Clinical Implications

The decreased FRC is usually of little concern to the normal parturient. However, conditions that decrease closing volume (otherwise unchanged in normal pregnancy), such as smoking, obesity, or kyphoscoliosis, may result in airway closure and increasing hypoxemia as pregnancy progresses.[18] The relationship between FRC and closing volume may be further aggravated by the positions assumed during birth (Trendelenburg, lithotomy, and supine) and by induction of general anesthesia.[19] One should therefore have a low threshold for administration of supplemental oxygen to the parturient in labor, particularly during episodes of fetal distress or prior to induction of general anesthesia. The decreased FRC implies that acute oxygenation (denitrogenation) can occur more rapidly in the parturient than in the nonpregnant woman, and indeed this is the case.[20] However, the marked increase in oxygen consumption contributes to the frighteningly rapid development of maternal hypoxemia during periods of apnea.[21] The decrease in dead space serves to enhance further the reliability of noninvasive respiratory monitoring (capnography and/or mass spectrometry), as the gap between end-tidal and arterial gas measurements narrows.[22]

GASTROINTESTINAL SYSTEM

Elevated levels of circulating progesterone decrease gastrointestinal motility, decrease food absorption, and lower esophageal sphincter pressure.[23] In addition, elevated gastrin levels (of placental origin) result in more acidic gastric contents.[24] The enlarged uterus increases intragastric pressure and decreases the normal oblique angle of the gastroesophageal junction.

Clinical Implications

These gastrointestinal tract alterations mean that the parturient should always be considered to have a full stomach, regardless of the actual number of hours elapsed since the last meal. Consequently, pregnant patients should always be considered at risk for aspiration of gastric contents (Mendelson syndrome), and measures should be taken to minimize this risk. Moreover, pain, anxiety, and treatment with narcotic analgesics serve to retard further gastric emptying during labor.[25] Maternal "bearing down" efforts and the lithotomy position during the second stage of labor and delivery, coupled with incompetence of the lower esophageal sphincter mechanism, make silent regurgitation and pulmonary aspiration more common than we often realize.

Our practice is to require oral administration of 30 ml of a nonparticulate antacid (0.3 mol/L sodium citrate or its equivalent) before the initiation of any anesthetic. This agent rapidly decreases the acidity of gastric contents and helps ameliorate the consequences of aspiration. Histamine receptor (H_2) antagonists such as cimetidine (Tagamet) or ranitidine (Zantac) may be administered orally the evening before, and orally or intravenously the morning of an elective procedure. Metoclopramide (Reglan) stimulates gastric emptying, increases lower esophageal sphincter tone, and serves as a centrally acting antiemetic. Metoclopramide has been very useful in parturients who have eaten a large meal shortly before arriving at the labor suite, as well as in diabetic patients, whose disease results in inherently slow gastric emptying.

HEMATOLOGIC SYSTEM

Both plasma volume and erythrocyte mass increase above prepregnant values, but the increase in the former far exceeds the increase in the latter. A "dilutional" anemia therefore ensues[3] (Table 4). Blood viscosity and

Table 1-4. Maternal Hematologic Alterations at Term

Variable	Change	Rate (%)
Blood volume	↑ ↑ ↑	35
Plasma volume	↑ ↑ ↑ ↑	45
Erythrocyte volume	↑ ↑	20
Blood urea nitrogen	↓ ↓ ↓	33
Plasma cholinesterase	↓ ↓	20
Total protein	↑	18
Albumin	↓	14
Globulin	±	0
AST, ALT, LDH	↑	
Cholesterol	↓	
Alkaline phosphatase (produced by placenta)	↑ ↑	

AST, aspartate aminotransferase; ALT, alanine aminotransferase; LDH, lactate dehydrogenase.
(From Skaredoff and Ostheimer,[56] with permission.)

Table 1-5. Coagulation Factors and Inhibitors during Normal Pregnancy

Factor	Nonpregnant	Late Pregnancy
Factor I (fibrinogen)	200–450 mg/dl	400–650 mg/dl
Factor II (prothrombin)	75–125%	100–125%
Factor V	75–125%	100–150%
Factor VII	75–125%	150–250%
Factor VIII	75–150%	200–500%
Factor IX	75–125%	100–150%
Factor X	75–125%	150–250%
Factor XI	75–125%	50–100%
Factor XII	75–125%	100–200%
Factor XIII	75–125%	35–75%
Antithrombin III	85–110%	75–100%
Antifactor Xa	86–110%	75–100%
Platelets		Slight ↑
Fibrinolysis		Slight ↓

(From Shnider and Levinson,[57] with permission.)

oxygen content both decrease. Platelet count is usually elevated, as are coagulation factors I, VII, X, and XII. Thrombocytopenia may, however, be seen in some normal pregnant patients in the absence of any other hematopathology.[26,27] Systemic fibrinolysis is slightly decreased from normal levels.

Clinical Implications

The physiologic "anemia of pregnancy" (normal hematocrit of 35 percent) is usually of little concern to the normal paturient, as increases in cardiac output serve actually to increase oxygen delivery to tissues. The increase in coagulation factors (Table 1-5) renders pregnancy a "hypercoagulable" state, with a consequent increase in the incidence of thrombotic events (e.g., deep venous and cortical vein thrombosis). Enhanced clotting, coupled with the expanded blood volume, affords teleologic protection to the parturient against the effects of bleeding at the time of delivery.

RENAL SYSTEM

Renal hemodyanamics undergo profound changes during gestation.[28] Marked increases in renal plasma flow (80 percent above normal) occur by the middle of the second trimester and then decline slightly by term. Glomerular filtration rate (GFR) increases to 50 percent above prepregnant values by the 16th gestational week and remains so until delivery (Fig. 1-3). Consequently, 24-hour creatine clearance values are elevated, a change discernible as early as the 8th week of gestation. Glycosuria is common in normal pregnancy, owing to both alterations in tubular reabsorptive capacity and the increased load of glucose presented by the increased GFR. While these changes are noted in early pregnancy, implying a hormonal stimulus, the exact mechanism is as yet unknown. Increased levels of aldosterone, cortisol, and human placental lactogen all contribute to the multifactorial renal adaptations to pregnancy. Progesterone causes dilation of the renal pelvis and ureters. Hence, the incidence of urinary tract infections is increased, particularly after instrumentation of the urinary bladder.[29]

Clinical Implications

Laboratory determinations of renal function are so altered that great care must be exercised when "normal" nonpregnant values are applied to the pregnant woman. For example, "normal" values of blood urea nitrogen and creatinine in a preeclamptic or diabetic patient may actually indicate serious renal compromise; in contrast such values may indicate hypovolemia in a parturient with otherwise normal renal function.

Although glucose excretion is enhanced during pregnancy, excessive administration of glucose to patients during labor may result in both maternal hyperglycemia and initial fetal hyperglycemia. Resultant fetal hyperinsulinemia persists after delivery, however, and a reactive neonatal hypoglycemia may ensue.[30]

Serum electrolyte values are unchanged during pregnancy. Expansion of plasma volume must therefore be accompanied by electrolyte retention. A primary resetting of thirst and vasopressin osmoreceptors allows the pregnant woman to maintain internal homeostasis during this volume-expanded state (i.e., the threshold for antidiuretic hormone secretion is reset at a lower level of plasma sodium, this allowing volume expansion without accompanying diuresis). The antecedent stimulus for this adaptation has yet to be elucidated.[28]

CENTRAL NERVOUS SYSTEM

Emotional, social, and cultural factors all contribute to the parturient's psychological milieu during labor and delivery.[31–34] Pregnancy is a stressful experience, and wide mood swings during gestation, delivery, and the postpartum period can be expected. A hormonal basis for this emotional lability has been proposed inasmuch as progesterone and endogenous endorphins act as both neurotransmitters and analgesics. Progesterone and endorphins also serve to decrease minimal alveolar concentration (MAC) of all inhaled anesthetic agents.[35,36] In addition, reduced enzymatic degradation of opioids at term contributes to elevated pain thresholds.[37]

Reduced doses of local anesthetic agents are required for spinal and epidural anesthesia compared with doses for nonpregnant patients.[38] Vascular congestion in the

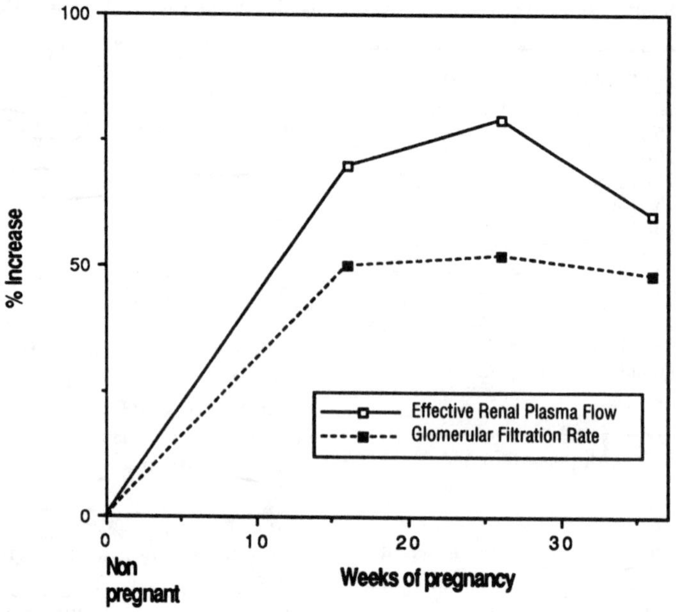

Fig. 1-3. Renal function during pregnancy. (Redrawn from Davison,[28] with permission.)

epidural space contributes to the decreased local anesthetic requirement through three mechanisms:

1. Reduced volume in the epidural space facilitates spread of a given dose of local anesthetic over a wider number of dermatomes.
2. Increased pressure within the epidural space facilitates dural diffusion and higher cerebrospinal fluid levels of local anesthetic.
3. Venous congestion of the lateral foramina decreases egress of local anesthetic via the dural root sleeves.

The respiratory alkalosis of pregnancy may enhance local anesthetic action by increasing the relative concentration of uncharged local anesthetic molecules, which facilitates penetration through neural membranes. This decreased requirement for local anesthetic is seen as early as the first trimester. Hormonal changes may be operative as well, since progesterone has been shown to correlate with enhanced conduction blockade in isolated nerve preparations.[39,40]

MISCELLANEOUS

Musculoskeletal

Placental production of the hormone relaxin stimulates generalized ligamentous relaxation.[41] Particularly notable is the widening of the pelvis in preparation for fetal passage. A resultant "head-down" tilt is seen when the parturient assumes the lateral position, and compensation should be made when the anesthesiologist performs regional anesthesia (Fig. 1-4).

Generalized vertebral collagenous softening, coupled with the burden of a gravid uterus, increases the lumbar lordosis. Technical difficulty with regional anesthesia may result. In addition, these changes account for the high incidence of back pain and sciatica during pregnancy, complaints which, per se, do not represent contraindications to regional anesthesia.[42] Stress fractures of the weight-bearing bony pelvis have also been noted, especially during difficult deliveries.[43]

Dermatologic

Hyperpigmentation of the face, neck (chloasma or "mask of pregnancy"), and abdominal midline (linea nigra) are due to the effects of melanocyte-stimulating hormone (MSH), a congener of adrenocorticotropic hormone (ACTH). Levels of MSH increase markedly during the first trimester and remain elevated until after delivery.[44]

Mammary

Breast enlargement is typical in normal pregnancy and is a result of human placental lactogen secretion. Enlarged breasts in an obese parturient with a short neck may lead to difficult laryngoscopy and intubation. Use of a short-handled laryngoscope can be extremely helpful in these patients[45] (Fig. 1-5).

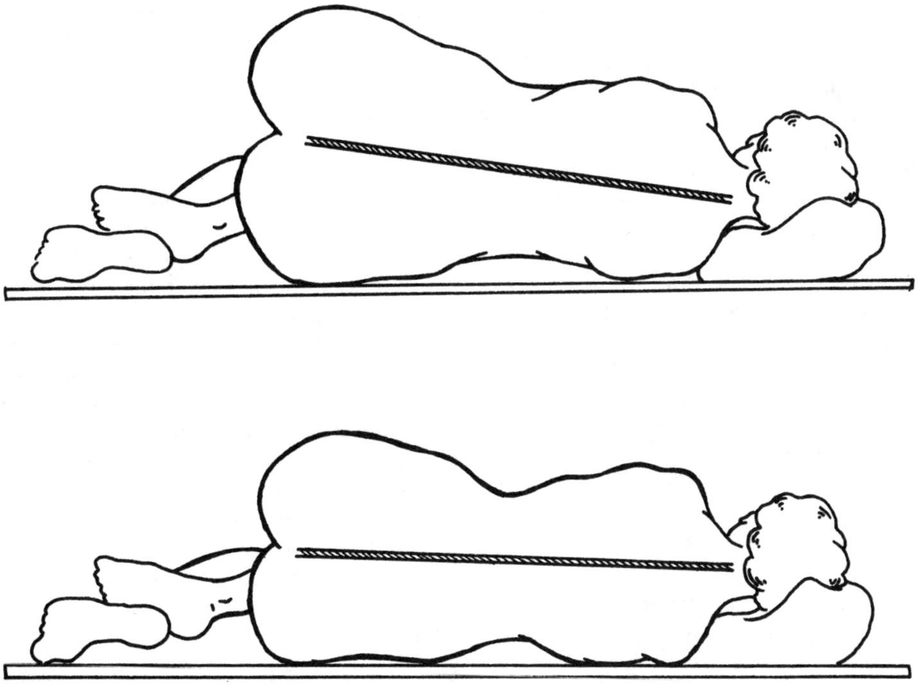

Fig. 1-4. Pelvic widening and resultant "head-down" tilt in the lateral position during pregnancy. (Upper panel, pregnant.)

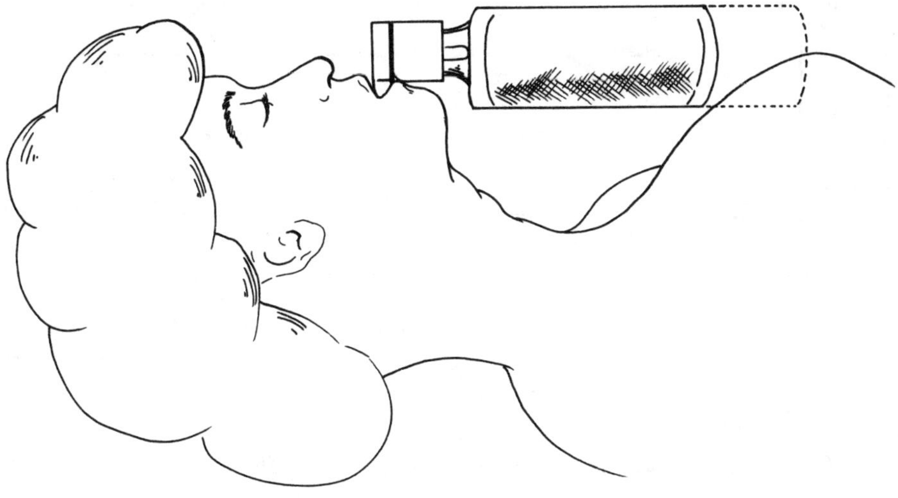

Fig. 1-5. Use of the short-handled laryngoscope for the large-breasted parturient. *Dotted line* indicates a traditional laryngoscope handle impinging on breast tissue.

Ocular

Conjunctival vasospasm and subconjunctional hemorrhage are occasionally seen, especially during maternal expulsive efforts and in preeclamptic patients.[46] The retina may manifest focal vascular spasm, detachment, and retinopathy associated with hypertensive disorders. Central serous choroidopathy, or a breakdown of the blood-retina barrier, may occur even in the absence of hypertension.

Intraocular pressure is lower during pregnancy—perhaps a result of progesterone and relaxin effects (which facilitate aqueous outflow) and human chorionic gonadotropin (which depresses aqueous humor production). Corneal thickening, a manifestation of the generalized edema of pregnancy, may produce mild visual disturbances and contact lens intolerance during gestation.[47]

INTRAPARTUM CHANGES

Active labor magnifies many of the physiologic variables already altered during gestation. Although the rigors of labor are usually well tolerated, the limited reserves of the term parturient may sometimes be stressed in ways not beneficial to mother or fetus.

Cardiovascular System

Cardiac output during active labor rises to approximately twice prelabor values, with the maximal increase seen in the immediate postdelivery period (Fig. 1-6). The rise in cardiac output is multifactorial. First, pain and anxiety during labor increase maternal circulating catecholamines, with a resultant tachycardia and increased stroke volume.[48] Second, uterine contractions result in cyclic autotransfusion and increased central blood volume. This augmentation of preload in the setting of normal (or hyperdynamic) ventricular function contributes to increased cardiac output via Frank-Starling mechanisms.

Adequate regional anesthesia can ameliorate many of the pain-mediated hemodynamic consequences of labor. Uterine contractions, however, will still cause transient autotransfusions of blood with elevation of central vascular pressures.

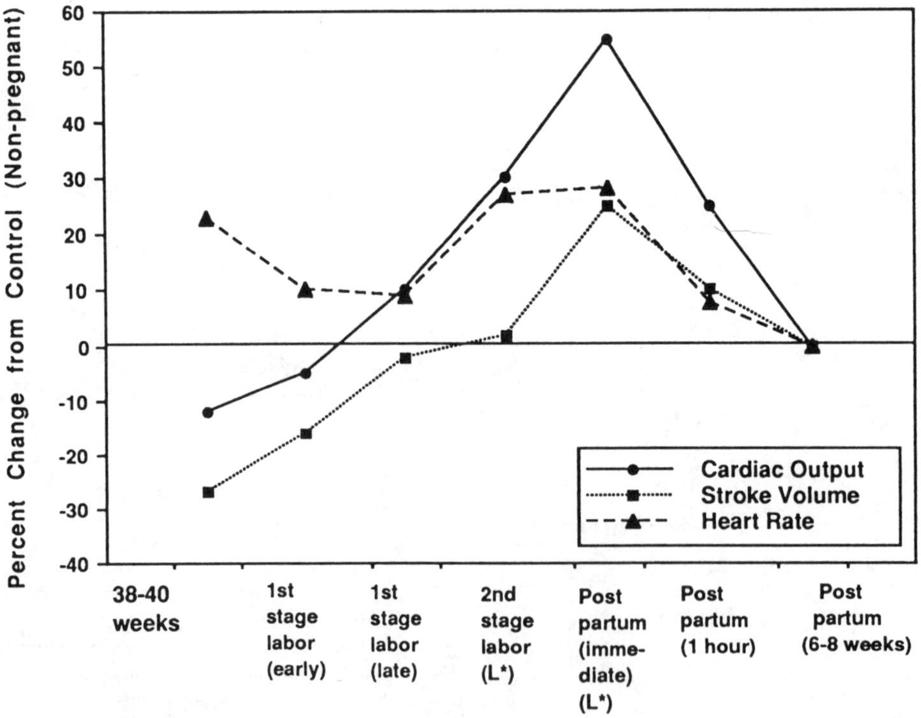

Fig. 1-6. Cardiovascular alterations during labor. (Redrawn from Shnider and Levinson,[57] with permission.)

Respiratory System

Hyperventilation is common during labor. This may be a natural response to pain or the result of various prepared childbirth methods in which repetitive, panting breathing techniques are used. Hyperventilation during labor in the setting of an already lowered maternal $PaCO_2$ at term may result in dangerous degrees of alkalemia. Women who have received narcotic analgesics during labor may alternate periods of hyperventilation with marked hypoventilation between contractions, resulting in wide swings in $PaCO_2$.[49] The uterine vascular response to hypocarbia is vasoconstriction and subsequent decreased placental perfusion.[50] Thus the potential for fetal hypoxemia exists during episodes of maternal alkalemia, particularly if a fetus is already compromised for other reasons.

Regional anesthesia during labor obviates the need for "breathing techniques" and eliminates pain-induced hyperventilation, so patients with marginal placental reserve (from preeclampsia, diabetes, postmature pregnancy, or small abruptio placentae, for example) are strong candidates for epidural anesthesia during labor.

Metabolic Effects

The homeostatic milieu that develops during gestation undergoes marked changes during labor. Metabolic acidosis may occur for several reasons. First, prolonged labor, especially in the setting of inadequate intravenous hydration, sometimes contributes to elevated lactate and pyruvate levels.[51] Second, muscular activity, due to pain, shivering, or respiratory muscle demands, adds to acidic metabolites in the maternal circulation. Third, maternal alkalemia may predispose to compensatory acid retention. Overall maintenance of normal acid-base status during labor is accomplished by the balance of what may be markedly altered (versus nonpregnant) levels of acidemic and alkalemic mediators. Thus, situations that further aggravate pH balance (e.g., dehydration, vomiting, ketoacidosis, hypothermia, hemorrhage) may be poorly tolerated by the gravida in labor.

The common markers of physiologic stress (epinephrine, norepinephrine, and cortisol) all increase during labor.[52,53] The magnitude of this increase is blunted by regional anesthesia.

PUERPERAL RESOLUTION

Cardiac output rises sharply immediately after birth, as sustained contraction of the emptied uterus results in autotransfusion of 500 to 750 ml of blood, coincident with elimination of the placental arteriovenous shunt. The immediate postpartum period is a high-risk time for decompensation in patients with certain cardiac disease states (particularly stenotic valvular lesions or pulmonary hypertension). Cardiac output gradually returns to nonpregnant levels by 2 to 4 weeks after delivery.[3]

Uterine evacuation and involution promote rapid resolution of many of the pulmonary changes induced by mechanical compression of the diaphragm and lungs by the gravid uterus. Thus, FRC and residual volume quickly return to normal. The gradual decline in blood progesterone levels is mirrored by a slow rise in arterial PCO_2, and alveolar ventilation returns to normal by 2 to 3 weeks post partum.[54]

Postpartum diuresis is common; this diuretic phase contributes to a gradual decline in plasma volume, although red cell mass remains constant. Thus, the "dilutional" anemia of pregnancy resolves, and the hematocrit rises to nonpregnant levels in 2 to 4 weeks. Excessive blood loss at delivery markedly alters the course of hematologic resolution. The GFR, blood urea nitrogen, and creatinine levels return to normal in 1 to 3 weeks.[28]

Mechanical effects on the gastrointestinal tract rapidly resolve by 2 to 3 days post partum. However, elevated levels of progesterone persist and may delay gastric emptying for several weeks. Precautions to minimize the risk and consequences of acid aspiration should therefore be taken if surgery with anesthesia is planned during this period.[55]

REFERENCES

1. Pernoll ML, Metcalf J, Schlenlser TL: Oxygen consumption at rest and during exercise in pregnancy. Respir Physiol 22:285, 1975
2. Mashini IS, Albazzaz SJ, Fadel HE: Serial noninvasive evaluation of cardiovascular hemodynamics during pregnancy. Am J Obstet Gynecol 156:1208, 1987
3. Ueland K: Maternal cardiovascular hemodynamics. VII. Intrapartum blood volume changes. Am J Obstet Gynecol 126:671, 1976
4. Schrier RW, Durr JA: Pregnancy: an overfill or underfill state. Am J Kidney Dis 9:284, 1987
5. Schrier RW: Pathogenesis of sodium and water retention in high-output and low-output cardiac failure, nephrotic syndrome, cirrhosis, and pregnancy. N Engl J Med 319:1127, 1988
6. Eckstein KL, Marx GF: Aortocaval compression: incidence and prevention. Anesthesiology 40:381, 1965
7. Enein M, Zina AA, Kassem M, et al: Echocardiography of the pericardium in pregnancy. Obstet Gynecol 69:851, 1987
8. Paller MS: Decreased pressor responsiveness in pregnancy:

studies in experimental animals. Am J Kidney Dis 9:308, 1987
9. Desimone CA, Leighton BL, Norris MC, et al: The chronotropic effect of isoproterenol is reduced in term pregnant women. Anesthesiology 69:626, 1988
10. Messih MNA: Epidural space pressures during pregnancy. Anaesthesia 36:775, 1981
11. Kirz DS, Dorchester W, Freeman RK: Advanced maternal age; the mature gravida. Am J Obstet Gynecol 152:7, 1985
12. Bletka M, Hlavat JV, Trakova M: Volume of whole blood and absolute amount of serum proteins in the early stages of late toxemia of pregnancy. Am J Obstet Gynecol 106:10, 1970
13. Knuttgen HG, Emerson K: Physiologic response to pregnancy at rest and during exercise. J Appl Physiol 36:549, 1975
14. Gilroy RJ, Mangura BT, Lavietes MH: Rib cage and abdominal volume displacements during breathing in pregnancy. Am Rev Respir Dis 137:668, 1988
15. Prowse CM, Gaenster EA: Respiratory and acid-base changes during pregnancy. Anesthesiology 26:381, 1965
16. Tyler JM: The effects of progesterone on the respiration of patients with emphysema and hypercapnea. J Clin Invest 39:34, 1960
17. Shankar KB, Moseley H, Vemula V, et al: Physiological dead space during general anesthesia for caesarean section. Can J Anaesth 34:373, 1987
18. Leontie EA: Respiratory disease in pregnancy. Med Clin North Am 62:111, 1974
19. Bevan DR, Holdcroft A, Loh L, et al: Closing volume and pregnancy. Br Med J [Clin Res] 1:13, 1974
20. Russell GN, Smith CL, Snowdon SL, et al: Preoxygenation and the parturient patient. Anaesthesia 42:346, 1987
21. Archer GW, Marx GF: Arterial oxygen tension during apnea in paturient women. Br J Anaesth 46:358, 1974
22. Bhavanishankaat K, Moseley H, Kumar Y, et al: Arterial to end-tidal carbon dioxide tension difference during anaesthesia for tubal ligation. Anaesthesia 42:482, 1987
23. Lind LJ, Smith AM, McIver DK, et al: Lower esophageal sphincter pressures in pregnancy. Can Med Assoc J 98:571, 1968
24. Attia RR, Ebeid AM, Fisher JE, et al: Maternal, fetal and placental gastrin concentrations. Anaesthesia 37:18, 1982
25. O'Sullivan GM, Sutton AJ, Thompson SA, et al: Noninvasive measurement of gastric emptying in obstetric patients. Anesth Analg 66:505, 1987
26. O'Brien WF, Saba HI, Knuppel RA, et al: Alterations in platelet concentration and aggregation in normal pregnancy and preeclampsia. Am J Obstet Gynecol 155:486, 1986
27. Burrows RF, Kelton JG: Incidentally detected thrombocytopenia in healthy mothers and their infants. N Engl J Med 319:142, 1988
28. Davison JM: Overview kidney function in pregnant women. Am J Kidney Dis 9:248, 1987
29. Bellina JH, Dougherty CM, Mickal A: Ureteral dilation in pregnancy. Am J Obstet Gynecol 108:356, 1970
30. Datta S, Kitzmiller JL, Naulty JS, et al: Acid-base status of diabetic mothers and their infants following spinal anesthesia for cesarean section. Anesth Analg 61:662, 1982
31. Stewart DE: Psychiatric symptoms following attempted natural childbirth. Can Med Assoc J 127:713, 1982
32. Lee RV, D'Alauro F, White LM, et al: Southeast Asian folklore about pregnancy and parturition. Obstet Gynecol 71:643, 1988
33. Senden IP, Wetering VD, Eskes TK, et al: Labor pain: a comparison of parturients in a Dutch and American teaching hospital. Obstet Gynecol 71:541, 1988
34. Colman AD: Psychological state during first pregnancy. Am J Orthopsychiatry 39:788, 1969
35. Palahniuic RJ, Shnider SM, Eger EI: Pregnancy decreases the requirement for inhaled anesthetic agents. Anesthesiology 41:82, 1974
36. Goland RS, Wordlaw SL, Stark RI, et al: Human plasma endorphin during pregnancy, labor and delivery. J Clin Endocrinol Metab 52:74, 1981
37. Lyrenas S, Nyberg F, Lindberg BO, et al: Cerebrospinal fluid activity of dynorphin-converting enzyme at term pregnancy. Obstet Gynecol 72:54, 1988
38. Datta S, Hurley RJ, Naulty JS, et al: Plasma and cerebrospinal fluid progesterone concentrations in pregnant and nonpregnant women. Anesth Analg 65:950, 1986
39. Datta S, Lambert DH, Gregus J, et al: Differential sensitivities of mammalian nerve fibers during pregnancy. Anesth Analg 62:1070, 1983
40. Flanagan HL, Datta S, Lambert DH, et al: Effect of pregnancy on bupivacaine-induced conduction blockade in the isolated rabbit vagus nerve. Anesth Analg 66:123, 1987
41. Kemp BE, Niall HD: Relaxin. Vitam Horm 41:79, 1985
42. Berg G, Hammar M, Moller J, et al: Low back pain during pregnancy. Obstet Gynecol 71:71, 1988
43. Moran JJ: Stress fractures in pregnancy. Am J Obstet Gynecol 158:1274, 1988
44. Diczfalusy E, Troen P: Endocrine functions of the human placenta. Vitam Horm 19:229, 1961
45. Datta S, Briwa J: Modified laryngoscope for endotracheal intubation of obese patients. Anesth Analg 60:120, 1981
46. Weinreb RN, Lu A, Key T: Maternal ocular adaptations during pregnancy. Obstet Gynecol Surv 42:471, 1987
47. Weinreb RN, Lu A, Besson C: Corneal thickness in pregnancy. Am J Ophthalmol 105:258, 1988
48. Jones CM, Greiss FC: The effect of labor on maternal and fetal circulating catecholamines. Am J Obstet Gynecol 194:149, 1982
49. Huch A, Huch R, Lindmark G, et al: Transcutaneous oxygen measurements in labor. J Obstet Gynaecol Br Commonw 81:608, 1974
50. Moya F, Morishima HO, Shnider SM, et al: Influence of maternal hyperventilation on the newborn infant. Am J Obstet Gynecol 90:76, 1965
51. Zador G, Willeck-Lund G, Nillson BA: Acid-base changes associated with labor. Acta Obstet Gynecol Scand [Suppl] 34:41, 1974

52. Lederman RP, McCann DS, Work B: Endogenous plasma epinephrine and norepinephrine in last trimester pregnancy and labor. Am J Obstet Gynecol 129:5, 1977
53. Maltau JM, Eielsen OV, Stotcke KT: Effect of stress during labor on the concentration of cortisol and estriol in maternal plasma. Am J Obstet Gynecol 134:681, 1979
54. Cugell DW: Pulmonary function in pregnancy. I. Serial observations in normal women. Am Rev Tuberc 67:568, 1953
55. James CF, Gibbs CP, Banner TE: Postpartum perioperative risk of pulmonary aspiration. Abstracts of scientific papers. Society for Obstetric Anesthesia and Perinatology. Vancouver, Canada, May, 1983
56. Skaredoff MN, Ostheimer GW: Physiological changes during pregnancy; effects of major regional anesthesia. Reg Anesth 6:28, 1981
57. Shnider S, Levinson G: Anesthesia for Obstetrics. 2nd ed. Williams & Wilkins, Baltimore, 1987

2

Understanding the Fetus

During the 9 months of pregnancy, the fetus develops in utero and is not accessible to direct evaluation. Monitoring the mother and fetus through this period of development has evolved considerably because of biochemical and technical advances, resulting in a more knowledgeable assessment of the fetus. Monitoring techniques are not only used for diagnostic purposes, thereby serving a preventive role, but are also necessary for treatment, should the fetus be stressed.

Stress to the fetus is defined in this chapter as either hypoxia or asphyxia, because the supply of oxygen to the fetus is crucial. Any diminution or cessation of oxygenation results in an immediate change in the biochemical status of the fetus that affects all organs, particularly the heart and brain. There are compensatory responses by the fetus, but these reserves are limited. Therefore, it is important to recognize the fetal response to stress, identify the cause of the stress, and treat it.

Anesthesia and analgesia, as an integral part of obstetric delivery, can have an impact on the outcome of delivery depending on the status of the fetus. For this reason, it is important to have an understanding of monitoring techniques, their results, and the interpretation of the underlying fetal pathophysiology, not only for labor and delivery, but also during pregnancy. This knowledge will serve as the basis for understanding what effects anesthesia and analgesia may have on the fetus, soon to be born, during the labor and delivery process.

THE FETAL REACTION TO STRESS

During labor and delivery, the main cause of stress for the fetus is hypoxia and asphyxia. Fetal hypoxia is due to the mother breathing a hypoxic mixture of gases and results in decreased oxygen tension presenting to the uteroplacental unit. Fetal asphyxia is secondary to a reduction of at least 50 percent in uterine blood flow. In addition to decreased oxygen tension, there is also increased carbon dioxide tension, producing both metabolic and respiratory acidosis. With prolonged asphyxia, the fetus switches to anaerobic metabolism and produces a buildup of lactate. Metabolic acidosis subsequently develops.

The fetal responses to hypoxia or asphyxia include the following:

1. Bradycardia (due to increased vagal activity) with systemic hypertension
2. Slight decrease in ventricular output
3. Redistribution of blood from the splanchnic bed to the heart, brain, placenta, and adrenals[1]
4. Decrease in fetal breathing movements (from 39 to 7 percent of the time)
5. Terminal gasping movements (with asphyxia)
6. Increased circulating catecholamine levels (demonstrated in fetal sheep)
7. Increased α-adrenergic activity

In chronically instrumented sheep, fetal oxygen consumption decreases as much as 60 percent from control values with hypoxia.[2] This is accompanied by fetal bradycardia, an increase in blood pressure, and progressive metabolic acidosis. The fetal sheep can tolerate this state for approximately 1 hour. These changes are rapidly reversed with restoration of oxygenation.[3] Fetal cerebral[4] and myocardial[5] oxygen consumption have been shown to remain constant. When hypoxia is prolonged or proceeds to asphyxia, these compensatory mechanisms are lost.

The ability to reverse the effects of hypoxia or asphyxia depends on recognition of the signs and symptoms. This is where fetal monitoring is crucial.

REFERENCES

1. Cohn HE, Piasecki GJ, Jackson BJ: Cardiovascular responses to hypoxemia and acidemia in fetal lambs. Am J Obstet Gynecol 129:817, 1974
2. Parer JT: The effect of acute maternal hypoxia on fetal oxygenation and the umbilical circulation in the sheep. Eur J Obstet Gynecol Reprod Biol 10:125, 1980
3. Mann LI: Effects in sheep of hypoxia on levels of lactate, pyruvate and glucose in blood of mothers and fetus. Pediatr Res 4:46, 1970
4. Jones MD, Sheldon RE, Peeters LL, et al: Fetal cerebral oxygen consumption at different levels of oxygenation. J Appl Physiol 43:1080, 1977
5. Fisher DS, Heymann MA, Rudolph AM: Fetal myocardial oxygen and carbohydrate consumption during acutely induced hypoxemia. Am J Physiol 242:H657, 1982

FETAL ASSESSMENT

DIAGNOSIS OF BIRTH DEFECTS

Between 3 and 5 percent of all births in the United States are afflicted with a major genetic defect. These include disorders of morphogenesis, chromosome abnormalities, and single-gene inherited diseases. Because these diseases are usually associated with decreased viability and/or significant physical handicaps, techniques are available during the first and second trimesters to diagnose some of these disorders.

Blood Tests

Maternal serum is sampled during the first trimester to assess the possibility of neural tube defects and Rh sensitization.

Neural Tube Defects. Neural tube defects are one of the most frequent congenital abnormalities, with an incidence of 1 to 2 per 1,000 live births in the United States. α-Fetoprotein (AFP) is elevated in the fetal serum during the first trimester when the neural tube fails to close, which results in anencephaly, meningomyelocoele, or encephalocoele. AFP passes through the placenta into the maternal serum and can be measured with a radioimmunoassay. AFP is also elevated in malformations of the gastrointestinal and genitourinary tracts, as well as fetal demise, decreasing the specificity of the test. Despite these shortcomings, it is still used as a general screening test. With any abnormal values, ultrasonography and an amniocentesis are performed to increase specificity and confirm the diagnosis.

Rh Sensitization. Rh sensitization occurs in Rh(D)-negative women who are carrying a Rh-positive fetus. Sensitization of the mother occurs from a prior delivery when fetal cells entered the maternal circulation and stimulated formation of maternal antibodies to fetal erythrocyte Rh antigens. With a subsequent pregnancy, the antibodies traverse the placenta and destroy fetal erythrocytes. This results in the syndrome of erythroblastosis fetalis, which is characterized by a severe hemolytic anemia that leads to edema, jaundice, and congestive heart failure. Rh titers are measured early and serially throughout the pregnancy in Rh-negative mothers. Rising or elevated maternal titers are assessed with an amniocentesis.

Amniocentesis

Amniocentesis is generally performed between the 12th and 16th weeks of gestation. An aliquot (20 to 30 ml) of amniotic fluid is removed by transabdominal aspiration with a needle. The fluid is used for biochemical determinations and fetal cells are cultured for karyotype. The indications for amniocentesis are listed in Table 2-1. An amniocentesis is usually preceded by an ultrasound examination of the uterus and fetus, which establishes gestational age and can identify certain gross disorders of morphogenesis. The ultrasound examination also reduces the risk of amniocentesis by locating the sac of amniotic fluid and the position of the placenta and the fetus for accurate needle placement.

Ultrasonography

Diagnostic ultrasonography is an integral part of obstetric care and has enhanced prenatal diagnosis during gestation. Recent advances in imaging and display techniques have provided insights into intrauterine life.

Table 2-1. Indications for Amniocentesis

Maternal age of 35 years or older at delivery
History of any chromosomal abnormality in a family member
Birth of a previous child with Down syndrome or other chromosomal disorder
Parents at risk for being carriers of X-linked disorders or inborn errors of metabolism
History of recurrent spontaneous abortions
Family history of neural tube defects

During the first trimester, this technique can accurately date a pregnancy by measuring fetal crown–rump length, establish fetal viability, and diagnose multiple gestation. Sometimes, an ectopic pregnancy can be visualized.

Ultrasonic techniques are available for the assessment of fetal gestational age and intrauterine growth during the second and third trimester. The method of estimation of gestational age most commonly used involves measurement of the biparietal diameter of the fetal skull. By comparing the measured biparietal diameter to a nomogram, an accurate estimation of gestational age can be made. This is most helpful when serial measurements are obtained. The accuracy of the technique is greatest in midtrimester. During this time, biologic variation in fetal head size is considerably smaller and the rate of growth of the fetal skull is greater than in the last trimester. This is important in the diagnosis of intrauterine growth retardation, which is associated with an increased risk of various complications in utero and after birth.

Ultrasonography is also able to diagnose certain kinds of congenital malformations in utero, including hydrocephaly, gastroschisis, various kinds of skeletal dysgenesis, and kidney dysplasia. Amniotic fluid volume can be assessed and cases of polyhydramnios or oligohydramnios identified. Delineation of placental position and structure is made by ultrasound, not only for amniocentesis but also in the evaluation of third-trimester uterine bleeding due to placenta previa and/or abruptio placentae.

ASSESSMENT OF FETAL MATURITY

Because fetal chronological age does not necessarily correlate with functional maturity, particularly in the pulmonary system, methods of assessing fetal maturity are important adjuncts in clinical decision-making. The majority of perinatal morbidity and mortality results from complications of premature delivery. The most frequently seen complication is the respiratory distress syndrome (RDS). This disorder is due to a deficiency of a surface-active agent (surfactant) that prevents alveolar collapse during expiration. Phospholipids produced by fetal alveolar cells are the major component of lung surfactant and are produced in sufficient amounts by 36 weeks gestation. The most commonly used technique to assess fetal lung maturity is to measure the lecithin:sphingomyelin (L:S) ratio. The concentration of lecithin, a component of surfactant, begins to rise in the amniotic fluid at 32 to 33 weeks gestation and continues to rise until term. The concentration of sphingomyelin remains relatively constant, so that the ratio of the two provides an estimate of surfactant production that is not affected by variations in the volume of amniotic fluid. The risk of neonatal RDS when the L:S ratio is greater than 2 is less than 1 percent, whereas if the ratio is less than 1.5, approximately 80 percent of neonates will develop RDS.

Some of the disadvantages in measuring the L:S ratio are a long turnaround time, use of toxic chemicals, dearth of technical expertise, and the inability to standardize the test. As a result, few hospitals are able to perform the test. Another method, the TDx fetal lung maturity test, is automated and avoids the technical involvement in sample preparation and measurement. The test relies on the fluorescence polarization of a dye added to a solution of amniotic fluid, which is then compared to values on a standard curve to determine the relative concentration of surfactant and albumin in a sample. The determined values are expressed in milligrams of surfactant per gram of albumin. With a cutoff of 50 mg/g for maturity, the TDx test was equal in sensitivity (0.96) and more specific (0.88 versus 0.83) when compared to the L:S ratio in one multicenter study.[1]

FETAL BIOPHYSICAL PROFILE

The fetal biophysical profile involves evaluation of immediate biophysical activities in the fetus (movement, muscle tone, breathing, and heart rate) as well as a semiquantitative assessment of amniotic fluid. The biophysical parameters reflect acute central nervous system activity and when present correlate positively with the lack of depression (secondary to asphyxia) of the central nervous system. Diminished amniotic fluid volume represents long-term or chronic fetal compromise.

The major indications for referral for biophysical profile are suspected intrauterine growth retardation, hypertension, diabetes, and postdates gestation.

The biophysical evaluation of the fetus is done by ultrasound with the purpose solely to detect changes in fetal activities due to asphyxia. As has been mentioned previously, changes in fetal breathing movements, heart rate, and body movements are indicators of the state of fetal oxygenation. Superimposed on these factors are the nonrandom pattern of central nervous system activity and the sleep state, the effects of which might be misconstrued for hypoxia. However, extending the period of observation to find a period of normal recovery for the latter conditions helps to differentiate asphyxia from normal variants.

The scoring of the fetal biophysical profile is an assessment of five variables (Table 2-2), four of which are monitored simultaneously by ultrasound. The vari-

Table 2-2. Fetal Biophysical Profile Scoring

Variable	Score = 2	Score = 0
Gross body movements	3 discrete body/limb movements in 30 min	<2 episodes in 30 min
Muscle tone	1 episode: extension/flexion of hand, limb, or trunk	Absent or slow movement
Breathing movements	1 episode, 30-sec duration in 30 min	Absent
Heart rate	2 episodes of acceleration with fetal movement in 30 min	<2 episodes
Amniotic fluid volume	1 pocket, measuring 1 × 1 cm	No amniotic fluid or a pocket < 1 × 1 cm

ables are said to be normal or abnormal and are assigned a score of 2 for normal and 0 for abnormal. The nonstress test (NST) is monitored after the biophysical evaluation. When the test score is normal, conservative therapy is indicated, with some exceptions:

1. Postdates gestation with a cervix favorable for induction
2. Growth-retarded fetus with mature pulmonary indices and a maternal cervix favorable for induction
3. Insulin-dependent diabetic woman at 37 weeks gestation or more with mature pulmonary indices
4. Class A (chemical diabetes diagnosed before pregnancy; managed by diet alone; any age of onset) diabetic woman at term with a cervix favorable for induction
5. Presence of medical disorders (asthma, hypertension, pregnancy-induced hypertension, etc.) that might pose a threat to maternal and fetal health.

Table 2-3 lists recommendations for management of biophysical profile scores.

Several prospective studies, summarized in Table 2-4, have shown that the majority of women studied (>97 percent) have normal test results and delivery outcome. Perinatal mortality varies inversely with the last score before delivery. In 1981[2] and 1985,[3] in large groups of patients, Manning found that the gross perinatal mortality rate decreased from 11.7 to 7.4 per 1,000 and the corrected value decreased from 5 to 1.9 per 1,000. In

Table 2-3. Interpretation and Management of Fetal Biophysical Profile Score

Score	Interpretation	Recommended Management
8–10	Normal infant	Repeat test in 1 week[a]
6	Suspect asphyxia	Repeat test in 4–6 hours[b]
4	Suspect asphyxia	If >36 weeks, deliver If <36 weeks, repeat in 24 hours If score <4, deliver
0–2	Strong suspicion for asphyxia	Deliver

[a] Repeat test twice per week if diabetic or greater than 42 weeks gestation.
[b] Deliver if oligohydramnios present.

Manitoba, since the use of this testing, the stillbirth rate has decreased by 30 percent. A stillbirth occurring within a week of a normal test result is defined as a false negative. This ranges from 0.41 to 1.01 per 1,000, with a mean of 0.64 per 1,000.

The false-negative rate, although small, directly reflects the negative predictive accuracy of the test. Manning et al.[4] calculated from a study of 19,221 pregnancies a negative predictive accuracy of 99.224 percent or the probability of fetal death after a normal test as 0.726 per 1,000 patients.

Because the ideal testing method would result in no false-negative deaths, the biophysical profile is not perfect. The cause of the imperfection is the probability of change in the fetal status from either a chronic condition or an acute variable. While more frequent testing of all patients would decrease the false-negative rate, this has not been tested due to the increased workload. The proper selection of patients requiring more vigilant monitoring, that is, those judged to be at risk (e.g., an immature fetus with growth retardation, pregnancy-induced hypertension, or diabetes), would render this more feasible.

Table 2-4. Biophysical Profile and Perinatal Mortality

Study	No. Patients	No. Deaths	Perinatal Mortality (Rate/1,000)
Manning[4]	19,221	141	1.92
Baskett[5]	5,034	32	3.10
Platt[6]	286	4	7.0
Schifrin[7]	158	7	12.6

NONSTRESS TESTING

Nonstress testing (NST) is the external detection of fetal heart rate (FHR) and fetal movement in relation to uterine contractions, noting accelerations of fetal heart rate with fetal movement. These assessments are predictors of fetal outcome.

Conduct of the Nonstress Test

With the patient recumbent in the semi-Fowler's position and the uterus displaced to the left by elevating the right hip (to displace the uterus from the aorta and inferior vena cava), 20 minutes of continuous FHR tracing is followed, along with measurement of uterine contractions using a tocodynamometer. Fetal movement is noted either by the patient using external palpation of the maternal abdomen or by changes in the tocodynamometer tracing.

The test is usually interpreted as one of the following[8,9]:

1. Reactive: at least two fetal movements in 20 minutes with acceleration of the FHR to at least 15 beats per minute (bpm) with long-term variability of at least 10 bpm and a baseline rate within the normal range (Fig. 2-1).
2. Nonreactive: no fetal movement or no acceleration of the FHR with movement and poor or no long-term variability and the baseline FHR within or outside the normal range (Fig. 2-2).
3. Uncertain reactivity: fewer than two fetal movements in 20 minutes or acceleration to less than 15 bpm; long-term variability amplitude less than 10 bpm and a baseline heart rate outside of normal limits.

Fetuses have sleep or inactive cycles that can last up to 80 minutes. One can either wait for a period of time or manually stimulate the infant and repeat the NST.

A reactive test is associated with survival of the fetus for 1 or more weeks in more than 99 percent of cases.[8,10] A nonreactive test is associated with poor fetal outcome in 20 percent of cases.[11] Although the false-

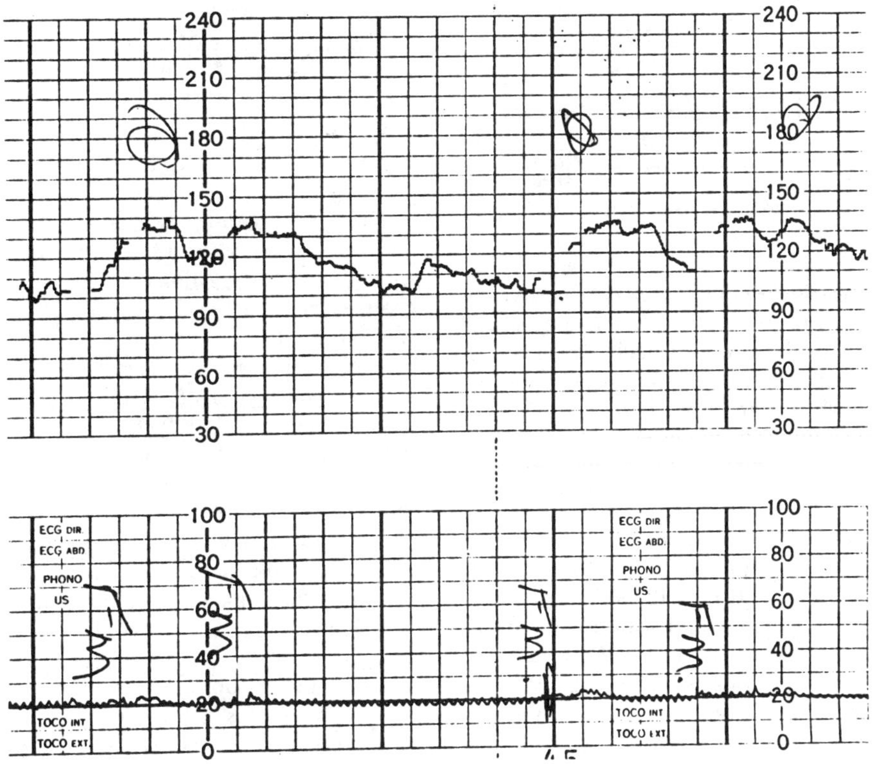

Fig. 2-1. Reactive nonstress test. Characterized by accelerations in the FHR with fetal movement (FM).

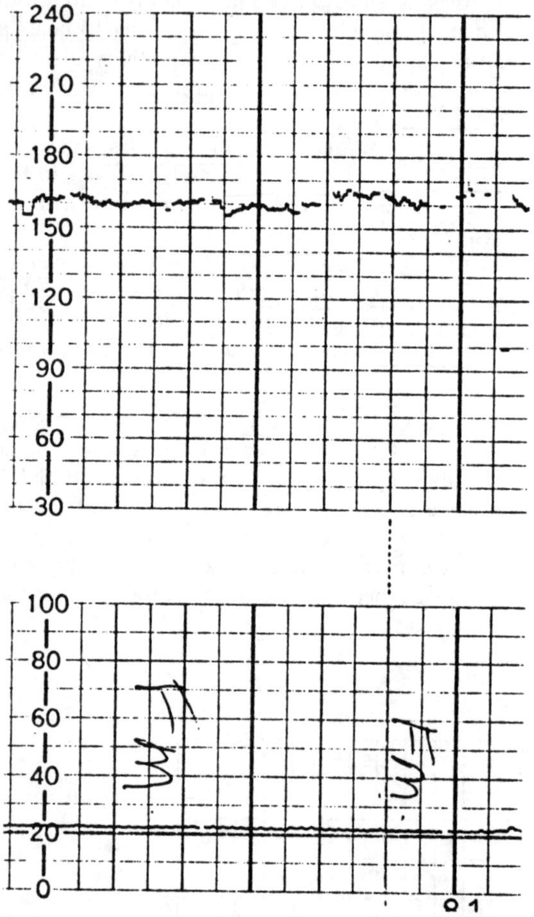

Fig. 2-2. Nonreactive nonstress test. No accelerations in FHR with fetal movement (FM).

positive rate of this technique is high (80 percent), further evaluation needs to be done when a nonreactive result is obtained. The next step is usually a contraction stress test (CST). Similarly, an uncertain reactive pattern needs to be followed up with either another NST or a CST.

CONTRACTION STRESS TESTING

As its name implies, the CST assesses the fetal response (heart rate pattern) to regular uterine contractions. Using the same technique as the NST, the CST requires three adequate contractions within a 10-minute period, each with a duration of 1 minute. If there are not enough spontaneous contractions, then augmentation with intravenous oxytocin is indicated. Beginning at a rate of 1.0 mU/min, the infusion is increased every 15 minutes until the requisite number of contractions are obtained. It is rarely necessary to exceed 10 mU/min.

Certain clinical situations present contraindications to CST: prior classic (vertical incision) cesarean delivery, placenta previa, and women at risk of premature labor (premature rupture of membranes, multiple gestation, incompetent cervix, and treatment for preterm labor).

The CST is interpreted as follows:

1. Negative: no late decelerations and normal baseline FHR
2. Positive: persistent late decelerations (even when the contractions are less frequent than three contractions within 10 minutes) and possible absence of FHR variability
3. Suspicious: intermittent late decelerations or variable decelerations and abnormal baseline FHR
4. Unsatisfactory: poor-quality recording or inability to achieve three contractions within 10 minutes
5. Hyperstimulation: excessive uterine activity (contractions closer than every 2 minutes or lasting longer than 90 seconds) resulting in late decelerations or bradycardia

A negative CST is associated with fetal survival for a week or more in 99 percent of cases,[8,9] whereas a positive CST is associated with poor fetal outcome in 50 percent of cases.[11] Like the NST, the CST also has a high-false positive rate (50 percent), but the treatment, if delivery is elected, can be a trial of induction of labor.

FETAL HEART RATE PATTERNS

The FHR pattern is characterized by its baseline between contractions and periodic changes in association with uterine contractions.[12] The baseline and periodic changes are further broken down into FHR and its variability.

Fetal heart rate is normal from 120 to 160 bpm between contractions (Fig. 2-3). Rates greater than 160 bpm are described as tachycardia (Fig. 2-4) and those less than 120 bpm as bradycardia (Fig. 2-5). If the alterations in rate are less than 2 minutes in duration, they are called accelerations and decelerations.

The usual initial response of the normal fetus to acute hypoxia or asphyxia is bradycardia. A heart rate between 100 and 120 bpm might signify either a compensated, mild hypoxic stress, or may be idiopathic and benign. Thus in many institutions, a fetal bradycardia is defined as less than 100 bpm. When the heart rate falls below 60 bpm the fetus is in distress and requires either reversal of the cause of the bradycardia or emergent delivery. Other causes of bradycardia that are nonasphyxic in origin are:

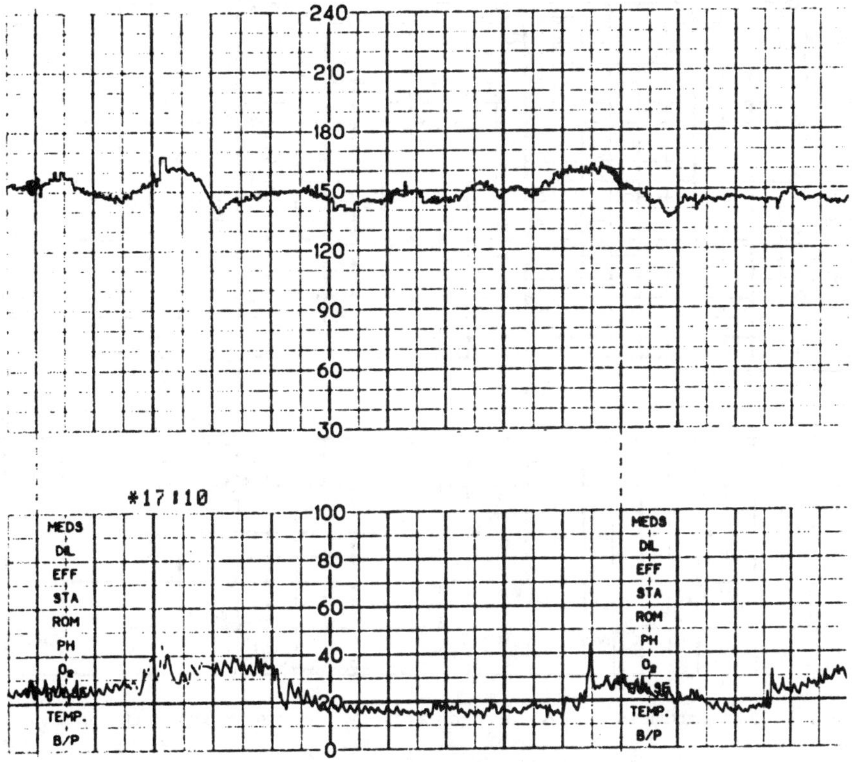

Fig. 2-3. Normal FHR pattern. The rate (140 bpm) and short- and long-term variability are normal. There are no periodic changes.

1. Bradyarrhythmias
2. Maternal drug ingestion (especially β-blockers)
3. Hypothermia

Tachycardia is occasionally seen with fetal asphyxia or with recovery from asphyxia, but is more likely seen secondary to:

1. Maternal or fetal infection, especially chorioamnionitis
2. Maternal ingestion of β-adrenergics or parasympathetic blockers
3. Tachyarrhythmias
4. Prematurity
5. Thyrotoxicosis

Variability in the FHR tracing describes the irregularity or the difference in interval from beat to beat. If the interval between heart beats were identical, then the FHR trace would be smooth (Fig. 2-6). The fact is that in most healthy fetuses, one notes an irregular tracing. This is thought to be secondary to an intact nervous pathway through the cerebral cortex, midbrain, vagus nerve, and the cardiac conduction system. It is thought that when asphyxia affects the cerebrum, there is decreased neural control of the variability. This is made worse by the failure of fetal hemodynamic compensatory mechanisms to maintain cerebral oxygenation. Therefore, with normal variability, irrespective of the fetal heart rate pattern, the fetus is not suffering cerebral anoxia.

Variability is described as being either short or long term. Short-term variability is the beat-to-beat difference and as such, it requires accurate detection of the heart rate. Because this can only be obtained with the fetal ECG, external monitors cannot be used to describe short-term variability, which is characterized as being either present or absent. Long-term variability looks at a wider window of the FHR, usually between 3 to 6 minutes. It can be detected using either internal or external methods of FHR monitoring and is described by the approximate amplitude range in bpm:

1. Normal: the amplitude range is 6 bpm or greater

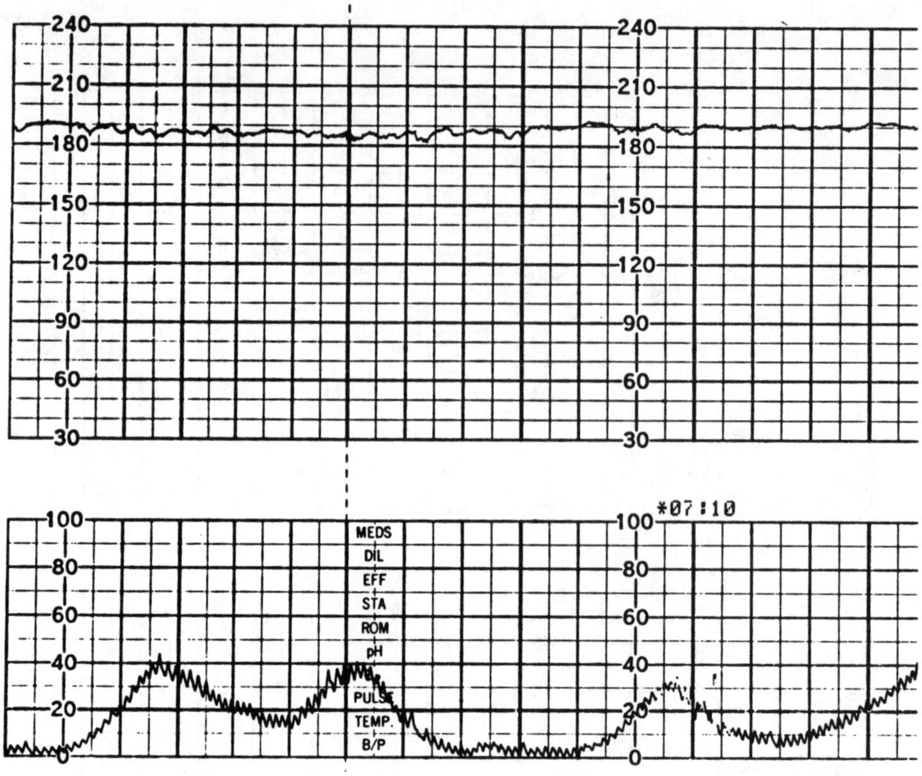

Fig. 2-4. Tachycardia. In this case there was a maternal fever secondary to chorioamnionitis.

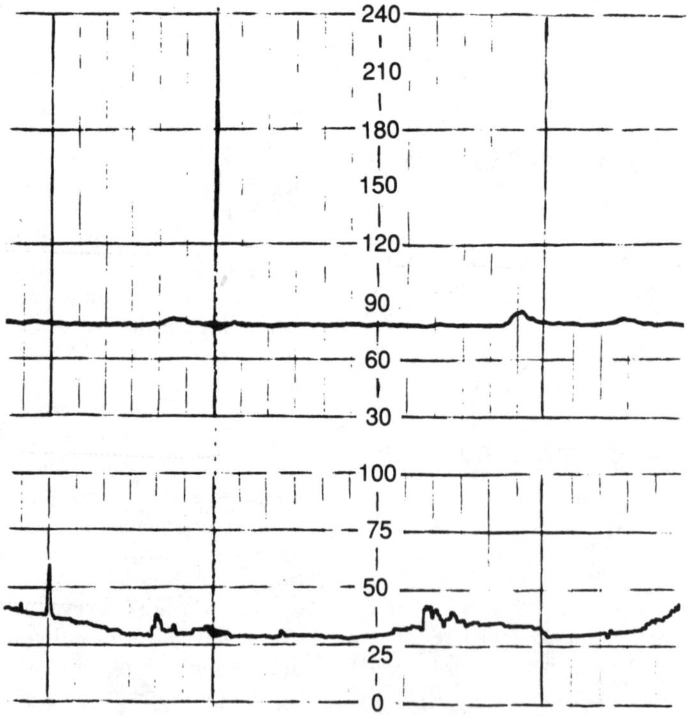

Fig. 2-5. Bradycardia, accompanied by absence of FHR variability.

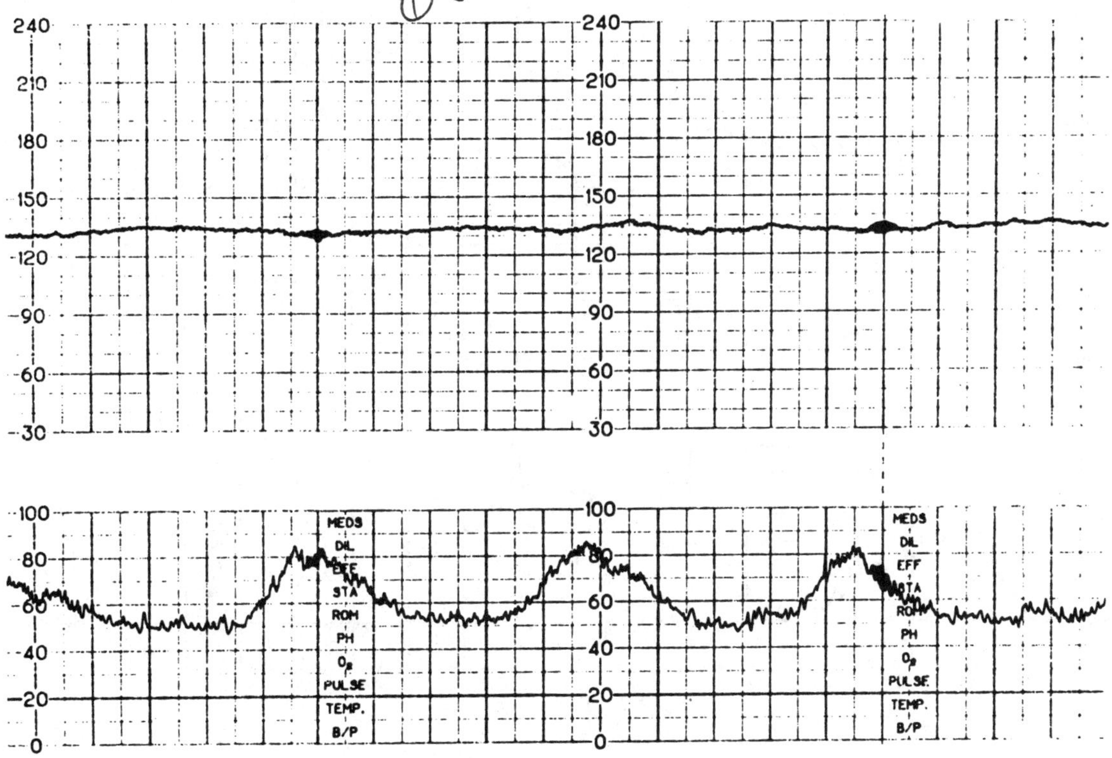

Fig. 2-6. Decreased variability of the FHR.

2. Decreased: the amplitude range is between 2 and 6 bpm
3. Absent: the amplitude range is less than 2 bpm
4. Saltatory: the amplitude is greater than 25 bpm.

In addition to asphyxia, there are other causes of altered variability: anencephaly, fetal drug effect (secondary to opioids, tranquilizers, magnesium sulfate, etc.), vagal blockade (due to atropine or scopolamine), and interventricular conduction delays (complete heart block).

Periodic changes in fetal heart rate occur in association with uterine contractions. *Early decelerations* occur concomitantly with a uterine contraction. They have a smooth contour and are a mirror image of the contraction (Fig. 2-7). The descent of the FHR is usually never more than 20 bpm below the baseline. The cause is presumed to be due to a vagal reflex caused by mild hypoxia but is not associated with fetal compromise. *Late decelerations* are also smooth in contour and mirror the contraction, but they begin 10 to 30 seconds after the onset of the contraction (Fig. 2-8). The depth of the decline is inversely related to the intensity of the contraction. Late decelerations have been classified as either reflex or nonreflex. The former is due to maternal hypotension, which acutely decreases uterine perfusion to an otherwise healthy fetus. A uterine contraction on top of this insult further reduces oxygen flow, causing cerebral hypoxia, which then leads to the deceleration. In between contractions the FHR returns to baseline with good variability. The nonreflex late deceleration is due to prolonged hypoxia that leads to myocardial depression. Cerebral function is also depressed. This is seen with pregnancy-induced hypertension, intrauterine growth retardation, and prolonged repetitive late decelerations. FHR variability is either decreased or absent.

Variable decelerations differ in duration, shape, and decrease in FHR from contraction to contraction. The abrupt onset and cessation of the deceleration is thought to be due to increased vagal firing in response to compression of either the umbilical cord (during early labor) or dural stimulation with head compression (during the second stage of labor). The vagal activity causes bradycardia, which decreases cardiac output as well as umbilical blood flow. Variable decelerations are described as severe when they fall to 60 bpm below the baseline FHR or last longer than 60 seconds (Fig. 2-9);

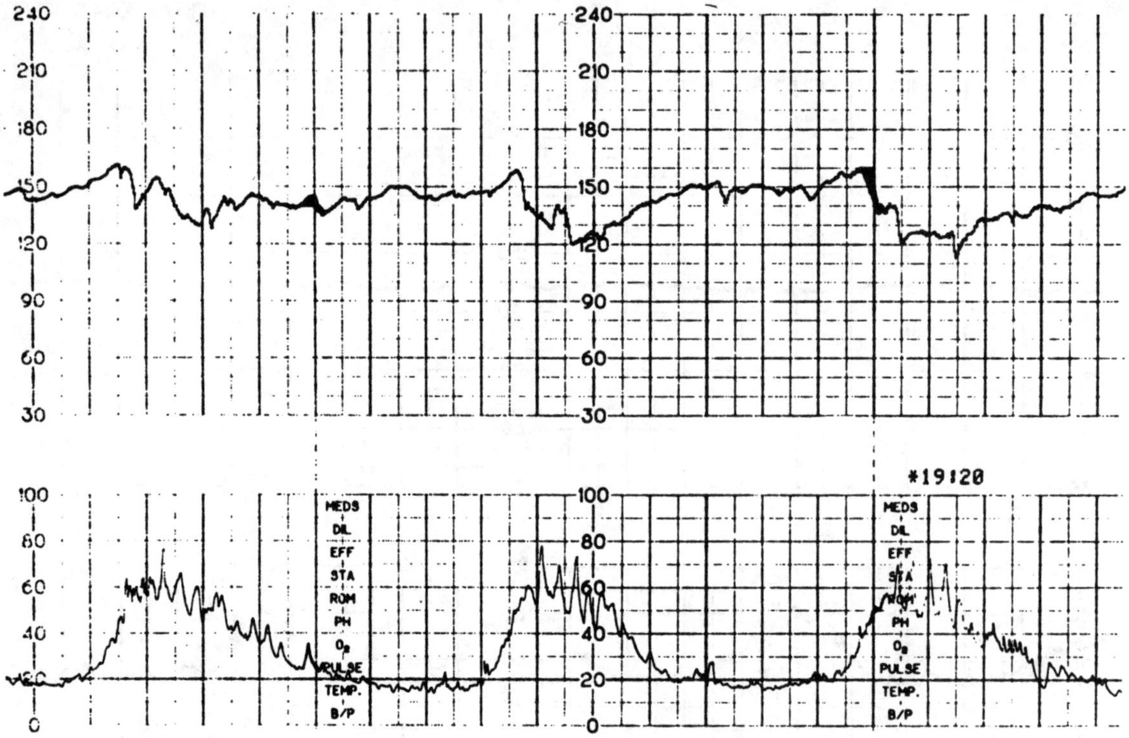

Fig. 2-7. Early decelerations.

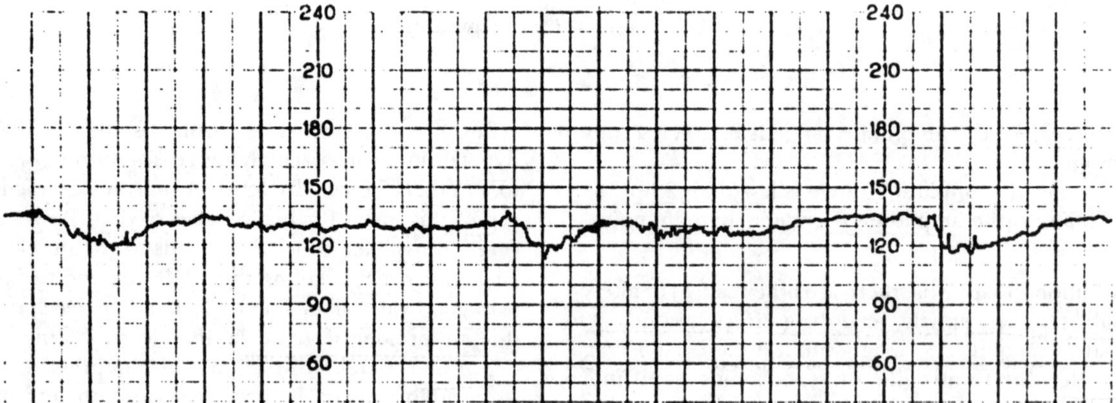

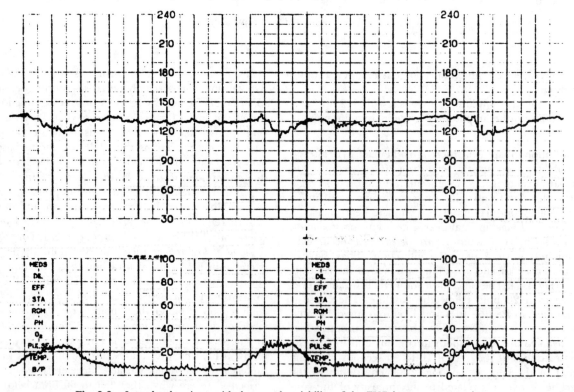

Fig. 2-8. Late decelerations, with decreased variability of the FHR between contractions.

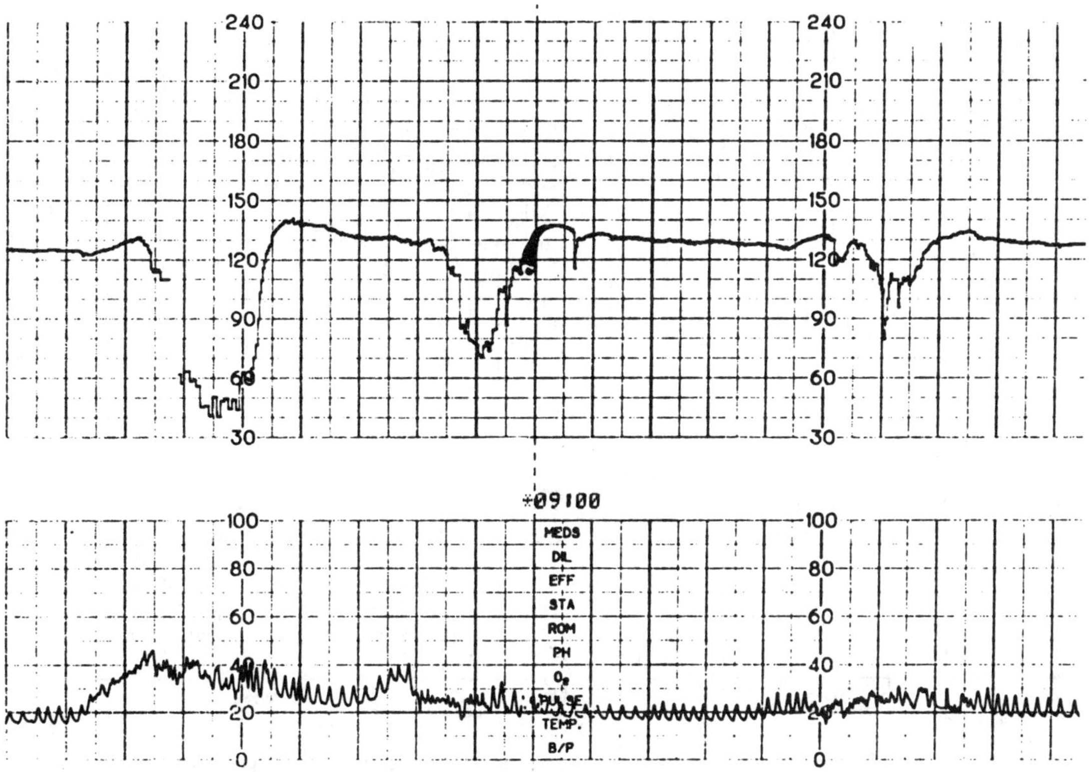

Fig. 2-9. Severe, deep variable decelerations, with decreased variability of the FHR between contractions.

otherwise, they are classified as mild to moderate (Fig. 2-10). The normal fetus is generally able to tolerate mild to moderate variable decelerations for prolonged periods of time; however, severe variable decelerations eventually result in fetal compromise unless reversed.

Accelerations with uterine contractions represent the greater effect of sympathetic activity over the parasympathetic nervous system (Fig. 2-11). They indicate a reactive, healthy fetus and have a good prognostic significance.

The above-described components of FHR comprise a normal pattern of a baseline rate of 120 to 160 bpm, which has a variability of greater than 6 bpm. One can see either no decelerations, early deceleration, or accelerations with contractions. This is associated with a good fetal outcome (i.e., an Apgar score of more than 7 at 5 minutes).[12,13] Depending on the severity and duration of the stress, there are other FHR patterns seen.

The acute stress pattern is a compensatory reaction in an otherwise healthy fetus to a short-lived period of asphyxia or hypoxia. The FHR usually demonstrates bradycardia, although tachycardia is also seen, but the most important fact noted is that variability remains normal. There can be either late or variable decelerations. The fetal outcome is generally good[14] because the impact of the asphyxia is brief, with possible depression from CO_2 narcosis, which is rapidly reversible.

When the stress persists, bradycardia is more profound, with decreased variability, as well as late and/or deep variable decelerations. This is a prolonged stress pattern that indicates mounting hypoxic damage to the heart and brain, resulting in the loss of compensatory mechanisms. Unless corrected, fetal death in utero can occur.

For a growth-retarded fetus, already compromised by a placenta with marginal function, persistent asphyxia results in a sinister pattern that is characterized by absent variability. The FHR displays severe variable or late decelerations, with a smooth rather than abrupt decrease and recovery in heart rate. Persistent bradycardia without variability is also called sinister.

Treatment of Abnormal Fetal Heart Rate Patterns

The first step in treatment is to recognize and describe an abnormal FHR pattern, then to identify the cause, and finally to correct it as quickly as possible. A list of

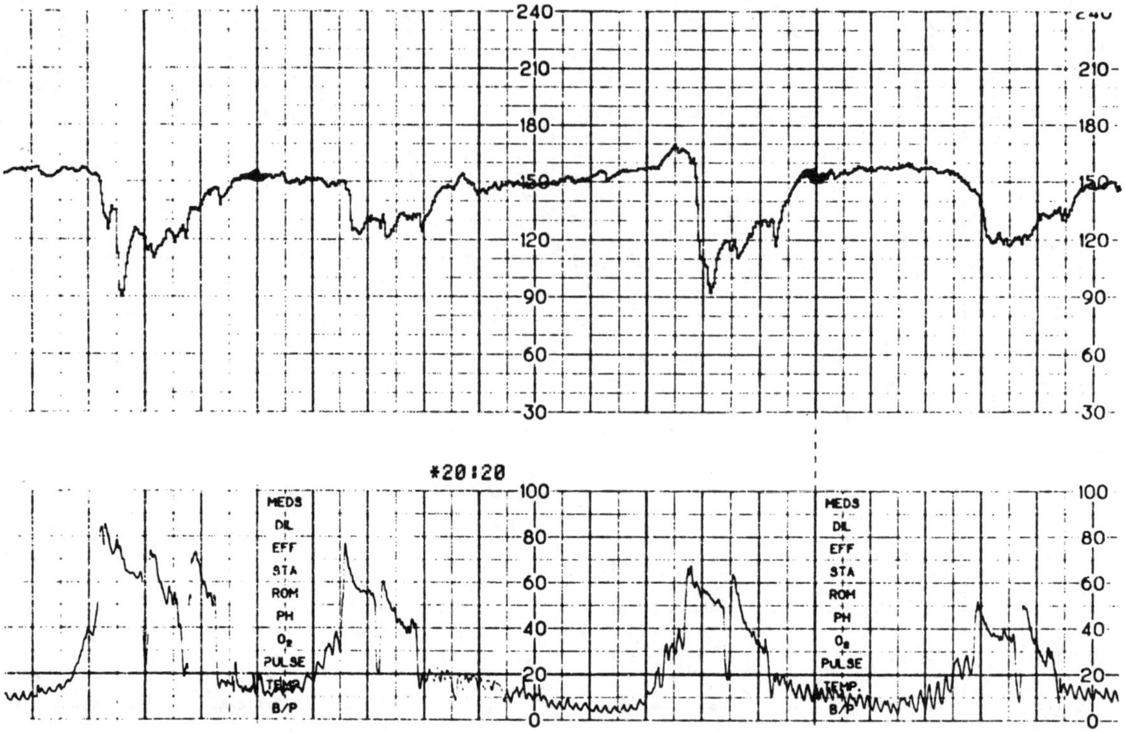

Fig. 2-10. Mild to moderate variable decelerations with pushing during the second stage of labor.

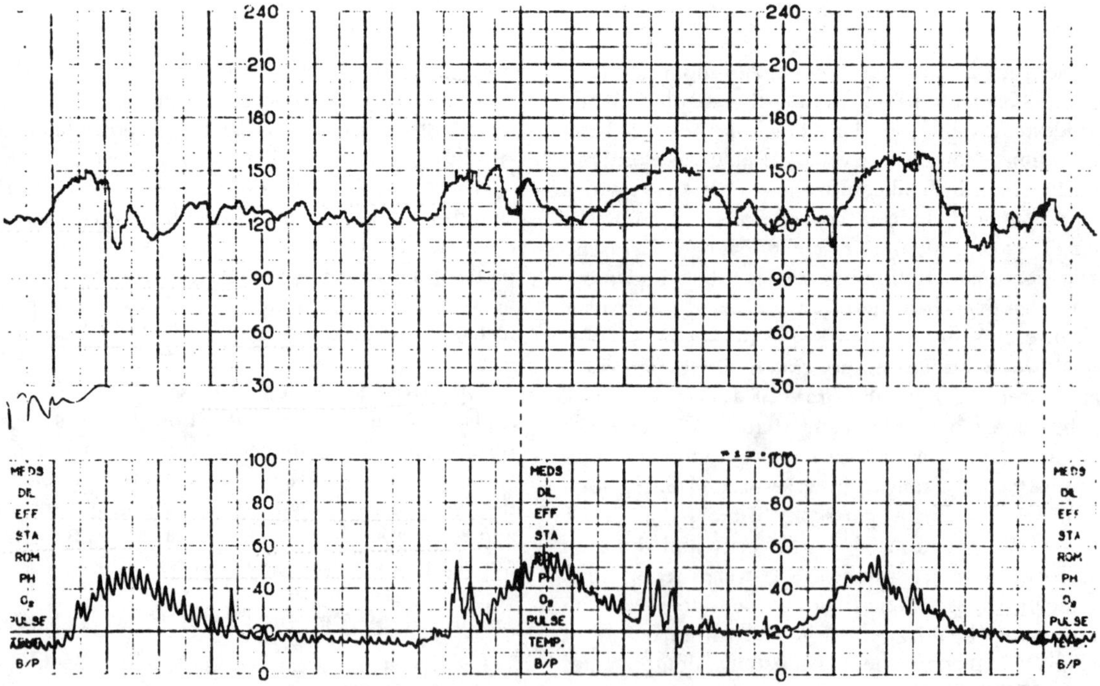

Fig. 2-11. Accelerations with uterine contractions.

Table 2-5. Causes and Treatment of Abnormal FHR Patterns

Pattern	Cause	Treatment
Bradycardia, late deceleration	Hypotension Uterine hyperstimulation	IV fluids, ephedrine, change position, decrease oxytocin
Variable decelerations	Umbilical cord compression, head compression	Change position Continue pushing if variability good
Late deceleration	Decreased uterine blood flow	Change position, O_2 for mother
Decrease in variability	Prolonged asphyxia	Change position, O_2 for mother

abnormal FHR patterns and their causes and treatment is given in Table 2-5. If the FHR pattern does not improve with these measures, then one needs to get more direct evidence of the fetal status (i.e., fetal capillary blood sampling) or deliver the fetus emergently.

FETAL CAPILLARY BLOOD SAMPLING

Since first introduced by Saling in 1967,[15] fetal blood sampling has become the final determinant in making a diagnosis of fetal hypoxia or asphyxia. The fetal blood sample is obtained from the presenting part (scalp or buttock) during labor. The instrumentation and technique of fetal blood collecting are described in standard obstetric textbooks. In this brief discussion, mention is made of the indications for sampling as well as the prognostic significance of values obtained.

Although a full set of blood gas determinations (pH, PCO_2 and PO_2) can be done on as little as 0.25 ml of blood, most institutions obtain the minimal amount of blood necessary for pH determination. However, having the pH value alone does not allow differentiation between metabolic and respiratory acidosis. Treatment of the causes of acidosis are theoretically different. Metabolic acidosis requires immediate delivery, whereas respiratory acidosis should respond to standard resuscitation. In reality, the initial resuscitative measures (oxygen for the mother, increased uterine displacement, and intravenous fluid bolus) are generally begun immediately following any severe deceleration. If a deceleration does not respond quickly to resuscitation, the clinical situation (stage of labor, presence of meconium, estimated fetal weight, gestational age, parity, etc.) will determine whether fetal capillary blood sampling is needed and/or if delivery is necessary immediately.

In human neonates, there is good correlation between the pH of fetal capillary blood taken shortly before delivery and that of umbilical cord samples. Beard et al.,[16] correlating fetal capillary blood pH and 2-minute Apgar scores, demonstrated that a pH above 7.25 was associated with an Apgar score more than 7 in 92 percent of cases. When the fetal capillary blood pH was less than 7.15, the Apgar score was less than 6 in 80 percent of cases. FHR decelerations have also been found to correlate with pH values (Table 2-6).[17] This correlation is not always close, therefore fetal capillary blood sampling is used when there is any question about the FHR tracing.

There are other FHR patterns that signal the need for fetal capillary blood sampling in addition to persistent late decelerations:

1. Absent or decreased short-term variability that might be due to central nervous system depressants given to the mother
2. Variable decelerations when combined with reduced or absent short-term variability
3. Severe, persistent variable decelerations

The clinical situation also provides indications for fetal capillary blood sampling, especially if there is decreased variability or severe decelerations.

Table 2-6. Correlation of Fetal Capillary Blood pH and Fetal Heart Rate Pattern

Deceleration Pattern	pH
Early, mild variable	7.30 ± 0.04
Moderate variable	7.26 ± 0.04
Mild, moderate late	7.22 ± 0.06
Severe late, variable	7.14 ± 0.07

(From Kubli et al.,[17] with permission.)

SUMMARY

This section has attempted to demonstrate the utility of the biochemical and technical advances in monitoring the fetus throughout pregnancy. Congenital malformation, chromosomal abnormalities, and Rh sensitization are perils to fetal health and can be diagnosed in utero. However, with the exception of cases of Rh sensitization, the chances for treatment are limited. The major focus of this section has been on maintaining oxygen supply to the fetus, because lack thereof quickly affects all fetal organs. More important is that reversal of hypoxia and asphyxia restores fetal well-being. The sooner the cause of distress is identified and treated, the less damage there is to the fetus. Therefore, the emphasis is on fetal monitoring for early identification of hypoxia and asphyxia.

The tests described monitor the status of the fetus externally during gestation and more directly, or internally, during labor. The data provide an assessment of the condition of the fetal neurologic and cardiovascular systems. But like any measurement, this information must fit into an overall clinical picture.

REFERENCES

1. Russell JC, Cooper CM, Ketchum CH, et al: Multicenter evaluation of TDx test for assessing fetal lung maturity. Clin Chem 35(6):1005, 1989
2. Manning, FA, Baskett TF, Morrison I, et al: Fetal biophysical profile scoring: a prospective study in 1184 high-risk patients. Am J Obstet Gynecol 140:289, 1981
3. Manning FA, Morrison I, Lange IR, et al: Fetal assessment based on fetal biophysical profile scoring: experience in 12,620 referred high-risk pregnancies. I. Perinatal mortality by frequent and etiology. Am J Obstet Gynecol 151:343, 1985
4. Manning FA, Morrison I, Harman CR, et al: Fetal assessment by fetal BPS: experience in 19,221 referred high-risk pregnancies. II. The false negative rate by frequency and etiology. Am J Obstet Gynecol 157:880, 1987
5. Baskett TF, Allen AC, Gray JH, et al: The biophysical profile score. Obstet Gynecol 70:357, 1987
6. Platt LD, Eglinton GS, Siopos L, et al: Further experience with the fetal biophysical profile score. Obstet Gynecol 61:480, 1983
7. Schifrin BS, Guntes V, Gergely RC, et al: The role of real-time scanning in antenatal fetal surveillance. Am J Obstet Gynecol 140:525, 1981
8. Schifrin BS: The rationale for antepartum fetal heart rate monitoring. J Reprod Med 23:213, 1979
9. Keegan KA, Paul RH: Antepartum fetal heart rate testing. IV. The nonstress test as a primary approach. Am J Obstet Gynecol 136:75, 1980
10. Evertson LR, Gauthier RJ, Collea JV: Fetal demise following negative contraction stress test. Obstet Gynecol 51:671, 1978
11. Ott WJ: Antepartum biophysical evaluation of the fetus. Perinatal Neonatol 2:11, 1978
12. Hon EH, Quilligan EJ: The classification of fetal heart rate. Conn Med 31:779, 1967
13. Schifrin BS, Dame L: Fetal heart rate patterns: prediction of Apgar score. JAMA 219:1322, 1972
14. Krebs HB, Petres RE, Dunn LJ, et al: Intrapartum fetal heart rate monitoring. I. Classification and prognosis of fetal heart rate patterns. Am J Obstet Gynecol 133:762, 1979
15. Saling E, Schneider D: Biochemical supervision of the foetus during labour. J Obstet Gynecaecol Br Commonw 74:799, 1967
16. Beard RW, Morris ED, Clayton SE: pH of foetal capillary blood as an indication of the condition of the foetus. J Obstet Gynaecol Br Commonw 74:812, 1967
17. Kubli FW, Hon EW, Khazin AF, et al: Observations on heart rate and pH in the human fetus during labor. Am J Obstet Gynecol 104:1190, 1969

PROGRESS OF LABOR

Labor is the progressive dilation of the cervix and descent of the fetal presenting part because of uterine contractions. The result is the expulsion of the fetus through the pelvis. The course of labor has been divided into three stages:

1. The *first stage* begins with the onset of regular contractions and concludes when the cervix is fully dilated.
2. The *second stage* spans the time period from full cervical dilation to the delivery of the infant.
3. The time from the delivery of the infant to the delivery of the placenta is called the *third stage*.

The first stage is further divided into latent and active phases. The latent phase is a preparatory phase of labor, where, despite regular contractions, there is little cervical dilation. The contractions do cause softening and thinning (or effacement) of the cervix. The active phase is characterized by rapid changes in cervical dilation, and has been further subdivided based on the slope of the curve of cervical dilation over time (Fig. 2-12).

Assessment of cervical dilation can only be made by periodic vaginal examinations, where, in addition to cervical dilation, effacement, consistency, and position (relative to the axis of the vagina) should be noted. In addition, each examination should supply information about the status of the membranes, fetal station and position, asynclitism, molding, and caput formation.

Table 2-7. Mean Values for the Progress of Labor

		Active Phase	
	Latent Phase Duration (Hours)	Rate of Cervical Dilation (cm/h)	Rate of Fetal Descent (cm/h)
Primipara	20	1.2	1
Multipara	14	1.5	2

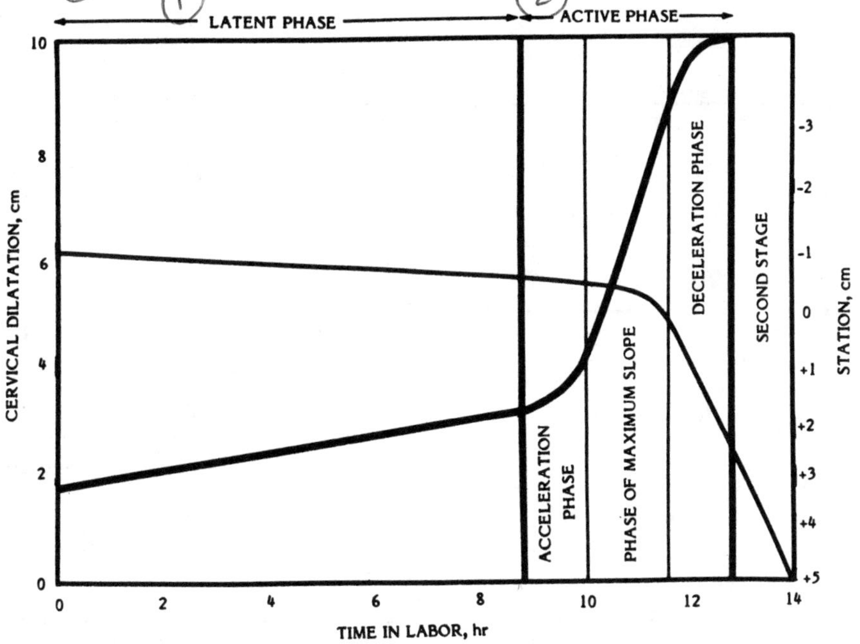

Fig. 2-12. Curves of cervical dilation and fetal descent, illustrating their interrelationship and component phases.

These data are then integrated with a graphic plot of cervical dilation and fetal station over time to provide a quantitative means of measuring the progress of labor. Friedman, after studying large numbers of parturients, generated a histogram and was able to define normal limits for these parameters (Table 2-7).[1] This is useful not only to define normal labor patterns, but more importantly, to recognize and describe aberrations from the norm that have implications for the outcome of labor.

LATENT PHASE

A prolonged latent phase (Fig. 2-13) is most commonly due to excessive narcotic-analgesic-sedative drugs or early use of epidural anesthesia. False labor, another cause, can only be diagnosed retrospectively. Treatment can be:

1. Stimulation of uterine activity with oxytocin. Thereupon, 85 percent of women will go into active labor.

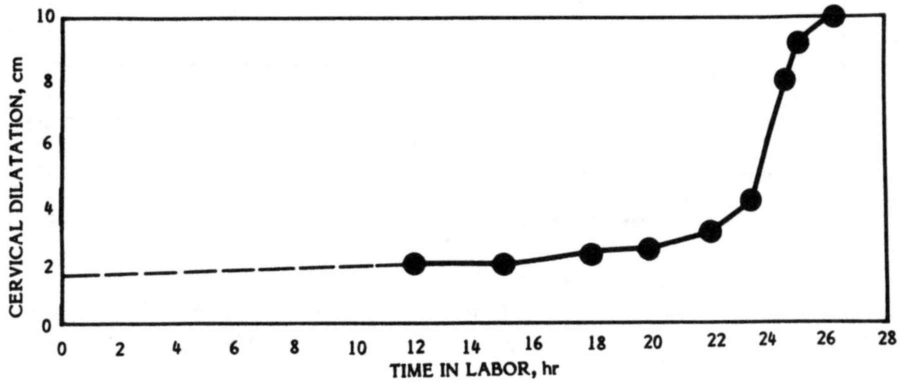

Fig. 2-13. Prolonged latent-phase pattern.

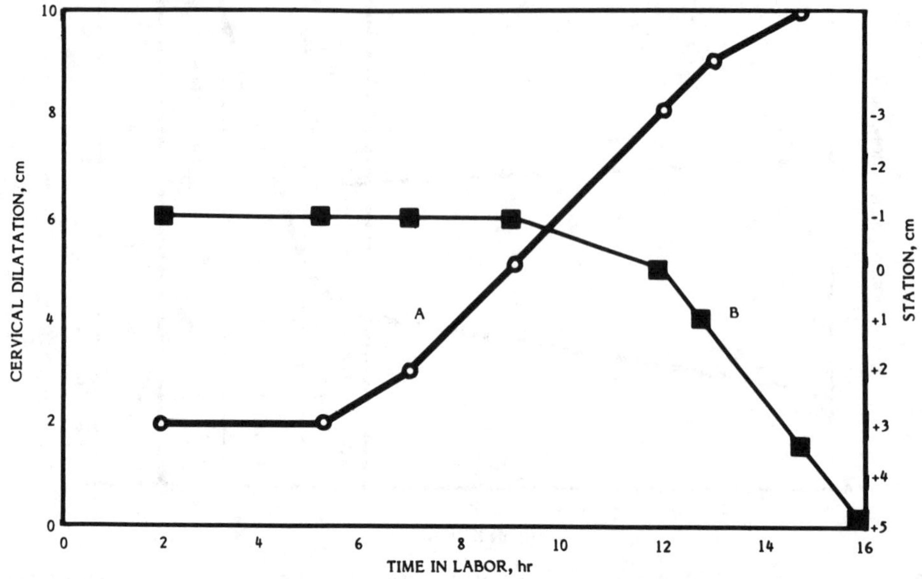

Fig. 2-14. Protracted active-phase dilation **(A)** and protracted descent **(B)** patterns are characterized by slow linear progress below established limits of normal.

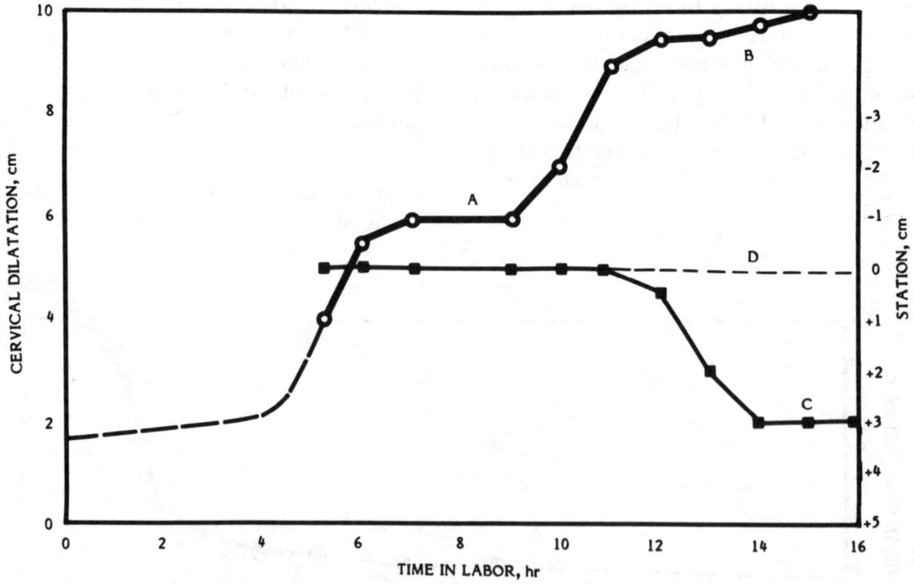

Fig. 2-15. Secondary arrest of dilation **(A)**, prolonged deceleration phase **(B)**, and arrest of descent **(C)**. Failure of descent **(D)** would have been diagnosed if descent had not begun to progress by the deceleration phase of dilation.

2. Resting the parturient with a narcotic-analgesic combination to induce sleep for 6 to 10 hours. Eighty-five percent of women will awaken in the active phase of labor. Ten percent, when awake, will have no contractions, and in retrospect can be said to have been in false labor. The remaining 5 percent will awaken with the same pattern of contractions and will benefit from oxytocin augmentation.

When the latent phase is prolonged, there is a higher incidence of cesarean delivery but the cause is not necessarily cephalopelvic disproportion.

ACTIVE PHASE

Protraction of the active phase (Fig. 2-14) places both the mother and fetus at increased risk of morbidity and mortality. One-third of women with this disorder have cephalopelvic disproportion, necessitating cesarean delivery. If disproportion is thought unlikely, then the parturient must be followed carefully, preferably with internal fetal heart rate monitoring. Frequent vaginal examinations are needed to make sure that descent is really occurring and not just deformational molding of the fetal scalp. If the fetal head becomes fixed in the pelvis, an extended second stage may cause intracranial damage, and there is the risk of uterine rupture from excessive distention and thinning of the lower uterine segment.[2]

If on two vaginal examinations, 1 hour apart, cervical dilation has stopped, the second stage is considered arrested (Fig. 2-15). Cephalopelvic disproportion, which is the cause in half the women who develop the arrest disorder, must be ruled out. If there is no disproportion, then oxytocin augmentation of uterine contractions is begun.

The term "failure to progress" is not well defined. It may mean different things under differing circumstances and the lack of specificity has no prognostic value for the outcome of labor. It is, therefore, preferable to define the stage or phase of labor and the problem, either protraction or arrest disorder.

REFERENCES

1. Friedman EA: Labor: Clinical Evaluation and Management. 2nd Ed. Appleton-Century-Crofts, New York, 1978
2. Cohen WR: Influence of the duration of second stage labor on perinatal outcome and puerperal morbidity. Obstet Gynecol 49:266, 1977

3

Perinatal Pharmacology

Perinatal pharmacology is the study of the physiologic and biochemical effects of both endogenous and exogenous compounds during the development of the human organism from conception through the first 28 days of neonatal life.

The obstetric anesthesiologist must care for patients who harbor a developing human organism at any stage of fetal development. The anesthesiologist is most often a part of the obstetric care team during parturition, which is the period leading to birth: the time of transition from fetal to neonatal life. The performance of the anesthesiologist's duties usually involves administration to the mother of compounds ordinarily foreign to the human body. These compounds are referred to as *xenobiotic substances* in the field of pharmacology, but are more commonly known to us as *drugs.*

A maternally administered drug may have drastic and far-reaching effects on the developing fetus. The fetus may be subject not only to the pharmacologic effects of the drug after it is transferred across the placenta, but also to alterations in its in utero environment because of the physiologic effects of the drug on the mother. Perinatal pharmacology must consider not only the fetus but also the mother, and the organs of gestation (uterus and placenta). In pharmacologic terms, these components are referred to as the *maternal–placental–fetal* unit. Therefore, it becomes important to the anesthesiologist to gain a basic understanding of the anatomy and physiology of the mother and fetus as well as an understanding of drug pharmacology.

ANATOMY OF THE MATERNAL–PLACENTAL–FETAL UNIT*

For the sake of simplicity, the maternal–placental–fetal unit can be separated into three components (Fig. 3-1). Constant interaction between the components is required for fetal well-being.

THE MATERNAL COMPONENT

Every maternal biologic system is dramatically altered during pregnancy. Most important to a discussion of perinatal pharmacology are the alterations in the maternal cardiovascular system and uterine anatomy.

Cardiovascular and Hemodynamic Changes

1. Increased total blood volume (25 to 40 percent) due to increased plasma volume (40 to 50 percent), and increased red cell mass (20 percent).
2. Increased cardiac output (30 to 50 percent) due to increased heart rate (12 to 15 beats/min) (bpm) increased stroke volume (30 percent), and decreased systemic vascular resistance (15 percent).
3. Increased uterine blood flow and a redistribution of uterine perfusion.

In the nonpregnant uterus, blood flow averages 50 ml/min, increasing with pregnancy to 500 to 700 ml/min. This change represents at least a 10-fold increase in blood flow. At term, 10 to 20 percent of maternal cardiac output is allotted to the uteroplacental circulation. The pattern of uterine perfusion must change with pregnancy because of the presence of the developing placenta and fetus. The placenta receives more than 80 percent of uterine perfusion, whereas the myometrium receives only 20 percent.

The cardiovascular and hemodynamic changes of pregnancy influence the pharmacologic characteristics of maternally administered drugs, including the volume of distribution and absorption from tissue depots.

Changes in Uterine Anatomy

The gravid uterus is an enlarging abdominal mass requiring an enlarging vascular supply.

An increase in vascular supply is necessitated by an increase in uterine weight from 70 to 1,100 g at term. This increase in weight does not include placental and fetal tissues; an increase in the mass of fibrous tissue and hypertrophy of uterine smooth muscle cells are responsible for uterine growth.

Arterial supply to the gravid uterus is provided by the uterine arteries, which arise from the hypogastric (internal iliac) and ovarian arteries. These vessels in turn arise from the abdominal aorta. The ovarian arteries may also contribute to the blood supply of the gravid uterus directly, although this contribution is variable and usually small.

Anastomoses occur between uterine and ovarian arteries along the lateral border of the gravid uterus in the broad ligament. Uterine vessels then penetrate the muscular layer of the uterus known as the *myometrium.* In the middle third of the myometrium, these vessels further divide to form a circular ring of vessels, the

* The opinions expressed herein are those of the author and are not to be construed as reflecting the views of the Navy Department, the Naval Service at large, or the Department of Defense.

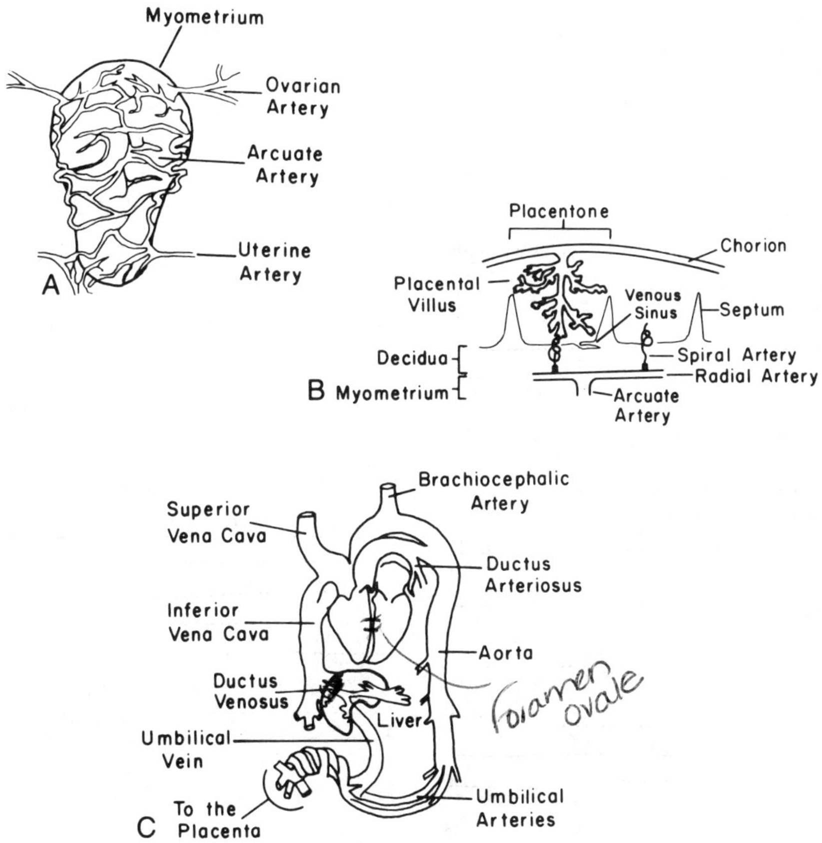

Fig. 3-1. The maternal-placental-fetal unit. **(A)** The maternal component. **(B)** The placental component. **(C)** The fetal component.

arcuate arteries. From this ring the radial arteries penetrate the remaining myometrium. The uterine mucosa, known as the *endometrium* (or *decidua* in the gravid uterus), contains the final branch of the uterine vasculature, the *spiral arteries* (named for their appearance). In the gravid uterus, the spiral arteries enter the placental tissue, ending in the intervillous space. There are 180 to 320 spiral arteries in the gravid uterus, each supplying one primary unit of the placenta (the *placentone*). The placentone consists of the spiral artery, surrounding intervillous space, and at least one fetal chorionic villus. As the uterine vascular supply subdivides, its characteristics change. The arcuate and radial arteries are muscular whereas the spiral arteries are not. For this reason, the spiral artery is more prone to occlusion. This fact becomes important in the discussion of the regulation of uteroplacental perfusion.

Venous drainage of the gravid uterus begins in decidual veins, which empty into larger conduits leading to the uterine and ovarian veins. They accompany the uterine and ovarian arteries. Ultimately, these veins join the inferior vena cava.

THE PLACENTAL COMPONENT

The placenta is an organ only present for gestation. It is composed of both maternal and fetal tissues. The placenta may be viewed as a semipermeable membrane that provides a junction for the maternal and fetal circulations. Its structure and function are, however, very complex. All substances necessary for fetal growth and development pass through this complicated interface.

Gross Anatomy

The human placenta resembles a disc. It can be viewed as two plates: a basal plate consisting of maternal tissue and a chorionic plate consisting of fetal tissue. These two plates join at the periphery to form a ring of connective tissue known as the *ring of Waldeyer.* In a normal gestation, the placenta weighs about one-sixth as much as the fetus (500 g).

Microscopic Anatomy

The basal plate of the placenta consists of the decidual tissue and vascular supply mentioned earlier. The chronic plate consists of three tissue layers and their supporting structures. These three tissue layers form the fetal chorionic villi, the structure of exchange for the fetus. The space separating the basal and chorionic plates is referred to as the *intervillous space.* The chorionic villi protrude into the intervillous space along with the spiral artery. The intervillous space is subdivided by a series of septa composed of decidual tissue. Each spiral artery with its accompanying decidual tissue, intervillous space, and chorionic villi constitute the functional unit of the placenta known as the placentone. The placenta is further divided by decidual tissue to form lobulations known as *cotyledons.* As gestation proceeds, the chorionic villi undergo a maturation process. Initially, the villi are smooth, consisting of an external layer of cuboidal cells (the *syncytiotrophoblast*) and an internal layer of cells (the *cytotrophoblast*). These two layers separate the intervillous space from the fetal umbilical capillaries. As maturation occurs, the villi become branched and the two cell layers flatten, reducing the distance between the intervillous space and the fetal umbilical capillaries. This maturation process becomes important in the discussion of placental transfer.

Pattern of Blood Flow

Maternal blood enters the intervillous space from the spiral artery and bathes the fetal chorionic villus. At the same time, fetal blood traverses the umbilical capillaries contained in the chorionic villus. Placental transfer from mother to fetus occurs across the chorionic membrane. This pattern of blood flow in the human placenta differs from other mammalian placentas, and is commonly referred to as the *villous stream pattern.* Although the mechanics of villous stream exchange are poorly understood, a simplified comparison can be drawn between the alveolus in the lung and the placentone in the placenta. Each placentone, like its structural counterpart the alveolus, may receive an unequal portion of the uteroplacental blood flow. At any one time, only approximately 100 spiral arteries out of the total 180 to 320 are patent. The placentone, like the alveolus, may be underperfused. Although shunt is a reality in the placenta as in the lung, its physiology remains unexplained.

THE FETAL COMPONENT

Fetal perfusion of the placenta (umbilical–placental perfusion) differs anatomically from maternal perfusion of the placenta (uteroplacental perfusion). The fetal cardiovascular system is designed to allow life in two radically different environments. An understanding of fetal cardiovascular anatomy is required for an understanding of perinatal pharmacology.

Blood Flow from the Fetus to the Placenta

Fetal blood enters the placenta via the two umbilical arteries, which arise from the internal iliac arteries. The umbilical arteries traverse the long umbilical cord to enter the placenta, where they subdivide to form smaller vessels and finally the umbilical capillaries. The umbilical capillaries traverse the chorionic villi surrounded by connective tissue and ultimately separated from maternal blood in the intervillous space by the two cellular layers, the cytotrophoblast and epitheloid syncytiotrophoblast. Poorly oxygenated fetal blood containing the by-products of metabolism enters the umbilical arteries, traverses the umbilical capillaries, and returns cleansed and oxygenated via the single umbilical vein.

Blood Flow from the Placenta to the Fetus

Well-oxygenated fetal blood returning to the fetus via the umbilical vein enters the fetus at the umbilicus, where approximately 50 percent of the blood enters the portal circulation perfusing the fetal liver. The remainder enters the inferior vena cava. The amount of fetal umbilical blood flow entering the fetal portal circulation may vary because of reactivity of the ductus venosus. Fetal acidosis has been shown to close the ductus venosus, shunting more umbilical blood flow into the inferior vena cava than the portal circulation. Eventually, all umbilical blood enters the inferior vena cava and flows into the right atrium. In the right atrium, blood from the inferior vena cava mixes with the poorly oxygenated blood from the head and upper extremities, returning to the right atrium via the superior vena cava. From the right atrium most of the blood is shunted across the forearm ovale into the left atrium. From the left atrium flow continues to the left ventricule and out into the aorta. A small fraction of right atrial flow proceeds through the right ventricle and out the pulmonary outflow tract to the fetal lungs. Since the fetal lungs do not have respiratory function in the fetus, their perfusion is not a priority. A significant portion of the blood flow to the lungs goes to the fetal aorta via a vascular shunt known as the *ductus arteriosus.* Ultimately, 40 to

50 percent of the fetal cardiac output returns to the placenta via the umbilical arteries.

PHYSIOLOGY OF THE MATERNAL–PLACENTAL–FETAL UNIT*

The organ of exchange in gestation, the placenta, differs hemodynamically from any other mammalian organ. The placenta provides a meeting for the maternal and fetal circulations—two dissimilar circulatory patterns. The coordinated function of these circulatory systems at the level of the placenta is tantamount to the survival of the developing fetus. Regulation of placenta circulation remains poorly understood.

Anesthetic drugs administered to the mother by a variety of different techniques may adversely affect the fetus by altering maternal circulation to the placenta (uteroplacental circulation) or fetal circulation to the placenta (umbilical–placental circulation). These effects may be referred to as *indirect* because they may significantly alter the in utero milieu and affect fetal outcome. An understanding of these indirect effects can lead to rapid identification, treatment, and resolution of fetal compromise.

UTEROPLACENTAL CIRCULATION

The Uterine Perfusion Equation

At term, 10 to 20 percent of the maternal cardiac output is dedicated to the maternal–placental–fetal unit. Of this 500 to 700 ml of blood flow per minute, 80 percent reaches the intervillous space for interface with the fetal circulation, and 20 percent perfuses the uterine myometrium. The vascular bed of the uterus is described as *maximally dilated,* without autoregulation. For this reason, blood flow is directly related to maternal blood pressure. Uteroplacental blood flow is described by the following relationship:

$$\text{UBF} = \frac{\text{MMAP} - \text{UVP}}{\text{UVR}}$$

where UBF is uteroplacental blood flow, MMAP is maternal mean arterial blood pressure, UVP is uterine venous pressure, and UVR is uterine vascular resistance.

Determinants of Uteroplacental Perfusion

The maternal mean arterial pressure for the resting uterus is the driving pressure for blood at the level of the spiral artery. It averages 80 mmHg.

Uterine venous pressure in the resting uterus is 6 to 8 mmHg. In addition to the above pressures, resting pressure in the intervillous space has been measured at 10 mmHg. Uteroplacental perfusion pressure in the resting state is therefore approximately 70 mmHg.

Uterine vascular resistance is influenced by two factors:

1. Tension in the myometrium, decreasing the caliber of the arcuate and radial arteries, which ultimately give rise to the spiral arteries.
2. Vasoconstriction of the uterine, ovarian, arcuate, and radial arteries. Although the uterine vasculature is considered maximally dilated in normal pregnancy, it actively responds to α stimulation; thus vascular resistance may be increased by any compound that causes a release of catecholamines.

Factors that Influence Uteroplacental Perfusion

Uteroplacental perfusion and the factors that affect it are very difficult to assess in humans at present. Advances in Scandinavia with radionuclide imaging offer a tool for noninvasive determination of uteroplacental perfusion. However, the risks to the fetus imposed by this technique have not been defined.

A promising noninvasive technique to assess trends in uterine and fetal umbilical artery flow is available. This technique relies on the transabdominal Doppler ultrasound measurement of velocity waveforms in these vessels. Risk to the fetus should be minimal with this technique. However, most investigations have been and continue to be conducted in laboratory animal models with the difficulties imposed by chronic instrumentation. The major factors influencing uteroplacental perfusion obtained from the animal models and sparse human data are detailed below.

Position. Compression of both the abdominal aorta and the inferior vena cava occurs in the supine pregnant patient as a result of mechanical compression by the gravid uterus. This phenomenon is referred to as *aortocaval compression.* Compression of the aorta occurs above the origin of the hypogastric (internal iliac) arter-

* The opinions expressed herein are those of the author and are not to be construed as reflecting the views of the Navy Department, the Naval Service at large, or the Department of Defense.

ies that supply the uterine arteries, reducing uteroplacental perfusion. Compression of the inferior vena cava leads to an increase in uterine venous pressure with a concomitant decrease in the perfusion pressure in the intervillous space and a decrease in maternal cardiac output.

Hypotension. Pressure in the uterine arteries equals maternal mean arterial pressure. A fall in maternal mean arterial pressure of 20 to 25 percent is associated with a significant reduction in uteroplacental blood flow. Maternal mean arterial pressure below 100 mmHg systolic severely compromises uteroplacental perfusion. For the obstetric anesthesiologist, the most common etiology of hypotension is sympathetic blockade from major regional anesthesia.

Alterations in Uterine Tone. Increases in uterine tone severely alter uteroplacental perfusion by raising the uterine venous pressure, reducing the intervillous perfusion pressure, and increasing uterine vascular resistance through compression of the arcuate and radial arteries. These changes decrease uteroplacental blood flow. Most commonly, uterine tone is altered during the physiologic process of parturition. However, certain drugs employed in obstetric anesthesia, such as ketamine, increase uterine tone in dosages greater than 1.5 mg/kg. The obstetric drug, oxytocin, used to induce or augment labor increases uterine tone. Pathologic conditions that lead to a tetanic uterine contraction, such as abruptio placentae, may also affect uteroplacental perfusion.

Maternal Respiratory Alterations. Severe hypoxia, hypercarbia, and hypocarbia are associated with a decrease in uteroplacental perfusion. Moderate alterations do not appear to affect uteroplacental blood flow.

Catecholamines. Exogenous or endogenous catecholamine stimulation decreases uteroplacental perfusion by augmenting uterine vascular resistance. Of the common vasopressors used in anesthetic practice, ephedrine and, more recently, phenylephrine have been shown to maintain uteroplacental perfusion. The increase in maternal mean arterial pressure with administration of ephedrine is presumed to be due to central nervous system (CNS) stimulation rather than primary catecholamine release.

UMBILICAL–PLACENTAL CIRCULATION

Fetal Blood Flow to the Placenta

In contrast to the maternal contribution to the uteroplacental circulation of 10 to 20 percent of cardiac output, the umbilical placental circulation receives 40 to 50 percent of the combined ventricular output of the fetus. The fetal contribution to the placenta is 75 ml/kg/min or 250 ml/min at term. In contrast to maternal uteroplacental flow, fetal umbilical–placental flow is much less. The two dissimilar circulatory patterns are also mismatched at the placenta. Placenta transfer is rapid, however. Although maternal uteroplacental perfusion may show marked variation in response to stimuli, the fetal umbilical–placental circulation is less variable. At present it appears that changes in umbilical–placental perfusion may, in most cases, be less predictable and less preventable.

The umbilical–placental circulation differs from the uteroplacental circulation in that the umbilical circulation is a low-pressure system and the uteroplacental circulation is a high-pressure system. In addition, the umbilical–placental circulation is dynamic throughout gestation, changing with fetal maturity as well as with alterations in maternal physiology. Therefore, the response of the fetal umbilical circulation to asphyxia and pharmacologic manipulation varies with the gestational age of the fetus.

Of the total umbilical flow to the placenta, approximately 20 percent is shunted and never functionally available for exchange with the uteroplacental circulation across the placenta.

Regulation of the Umbilical–Placental Circulation

Control of the umbilical–placental circulation is poorly understood. Two major mechanisms are cited in the regulation of umbilical–placental circulation: physiologic reflex changes in the fetus and alterations in the neuroendocrine axis of the fetus. Because the umbilical–placental circulation provides a wide margin of safety for the fetus, a challenge to fetal survival (most commonly asphyxia) must be present for these mechanisms to be obvious without monitoring of the fetal heart rate (FHR). Continuous FHR monitoring is useful in detecting changes in umbilical–placental circulation.

Reflex Changes in the Fetal Circulation. The fetal circulation is a low-resistance system that relies on fetal cardiac output to maintain umbilical–placental circulation. In the developing fetus, cardiac output is determined primarily by the FHR since alterations in stroke volume are not possible. In the immature fetus, peripheral resistance is not usually responsive. As the fetus matures, however, FHR declines and fetal blood pressure rises, indicating a transition of the circulatory pattern and a maturation of peripheral resistance control. The transition corresponds closely to development of the aortic chemoreceptors. In early gestation, the fetus responds to asphyxia by increasing heart rate without changing blood pressure. As the fetus matures, the response to asphyxia is bradycardia with a concomitant increase in blood pressure, suggesting a reflex mechanism. CNS control and/or catecholamine release is presumed to be responsible for the regulation of these circulatory responses in the immature fetus, whereas the aortic chemoreceptors are responsible in the more mature fetus.

Alterations in the Neuroendocrine Axis. Although reflex changes contribute significantly to the regulation of umbilical–placental perfusion in the mature fetus, they are not entirely responsible. In the immature as well as the mature fetus, certain substances found in the neuroendocrine system, such as vasopressin, prostaglandins, endorphins, and catecholamines, have been implicated in the regulation of umbilical–placental perfusion.

Factors That Influence the Umbilical–Placental Circulation

The factors below are known to influence the umbilical–placental circulation.

Direct Effects on Umbilical Vessels. The umbilical vessels are lengthy, redundant, and muscular with sparse innervation (prior to entry into the fetal abdomen). Umbilical–placental perfusion may be altered by:

1. Mechanical compression secondary to cord prolapse or compression by fetal parts.
2. Vasospasm secondary to placental transfer of local anesthetics, vasopressors, maternal hypocarbia, or norepinephrine release.
3. An increase in intervillous pressure (most commonly due to uterine hypertonus) limiting blood flow through the chorionic villi in the intervillous space (Starling resistor effect).

Alterations in the Fetal Neuroendocrine Axis by Drugs. The administration of certain drugs may produce changes in the fetal neuroendocrine system. Although these changes are well documented, their etiology and specific mechanism of action are unclear. For example, administration of morphine and diazepam to the mother results in a decrease in the variability of the FHR. Similarly, adrenergic agents used to halt labor may lead to fetal tachycardia, presumably through an autonomic nervous system mechanism.

A MODEL FOR THE PLACENTAL TRANSFER OF ANESTHETICS*

IMPORTANCE OF THE CONCEPT OF PLACENTAL TRANSFER

All drugs administered to the mother will pass to the fetus to some extent, potentially affecting either fetal development or neonatal behavior (Fig. 3-2). The administration of diethylstilbesterol to mothers in the 1960s to prevent abortion and the subsequent development of vaginal carcinoma in many of their female progeny in later life remains a painful remainder of the far-reaching effects of drugs administered to the maternal–placental–fetal unit. More recently, neurobehavioral testing of the neonate has detected behavioral changes secondary to the maternal administration of drugs commonly used as anesthetics. These behavioral changes have proven to be evanescent. Behavioral and developmental changes noted in the fetus or neonate that can be ascribed to a particular compound are direct effects of that compound because it is assumed that the quantitative transfer of the drug or its metabolites across the placenta and its ultimate disposition in the neonate are responsible. Utilizing the principles of placental transfer, we can predict the extent of drug transfer from mother to fetus and uncover the direct effects of drugs on the fetus.

THE PLACENTAL TRANSFER EQUATION (FICK EQUATION)

Placental transfer may occur by several mechanisms, including simple diffusion, active transport, bulk flow, facilitated diffusion, and breaks in the chorionic membrane. Anesthetic compounds and inhaled gases cross the placenta primarily by simple diffusion. The concept of simple diffusion is described by a general equation known as the *Fick equation.* This equation describes a perfect relationship in an imperfectly related biologic system. For this reason the equation is used only to demonstrate the principles of placental transfer:

$$Q/t = \frac{K \times A \times (Cm - Cf)}{D}$$

* The opinions expressed herein are those of the author and are not to be construed as reflecting the views of the Navy Department, the Naval Service at large, or the Department of Defense.

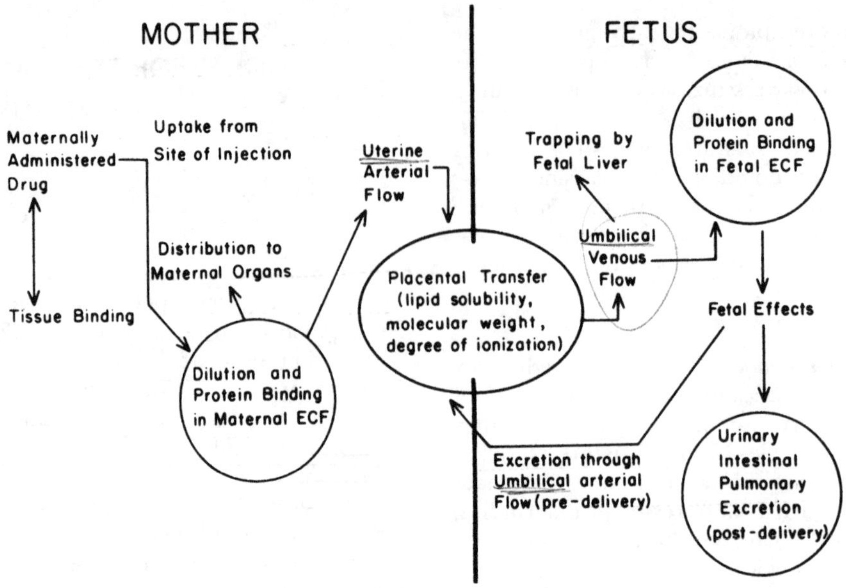

Fig. 3-2. Perinatal drug transfer.

Q/t is the quantity of "free" drug (nonionized and non-protein-bound) transferred in a unit of time; K is the diffusion coefficient of the drug being studied (a constant value that varies for each compound); A is the total area of the membrane (in this case the chorionic membrane) available for transfer; Cm is the maternal concentration of "free" drug (usually expressed in μg/ml); Cf is the fetal concentration of "free" drug (in μg/ml); and D is the distance across the membrane (the chorionic membrane) (expressed in μm).

Assumptions for the Fick Equation

As is most mathematical models for a complex biologic system, certain assumptions must be allowed:

1. Compounds that are transferred by facilitated diffusion (e.g., glucose) or those transferred by active transport (e.g., amino acids) may not be described by the model.
2. Only drug in the nonionized, non-protein-bound form ("free" drug) is described by the model.
3. The mathematical model is dynamic and cannot be used to predict "free" drug levels at equilibrium.

Relation of the Fick Equation to the Maternal–Placental–Fetal Unit

Variables in the Fick equation may be divided into four categories:

1. Drug factors, described by the diffusion constant (K).
2. Maternal factors, described by the term for the maternal concentration of "free" drug (Cm).
3. Placental factors, described by the terms for area of transfer (A) and diffusion distance (D).
4. Fetal factors, described by the term for the fetal concentration of "free" drug (Cf).

DRUG FACTORS

The term K in the placental transfer equation is the diffusion coefficient of the drug. It is a constant, but varies with the individual drug being addressed. The value of K is dependent on:

1. Molecular weight: as the molecular weight increases K decreases
2. Spatial configuration: the smaller the molecules, the greater the K
3. Degree of ionization (or pK_a, the dissociation constant): at body pH the more drug in the unionized form, the higher the K value
4. Lipid solubility: the greater the lipid solubility, the greater the K value

Thus, K is directly proportional to all but molecular weight, to which it is inversely proportional. Since most drugs in anesthesia have molecular weights of less than 600 and are highly lipid soluble, their K values and thus their rates of placental transfer are high.

PLACENTAL FACTORS

The rate of drug transfer increases with an increasing area of transfer and decreases as the distance for diffusion increases. The situation here is analogous to the lung.

Area

Similarly to the lung, the placenta possesses certain regions of physiologic shunt. Of the 180 to 320 spiral arteries supplying a placentone only about 100 are patent at any one time. It is reasonable to assume that under conditions of decreased placental perfusion, this number may fall even further. The area over which diffusion occurs is constantly varying in the placenta and the mechanism for regulation remains unclear.

Distance

The distance over which diffusion occurs is related to the maturity of the chorionic villi. As the maternal–placental–fetal unit approaches term, the villi become more mature and the average distance across the villi approximates 2 μm. Certain diseases of pregnancy may increase the diffusion distance (e.g., pregnancy-induced hypertension).

Metabolism

Evidence does exist that placental tissue may have a limited ability to metabolize some drugs (i.e., thiopental); however, it is unlikely that placental metabolism actually affects the rate of transfer by decreasing the concentration of "free" drug available for transfer across the placenta.

MATERNAL DRUG CONCENTRATION

The maternal concentration of "free" drug in the blood is dependent on several factors.

Site of Administration

Peak blood levels of drug are greatest in areas of dense vascularity. Peak blood levels from greatest to least are as follows: intravenous > caudal epidural > paracervical block > lumbar epidural > intramuscular > subarachnoid block. With epidural block, peak blood levels may be decreased by the addition of a vasoconstrictor substance (i.e., epinephrine or phenylephrine). The vasoconstrictor effect may be attenuated by the inherent vasodilating action of the drug itself, as is seen with etidocaine and bupivacaine.

Total Dosage

As the dosage administered increases, the plasma concentration also increases. Beyond a certain point, plasma binding sites may become saturated, causing "free" drug concentration to increase and making more drug available for transfer across the placenta.

Protein Binding

Within the blood an equilibrium is established, with the total amount of drug divided between the protein-bound portion and "free" drug. Protein binding, however, is not a static condition. As "free" drug concentration decreases because of redistribution and placental transfer, more drug enters the "free" drug compartment from the protein-bound compartment. Therefore, protein binding does little to limit the placenta transfer of a drug.

Redistribution

The circulation redistributes drug to new areas, where it is taken up. Tissue redistribution is a major factor in decreasing maternal drug concentration.

Clearance and Metabolism

Clearance and *metabolism* describe removal of a drug from the circulation and therefore from transfer. Metabolism of a drug, however, may yield other active compounds that transfer to and affect the fetus.

Blood pH

Maternal intravascular pH may affect the amount of "free" drug available for transfer by increasing the amount of nonionized drug and altering the portion bound to plasma protein.

FETAL DRUG CONCENTRATION

The concentration of "free" drug in the blood is dependent on several factors.

Concentration of the Drug at the Chorionic Villi

Drug concentration at the site of transfer in the placenta may vary because of:

1. Time of injection with regard to uterine contraction. Maternal intravascular injection at the time of uterine contraction may lead to a decrease in the con-

centration of drug in the placenta since placental blood flow may be decreased or halted at that time.

2. Placental shunting of blood. The number of placentones receiving maternal blood may vary at any time. The regulation of this variable is unclear.

Alterations in Fetal Circulation

Ordinarily, more than 50 percent of the fetal blood returning via the umbilical vein passes through the portal circulation and is filtered by the liver before entering the systemic circulation. The remainder passes through the ductus venosus. Via this route, many drugs are substantially removed from the fetal circulation and sequestered in the liver. During periods of fetal asphyxia and subsequent acidosis, flow through the ductus venosus may increase, allowing more drug to pass into the central circulation and affect target organs (i.e., the brain and heart). Additionally, at times of compromise, blood flow to the vital organs may also increase, leading to augmented delivery of drug to these tissues.

Fetal pH

The acid–base balance of fetal blood may affect the concentration of "free" drug in two ways. In drugs that are weak bases (e.g., local anesthetics) a decrease in fetal pH may lead to an increase in the concentration of "free" drug in the ionized form, thus preventing back-transfer across the placenta to the maternal circulation as maternal concentrations fall. This phenomenon is known as *ion trapping* and has been documented to occur in humans as well as in animal models. A decrease in serum pH in the fetus may also cause a decrease in plasma protein affinity for the drug, leading to increased concentration of "free" drug.

Plasma Protein Binding

Plasma proteins in the fetus possess a lesser drug-binding capacity than those of the mother, leading to an increase in the fraction of "free" drug in fetal serum.

Fetal Metabolism

Although the fetus has been shown to possess many of the metabolic pathways present in the mother, these pathways are not as developed and may easily be saturated. For this reason, the half-lives of many drugs are prolonged in the fetus and also in the neonate. Evidence exists that the relative maturity of the enzyme systems parallels fetal maturity (i.e., the younger the fetus, the more immature the enzyme system). Although fetal metabolism usually decreases the toxicity of a compound, in some instances (e.g., with lidocaine and meperidine), metabolites are as toxic as or more toxic than the parent compounds, and their metabolism may be limited.

Maternal Transfer

As maternal drug concentration in plasma falls below fetal drug concentration in plasma, transfer of drug from the fetus to the mother may occur, decreasing fetal concentration. The maternal circulation changes from a reservoir to a sink for fetal drug elimination.

Tissue Binding

Uptake of drug by fetal tissues also tends to decrease fetal drug concentration. Tissue binding in a specific target organ in the fetus is governed by a host of factors, including tissue blood flow, arterial-to-venous gradient, and lipid solubility of the drug. The relevance of tissue binding to ultimate fetal outcome is poorly understood at present and requires investigation.

To understand placental transfer of drugs one must realize that the maternal–placental–fetal unit is pharmacologically dynamic. Although the fetus receives a portion of virtually everything administered to the mother, the size of that portion and the ultimate effect is subject to many variables. At present, the relative importance of these variables remains unknown.

RESEARCH IN PERINATAL PHARMACOLOGY*

Although perinatal pharmacology has been avidly studied for the past 30 years, research in this dynamic, complex field has been and continues to be fraught with difficulty. The material presented in this introduction is accepted by many investigators in this field. Future study may, however, demonstrate our ignorance. An outline of the difficulties encountered in research in perinatal pharmacology follows.

LIMITATIONS OF ANIMAL STUDIES

Other than the Scandinavian studies of human placental perfusion using the radioactive xenon clearance technique and the recent introduction of Doppler ultra-

* The opinions expressed herein are those of the author and are not to be construed as reflecting the views of the Navy Department, the Naval Service at large, or the Department of Defense.

sound techniques to assess human placental function, most research has been conducted in animal models, usually the gravid ewe.

1. Most animal model studies as well as the in vivo human studies involve chronic instrumentation of the maternal–placental–fetal unit. Instrumentation certainly introduces error into studies by altering both anatomy and physiology.
2. Variables known to alter the physiology of the maternal–placental–fetal unit have not been standardized. As a result, data obtained may vary greatly from one study to another.
3. Most studies in the animal models have required general anesthesia or heavy sedation to complete. Drugs do, as we have seen, alter the physiology of the maternal–placental–fetal unit.
4. Although animal models are selected for their similarity to the human, none is a perfect replica of the humans (e.g., their size or placental structure differs from that of the human).

In order to minimize these problems, it is imperative that current noninvasive methods (i.e., xenon clearance) or new noninvasive methods be applied to the study of perinatal pharmacology.

UTILITY OF THE FETAL/MATERNAL RATIO

The placental transfer of drugs in both human and animal models studies is difficult to determine. The maternal–placental–fetal unit is pharmacologically dynamic and multicompartmented. A simple approach to determining the ease with which a drug crosses the placenta as well as its uptake by the fetus has been to administer the drug maternally and obtain serum concentrations of the drug in the mother (either arterial or venous samples) and in the fetus (usually umbilical venous and arterial samples at delivery) at an arbitrary time. Given the dynamic nature of placental transfer and the many variables involved, the validity of this technique must be questioned. Past studies utilizing this technique have demonstrated the following inadequacies.

1. Any one-time determination of fetal and maternal serum drug levels does not reflect the dynamic nature of placental transfer.
2. Maternal venous and arterial concentrations as well as umbilical venous and arterial concentrations are not equivalent if any equilibrium state has not been achieved. Present studies are not frequently done at equilibrium.
3. Because of differences in fetal and maternal protein binding and tissue/blood partition characteristics, fetal sequestration of a drug may not be reflected by the fetal/maternal ratio.

These inadequacies raise the question of the utility of the fetal/maternal ratio as a tool in perinatal pharmacologic research.

NEUROBEHAVIORAL STUDIES

Neonatal neurobehavioral changes have long been suspected to occur when drugs are administered to the maternal component of the maternal–placental–fetal unit. However, the scoring system developed by Apgar was not sensitive enough to demonstrate many of these changes. The Neonatal Behavioral Assessment Scale (NBAS) developed by Brazelton was sensitive to these changes but time-consuming to perform. The advent of two sensitive and easily performed scoring systems, the Early Neonatal Neurobehavioral Scale (ENNS) of Scanlon and co-workers and the Neurologic and Adaptive Capacity Score (NACS) of Amiel-Tison and co-workers ushered in a new approach to research in perinatal pharmacology. Carefully controlled studies using these neurobehavioral tools provides very useful information to illuminate perinatal pharmacology.

In the discussions that follow, a detailed description of the pharmacology, methods of use, and untoward effects of commonly used obstetric anesthetic drugs is presented. For all agents discussed, a profile of the direct effects (fetal neurobehavioral and developmental alterations) and the indirect effects (alterations in the physiology of the maternal–placental–fetal unit) should be constructed by the reader. An understanding of these effects will lead to the safe conduct of obstetric anesthesia.

SUGGESTED READINGS

1. Chamberlain GVP, Wilkinson AW (eds): Placental Transfer. Pitman Medical Publishers, Kent, England, 1979
2. Wheeler AS, Harris BA: The Uterus, Placenta, and Fetus. Semin Anesth 1:101, 1982

OBSTETRIC ANESTHESIA AND UTEROPLACENTAL BLOOD FLOW

As anesthesiologists, clearly we need to have an understanding of uteroplacental perfusion because many clinical situations and the administration of various agents may have profound effects on uterine and, ultimately, umbilical blood flow.

PHYSIOLOGY OF UTEROPLACENTAL BLOOD FLOW

Uterine blood flow is determined by the following relationship:

$$\text{uterine blood flow} = \frac{\text{Uterine arterial pressure} - \text{Uterine venous pressure}}{\text{Uterine vascular resistance}}$$

The rate of blood flow to the gravid uterus at term is approximately 700 ml/min, about 10 percent of the maternal cardiac output. Under normal conditions, the uterine vascular bed is maximally dilated. There is no autoregulation and flow is dependent on perfusion pressure.[1]

Seventy to 90 percent of uterine blood flow passes through the intervillous space. Investigations in animals suggest that the normal placenta has a 50 percent "safety factor," that is, uterine blood flow can decrease to 50 percent of normal before fetal hypoxia and acidosis develop.[2] This safety factor is generally adequate to protect the fetus from the stresses of normal pregnancy, labor, and delivery. However, this only applies to the normal placenta and is not the case in parturients with a pathology such as pregnancy-induced hypertension or diabetes (Fig. 3-3).

Uteroplacental Circulation and Respiratory Gas Exchange

Oxygen. Fetal oxygen delivery is determined by factors that affect umbilical blood flow and umbilical vein oxygen content. Studies in animals suggest that reduc-

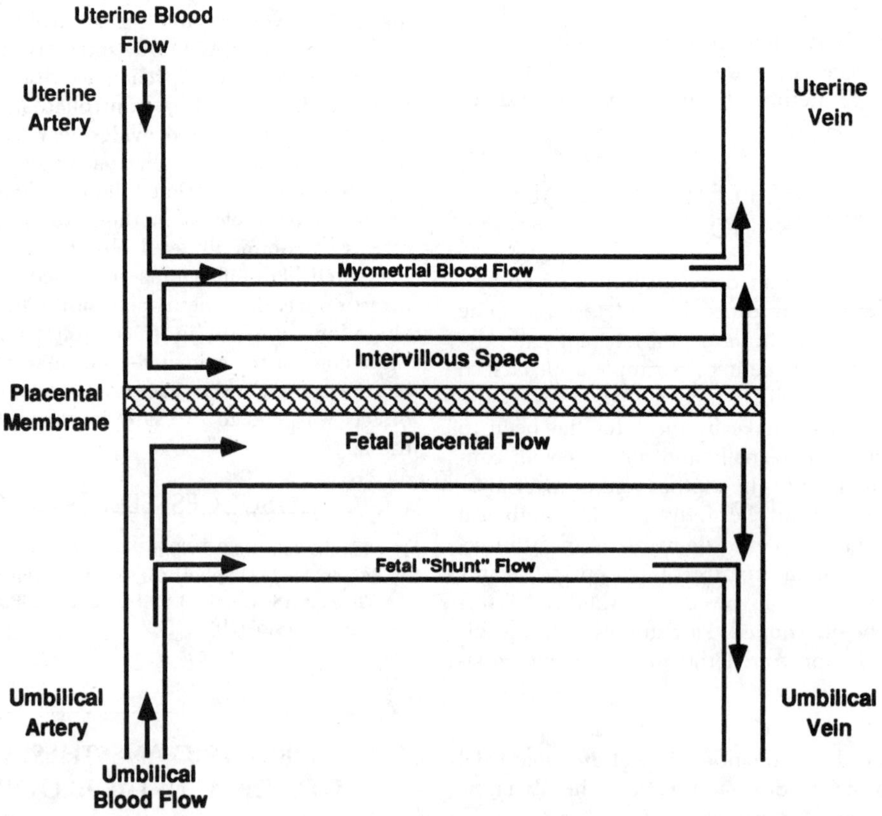

Fig. 3-3. Diagrammatic representation of uteroplacental perfusion. (From Parer JT: Ureteroplacental circulation and respiratory gas exchange. p. 14. In Shnider SM, Levinson G (eds): Anesthesia for Obstetrics. 2nd Ed. Williams & Wilkins, Baltimore, 1987, with permission.)

tions in oxygen delivery of as much as 40 to 50 percent are tolerated by the fetus without adverse effects on fetal oxygen consumption.[3] This suggests the existence of a fetal reserve as well as other compensatory mechanisms.[4] In animals, fetal oxygen delivery averages 24 ml/min/kg and oxygen consumption averages 8 ml/min/kg. A reduction in oxygen delivery is compensated for by an increase in oxygen extraction. When oxygen delivery drops below 12 to 14 ml/min/kg, fetal oxygen consumption decreases and the fetus incurs an oxygen debt, which results in an increased base deficit. Redistribution of blood flow to vital organs occurs.

Carbon Dioxide. Carbon dioxide elimination is dependent on blood flow. In the fetus, a condition analogous to "respiratory acidosis" develops when there is a decrease in either uterine or umbilical blood flow. In such circumstances, carbon dioxide acutely rises and the pH decreases without changes in fixed acid.

Maternal hypocapnia may result in fetal hypocarbia ("respiratory alkalosis"), lower fetal PO_2, and increased base deficit. It is postulated that maternal hypocapnia may cause uterine arterial vasoconstriction, which leads to a decrease in uterine blood flow.[5,6] Additionally, maternal–fetal alkalosis results in a shift to the left of the oxygen-hemoglobin dissociation curve, which leads to decreased oxygen delivery to fetal tissues.

Factors That Contribute to a Decrease in Uteroplacental Blood Flow

1. Uterine contraction leads to a decrease in blood flow; this occurs in response to the increase in uterine venous pressure caused by the increase in transuterine pressure. There may also be decreases in uterine arterial pressure with contractions. Uterine hypertonus results in a decrease in uteroplacental blood flow by the same mechanism.
2. Uterine blood flow is dependent on perfusion pressure, thus any condition that results in hypotension, such as sympathetic block, hypovolemic shock, and supine hypotensive syndrome (aortocaval compression), causes decreased uteroplacental blood flow.
3. Hypertension, either essential or pregnancy induced, results in a decrease in uteroplacental blood flow due to high vascular resistance in the uterine vessels and narrowing of placental vascular beds.
4. Vasoconstrictors, either endogenous or exogenously administered, increase uterine vascular resistance, leading to a decrease in uteroplacental blood flow.
5. Uteroplacental blood flow is decreased in postmature pregnancy and is potentially compromised in diabetic mothers.

MEASUREMENT OF UTEROPLACENTAL BLOOD FLOW

There is no practical direct method of monitoring uteroplacental blood flow in humans. In clinical practice we infer changes in uteroplacental blood flow by monitoring fetal heart rate (FHR) and acid-base status, an abnormal scalp blood pH being less than 7.20 and normal being greater than 7.25. In the late 1970s, Rekonen et al. developed a quantitative method of measuring intervillous and myometrial flow based on the clearance of xenon 133 (^{133}Xe) administered intravenously with less than 1 mrad exposure.[7] For obvious reasons, this technique has not become popular in this country. Two millicuries of ^{133}Xe in saline is injected intravenously and the patient is instructed to hold her breath for about 20 seconds, as ^{133}Xe is freely diffusible with complete clearance during passage through the lung. This allows the isotope to enter the systemic circulation as a bolus. The clearance of the isotope is measured with a scintillation detector positioned over the area of the placenta. A biexponential curve ($A_1e^{-k1t} + A_2e^{-k2t}$) is obtained. F_1 on the curve represents intervillous blood flow and F_2 represents myometrial blood flow. F_2 is determined from the equation $F_2 = 0.7{*}K_2$, where 0.7 is the partition coefficient of xenon between blood and myometrial tissue. The intervillous blood flow (F_1) is determined from the equation $F_1 = 100{*}k_1$. This technique has been found to be highly reproducible[8] (Fig. 3-4).

More recently, investigators have been studying Doppler ultrasound examinations of maternal uterine and fetal umbilical arterial velocity waveforms.[9,10] A 4-MHz Doppler probe is positioned over the abdomen and the vessel of interest is identified; an amplitude versus frequency characteristic of the Doppler return is calculated and displayed as amplitude and frequency versus time. The ratio of the systolic peak of this waveform to the diastolic trough of the blood velocity (S/D) is thought to be reflective of the vascular resistance distal to the measurement[11]—in other words, an indirect assessment of perfusion. A high S/D ratio is thought to correlate with poor perfusion.

Most information regarding uteroplacental blood flow is extrapolated from animal studies. Animals are chronically instrumented, which allows precise measurement of changes in uterine and placental blood flow and their effect on fetal acid-base status. Uterine blood flow is measured by one of many techniques, including electromagnetic flow probes, steady-state diffusion techniques (Fick principle), and injection of radioactive tracers (Fig. 3-5).

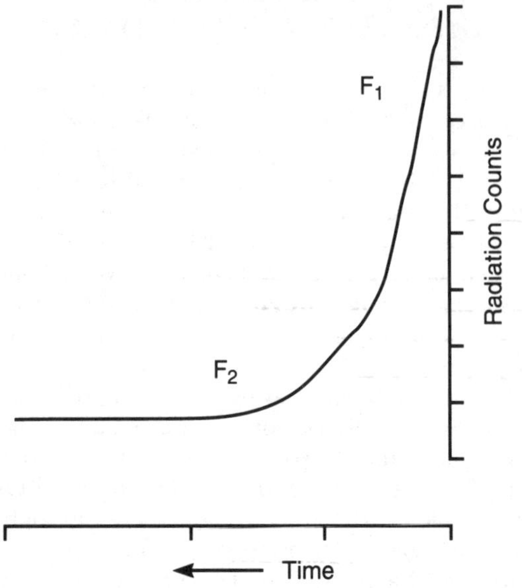

Fig. 3-4. Measurement of intervillous (F_1) and myometrial (F_2) blood flow by the intravenous ^{133}Xe method. (Modified from Jouppila R, Jouppila P, Hollmen A, Kuikka J: Effect of segmental extradural analgesia on placental blood flow during normal labour. Br J Anaesth 50:563, 1978, with permission.)

ANESTHETIC AGENTS AND UTEROPLACENTAL BLOOD FLOW

General Anesthesia

Barbiturates. Animal studies with thiopental and thiamylal in clinical doses (4 mg/kg) demonstrated reduced maternal systolic and diastolic blood pressure as well as uterine blood flow.[12] The onset, as one might expect, was within 20 to 30 seconds of injection and the effect lasted from 3 to 8 minutes. These changes were associated with transient fetal hypoxia and acidosis. Methohexital showed similar findings, although these effects were smaller in magnitude and of shorter duration and were not associated with changes in fetal PaO_2 or acid-base status.

Shnider et al. studied thiopental induction in sheep followed by administration of succinylcholine, direct laryngoscopy, and endotracheal intubation.[13] They observed a 65 percent increase in blood pressure but a 24 percent decrease in uterine blood flow. This was thought to be due to maternal catecholamine increases in norepinephrine to 89 percent above control. These hemodynamic changes resolved quickly after terminating the airway manipulation.

Thiopental has also been studied in humans. Ten healthy women undergoing elective cesarean delivery were induced with thiopental 4 mg/kg and succinylcholine 1 mg/kg followed by laryngoscopy and intubation. Intervillous blood flow was determined pre- and postinduction and a decrease in intervillous blood flow averaging 35 percent ($P < .001$) was demonstrated.[14] All neonates had a 1-minute Apgar score of 7 or greater and only one neonate had an umbilical vein blood gas analysis that showed signs of respiratory and metabolic acidosis.

Ketamine. In the near-term ewe, ketamine administered intravenously at doses of 5 mm/kg produced a 15 percent increase in mean blood pressure with a concomitant 10 percent increase in uterine blood flow.[15] In laboring sheep, doses of ketamine from 0.9 to 5 mg/kg demonstrated an increase in uterine tone with a concomitant decrease in uterine blood flow. This phenomenon was dose related and accompanied by fetal acidosis.[16] Intrauterine pressures in postpartum humans demonstrate a dose-related increase in uterine tone with increasing doses of ketamine.[17] For general anesthesia, induction doses of ketamine up to 1 mg/kg appear to have little effect on uterine blood flow.

Volatile Anesthetics. The volatile agents are potent uterine relaxants. Uteroplacental flow with halothane at 1 to 1.5 MAC (minimal alveolar concentration) is essentially unchanged; however, at 2 MAC, there is a resultant decrease in cardiac output and blood pressure, leading to a decrease in uteroplacental blood flow. Isoflurane and enflurane are essentially identical to halothane in their effects on uterine blood flow. Light planes of anesthesia do not decrease uterine blood flow, but deeper planes do.[18]

Enflurane, when studied in acidotic fetuses at concentrations of 1 percent or higher, produced a dose-related maternal and fetal bradycardia, a decrease in uterine blood flow, and fetal acidosis.[19]

Nitrous Oxide. Nitrous oxide can increase sympathetic activity, which theoretically can lead to a decrease in placental perfusion. However, when combined with volatile anesthetics, as is our clinical practice, the increases in sympathetic activity are blunted. There is some evidence from animal studies that suggests this.[20]

Local Anesthesia

Greiss studied local anesthetics and their effects on uteroplacental blood flow[21] (Fig. 3-6).

Local anesthetic was infused directly into the uterine artery of nonpregnant ewes. The threshold level at

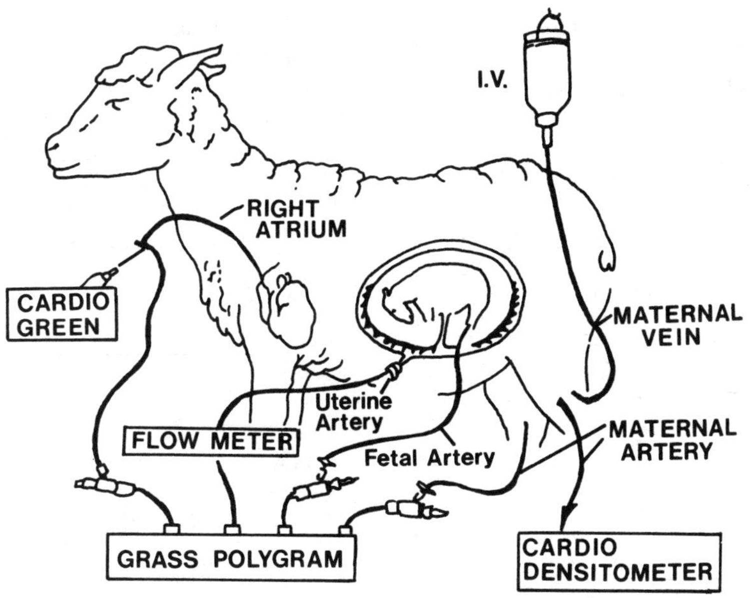

Fig. 3-5. Animal model with chronically implanted maternal and fetal intravascular catheters and an electromagnetic flow probe around a branch of the uterine artery. (From Ralston et al.,[2] with permission.)

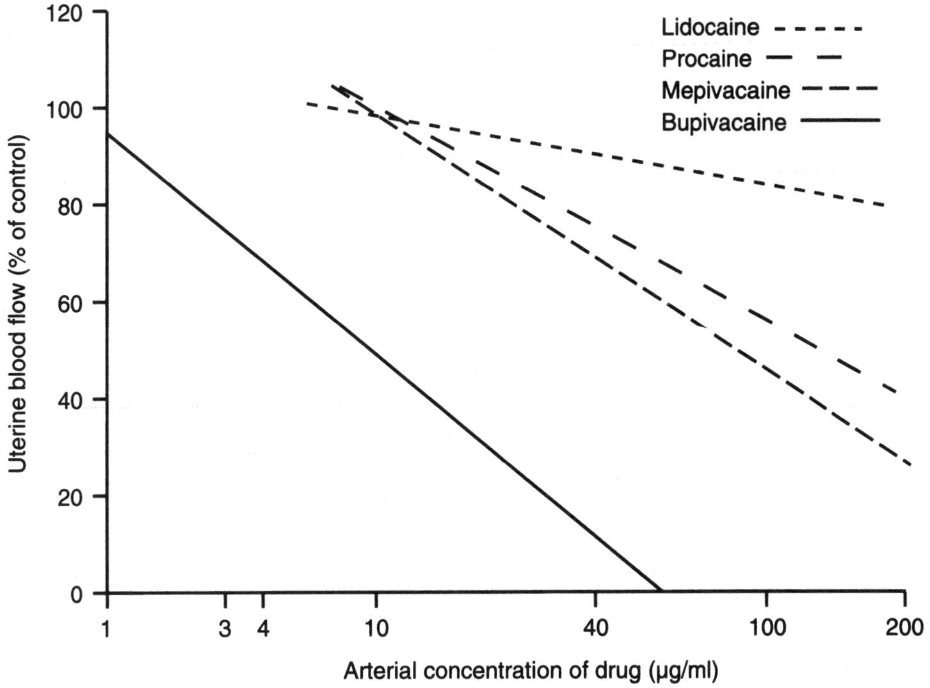

Fig. 3-6. Effects of local anesthetics on ureteroplacental blood flow. (From Greiss et al.,[21] with permission.)

which uterine blood flow was first noted to decrease was 1 μg/ml for bupivacaine and 3 to 4 μg/ml for lidocaine, mepivacaine, and procaine. The point at which there are severe reductions in uterine blood flow is much higher than would be expected clinically with epidural or subarachnoid anesthesia, unless associated with an intravascular injection.

Concentrations of this magnitude, however, can be seen locally with a paracervical block. Some investigators have suggested that the fetal bradycardia associated with paracervical block is due to decreases in oxygenation secondary to vasoconstriction of uterine arteries[22] and possibly uterine hypertonus,[23] resulting in diminished uteroplacental blood flow.

Regional Anesthesia

Epidural anesthesia in pregnant sheep has been shown not to affect uteroplacental perfusion unless associated with decreases in systemic blood pressure.

In a classic study in humans during normal labor, increases in intervillous blood flow were demonstrated after epidural anesthesia.[24]

Preeclamptic patients appear to benefit greatly from epidural anesthesia, with some studies showing an increase in intervillous blood flow of as much as 77 percent after epidural anesthesia.[25]

In the absence of intravascular injection, epinephrine-containing local anesthetics seem to have little or no effect on uteroplacental perfusion.[26] However, when studied in animals, as little as 15 μg of epinephrine injected intravascularly can result in a 50 percent decrease in uterine blood flow.[27] Since it is not uncommon to unintentionally enter an epidural vessel in gravid patients during the placement of an epidural catheter, these data suggest epinephrine-containing local anesthetics should be administered carefully when initiating an epidural block in these patients.

Vasopressors

Vasopressors may have a primary α, β, or mixed effect:

	α	β
Ephedrine	++	+++
Mephentermine	+	++
Metaraminol	+++	+
Methoxamine	+++++	0
Phenylephrine	+++++	0

In their classic study, Ralston and Shnider demonstrated that ephedrine affected uterine blood flow the least when administered to normotensive pregnant ewes as compared to other vasopressor agents.[2] Phenylephrine was not evaluated in this study.

More recently investigators have studied the use of ephedrine versus phenylephrine in treating hypotension secondary to epidural and spinal anesthesia.[28,29] Studies in healthy women undergoing elective cesarean delivery detected no abnormalities in fetal acid-base status.

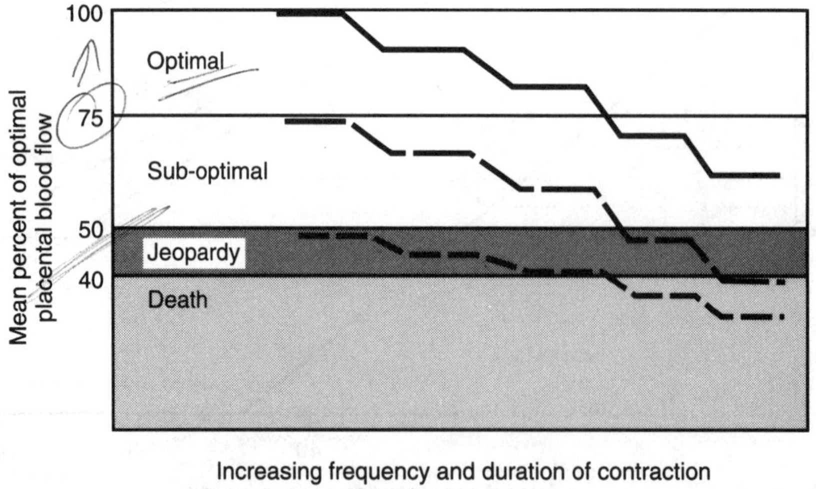

Fig. 3-7. Hypothetical relationship between fetal condition and placental blood flow in labor. (Redrawn from Greiss FC, Jr.. Obstet Gynecol Annu 2:55, 1973, with permission.)

In patients with normal placental reserve who are not in labor, decreases in blood pressure are generally well tolerated by the fetus in terms of changes in uteroplacental blood flow. Most measures used to increase maternal blood pressure will, for the most part, restore uteroplacental blood flow to an adequate level. The fetus should be little affected because there is significant fetal reserve.

If there is pre-existing placental insufficiency or superimposed labor, particularly if contractions are prolonged, the decreases in maternal blood pressure may have very adverse affects on uterine blood flow, and agents used to restore blood pressure may have differential effects in terms of efficacy. In these situations it may be more efficacious to use a β-specific agent rather than an α-specific agent to increase maternal blood pressure (Fig. 3-7).

REFERENCES

1. Assali NS, Brinkman CR III: The uterine circulation and its control. p. 121. In Longo LD, Bartels H, (eds): Respiratory Gas Exchange and Blood Flow in the Placenta. US Department of Health, Education and Welfare, Washington, DC, 1972
2. Ralston DH, Shnider SM, deLorimer AA: Effect of equipotent ephedrine, metaraminol, mephentermine, and methoximime on uterine blood flow in the pregnant ewe. Anesthesiology 40:354, 1974
3. Wilkening RB, Meschia G: Fetal oxygen uptake, oxygenation, and acid base balance as a function of uterine blood flow. Am J Physiol 244 (Heart Circ Physiol 13):H749, 1983
4. Edelstone DI: Fetal compensatory response to reduced oxygen delivery. Semin Perinatol 8:184, 1984
5. Motoyama EK, Rivard G, Acheson F, et al: Adverse effect of maternal hyperventilation on the foetus. Lancet 1:286, 1966
6. Peng ATC, Bancato LS, Motoyama EK: Effect of maternal hypocapnia v. eucapnia on the foetus during caesarian section. Br J Anaesth 44:1173, 1972
7. Rekonen A, Luotola H, Pitanen M, et al: Measurement of intervillous and myometrial blood flow by intravenous ^{133}Xe method. Br J Obstet Gynaecol 83:723, 1976
8. Jouppila R, Jouppila P, Kuikka J, Hollmen A: Placental blood flow during caesarean section under lumbar extradural analgesia. Br J Anaesth 50:275, 1978
9. Mark GF, Patel S, Berman J, et al: Umbilical blood flow velocity waveforms in different maternal positions and with epidural analgesia. Obstet Gynecol 68:61, 1986
10. Giles WB, Lah FX, Trudinger BJ: The effect of epidural anesthesia for caesarean section on maternal uterine and fetal umbilical artery blood flow velocity waveform. Br J Obstet Gynaecol 94:55, 1987
11. O'Rourke MF: Vascular impedance in studies of arterial and cardiac function. Physiol Rev 62:570, 1982
12. Cosmi EV, Condorelli S, Scarpelli EM: Fetal asphyxia induced by sodium thiopental, thiamylal and methohexital. In Proceedings, 4th European Congress of Perinatal Medicine, Praha, 1974, Abstract No. IV, 3/12
13. Shnider SM, Wright RG, Levinson G, et al: Plasma norepinephrine and uterine blood flow changes during endotracheal intubation and general anesthesia in the pregnant ewe. p. 115. In Abstracts of Scientific Papers, Annual Meeting, American Society of Anesthesiologists, Chicago, 1978
14. Jouppila P, Kuikka J, Hollmen A: Effect of induction of general anesthesia for cesarean section on intervillous blood flow. Acta Obstet Gynaecol Scand 58:249, 1979
15. Levinson G, Shnider SM, Gildea JE, deLorimer AA: Maternal and foetal cardiovascular and acid base changes during ketamine anaesthesia in pregnant ewes. Br J Anaesth 45:1111, 1973
16. Cosmi EV: Drugs, anesthetics and the fetus. p. 191. In Scarpelli EM, Cosmi EV (eds): Reviews in Perinatal Medicine. Vol. 1. University Park Press, Baltimore, 1976
17. Marx GF, Hwang HS, Chandra P: Postpartum uterine pressures with different doses of ketamine. Anesthesiology 50:163, 1979
18. Palahniuk RJ, Shnider SM: Maternal and fetal cardiovascular and acid base changes during halothane and isoflurane anesthesia in the pregnant ewe. Anesthesiology 41:462, 1974
19. Cosmi EV: Drugs, anesthetics and the fetus. p. 191. In Scarpelli EM, Cosmi EV (eds): Reviews in Perinatal Medicine. Vol. 1. University Park Press, Baltimore, 1976
20. Fujinaga M, Baden JM, Yhap EO, et al: Reproductive and teratogenic effects of nitrous oxide, isoflurane and their combination in Sprauge-Dawley rats. Anesthesiology 67:960, 1987
21. Griess F, Still JG, Anderson SG: Effects of local anesthetic agents on the uterine vasculatures and myometrium. Am J Obstet Gynecol 124:889, 1976
22. Gibbs CP, Noel SC: Human uterine artery response to lidocaine. Am J Obstet Gynecol 126:313, 1976
23. Morishima HO, Covin BG, Yeh MN, et al: Bradycardia in the fetal baboon following paracervical block anesthesia. Am J Obstet Gynecol 140:775, 1981
24. Hollmen AI, Jouppila R, Jouppila P, et al: Effect of extradural analgesia using bupivacaine and 2-chloroprocaine on intervillous blood flow during normal labor. Br J Anaesth 54:837, 1982
25. Jouppila P, Jouppila R, Hollmen AI, et al: Lumbar epidural analgesia to improve intervillous blood flow during labor in severe preeclampsia. Obstet Gynecol 59:158, 1982
26. Albright GA, Jouppila R, Hollmen AI, et al: Epinephrine does not alter human intervillous blood flow during epidural anesthesia. Anesthesiology 54:131, 1985
27. Hood DD, Dewan DM, James FM III: Maternal and fetal effects of epinephrine in gravid ewes. Anesthesiology 64:610, 1986
28. Ramanathan S, Grant GJ: Vasopressor therapy for hypotension due to epidural anesthesia for cesarean section. Acta Anesth Scand 32:559, 1988
29. Moran DH, Perillo M, LaPorta RF, et al: Phenylephrine in

prevention of hypotension following to spinal anesthesia for cesarean delivery. J Clin Anes 3:301, 1991

CLINICAL IMPLICATIONS OF THE PLACENTAL TRANSFER OF DRUGS

Placental transfer of drugs can occur by several mechanisms, including simple diffusion, facilitated diffusion, active transport, bulk flow, and direct diffusion through breaks in the placental or, more accurately, the chorionic membrane. Factors related to drug transfer across this membrane include the diffusion constant for the particular drug, the surface area and the thickness of the chorionic membrane across which the drug will diffuse, and the diffusion gradient from maternal to fetal tissues.[1] This can be summarized in the equation:

$$Q/t = \frac{K \times A \times (Cm - Cf)}{D}$$

where Q/t is the amount of drug transferred per unit of time;

K is the diffusion coefficient or constant of the drug studied;

A is the total surface area of the chorionic membrane available for transfer;

(Cm − Cf) is the diffusion gradient (maternal drug concentration minus fetal drug concentration); and

D is thickness of the chorionic membrane.

The diffusion coefficient (K) is dependent on several variables including the molecular weight, lipid solubility, and protein binding of the drug. A molecular weight of 1,000 appears to be the maximal size for drugs to cross the placenta by simple diffusion. The analgesic and anesthetic drugs have molecular weights below 500 (see Table 3-1). They cross the placenta by simple diffusion. Many of these drugs exist in both ionized and nonionized forms. The nonionized form is more lipid soluble and passes through the membrane more readily. Because the neonate's blood is more acidotic than the mother's blood, basic drugs may achieve a higher blood concentration in the neonate. This can occur as a result of ion trapping and occurs more frequently if the fetus develops distress with a very low blood pH. Increased protein binding may decrease drug transfer, as only the unbound drug can pass the placenta. However, this may not be significant, as binding is a reversible process and any unbound drug that crosses the placenta will promote drug release from the bound form.

The important factor of time must be kept in mind when evaluating drug transfer. The more time allowed, the more drug is transferred. Finally, one must bear in mind that placental transfer is a dynamic process that continues in both directions across the chorionic membrane until birth.

Table 3-1. Molecular Weight of Several Drugs Used in Obstetrics

Drug Classification	Molecular Weight
Induction agents	
Etomidate	244
Ketamine	238
Propofol	178
Sodium thiopental	264
Neuromuscular drugs	
Succinylcholine chloride	361
Gases	
Enflurane	184
Halothane	197
Isoflurane	184
Nitrous oxide	44
Oxygen	32
Anticoagulants	
Sodium warfarin	330
Heparin	6,000+
Local anesthetics	
Bupivacaine	288
Chloroprocaine	271
Etidocaine	276
Lidocaine	234
Mepivacaine	246
Prilocaine	220
Procaine	236
Tetracaine	264
Narcotics	
Fentanyl	336
Meperidine	247
Methadone	309
Morphine	285
Tranquilizers	
Midazolam	325

REFERENCES

1. Burger GA: Principles of perinatal pharmacology. p. 47. In Ostheimer GW (ed): Manual of Obstetric Anesthesia. Churchill Livingstone, New York, 1984

Table 3-2. The Apgar Score

Score	0	1	2
Heart rate	Absent	<100	>100
Respiratory effort	Absent	Irregular, shallow	Good, crying
Reflex irritability	No response	Grimace	Cough, sneeze
Muscle tone	Flaccid	Good tone	Spontaneous flexed arms/legs
Color	Blue, pale	Body pink, extremities blue	Entirely pink

(From Apgar,[1] with permission.)

NEONATAL EVALUATION

There are many ways to evaluate the neonate at birth. Early in the systematic evaluation of the neonate, breathing time (time to the beginning of spontaneous respiration) was used. In 1952, the Apgar score[1] was introduced and continues to be widely used. Because extrinsic uterine events can affect uteroplacental blood flow, umbilical blood gas data at the time of delivery has been utilized. To detect more subtle changes in the neonate's adaptation to extrauterine life, neurobehavioral tests were developed. This section presents an overview of these methods of neonatal evaluation.

RESPIRATORY TIMES

Breathing time is defined as the time from delivery of the head to the first breath (normally within 30 seconds of delivery). Time to sustained respiration (TSR) occurs when breathing becomes sustained (normally by 90 seconds after delivery). Crying time is the time until the establishment of a satisfactory cry.

Dr. Virginia Apgar[1] pointed out some problems with breathing and crying times. She noted that breathing time can be difficult to interpret when the mother has received excessive amounts of depressant drugs in the antepartum period, as the neonate may take a breath and then become apneic for several minutes. Crying time may also be difficult to interpret, as a satisfactory cry may not be established in a particular neonate by the time the infant leaves the delivery room. Because of the difficulty in interpreting the meaning of these times, they are not widely used today but are presented for historical interest.

APGAR SCORE

Since Dr. Apgar[1] introduced the scoring system in 1952, the Apgar score has become the most frequently used method for evaluating the well-being of the neonate and the effects of maternally administered medications. Although subjective, her scoring system proved to be rapid and reproducible. A summary of her scoring system of five evaluations (heart rate, respiratory effort, reflex irritability, muscle tone, and color) is presented in Table 3-2. Each evaluation is given a score (0, 1, or 2) and the scores are totaled (0 to 10) to obtain the Apgar score.

The five evaluations used are essentially a set of vital signs that can be used to describe the healthy neonate's condition and can serve as a guide to success during neonatal resuscitation. Care of the neonate, however, begins at the time of delivery and not after a score is performed. Scoring is performed on all neonates at 1 and 5 minutes after birth, and if the neonate is depressed, also at 10, 15, and 20 minutes. Table 3-3 shows typical percentages of neonatal scores.

Of the five scores, Dr. Apgar[2] stated that heart rate and respiratory effort are much more important than reflex irritability and muscle tone. Color has the least significance. As a result, some researchers use an Apgar minus Color (A-C) score.[3]

The scoring is easy to perform, however, given the same neonate different scores may be given by different examiners.[4–6] This makes interpretation of the results more difficult.

The 1-minute score is thought to be a reflection of the acid-base status of the neonate. However, this correlation is not strong.[3] In 1982, Sykes et al.[7] showed that only 21 percent of neonates with a 1-minute Apgar score of <7 had severe acidosis (umbilical artery pH ≤7.10 and base deficit ≥13 mmol/L), whereas 73 percent of neonates with severe acidosis had a 1-minute Apgar score of ≥7. In premature infants, this correlation is particularly poor. In 1984, Goldenberg et al.[8] showed that "the more premature the infant, the more likely

Table 3-3. Normal Distribution of Apgar Scores

Score	1 Minute (%)	5 Minutes (%)
0–3 (severely depressed)	6.7	1.8
4–6 (moderately depressed)	14.5	3.5
7–10 (normal)	78.9	94.8

(From Drage and Berendes,[9] with permission.)

Date Hour

Infants's name ______ Sex ______ Age ______ Born ______
Mother's age ______ Father's age ______ Father's S.E.S. ______
Apparent race ______
Examiner(s) ______ Place of examination ______
Conditions of examination ______ Date of examination ______
Birth weight ______ Current weight ______ Length ______ Head circ. ______
Time examined ______ Time last fed ______ Type of feeding ______
Type of delivery ______ Apgar ______
Length of labor ______ Birth order ______
Type, amount and timing of medication given mother ______

Anesthesia? ______
Abnormalities of labor ______

Initial state: observe 2 minutes

1	2	3	4	5	6
deep	light	drowsy	alert	active	crying

Predominant states (mark two)

1	2	3	4	5	6

Elicited Responses

	O*	L	M	H	A†
Platar grasp		1	2	3	
Hand grasp		1	2	3	
Ankle clonus		1	2	3	
Babinski		1	2	3	
Standing		1	2	3	
Automatic walking		1	2	3	
Placing		1	2	3	
Incurvation		1	2	3	
Crawling		1	2	3	
Glabella		1	2	3	
Tonic deviation of head and eyes		1	2	3	
Nystagmus		1	2	3	
Tonic neck reflex		1	2	3	
Moro		1	2	3	
Rooting (intensity)		1	2	3	
Sucking (intensity)		1	2	3	
Passive movement					
Arms R		1	2	3	
L		1	2	3	
Legs R		1	2	3	
L		1	2	3	

Descriptive Paragraph (optional)

Attractive	0	1	2	3
Interfering variables	0	1	2	3
Need for stimulation	0	1	2	3

What activity does he use to quiet self?
hand to mouth
sucking with nothing in mouth
locking onto visual or auditory stimuli
postural changes
state change for no observable reason

COMMENTS:

*O = response not elicited (omitted)
†A = asymmetry

A

Fig. 3-8. **(A)** Brazelton Neonatal Behavior Assessment Scale. (*Figure continues.*)

the Apgar score was low in the presence of a pH ≥7.25." This may be related to the premature infant not being strong enough to elicit the responses recorded on the Apgar score.

The 5-minute score is thought to be a predictor of both survival and neurologic abnormalities.[4] In 1966, Drage et al.[9] showed that a 5-minute Apgar score of 0 or 1 was associated with a 49 percent incidence of neonatal death. They also reported a correlation between the 5-minute Apgar scores and neurologic abnormalities in infants at 1 year of age. Infants with a 5-minute Apgar score of 0 to 3 had a higher incidence of neurologic abnormalities when compared to those infants with a score of 7 to 10 (7.4 percent versus 1.7 percent). Thus, over 90 percent of surviving infants with low Apgar scores (0 to 3) were neurologically normal at 1 year of age! In 1975, Niswander et al.[10] failed to show a correlation between Apgar score and neurologic abnormalities in 4-year-olds. Perhaps this is due to the enormous growth of nervous tissue that occurs after birth. In 1983, Paneth et al.[11] noted that the majority of infants with cerebral palsy had no evidence of depression at birth (73 percent of the subjects had a 5-minute Apgar score of ≥7).

Scale (Note State)	*Inital State* .... *Predominant State* 1 2 3 4 5 6 7 8 9
1. Reponse decrement to light (2. 3)	
2. Response decrement to rattle (2, 3)	
3. Response decrement to bell (2, 3)	
4. Response decrement to pinprick (1, 2, 3)	
5. Orientation inanimate visual (4 only)	
6. Orientation inanimate auditory (4, 5)	
7. Orientation animate visual (4 only)	
8. Orientation animate visual (4, 5)	
9. Orientation animate visual & auditory (4 only)	
10. Alertness (4 only)	
11. General tonus (4,5)	
12. Motor maturity (4,5)	
13. Pull-to-sit (3,5)	
14. Cuddliness (4,5)	
15. Defensive movements (4)	
16. Consolability (6 to 5, 4, 3, 2)	
17. Peak of excitement (6)	
18. Rapidity of buildup (from 1, 2 to 6)	
19. Irritability (3, 4, 5)	
20. Activity (alert states)	
21. Tremulousness (all states)	
22. Startle (3, 4, 5, 6)	
23. Liability of skin color (from 1 to 6)	
24. Liability of states (all states)	
25. Self-quieting acitvity (6, 5 to 4, 3, 2, 1)	
26. Hand-mouth facility (all states)	
27. Smiles (all states)	

B

Fig. 3-8. *(Continued)* **(B)** Brazelton Neonatal Behavior Assessment Scale. (From Brazelton,[16] with permission.)

Thus, the Apgar score has encouraged us to look more objectively at the neonate in a quick, systematic, and inexpensive manner. The value of the Apgar score to predict neonatal acidosis and neurologic abnormalities is poor. By itself, a low score indicates neonatal depression. However, the reason for a low score may include inaccurate scoring, prematurity, drug effects, congenital abnormalities, endotracheal intubation, nasopharyngeal suctioning, and/or asphyxia. Recently, it has been suggested that the Apgar score should be abandoned because of its misuse and inaccuracies.[12] Many,[13] including this author (and the editor), still

NAME: ______________________________ UNIT NUMBER: ____________
TIME: ______________ BLOOD GASES PO_2 ______ PCO_2 ______ *p*H ______
ANESTHETIC LEVEL ____________ TYPE __________ BODY TEMP ____________
APGAR HR ____ RESP EFF ____ TONE ____ IRRIT ____ COLOR _____ TOTAL _____

NEURO EXAM

STATE: __________ 1. Response to pin prick 0 1 2 3
Habituation no. __________
__________ 2. Resistance against passive motion
A. Pull to sitting 0 1 2 3
B. Arm recoil 0 1 2 3
C. Truncal tone 0 1 2 3
D. General body tone 0 1 2 3
__________ 3. Rooting 0 1 2 3
__________ 4. Sucking 0 1 2 3
__________ 5. Moro response 0 1 2 3
Threshold (# of attempts)
Extinguishment
__________ 6. Habituation to light in eyes. No. ______
__________ 7. Response to sound 0 1 2 3
Habituation no. ______
__________ 8. Placing 0 1 2 3
__________ 9. Alertness 0 1 2 3
__________ 10. General assessment A B N S
(circle)
Reasons
STATE ______________________________
LIABILITY OF STATE ______________________
COMMENTS:

Fig. 3-9. Scanlon Early Neonatal Neurobehavioral Assessment Scale. (Redrawn from Scanlon et al.,[18] with permission.)

believe that its use is important, if for no other reason than to give a common reference for evaluating how the neonate is adapting to extrauterine life.

UMBILICAL BLOOD GAS DATA

To appreciate placental perfusion, umbilical blood gas studies are often performed. Chronic fetal asphyxia is associated with neonatal metabolic acidosis (i.e., low pH, normal or high PCO_2, and high base deficit), whereas brief asphyxia is associated with the more common respiratory acidosis (i.e., low pH, high PCO_2, and normal base deficit).[14,15] Umbilical cord blood gas analysis can be performed to determine how well the fetus adapted to the intrauterine environment (Table 3-4).

Table 3-4. Normal Term Neonate Blood Gas Data (± 1 SD)

	Umbilical Vein	Umbilical Artery
PO_2 (mmHg)	29.2 ± 5.9	18.0 ± 6.2
PCO_2 (mmHg)	38.2 ± 5.6	49.2 ± 8.4
pH	7.35 ± 0.05	7.28 ± 0.05
Bicarbonate (mEq/L)	20.4 ± 2.1	22.3 ± 2.5

(From Yeomans et al.,[20] with permission.)

NEUROBEHAVIORAL TESTS

One problem with the Apgar score is that only the most severe neonatal depression from excessive or poorly timed maternal medications can be detected by the score at birth. To better evaluate the more subtle effects of maternally administered drugs, neurobehavioral tests were developed. Neurobehavioral assessment is not a standard part of the neonatal examination but has been used to assess the neonate's response to its environment. Although there are several neurobehavioral tests, three are more commonly used: Brazelton's Neonatal Behavior Assessment Scale, Scanlon's Early

Name ______________________ Date of Birth ____________ Chart Number ____________

Category	Item	Score	0	1	2
Adaptive Capacity	1. Response to sound		absent:	mild:	vigorous:
	2. Habituation to sound		absent:	7–12 stimuli:	≤ 6 stimuli:
	3. Response to light		absent:	mild:	brisk blink or startle:
	4. Habituation to light		absent:	7–12 stimuli	≤ 6 stimuli
	5. Consolability		absent:	difficult:	easy:
	Total	☐	Adaptive Capacity		

Category	Item	Score	0	1	2
Passive Tone	6. Scarf sign		encircles the neck:	elbow slightly passes midline:	elbow does not reach midline:
	7. Recoil of elbows		absent:	slow: weak:	brisk: reproducible:
	8. Popliteal angle		>110°	100°–110°	≤ 90°
	9. Recoil of lower lines		absent:	slow: weak:	brisk: reproducible:
Active Tone	10. Active contraction of neck flexors (from lying position)		absent or abnormal:	difficult:	good: head is maintained in the axis of the body:
	11. Active contraction of neck extensors (from leaning forward position)		absent or abnormal:	difficult:	good: head is maintained in the axis of the body:
	12. Palmar grasp*		absent:	weak:	excellent: reproducible:
	13. Response to traction (following palmar grasp)		absent:	lifts part of the body weight:	lifts all of the body weight:
	14. Supporting reaction (upright position)		absent:	incomplete: transitory:	strong: supports all body weight:
*Primary Reflexes	15. Automatic walking*		absent:	difficult to obtain:	perfect: reproducible:
	16. Moro reflex*		absent:	weak: incomplete:	perfect: complete:
	17. Sucking*		absent:	weak:	perfect: synchronous with swallowing
General Assessment	18. Alertness		coma:	lethargy:	normal:
	19. Crying		absent:	weak: high pitched: excessive:	normal:
	20. Motor activity		absent or grossly excessive:	diminished or mildly excessive:	normal:
	Total	☐	Neurological		
	Total Score	☐	At ________ minutes of life		

Fig. 3-10. Neurologic and Adaptive Capacity Scores. Asterisks signify primary reflexes. (From Amiel-Tison,[19] with permission.)

Neonatal Neurobehavioral Scale, and the Neonatal Neurologic and Adaptive Capacity Score of Amiel-Tison et al.

Brazelton states: "The neonate and his behavior cannot be assumed to be purely of genetic origin. Intrauterine influences are powerful and have already influence the physiologic and behavioral reactions of the baby at birth."[16] Because intrauterine influences such as nutrition, infection, hormones, and medications may affect the fetus, a behavioral scale to evaluate the neonate was proposed.

The baby's state of consciousness (deep sleep, light sleep, drowsy, alert, active, crying) is probably the most important element of the behavioral examination, since the neonate's responses to external stimuli depend on his or her state of consciousness. The Neonatal Behavioral Assessment Scale includes 27 behavioral items (9-point scale) and 20 elicited responses (3-point scale). The midpoint of the scale is the norm. Brazelton states[16]: "This mean is related to the expected behavior for an 'average' 7+ pound, full-term (40-week gestation), normal Caucasian infant, whose mother has had not more than 100 mg of barbiturates and 50 mg of other sedative drugs prior to delivery, whose Apgar scores were no less than 7 at 1, 8 at 5 and 8 at 15 minutes after delivery, who needed no special care after delivery, and who had an apparently normal intrauterine experience." The score is based on the neonate's best performance. Tests repeated on several days in the neonatal period are more valuable than one examination. Because many infants are discoordinated during the first 48 hours after delivery, the behavior on the third day is the expected norm (Fig. 3-8).

A period of 3 to 4 weeks of training is needed in order to become adequately trained in performing the Brazelton examination. About 45 minutes is required to perform each test.[17] As a result of the amount of training needed and the time required to perform this test, the Brazelton examination is not as widely used today as the other tests discussed below. It is, however, considered the "gold standard" for neurobehavioral evaluations, particularly in the research setting.

Scanlon et al.[18] in 1974, developed a neurobehavioral examination called the Early Neonatal Neurobehavioral Scale (ENNS) in an attempt to simplify neurobehavioral testing and to assess the neonatal effects of epidural anesthesia. The main advantages of this examination are that it is simple and rapid to perform (it takes only 5 to 10 minutes) and personnel can be trained to 85 percent reliability in only 2 to 3 days.

The examination begins with the evaluation of the neonate's state of consciousness (four awake and two sleep states). It is then followed by specific tests. Tests 1 to 9 are scored on a 0, 1, 2, 3 scale. Test 10 is scored as abnormal, borderline, normal, or superior. Again, an important aspect of the ENNS is the assessment of state and its changes during the examination (Fig. 3-9).

In regard to statistical analysis for the ENNS, it should be noted that none of the items is a continuous scale. For several scores (tone in particular), both extremely high and low scores may be abnormal; a summation of "total score" can therefore be misleading. Statistical techniques should attempt to measure differences in median scores. Several nonparametric tests are useful, such as chi-square and the Fisher exact test. F-testing and matched-pair median subtest covariance analysis are also appropriate.[17]

Amiel-Tison, Barrier, and Shnider, and co-workers,[19] in 1982, introduced another neurobehavior test called the Neonatal Neurologic and Adaptive Capacity Score (NACS), also called the ABS score. This examination takes less time than the ENNS (4.4 minutes versus 7.2 minutes), places greater emphasis on motor tone, and avoids the use of noxious stimuli. It is divided into five sections and includes 20 criteria. Each criteria is scored 0, 1, or 2. The scores of each criterion can be added together to give a maximum score of 40. A score of 35 to 40 denotes a vigorous neonate (Fig. 3-10).

These neurobehavioral assessments were designed only to evaluate the neonate in the first few hours to days after delivery. If abnormal behavior is identified in the early neonatal period, it may influence the interaction between the caregiver and the infant, which in turn may set the stage for abnormal interactions throughout childhood.

The Apgar score, which looked at dramatic depressive effects of drugs on the neonate for the first few minutes after delivery, has proved to be of little predictive value for long-term neurologic behavior. Will the neurobehavioral evaluations, which look at more subtle effects of drugs on the neonate over a few days, be of better predictive value? The answer to that question is still unanswered, as there are precious few long-term evaluations of infants originally tested with a neurobehavioral assessment.

REFERENCES

1. Apgar V: A proposal for a new method of evaluation of the newborn infant. Anesth Analg 32:260, 1953
2. Apgar V, Holaday DA, James S, et al: Evaluation of the newborn infant—second report. JAMA 168:1985, 1958
3. Marx GF, Mahajan S, Miclat MN: Correlation of biochemical data with Apgar scores at birth and at one minute. Br. J Anaesth 49:831, 1977
4. Apgar V: The newborn (Apgar) scoring system—reflections and advise. Pediatr Clin North Am 13:645, 1966
5. Clark DA, Hakanson DO: The inaccuracy of Apgar scoring. J Perinatol 8:203, 1988
6. Schifrin BS: Polemics in perinatology—the Apgar score—what should we call it? J Perinatol 9:331, 1989
7. Sykes GS, Hohnson P, Ashworth F, et al: Do Apgar scores indicate asphyxia? Lancet 1:494, 1982
8. Goldenberg RL, Huddleston JF, Nelson KG: Apgar scores and umbilical arterial pH in preterm newborn infants. Am J Obstet Gynecol 149:651, 1984
9. Drage JS, Berendes H: Apgar scores and outcome of the newborn. Pediatr Clin North Am 13:635, 1966
10. Niswander KR, Gordon M, Drage JS: The effect of intrauterine hypoxia on the child surviving to 4 years. Am J Obstet Gynecol 121:892, 1975
11. Paneth N, Stark RI: Cerebral palsy and mental retardation in relation to indicators of perinatal asphyxia. An epidemiologic overview. Am J Obstet Gynecol 147:960, 1983
12. Is the Apgar score outmoded? Lancet 1:591, 1989
13. Editorial Board: Point-counterpoint—the Apgar score . . . revisited. J Perinatol 9:338, 1989
14. James LS, Weisbrot IM, Prince CE, et al: The acid-base status of human infants in relation to birth asphyxia and the onset of respiration. J Pediatr 52:379, 1958
15. Wilbe JL, Petrie RH, Koons A, et al: The clinical use of umbilical cord acid-base determinations in perinatal surveillance and management. Clin Perinatol 9:387, 1982
16. Brazelton TB: Neonatal behavioral assessment scale. Clincs in Developmental Medicine, No. 50. Spastics Int Med Publ., London, 1973
17. Ostheimer GW: Neurobehavioral effects of local anesthesia and fetal resuscitation. Reg Anesth 6:136, 1981
18. Scanlon JW, Brown WU Jr, Weiss JB, et al: Neurobehavioral responses of newborn infants after maternal epidural anesthesia. Anesthesiology 40:121, 1974
19. Amiel-Tison C, Barrier G, Shnider SM, et al: A new neurologic and adaptive capacity scoring system for evaluation obstetric medications in full term newborns. Anesthesiology 56:340, 1982
20. Yeomans ER, Hauth JC, Gilstrap LC III, et al: Umbilical

cord pH, PCO_2, and bicarbonate following uncomplicated term vaginal deliveries. Obstet Gynecol 151:798, 1985

PAIN RELIEF AND VAGINAL DELIVERY

In 1984, Melzack[1] studied labor pain and stated: "While the average intensity of labor pain is extremely high, there is a wide range of pain scores." For primiparous women, 9.2 percent perceived the pain as mild; 29.5 percent, moderate; 37.9 percent, severe: and 23.4 percent, extremely severe. The multiparous women perceived the pain as less: 24.1 percent as mild; 29.6 percent moderate; 35.2 percent severe; and 11.1 percent, extremely severe.

In 1986, Gibbs et al.[2] reviewed the pain relief used in approximately 1,200 hospitals in the United States for the year 1981. The results are summarized in Table 3-5.

Because of the wide variation in the perception of pain and the several methods of relieving pain available, one should individualize the type and amount of analgesics administered and should understand the effects of analgesia on the mother as well as the fetus and neonate. In the previous section, the methods for evaluation of the neonate were reviewed. This section reviews the methods of pain relief used for vaginal delivery and the effects on the mother and the neonate.

Table 3-5. Obstetric Anesthesia—A National Survey

Anesthetic Procedure	Labor (%)	Vaginal Delivery (%)	Cesarean Delivery (%)
None	32	15	—
Narcotic/ barbiturate/ tranquilizer	49	—	—
Inhalational	0	6	—
Paracervical block	5	—	—
Infiltration/ pudendal block	—	59	—
Epidural	16	14	21
Spinal	—	9	34
General	—	3	41

Note: The sum is not 100 percent because some patients received more than one modality of pain relief, or the respondents did not fill in the forms completely.

(From Gibbs et al.,[2] with permission.)

METHODS OF PAIN RELIEF FOR VAGINAL DELIVERY

No Analgesics

Some women choose not to receive analgesics for labor and delivery. Their reasons include mild pain, rapid labor, and a short duration of pain; the wish to deliver naturally; or fear that the drugs used may be harmful. For these women, we must look at the effects of labor pain on the fetus and neonate.

The pain of uterine contractions causes maternal hyperventilation and an increase in maternal oxygen consumption.[3] Hyperventilation will further lower the mother's normally low $PaCO_2$ of 32 to 34 mmHg, and will also decrease fetal PaO_2.[4–6] The average PCO_2 in laboring women is 25.3 ± 8.0 mmHg, with 7 percent of women having a PCO_2 below 15 mmHg.[7] The decrease in fetal PaO_2 seen with maternal hyperventilation may be due to a decrease in uterine blood flow and/or a shift to the left in the maternal oxygen-hemoglobin dissociation curve (allowing maternal hemoglobin to bind oxygen more readily).[4,8] A decrease in maternal $PaCO_2$ from 34 to 17 mmHg will decrease fetal PaO_2 from 18 to 13 mmHg (oxygen saturation from 49 to 38 percent).[4] The increase in oxygen consumption and hyperventilation during contractions can be mitigated with effective analgesia.[3,9]

In pregnant ewes, nonpainful as well as painful stimuli have been demonstrated to raise the level of circulating catecholamines, especially norepinephrine. Catecholamines can raise maternal blood pressure 45 to 50 percent and diminish uterine blood flow 30 to 50 percent.[10] Effective analgesia can decrease maternal catecholamines[11] and maintain, and in some cases improve, intervillous blood flow.[12,13]

In addition, "bearing down" in the second stage of labor can also diminish uterine blood flow.[14]

Thus, in some women who experience labor pain, the physiologic effects of pain can biochemically affect and possibly jeopardize the fetus even though no medications were administered. When looking at the effects of drugs, we must consider the effects of not having analgesia on the fetus and newborn as well.

Prepared Childbirth

Prepared childbirth classes are designed to educate the parturient and her significant other as to the events that will occur during pregnancy, labor and delivery. To decrease the pain and stress of labor, the parturient is taught to breathe in a specific pattern until the contraction is over. The breathing exercises do not reduce the pain but act as a distraction and a means of control to help the parturient endure the contractions. In addition, most classes today inform the parturients of other available options for analgesia, such as narcotics and regional anesthesia. By attending the classes, it is hoped that the parturient will have less anxiety and fear associated with labor and delivery.[15]

Scott et al.[15] examined the effect of prepared childbirth (Lamaze) classes on outcome. They compared 129 primiparous women who attended classes with 129 women who did not. They noted that less medication was used in the prepared group (although the majority of women in both groups required pain medications, most often narcotics). There was no difference in neonatal outcome between the groups with respect to 1-minute and 5-minute Apgar scores, frequency of fetal distress, and neonatal problems.

Nelson et al.[17] compared the Leboyer approach to delivery with conventional delivery. They randomized 54 patients into a Leboyer group (28 patients) and a control group (26 patients). They evaluated several variables, including the Apgar score, the Brazelton neurobehavioral assessment at 24 to 72 hours, and an 8-month developmental examination. They found no significant differences between the two groups.

Parenteral Medications

Several types of parenteral medications have been used to ease the discomfort of labor. These include for analgesia, the narcotics and the anesthetic agent ketamine; and to decrease anxiety and produce sedation, the tranquilizers and the barbiturates.

Opioids (and the Opioid Antagonist, Naloxone). Opioids are still the primary form of pain relief used in obstetrics today. Although they are effective analgesics, they have several significant side effects that limit their dosage and effectiveness. These side effects for the mother include drowsiness, nausea and vomiting, orthostatic hypotension, decreased gastric motility, and respiratory depression. Fetal effects include variations of the fetal heart rate (FHR), such as a decrease of beat-to-beat variability and, occasionally, a benign sinusoidal pattern. The neonate can have decreased Apgar scores and respiratory acidosis, as well as neurobehavioral alterations. Because of their adverse effects on the neonate, narcotics are being used in low doses early on in the first stage of labor. See Table 3-6 for narcotic dosages.

In 1803, morphine was the first opioid to be isolated from opium. It was first used in labor in 1837. In 1902, Steinbuckel first recommended the use of scopolamine–morphine amnesia, more commonly known as "twilight sleep." In this technique, the parturient received a single dose of morphine and scopolamine, followed most commonly by scopolamine alone. In long labors morphine was sometimes repeated. Twilight sleep was often accompanied by protracted labor, a restless parturient, and respiratory depression of the neonate. This technique was commonly used until World War II.[21] In 1961, Campbell et al.[22], compared pentobarbital, meperidine, and morphine in 212 patients in labor and found only minimal differences in Apgar scores and no significant depression in any infant group. The average dose of pentobarbital was 215 mg; for meperidine, 120 mg; and for morphine, 11 mg. In 1965, Way et al.[23] administered morphine 0.05 mg/kg to four infants and meperidine 0.5 mg/kg to four infants and found greater respiratory depression with morphine. This may be related to the greater permeability of the neonate's blood-brain barrier to morphine. Because of the greater respiratory depression that may be produced by morphine, many clinicians prefer meperidine (currently the most popular narcotic administered for labor analgesia).[24] Some clinicians still use morphine, in a maximum dose of 15 to 20 mg.[25] The duration of analgesia is about 4 hours.[20]

Meperidine was synthesized in 1939 and was first used in obstetrics in 1940.[21] The peak analgesic effect occurs 5 to 10 minutes after intravenous administration and 40 to 50 minutes after intramuscular injection. The duration of maternal analgesia is 2 to 4 hours.[20] The adverse effects may be related to either meperidine or the active metabolite, normeperidine. Meperidine reaches the fetus within 2 minutes of maternal intravenous administration, and has been found in the neonate for up to 6 days after maternal administration for

Table 3-6. Opioids Used for Labor Analgesia and Common Doses

Narcotic	Comparative Dose	Intravenous Dose	Intramuscular Dose
Morphine	10 mg	2.5–5 mg	5–10 mg
Meperidine or pethidine (Demerol)	100 mg	25–50 mg	50–100 mg
Fentanyl (Sublimaze)	100 μg	25–50 μg	50–100 μg
Pentazocine (Talwin)	30 mg	10–20 mg	20–30 mg
Butorphanol (Stadol)	2 mg	1–2 mg	1–2 mg
Nalbuphine (Nubain)	10 mg	5–10 mg	10–20 mg

(Data from Paddock et al.,[18] Physicians' Desk Reference,[19] and Wood and Wood.[20])

labor.[26,27] The half-life of meperidine is 3 to 7 hours in the mother and 13 to 23 hours in the neonate.[28–30] The half-life of normeperidine is longer: 21 hours in the mother and 63 hours in the neonate.[29,30] Adverse effects include decreased Apgar scores (especially if delivery occurs in the second or third hour after drug administration),[29] decreased pH associated with an increase in PCO_2,[32] and changes in neurobehavioral tests for up to 3 days of life.[33–35]

Fentanyl, a short-acting opioid, was synthesized in 1960. The peak analgesic effect occurs 3 to 5 minutes after intravenous injection and lasts 30 to 60 minutes. After intramuscular injection, peak analgesia occurs within 20 to 30 minutes and lasts 1 to 2 hours. Because of its short duration of analgesia, it is not widely used to control labor pain. Use of fentanyl is not recommended by the manufacturer, as insufficient data exist to support its safe use during labor.[19]

Pentazocine is a opioid agonist with some weak antagonist activity. Analgesia occurs within 2 to 3 minutes after intravenous injection and 10 to 20 minutes after intramuscular injection. Duration of analgesia is 3 to 4 hours. Pentazocine has an elimination half-life of about 2 hours.[20] Umbilical: maternal blood concentration is 0.4:0.7 and is less than that of meperidine if time from injection to delivery is the same.[36,37] In 1969, Duncan et al.[37] reported no difference in Apgar scores between neonates whose mothers received pentazocine (48 mg) and mothers who received meperidine (120 mg). A control group of neonates whose mothers did not receive either opioid had higher Apgar scores. In 1980, Refstad,[38] in a double-blind randomized study of 85 patients, reported better 1- and 5-minute Apgar scores when pentazocine (45 mg) was used compared with meperidine (100 mg). Two neonates in the pentazocine group and four neonates in the meperidine group required naloxone. Umbilical artery blood gas data were similar between the groups.

Butorphanol, a opioid agonist–antagonist, was introduced in 1974. Analgesia occurs within 2 to 3 minutes after intravenous injection and 30 minutes after intramuscular injection. Duration of analgesia is 3 to 4 hours. Excretion of butorphanol is primarily in the urine (70 percent) and the elimination half-life is 2.5 to 3.5 hours.[20] In 1979, Hodgkinson et al.[39] looked at 200 parturients in labor and compared intravenous doses of butorphanol 1 mg with meperidine 40 mg and butorphanol 2 mg with meperidine 80 mg. They reported no significant differences in maternal analgesia, in FHR during labor, in the Apgar scores, or in neurobehavioral scores [the Early Neonatal Neurobehavioral Scale (ENNS)]. They did find fewer maternal side effects with butorphanol (2 percent) compared to meperidine (13 percent). When larger doses are needed, butorphanol may be better than meperidine because less respiratory depression is thought to occur with butorphanol.[40]

Nalbuphine is a opioid agonist–antagonist. Its maternal half-life is 2.4 hours.[41] The duration of analgesia is 3 to 6 hours.[20] Maximal adult respiratory depression occurs after administration of 30 mg.[42] In one study in which 15 to 20 mg was injected intravenously for analgesia during labor, Apgar scores were normal and neonatal drug concentrations varied between one-third and six times the maternal concentration.[41] In 1987, Frank et al.[43] failed to note any significant difference in Apgar scores or neurobehavioral evaluations [the Neonatal Neurologic and Adaptive Capacity Score (NACS)] between nalbuphine and meperidine. They administered the narcotics by patient-controlled analgesia (PCA) pumps.

Naloxone (Narcan) is a pure opioid antagonist. The question has been raised as to whether naloxone should be given prior to delivery in order to avert the possible respiratory depression seen in the neonate after maternal narcotic administration. Naloxone should *not* be administered to the mother just prior to delivery in an attempt to prevent neonatal depression from maternal narcotic administration. This will only reverse the analgesia at a time when it is needed most. In addition, reversal of neonatal opioid depression will be unpredictable at best and may not even be necessary. Thus, naloxone should be administered to the neonate after delivery only if clinically indicated. After naloxone administration, the neonate should be observed for at least 4 hours before transfer to the regular nursery, since the longer-acting opioids may outlast the antagonist.[44] Dosage of naloxone has recently been increased from 0.01mg/kg to 0.1 mg/kg given intravenously, intramuscularly, subcutaneously, or via the endotracheal tube.[45,46] The use of the dilute neonatal naloxone concentration (0.02 mg/ml) is no longer recommended because unacceptable fluid volumes may be given. The adult concentrations (0.4 mg/ml or 1 mg/ml) are the recommended concentrations.[46]

Ketamine. Ketamine (Ketalar) is an intravenous anesthetic that produces intense analgesia and a dissociative state regarded as sleep. Its use for vaginal delivery is controversial. It has the advantage of being a powerful analgesic as well as a good induction agent for general anesthesia for cesarean delivery (see the next section). Ketamine, however, tends to produce amnesia, which may be undesirable. Once thought to preserve laryngeal or pharngeal reflexes in the anesthetized patient, this has proved untrue.[47–49] Another disadvantage is the production of unpleasant dreams. If ketamine is given in a dose of 2 mg/kg for anesthesia for forceps delivery, over half of the parturients will report unpleasant dreams, which could conceivably adversely affect the mother–child relationship.[50]

In 1974, Janeczko et al.[48] reported the use of high doses of ketamine (0.7 mg/kg and 2.2 mg/kg) for many women who also received nitrous oxide analgesia by mask for vaginal delivery. In the 0.7-mg/kg group, 9.4 percent of neonates had low Apgar scores (≤6). In the 2.2-mg/kg group, 29 percent had low Apgar scores. This was compared with a group who delivered under epidural or spinal anesthesia with 6 percent low Apgar scores and a group who delivered under general endotracheal anesthesia with 13.5 percent low Apgar scores. They did have one patient in their 0.7-mg/kg ketamine group who vomited and aspirated.

In 1974, Akamatsu et al.[51] reported the use of low-dose ketamine (12.5 to 25 mg or 0.2 to 0.4 mg/kg, repeated as needed to 100 mg) for vaginal delivery in 80 patients. Complete analgesia occurred in 78 patients, with partial or no analgesia occurring in the remaining 2 patients. Apgar scores were ≥7 for all neonates.

Thus, low doses of ketamine are not overly depressant to the neonate, whereas large doses may be. One must always keep in mind the ever-present risk of aspiration when this drug is administered intravenously to a parturient, as she may subsequently become unresponsive. The induction dose for general anesthesia is 1 mg/kg. In my practice, ketamine is only used as an induction agent for general endotracheal anesthesia for emergency delivery—usually in the circumstances of maternal hypotension from hemorrhage, since sympathetic tone is well maintained.

Tranquilizers. Tranquilizers have been used in obstetrics to decrease the anxiety experienced by parturients during labor and delivery, as well as to potentiate the analgesic properties of opioids. Diazepam, the most studied of the tranquilizers, has anticonvulsant activity and has been used to prevent and treat toxemic seizures. Tranquilizers fall into three groups (see Table 3-7).

Diazepam was synthesized in 1959. It has been shown to decrease anxiety as well as produce amnesia in the parturient.[52,53] It also has the advantage of decreasing the need for narcotics as well as the total dosage of narcotics used during labor.[52–54] The drug rapidly crosses the placenta and achieves fetal/maternal blood levels often exceeding 1.0.[55–60] With the use of 5 to 20-mg doses, fetal monitoring shows an increase in FHR[58] and a decrease in beat-to-beat variability.[59,60] This decrease in variability is not associated with changes in fetal pH, PO_2, PCO_2, or base deficit and thus does not signify fetal asphyxia.[60] The metabolism of diazepam in the neonate is slow, with a mean half-life of about 31 hours.[57] Diazepam and its active metabolites have been detected in the neonate up to 8 to 10 days after birth.[55,61] Thus, effects of this drug on the neonate may last several days. When mothers receive diazepam 20 mg or less, the Apgar scores do not appear to be affected.[52,54,56,59,60] Neonates whose mothers have received larger doses often demonstrate low Apgar scores, lethargy, apnea, hypotonia, hypothermia, poor feeding, and an inability to respond to their environment for up to 3 days after delivery.[53,55,57,58,61]

Table 3-7. Tranquilizers Used during Labor

Group	Drug	Brand Name
Benzodiazepines	Diazepam	Valium
	Lorazepam	Arivan
	Midazolam	Versed
Antihistamine	Hydroxyzine	Vistaril
Phenothiazines	Promethazine	Phenergan
	Promazine	Sparine
	Chlorpromazine	Thorazine
	Prochlorperazine	Compazine

Lorazepam has pharmacologic actions similar to diazepam. A 1- to 2-mg dose of lorazepam is similar to a 10-mg dose of diazepam. Although lorazepam has a shorter elimination half-life (10 to 24 h) when compared to diazepam, its clinical effects are of longer duration. This may be related to tighter binding of lorazepam to the benzodiazepine receptor.[62] Onset of action is slow, occurring 20 to 40 minutes after intravenous administration.[20] Lorazepam crosses the placenta and produces a fetal/maternal blood concentration that is usually less than 1.0. With large doses, the depressant effects are similar to those of diazepam, namely low Apgar scores, depressed respiration, hypothermia, and poor feedings. These effects are more pronounced in the preterm neonate.[3] With the slow onset of action and depressant effects similar to diazepam, the use of lorazepam is limited in labor.

Midazolam was synthesized in 1976. It has a rapid onset and a short duration of action. A 3- to 5-mg dose of midazolam is approximately equal to a 10-mg dose of diazepam. Midazolam has a short half-life of 1 to 2 hours.[20] Looking at placental transfer in pregnant ewes, the fetal/maternal drug concentration for midazolam is less (about 0.6) than with diazepam (about 0.8), suggesting the lesser placental permeability of midazolam.[64] When used as a premedication both orally and intramuscularly for elective cesarean delivery, midazolam was effective as an anxiolytic. When given as a single

15-mg dose orally the night before surgery, midazolam was virtually undetectable in maternal or umbilical cord serum the next morning. Midazolam was detectable in maternal and umbilical cord serum if administered in a 15-mg intramuscular dose just prior to surgery. Apgar scores were unaffected with the 15-mg dose given preoperatively either orally or intramuscularly.[65] Although midazolam appears to be a good anxiolytic, it is also a good amnesic. When used for sedation after delivery under regional anesthesia for cesarean delivery in doses of 2 to 7 mg intravenously, some parturients complained of having no recall of the birth of their babies.[66] Thus, one must be cautious about its use as a sedative if one wants to preserve recall. In addition, the manufacturer recommends, "the initial intravenous dose for conscious sedation may be as little as 1 mg, but should not exceed 2.5 mg in a normal healthy adult," because respiratory depression and respiratory arrest has been reported with its use. The manufacturer does not recommend its use in labor because of possible central nervous system depression of the neonate and the lack of adequate clinical study.[19]

Hydroxyzine is rapidly transferred across the placenta. In doses of 1.5 mg/kg, up to a maximum of 100 mg, given as a premedicant 1 hour before elective cesarean delivery under spinal anesthesia, Apgar scores and neurobehavioral evaluations (NACS) were normal.[67] Hydroxyzine can be combined with narcotics to reduce anxiety and potentiate narcotic analgesia in a manner similar to diazepam. When used in conjunction with meperidine during labor, no adverse effects on the 1-minute Apgar scores have been reported.[68]

Promethazine has also been used in conjunction with meperidine during labor to relieve anxiety and provide sedation in labor with no adverse effects on the 1-minute Apgar scores.[68] A combination of promethazine 25 mg with meperidine 25 mg per ml is currently available as Mepergan.[19] It also has antihistaminic, antiemetic, and anticholinergic effects.

Promazine, chlorpromazine, and prochlorperazine are not widely used in obstetrics because they have significant adrenergic blocking properties that may result in maternal hypotension.[24] Corke, in 1977,[69] reported poorer neurobehavioral scores in neonates whose mothers received promazine and meperidine for labor analgesia when compared to neonates whose mothers received no analgesia or epidurally administered bupivacaine.

Barbiturates. Barbiturates, such as pentobarbital (Nembutal) and secobarbital (Seconal), have continued to lose popularity, as it has become increasingly apparent that they have prolonged depressant effects on the neonate.[70,71] These sedative-hypnotics possess amnesic properties but no analgesic properties, and in agitated parturients with pain, may produce an antianalgesic effect that makes management more difficult. In one study in which the average dose of pentobarbital was 215 mg, 41 percent of the mothers were difficult to manage, 54 percent reported amnesia for the entire labor, and 89 percent were satisfied with their care.[22] At the present time, barbiturates are used to produce overnight sedation for parturients who require a stepwise induction of labor that may take 2 or 3 days. The doses commonly used are 100 to 200 mg of pentobarbital or secobarbital orally. Intramuscular injection is painful. (Midazolam may prove to be safer for the neonate because of its faster metabolism.)

Inhaled Anesthetics

The use of inhaled anesthetics in obstetrics dates back to January 1847, when Dr. Simpson of Edinburgh "administered the vapour [ether] in a case of labour, and ascertained that it was capable of removing the sufferings of the patient without interfering with the process of parturition." Since then, several other agents have been used in obstetrics. These include chloroform (November 1847); nitrous oxide (1880); cyclopropane (1935); trichloroethylene (1942); methoxyflurane (1962); and recently halothane, enflurane, and isoflurane.[21]

The inhaled anesthetics may be used in two ways: as analgesics and as anesthetics. Inhalational analgesia is the administration of a low concentration of the inhaled anesthetic either continuously or intermittently with contractions to provide partial relief of pain. The parturient remains awake and has intact laryngeal reflexes so that the risk of aspiration is minimized. Inhalational anesthesia is the administration of slightly higher concentrations of inhaled agents to produce maternal unconsciousness. With the loss of consciousness, there is an ever-present risk of maternal aspiration unless the larynx is protected. Thus, if inhalational anesthesia (general anesthesia) is needed, a rapid-sequence induction with the placement of an endotracheal tube is mandatory.

Volatile agents have dose-related uterine muscle relaxant properties. The effects of volatile anesthetic agents are described in terms of the minimal alveolar concentration, or MAC, at which point 50 percent of patients do not move when exposed to a noxious stimulus. At levels of 0.5 (50 percent) MAC, spontaneous uterine activity is depressed. At 0.8 to 0.9 MAC, the uterine response to oxytocin is suppressed. The MAC for nonpregnant adult patients is 0.76 percent for halothane, 1.12 percent for isoflurane, and 1.68 percent for enflurane. The MAC is decreased about 25 to 40 percent for the pregnant patient.[72]

In 1981, Abboud et al.[73] compared 0.25 to 1.25 percent enflurane in oxygen (55 patients) with 30 to 60 percent nitrous oxide in oxygen (50 patients) for analgesia during the second stage of labor. About 40 percent of the mothers also received a narcotic during labor and about 45 percent of mothers received a local anesthetic for delivery. The anesthetic concentration was adjusted to keep the patient awake, cooperative, and oriented. The duration of analgesia was most often 11 to 20 minutes. The neonates were vigorous and had similar Apgar scores and blood gas data.

In 1982, Stefani et al.[74] investigated the administration of inhalational analgesia during the second stage of labor. They compared 0.3 to 0.8 percent enflurane in oxygen (22 patients) with 30 to 50 percent nitrous oxide in oxygen (18 patients) and a control group that received no inhaled agent (21 patients). The mean duration of inhalational analgesia was 16.5 minutes in the enflurane group and 14.8 minutes in the nitrous oxide group. Over 50 percent of the mothers also received a narcotic and over 50 percent of the mothers received a local anesthetic (pudendal block and/or infiltration) just before delivery. These investigators found no differences among neonates with regard to the time to sustained respirations, Apgar scores, blood gas values, the neurobehavioral scores (ENNS and NACS) performed at 2 and 24 hours after birth.

In 1989, Abboud et al.[75] compared 0.2 to 0.7 percent isoflurane in oxygen (30 patients) with 30 to 60 percent nitrous oxide in oxygen (30 patients) for analgesia during the second stage or labor. The mean duration of inhalational analgesia was 13 minutes in the isoflurane group and 14.7 minutes in the nitrous oxide group. They found no difference in 1- or 5-minute Apgar scores, blood gas results, or neurobehavioral scores (NACS) performed at 15 minutes, 2 hours, and 24 hours of age.

Inhalational analgesia appears to have minimal effects on the neonate. Even though volatile analgesics allow a higher inspired oxygen concentration to be administered compared to nitrous oxide, umbilical cord PaO_2 values are not significantly different.

Although inhalational analgesia appears safe for the neonate, inhalational analgesia may occasionally become inhalational mask anesthesia. The resultant loss of consciousness in the mother, who often has a full stomach, may lead to aspiration of gastric contents and resultant maternal morbidity. Because of this risk of aspiration, the safety of inhalational pain relief for labor is questioned and many obstetric anesthesiologists do not offer this type of analgesia.

Regional Analgesia and Anesthesia

Regional, or local, anesthesia has become a popular method of obtaining pain relief, as it is effective in providing pain relief without producing sedation. Although local anesthetics are most often used, narcotics recently have been injected epidurally and subarachnoid for analgesia either alone and in combination with local anesthetics.

Local anesthetics are commonly divided into three groups according to their duration of action[76] (Table 3-8).

Local anesthetics may affect the neonate directly or indirectly. The direct mechanism is related to the amount of local anesthetic that crosses the placenta to the fetus. The indirect effects of local anesthetics are related to a decrease in maternal blood pressure (driving force) or an increase in uterine artery tone (resistance) that can occur with high levels of local anesthetic, as seen in paracervical block.

The direct effects of the drug can be assessed by measuring the amount of drug in the neonate. Many studies have measured the blood concentration (an indirect measurement of the amount of drug at the neonate's drug receptor). The toxic blood levels that produce a higher incidence of depression in neonates have been determined for several drugs. For lidocaine[78] and mepivacaine,[79] the toxic levels above which neonates appear depressed is 3μg/ml. Because chloroprocaine is broken down so rapidly in the maternal and fetal blood (after about 21 seconds in the mother and 43 seconds in the fetus[80]), direct effects with this drug probably are minimal, if present at all.

Because local anesthetics cross the placenta by passive diffusion, attempts have been made to determine

Table 3-8. Parenteral Local Anesthetics and Year Synthesized

Short Duration of Action and Low Anesthetic Potency	
Procaine (Novacain)	1904
Chloroprocaine (Nesacaine)	1951
Intermediate Duration of Action and Intermediate Anesthetic Potency	
Lidocaine (Xylocaine)	1943
Mepivacaine (Carbocaine, Polocaine)	1956
Prilocaine (Citanest)	1959
Long Duration of Action and High Anesthetic Potency	
Tetracaine (Pontocaine)	1928
Bupivacaine (Marcaine, Sensorcaine)	1957
Etidocaine (Duranest)	1971

(Data from Physicians' Desk Reference,[19] Covino,[76] and Fink.[77])

Table 3-9. Fetal/Maternal (UV/MV) Ratio for Amide Local Anesthetics

Lidocaine	0.45–0.7	
Mepivacaine	0.45–0.7	
Prilocaine	1.0–1.2	
Bupivacaine	0.20–0.45	(paracervical 0.60)
Etidocaine	0.15–0.40	

(Data from Refs. 78, 79, 81, 83–87.)

Table 3-10. Half-Life of Local Anesthetics

	Neonatal	Adult
Chloroprocaine	15–43 s	11–25 s
Lidocaine	3–4 h	1.5–2 h
Mepivacaine	8–10 h	2–3 h
Bupivacaine	8–18 h	1.25–4 h

(Data from Physicians' Desk Reference,[19] O'Brien et al.,[80] Brown et al.,[83] Caldwell et al.,[91] Kuhnert et al.,[92] and Scanlon et al.[93])

whether some drugs diffuse more slowly than others and thus produce less direct effect on the fetus and neonate. Early attempts looked at the ratio of drug in the fetus (umbilical vein) to the drug in the mother (maternal vein) (the UV/MV ratio). The UV/MV ratio for each drug does not appear to depend on the route of administration, except for paracervical block, in which the ratio is higher. With paracervical block, the local anesthetic is deposited near the uterine arteries. This permits diffusion of the drug directly into these vessels, producing a high local blood level in the placental intervillous space.[81,82] Table 3-9 lists the fetal/maternal blood ratio for amide local anesthetics after the common obstetric regional blocks except for paracervical blocks, for which the ratio is listed only for bupivacaine.

If the fetus becomes acidotic, ion trapping of the local anesthetic is possible and may produce a high fetal/maternal ratio.[88,89] For example, Brown et al.[89] reported a UV/MV ratio of 2.91 for a parturient who received a mepivacaine epidural anesthetic and whose child had a fetal umbilical vein pH of 7.03.

The lower UV/MV ratio for bupivacaine and etidocaine as compared with lidocaine and mepivacaine may be related to the higher maternal protein binding that exists with these long-acting agents. As a result of this finding, many believe that the effects on the neonate may be less with bupivacaine and etidocaine as compared with lidocaine or mepivacaine. Some studies suggest that this may not be the case. The lower UV/MV ratios may be due to the higher lipid solubility of these long-acting agents, making distribution greater to fetal lipid tissues, such as the brain.[90]

The duration of effects of any local anesthetic that exists in the neonate will depend on the half-life of the drug. The duration of action is longer in neonates than adults. This may be related to slower hepatic metabolism or slower renal excretion of the drugs (Table 3-10).

Because the metabolic product of prilocaine is o-toluidine, which can cause methemoglobinemia in the mother and the fetus and neonate, this drug is not commonly used today, even though the maternal cyanosis caused by methemoglobin can be reversed with methylene blue and produces no adverse effects on the neonate.[84]

Routes of Administration for Local Anesthetics.

Paracervical Block. A paracervical block involves the injection of local anesthetic around the rim of the cervix for relief of pain in the first stage of labor. It is easy to perform and has an almost immediate onset of analgesia. It has the advantage of not producing sympathetic blockade; thus, maternal hypotension is not associated with paracervical block. However, fetal bradycardia with fetal distress and sometimes fetal death can occur.[94–97] In a study by Shnider et al.,[96] the incidence of FHR changes were higher in primiparous parturients and in fetuses that were premature or had pre-existing fetal distress.

Typically when bradycardia occurs, the FHR decreases within 20 minutes after the block (median 4.6 minutes) and persists for less than 30 minutes (median 3.3 minutes).[96]

In 1981, Morishima et al.[98] demonstrated that fetal bradycardia is not due to direct toxic effects from a high fetal blood concentration of local anesthetic; the fetal levels obtained are much lower than the levels needed for direct cardiovascular toxicity. (*Note*: a direct toxic effect could occur if the injection is made directly into the fetus.) The bradycardia seen after paracervical block is, in part, due to a decrease in oxygen delivery to the fetus secondary to an increase in uterine activity and a decrease in uterine artery blood flow. The decrease in oxygen delivery may produce fetal hypoxia, acidosis, and cardiac depression. The increase in uterine tone may decrease uterine arteriolar blood flow. The decrease in uterine artery blood flow may be caused by uterine artery vasoconstriction associated with high concentrations of local anesthetics that exists near the arteries.[99,100]

In 1983, Weiss et al.[101] compared 1 percent lidocaine to 2 percent chloroprocaine in a double-blind randomized study of 60 parturients receiving paracervical blocks. The total volume injected was 20 ml, 10 ml each side. They showed a lower incidence of bradycardia with chloroprocaine (1 of 29) compared to lidocaine (5 of 31). This was not statistically significant. The bradycardias subsided within 6 minutes. One neonate in each group had a low 1-minute Apgar score (5 and 6) without having bradycardia during labor. One other neonate, in the lidocaine group, had bradycardia during labor and a 1-minute Apgar score of 5 associated with an umbilical artery pH of 7.14 and an umbilical venous pH of 7.27. Mean umbilical cord pHs were no different between the groups. A low incidence of bradycardia with chloroprocaine has also been reported by others.[102,103]

It has been suggested that lower volumes of local anesthetic (3 to 5 ml) may produce fewer episodes of bradycardia than larger volumes of local anesthetic (10 to 15 ml) and still produce effective analgesia.[103–105]

In 1988, Kangas-Saarela et al.[104] found no difference in Apgar scores and neurobehavioral examinations (ENNS) at 1, 2, and 4 to 5 days after delivery in 22 healthy parturients (10 paracervical and 12 control [no analgesia]). They used a low dose of bupivacaine.

In the United States, chloroprocaine, lidocaine, and etidocaine are approved for use in paracervical blocks. Bupivacaine is not approved.[19]

Continuous FHR monitoring is now considered mandatory if paracervical block is administered. If signs of fetal distress appear, capillary blood sampling from the fetal scalp should be done to evaluate the pH of the fetus.[97] If deterioration is progressive, delivery is indicated.

Infiltration. Infiltration of the perineum can affect the fetus by the direct mechanism of drug toxicity.

In 1984, Philipson et al.[106] detected lidocaine in maternal blood as early as 1 minute after perineal infiltration, with peak levels within 3 to 12 minutes. The highest umbilical venous level was 1.38 μg/ml. In addition, they demonstrated lidocaine and the active metabolites in neonatal urine for 48 hours after delivery. Apgar scores were normal in all neonates.

In 1987, Philipson et al.[107] were unable to detect chloroprocaine in the cord blood of 16 of 17 neonates whose mothers received local perineal infiltration with an average dose of 82 mg. The one neonate in whom chloroprocaine was demonstrated had a level of 4.84 ng/ml, an extremely low level.

Since the injection to delivery time is usually much less with perineal infiltration as compared with an epidural anesthetic, the total amount of drug transferred is less (especially with chloroprocaine), and presumably the direct neonatal effects would be minimal.

Pudendal Block. In 1980, Merkow et al.[108] compared 3 percent chloroprocaine (900 mg) with 1 percent mepivacaine (300 mg) and (150 mg) bupivacaine 0.5 percent in paturients having a pudendal block for delivery. Of the 54 parturients, 36 were also given 20 to 30 mg of alphaprodine (a narcotic no longer available in the United States) a mean of 2 hours before delivery. The umbilical vein level of mepivacaine was 0.94 μg/ml and of bupivacaine was 0.35 μg/ml. No difference was found in Apgar scores or blood gas data in the neonates between the different drug groups. When the neurobehavioral evaluation (ENNS) was performed at 4 and 24 hours of age, all results were similar, except that some infants who received mepivacaine scored better at 4 hours in the response decrement to pinprick (noxious stimuli).

Thus, pudendal nerve block performed shortly before delivery does not adversely affect the neonate if reasonable doses are administered and intravascular injection does not occur.

Epidurally Administered Local Anesthetics. Epidural anesthesia with local anesthetics can affect the fetus by a direct effect of the anesthetic and also by an indirect effect if maternal blood pressure decreases secondary to sympathetic blockade, resulting in decreased uteroplacental perfusion. (Transient hypotension with epidural anesthesia for vaginal delivery occurs in only about 4 percent of patients, if acute hydration and left uterine displacement are used.[109] Lidocaine[78] and bupivacaine[81] have been detected in the maternal bloodstream within 3 minutes of epidural injection and peak concentrations occur between 10 and 30 minutes after injection. If the blood pressure is maintained, effective anesthesia can decrease maternal catecholamines[11] and, in some cases, may improve intervillous blood flow.[12,13]

In 1974, Scanlon et al.[93] compared neonates of women who received epidural lidocaine (9 patients) or mepivacaine (19 patients) with a control group of neonates whose mothers did not receive an epidural (13 patients). The mean dose of lidocaine was 423 mg and of mepivacaine was 374 mg. The mean time from last dose of local anesthetic to delivery was 22 minutes for lidocaine and 27 minutes for mepivacaine. The mean umbilical artery blood levels were 0.48 μg/ml in the lidocaine group and 1.68 μg/ml in the mepivacaine group. Alphaprodine and/or secobarbital was given to 11 of 28 of the epidural group and to 4 of 13 of the control group 6 or more hours prior to delivery. They found Apgar scores of ≥7 in all neonates. Upon neurobehavioral evaluation (ENNS), the neonates in the epidural group demonstrated a decrease in motor strength and tone during the first few hours of life; they characterized these neonates as "floppy but alert."

In 1976, Scanlon et al.[86] compared neonates of women who received epidural bupivacaine (20 patients) with the control group infants in the 1974 study.[93] The mean dose of bupivacaine during labor was 112 mg. The time from last dose of local anesthetic to delivery was 71 minutes, which was well into the redistribution phase of bupivacaine. The mean umbilical artery blood level was 0.10 μg/ml. Apgar scores, umbilical blood pH values, and neurobehavioral scores (ENNS) between 2 and 4 hours of life were all normal.

In 1976, Tronick et al.,[110] using the neurobehavioral evaluation (ENNS), compared neonates whose mothers received minimal medication (no analgesia, subarachnoid infiltration anesthesia), analgesics (alphaprodine and/or promazine), or epidural local anesthetics (lidocaine or mepivacaine with and without analgesics). The neurobehavioral effects (as measured by the ENNS) of epidural anesthesia were minimal and of doubtful significance.

In 1977, Corke et al.[69] compared neonates of women who received sedation with meperidine and promazine (22 neonates), epidural anesthesia with 0.25 to 0.5 percent bupivacaine (15 neonates), and a control group who received no analgesics (14 neonates). Utilizing the neurobehavioral evaluation (ENNS) within 4 hours of birth, the neonates whose mothers received meperidine and promazine scored significantly worse than those in the epidural or control groups.

In 1981, Rosenblatt et al.[111] reported significant neurobehavioral alterations after the use of maternal epidural anesthesia with bupivacaine. They make several controversial statements, including "infants with greater exposure to bupivacaine in utero were more likely to be cyanotic and unresponsive to their surroundings." I have never seen cyanosis directly attributed to the use of bupivacaine nor can I understand how it would occur with the doses used clinically. A careful look at their paper is essential for two reasons. First, advocates of no pain relief during childbirth will take material such as this as evidence to further their cause. Second, one must realize that some papers are published that are not adequately peer reviewed. Significant problems with their report include misquoting other papers, such as Tronick et al.[110] (see above); lack of any obstetric information (were the neonates born vaginally or by cesarean delivery?); absence of any information of the fetus during labor (was fetal monitoring used? If so, was fetal distress present?); no neonatal information such as gestational age or weight; and no information on the common neonatal examinations such as Apgar scores or acid-base data. Furthermore, their technique of epidural anesthesia was poor; they made no attempt to prevent maternal hypotension (i.e., acute hydration wasn't used) and did not mention whether hypotension occurred and, if so, how it was treated. Perhaps their findings relate to the effects of hypotension on the neonate instead of the neonatal effects of bupivacaine. The mean umbilical artery level of bupivacaine was 0.08 μg/ml (lower than the level seen in Scanlon's 1976 study[86]). This paper is included as an example to point out that one must not only read the summary, but analyze the contents of papers as well. Interestingly, no anesthesiologist is included among the eight authors.

In 1982, Abboud et al.[109] compared neonates of women who received intermittent boluses of epidural 2 percent chloroprocaine (50 patients), 1.5 percent lidocaine (50 patients), or 0.5 percent bupivacaine (50 patients) with a control group who received no maternal analgesics (20 patients). The mean umbilical artery plasma levels were 0.01 μg/ml for chloroprocaine, 0.70 μg/ml for lidocaine, and 0.13 μg/ml for bupivacaine. Apgar scores, cord blood gas values, and neurobehavioral scores (ENNS) at 2 and 24 hours of life were all normal and showed no significant differences between the four groups.

In 1983, Abboud et al.[112] compared neonates of women who received intermittent boluses of epidural 1.5 percent lidocaine (22 patients) with a control group (17 patients). The mean dose of lidocaine in this study was larger, 446 mg, compared to 240 mg in the previous study.[109] The umbilical artery plasma lidocaine level was higher, 0.91 μg/ml. Again, Apgar scores, cord blood gas values, and neurobehavioral evaluations (ENNS) were normal.

In 1984, Abboud et al.[113] again looked at epidural local anesthetics. This time they administered the local anesthetic by continuous infusion after the loading dose: 2 Chloroprocaine (a 2 percent infusion followed by a 0.75 percent infusion; mean dose 852 mg), lidocaine (a 1.5 percent infusion followed by a 0.75 percent infusion; mean dose 623 mg), and bupivacaine (a 0.5 percent infusion followed by a 0.125 percent infusion; mean dose 182 mg). The mean umbilical artery plasma levels were 0.02 μg/ml for chloroprocaine, 1.16 μg/ml for lidocaine, and 0.15 μg/ml for bupivacaine. Again, Apgar scores, cord blood gas values, and neurobehavioral evaluations (NACS) were normal.

In 1986, Abboud et al.[114] compared neonates of women who received intermittent boluses of epidural 1.5 percent mepivacaine (20 patients) with a control group that did not receive any analgesics (16 patients). The mean mepivacaine dose was 154 mg (less than half the dose used in Scanlon's 1974 study). The mean umbilical artery plasma levels was 2.2 μg/ml for mepivacaine. Apgar scores, cord blood gas values, and neurobehavioral scores (ENNS) were similar.

Epidurally Administered Opioids. The subarachnoid

and epidural use of opioids in humans began in 1979.[115] Advantages include localized and prolonged pain relief without blocking proprioception, light touch, or autonomic or motor function. Disadvantages include respiratory depression, nausea and vomiting, pruritus, and urinary retention.[116,117]

In obstetrics, subarachnoid and epidural opioids are used in three settings: to supplement local anesthesia during cesarean delivery (see the next section), for postcesarean delivery analgesia, and for labor pain. As this section deals with vaginal delivery, we will limit our discussion to labor analgesia.

Blood levels obtained after epidural administration of morphine are similar to those obtained after intramuscular administration of morphine.[118] In the parturient, absorption is faster with epidural than with intramuscular administration. One might suspect similar effects on the neonate with similar doses of intramuscular and epidural morphine.

In 1981, Nybell-Lindahl et al.[119] reported rapid absorption and rapid placental transfer after epidural administration of morphine 4 to 6 mg. They also found a close correlation between the fetal and maternal blood concentrations. One case of respiratory depression was noted in a 36-week neonate who was delivered 110 minutes after epidural administration of morphine 5 mg.

In 1984, Hughes et al.[120] compared the epidural administration of 0.5 percent bupivacaine with morphine 2, 5, and 7.5 mg. Better analgesia was obtained with bupivacaine. Morphine 2 and 5 mg proved inadequate for labor pain, although 7.5 mg was adequate. A period of 20 to 45 minutes was needed for the onset of analgesia. All patients required local anesthetic if instrumentation or episiotomy was needed. No effects on the FHR were noted with epidural morphine. The neonates were normal with respect to Apgar scores, umbilical blood gas values, and neurobehavioral scores (NACS) at 2 and 24 hours of life.

Some evidence suggests that low levels of fentanyl appear in the blood after maternal epidural administration. This may be related to the faster penetration of the dura by fentanyl when compared with morphine due to the shape and higher lipid solubility of fentanyl.[121]

In 1981, Carrie et al.[122] gave relatively large doses of epidural fentanyl (150 to 200 μg) to 38 paturients. Analgesia was excellent for most of the first stage but inadequate for the second stage. Maternal plasma levels were a median of 0.30 ng/ml. Umbilical artery plasma fentanyl levels were 0.18 ng/ml. All neonates had an Apgar score of ≥7 except one neonate, who had an Apgar score of 3 and required intubation, oxygen, and naloxone. The plasma fentanyl level in this neonate was 0.25 ng/ml, similar to many nondepressed neonates.

In 1987, Heytens et al.[123] compared epidural alfentanil (a short-acting fentanyl-like analgesic) to a control group. Alfentanil was administered in a bolus of 30 μg/kg followed by an infusion of 30 μg/kg/h. If needed, a repeat bolus of alfentanil was given, with 0.2 percent bupivacaine given if analgesia was inadequate. The control group did not receive any analgesics. About half of the mothers reported drowsiness with the alfentanil. Alfentanil produced excellent first-stage analgesia, but inadequate second-stage analgesia. Although the Apgar scores were similar between the groups, the neurobehavioral evaluation (NACS) showed neonatal hypotonia in the alfentanil group.

Epidural opioids alone for labor have not been as effective as local anesthetics in relieving pain.[120,124] To be effective moderate doses of epidural narcotics are needed. These doses can give good to excellent analgesia for the first stage of labor but in general give poor second-stage analgesia. The second stage usually requires local anesthetic supplementation. Because of the larger doses needed, neonatal depression may result.

Epidurally Administered Local Anesthetics with Narcotics. By combining epidural administration of local anesthetics with opioids, one can decrease the total dose of each drug needed to produce adequate pain relief. The effects on the neonate would reflect the additive effects of the local anesthetics and the opioids. However, with the lower doses used, the clinical effects would be expected to be less.

In 1987, Cohen et al.[125] compared 0.25 percent bupivacaine alone to bupivacaine with fentanyl in various combinations. They noted no differences between the various groups in time to sustained respirations, 1- and 5-minute Apgar scores, umbilical cord blood gas values, or neurobehavioral scores (NACS).

In 1988, Phillips[126] compared bupivacaine alone (0.25 percent bolus plus infusion of 0.125 percent) to 0.125 percent bupivacaine with sufentanil (2-μg/ml bolus plus 1 μg/ml in infusion). Sufentanil is a opioid with greater lipid solubility than fentanyl. Apgar scores and respiratory rates at 1, 2, and 3 hours after birth were similar in the neonates. Plasma sufentanil levels were too low to be detected (less than 0.2 ng/nl) in all maternal and cord blood samples.

In 1989, Abboud et al.[127] compared bupivacaine alone to bupivacaine with butorphanol 1 mg, butorphanol 2 mg, morphine 2 mg. They found no difference in Apgar scores, umbilical blood gas values, or neurobehavioral evaluations (NACS) between the groups.

In 1989, Hunt et al.[128] compared 0.25 percent bupivacaine alone and with butorphanol 1, 2, or 3 mg. Four of six neonates in the bupivacaine plus butorphanol 3 mg group had benign sinusoidal heart rate changes. They found no difference in Apgar scores, umbilical blood gas values, or neuorbehavioral evaluations (ENNS) between the groups.

Subarachnoid Local Anesthetics. Spinal anesthesia can affect the fetus by the indirect effect of a decrease in maternal blood pressure secondary to sympathetic block producing a decrease in intervillous blood flow. The lack of direct effect is attributed to the small amounts of local anesthetic injected and the negligible blood levels measured in the mother (see the next section).

Subarachnoid Opioids. Subarachnoid opioids can produce prolonged analgesia in small doses (e.g., morphine 0.5 to 2 mg). The blood levels obtained are very small and are unlikely to produce systemic analgesia.[129,130] These low blood levels should not have a significant effect on the fetus or neonate.

In 1981, Srinivasan[131] reported results in 16 parturients using morphine 1.5 mg for labor. Onset occurred in 10 minutes with a maximal duration of 19 hours. Analgesia was adequate for all first-stage labor pain but inadequate in three patients for second-stage pain. Apgar scores were excellent in all neonates.

In 1981, Baraka et al.[132] reported excellent maternal analgesia in 20 primiparous women administered morphine 1 to 2 mg and no adverse effects on the neonates assessed by Apgar scores and neurobehavioral evaluation (ENNS). The average onset of pain relief was 32 to 36 minutes and it lasted for 8 to 11 hours. Lidocaine was needed as a supplement (14 infiltration, 2 pudendal, 4 epidural) for the second stage of labor and delivery.

In 1982, Bonnardot et al.[129] reported effective labor analgesia in 25 parturients given subarachnoid morphine 1 to 1.75 mg. They measured maternal and fetal plasma levels of morphine and found all levels below 6 ng/ml (sedation is noted when the levels are greater than 30 ng/ml). Apgar scores were normal in all neonates except one who had a "misplaced umbilical cord" and an Apgar score of 5.

In 1989, Leighton et al.[133] administered subarachnoid fentanyl 25 μg with morphine 0.25 mg to 15 parturients. Analgesia developed within 5 minutes. Two neonates had a 1-minute Apgar score of 6; all others had a 1-minute Apgar score of 7 or greater. All neonates had 5-minute Apgar scores of 7 or greater.

Although subarachnoid narcotics can produce adequate first-stage analgesia, most parturients have inadequate perineal pain relief for the second stage and need supplemental analgesia. Even though the studies of subarachnoid opioids are encouraging, the possibility of delayed maternal respiratory depression, occurring up to 10 to 12 hours after injection of morphine, makes subarachnoid narcotic less attractive for routine obstetric practice, since the postpartum wards are often are understaffed at night and adequate respiratory monitoring of the mothers cannot be assured.[134]

General Anesthesia

If general anesthesia is needed for vaginal delivery, the induction and maintenance of anesthesia would be the same as a general anesthetic for a cesarean delivery. If uterine relaxation is also needed, one simply increases the concentration of the volatile anesthetic. General anesthesia is described in the next section.

REFERENCES

1. Melzack R: The myth of painless childbirth (The John J. Bonica Lecture). Pain 19:321, 1984
2. Gibbs CP, Krischer J, Peckham BM, et al: Obstetric anesthesia—a national survey. Anesthesiology 65:298, 1986
3. Hagerdal M, Morgan CW, Sumner AE, et al: Minute ventilation and oxygen consumption during labor with epidural analgesia. Anesthesiology 59:425, 1983
4. Levinson G, Shnider SM, deLorimier AA, et al: Effects of maternal hyperventilation on uterine blood flow and fetal oxygenation and acid-base status. Anesthesiology 40:340, 1974
5. Motoyama EK, Rivard G, Acheson F, et al: Adverse effect of maternal hyperventilation on the foetus. Lancet 1:286, 1966
6. Prowse CM, Gaensler EA: Respiratory and acid-base changes during pregnancy. Anesthesiology 26:381, 1965
7. Saling E, Ligdas P: The effect on the fetus of maternal hyperventilation during labor. J Obstet Gynaecol Br Commonw 76:877, 1969
8. Ralston DH, Shnider SM, deLorimier AA: Uterine blood flow and fetal acid-base changes after bicarbonate administration to the pregnant ewe. Anesthesiology 40:348, 1974
9. Sangoul F, Fox GS, Houle GL: Effect of regional analgesia on maternal oxygen consumption during the first stage of labor. Am J Obstet Gynecol 121:1080, 1975
10. Shnider SM, Wright RG, Levinson G, et al: Uterine blood flow and plasma norepinephrine changes during maternal stress in the pregnant ewe. Anesthesiology 50:524, 1979
11. Shnider SM, Abboud TK, Artal R, et al: Maternal catecholamines decrease during labor after lumbar epidural anesthesia. Am J Obstet Gynecol 147:13, 1983
12. Hollmen AI, Jouppila R, Joupilla P, et al: Effect of extradural analgesia using bupivacaine and 2-chloroprocaine on intervillous blood flow during normal labor. Br J Anaesth 54:837, 1982
13. Jouppila R, Jouppila P, Hollmen A, et al.: Effect of

segmental extradural analgesia on placental blood flow during normal labour. Br J Anaesth 50:563, 1978
14. Bassell GM, Humayun SG, Marx GF: Maternal bearing down efforts—another fetal risk? Obstet Gynecol 56:39, 1980
15. Chantigian RC: Non-pharmacological methods for pain relief in obstetrics. Clin Anaesthesiol 4:197, 1986
16. Scott JR, Rose NB: Effect of psychoprophylaxis (Lamaze preparation) on labor and delivery in primiparas. N Engl J Med 294:1205, 1976
17. Nelson NM, Enkin MW, Saigal S, et al: A randomized clinical trial of the Leboyer approach to childbirth. N Engl J Med 302:655, 1980
18. Paddock R, Beer EG, Bellville JW, et al: Analgesic and side effects of pentazocine and morphine in a large population of postoperative patients. Clin Pharmacol Ther 10:355, 1969
19. Physicians' Desk Reference, 44th Ed. Medical Economics Company Inc., Oradell, NJ, 1990
20. Wood M, Wood AJJ: Drugs and Anesthesia—Pharmacology for Anesthesiologists. Williams & Wilkins, Baltimore, 1982
21. Schaer HM: History of pain relief in obstetrics. p.1. In Marx GF, Bassell M (eds): Obstetric Analgesia and Anaesthesia. Elsevier, New York, 1980
22. Campbell C, Phillips OC, Frazier TM: Analgesia during labor: a comparison of pentobarbital, meperidine and morphine. Obstet Gynecol 17:714, 1961
23. Way WL, Costley EC, Way EL: Respiratory sensitivity of the newborn infant to meperidine and morphine. Clin Pharmacol Ther 6:454, 1965
24. Shnider SM, Levinson G: Anesthesia for Obstetrics. 2nd Ed. Williams & Wilkins, Baltimore, 1987
25. Lavery JP: Morphine for obstetric analgesia? Contemp Obstet Gynecol April: 95, 1985
26. Cooper LV, Stephen GW, Aggett PJA: Elimination of pethidine and bupivacaine in the newborn. Arch Dis Child 52:638, 1977
27. Crawford JS, Rudofsky S: The placental transmission of pethidine. Br J Anaesth 37:929, 1965
28. Caldwell J, Wakile LA, Notarianni LJ, et al: Maternal and neonatal disposition of pethidine in childbirth—a study using quantitative gas chromatography-mass spectrometry. Life Sci 22:589, 1978
29. Kuhnert BR, Kuhnert PM, Philipson EH, et al: Disposition of meperidine and normeperidine following multiple doses during labor. II. Fetus and neonate. Am J Obstet Gynecol 151:410, 1985
30. Kuhnert BR, Philipson EH, Kuhnert PM, et al: Disposition of meperidine and normeperidine following multiple doses during labor. I. Mother. Am J Obstet Gynecol 151:406, 1985
31. Shnider SM, Moya F: Effects of meperidine on the newborn infant. Am J Obstet Gynecol 89:1009, 1964
32. Koch G, Wendel H: The effect of pethidine on the postnatal adjustment of respiration and acid base balance. Acta Obstet Gynecol Scand 47:27, 1968
33. Hodgkinson R, Bhatt M, Wang CN: Double-blind comparison of the neurobehaviour of neonates following the administration of different doses of meperidine to the mother. Can Anaesth Soc J 25:405, 1978
34. Hodgkinson R, Husain R: The duration of effect of maternally administered meperidine on neonatal behavior. Anesthesiology 56:51, 1982
35. Kuhnert BR, Linn PL, Kennard MJ: Effects of low doses of meperidine on neonatal behavior. Anesth Analg 64:335, 1985
36. Beckett AH, Taylor JF: Blood concentrations of pethidine and pentazocine in mother and infant at time of birth. J Pharm Pharamacol 19:50S, 1967
37. Duncan SLB, Ginsburg J, Morris NF: Comparison of pentazocine and pethidine in normal labor. Am J Obstet Gynecol 105:197, 1669
38. Refstad SO, Lindbaek E: Meperidine or pentazocine for labor pain? Br J Anaesth 52:265, 1980
39. Hodgkinson R, Huff RW, Hayashi RH, et al: Double-blind comparison of maternal analgesia and neonatal neurobehaviour following intravenous butorphanol and meperidine. J Int Med Res 7:224, 1979
40. Quilligan EJ, Keegan KA, Donahue MJ: Double-blind comparison of intravenously injected butorphanol and meperidine in parturients. Int J Gynaecol Obstet 18:363, 1980
41. Wilson SJ, Errick JK, Balkon J: Pharmacokinetics of nalbuphine during parturition. Am J Obstet Gynecol 155:340, 1986
42. Romangnoli A, Keats AS: Ceiling effect for respiratory depression by nalbuphine. Clin Pharmacol Ther 27:478, 1980
43. Frank M, McAteer EJ, Cattermole R, et al: Nalbuphine for obstetric analgesia. A comparison of nalbuphine with pethidine for pain relief in labour when administered by patient-controlled analgesia (PCA). Anaesthesia 42:697, 1987
44. Ostheimer GW: Newborn resuscitation. Clin Obstet Gynecol 24:635, 1981
45. American Heart Association, American Academy of Pediatrics: Textbook of Neonatal Resuscitation. American Heart Association, Dallas, 1987
46. Emergency drug doses for infants and children and naloxone use in newborns—clarification. Pediatrics 83:803, 1989
47. Carson IW, Moore J, Balmer JP, et al: Laryngeal competence with ketamine and other drugs. Anesthesiology 38:128, 1973
48. Janeczko GF, El-Etr AA, Younes S: Low-dose ketamine anesthesia for obstetrical delivery. Anesth Analg 53:828, 1974
49. Penrose BH: Aspiration pneumonitis following ketamine induction for general anesthesia. Anesth Analg 51:41, 1972
50. Ellingson A, Haram K, Sagen N: Ketamine and diazepam as anaesthesia for forceps delivery. A comparative study. Acta Anaesth Scand 21:37, 1977
51. Akamatsu TJ, Bonica JJ, Rehmet R, et al: Experiences with the use of ketamine for parturition. I. Primary

anesthesia for vaginal delivery. Anesth Analg 53:284, 1974

52. Bepko F, Lowe E, Waxman B: Relief of the emotional factor in labor with parenterally administered diazepam. Obstet Gynecol 26:852, 1965
53. Flowers CE, Rudolph AJ, Desmond MM: Diazepam (Valium) as an adjunct in obstetric analgesia. Obstet Gynecol 34:68, 1969
54. Niswander KR: Effect of diazepam on meperidine requirements of patients during labor. Obstet Gynecol 34:62, 1969
55. Cree JE, Meyer J, Hailey DM: Diazepam in labour: its metabolism and effect on the clinical condition and thermogenesis of the newborn. Br Med J 4:251, 1973
56. Kanto J, Erkkola R, Sellman R: Accumulation of diazepam and N-demethyldiazepam in the fetal blood during the labour. Ann Clin Res 5:375, 1973
57. Mandelli M, Morselli PL, Nordio S, et al: Placental transfer of diazepam and its disposition in the newborn. Clin Pharmacol Ther 17:564, 1975
58. Owen JR, Irani SF, Blair AW: Effect of diazepam administered to mothers during labor on temperature regulation of neonate. Arch Dis Child 47:107, 1972
59. Scher J, Hailey DM, Beard RW: The effects of diazepam on the fetus. J Obstet Gynaecol Br Commonw, 79:635, 1972
60. Yeh SY, Paul RH, Cordero L, et al: A study of diazepam during labor. Obstet Gynecol 43:363, 1974
61. McCarthy GT, O'Connell B, Robinson AE: Blood levels of diazepam in infants of two mothers given large doses of diazepam during labour. J Obstet Gynaecol Br Commonw 80:349, 1973
62. White PF: Pharmacologic and clinical aspects of preoperative medication. Anesth Analg 65:963, 1986
63. Whitelaw AGL, Cummings AJ, McFadyen IR: Effect of maternal lorazepam on the neonate. Br Med J 282:1106, 1981
64. Conklin KA, Graham CW, Murad S, et al: Midazolam and diazepam: maternal and fetal effects in the pregnant ewe. Obstet Gynecol 56:471, 1980
65. Kanto J, Sjovall S, Erkkola R, et al: Placental transfer and maternal midazolam kinetics. Clin Pharmacol Ther 33:786, 1983
66. Camann W, Cohen MB, Ostheimer GW: Is midazolam desirable for sedation in parturients? Anesthesiology 65:441, 1986
67. Abouleish EI: Placental transfer of hydroxyzine hydrochloride and its effect on the human neonate. Anesth Analg Abstr 63:176, 1984
68. Malkasian GD Jr, Smith RA, Decker DG: Comparison of hydroxyzine-meperidine and promethazine-meperidine for analgesia during labor. Obstet Gynecol 30:568, 1967
69. Corke BC: Neurobehavioural responses of the newborn—the effect of different forms of maternal analgesia. Anaesthesia 32:539, 1977
70. Brazelton TB: Effect of prenatal drugs on the behavior of the neonate. Am J Psychiat 126:1261, 1970
71. Kron RE, Stein M, Goddard KE: Newborn sucking behavior affected by obstetric sedation. Pediatrics 37:1012, 1966
72. Palahniuk RJ, Shnider SM, Eger EI II: Pregnancy decreases the requirement for inhaled anesthetic agents. Anesthesiology 41:82, 1974
73. Abboud TK, Shnider SM, Wright RG, et al: Enflurane analgesia in obstetrics. Anesth Analg 60:133–137, 1981
74. Stefani SJ, Hughes SC, Shnider SM, et al: Neonatal neurobehavioral effects of inhalation analgesia for vaginal delivery. Anesthesiology 56:351, 1982
75. Abboud TK, Gangolly J, Mosad P, et al: Isoflurane in obstetrics. Anesth Analg 68:388, 1989
76. Covino BG: Pharmacology of local anesthetic drugs. p. 99. In Ostheimer GW (ed): Manual of Obstetric Anesthesia. Churchill Livingstone, New York, 1984
77. Fink BR: History of neural blockade. p. 3. In Cousins MJ, Bridenbaugh PO (eds): Neural Blockade in Clinical Anesthesia and Management of Pain. 2nd Ed. JB Lippincott, Philadelphia, 1988
78. Shnider SM, Way EL: Plasma levels of lidocaine (Xylocaine) in mother and newborn following obstetrical conduction anesthesia: clinical applications. Anesthesiology 29:951, 1968
79. Morishima HO, Daniel SS, Finster M, et al: Transmission of mepivacaine hydrochloride (Carbocaine) across the human placenta. Anesthesiology 27:147, 1966
80. O'Brien JE, Abbey V, Hinsvark O, et al: Metabolism and measurement of chloroprocaine, an ester-type local anesthetic. J Pharmaceut Sci 68:75, 1979
81. Hyman MD, Shnider SM: Maternal and neonatal blood concentrations of bupivacaine associated with obstetrical conduction anesthesia. Anesthesiology 34:81, 1971
82. Steffenson JL, Shnider SM, DeLorimier AA: Transarterial diffusion of mepivacaine. Anesthesiology 32:459, 1970
83. Brown WU Jr, Bell GC, Lurie AO, et al: Newborn blood levels of lidocaine and mepivacaine in the first postnatal day following maternal epidural anesthesia. Anesthesiology 42:698, 1975
84. Poppers PJ, Finster M: The use of prilocaine hydrochloride (Citanest) for epidural analgesia in obstetrics. Anesthesiology 29:1134, 1968
85. Ralston DH, Shnider SM: The fetal and neonatal effects of regional anesthesia in obstetrics. Anesthesiology 48:34, 1978
86. Scanlon JW, Ostheimer GW, Lurie AO, et al: Neurobehavioral responses and drug concentrations in newborns after maternal epidural anesthesia with bupivacaine. Anesthesiology 45:400, 1976
87. Tucker GT, Boyes RN, Bridenbaugh PO, et al: Binding of anilide-type local anesthetics in human plasma: II. Implications in vivo, with special reference to transplacental distribution. Anesthesiology 33:304, 1970
88. Biehl D, Shnider SM, Levinson G, et al: Placental transfer of lidocaine: effects of fetal acidosis. Anesthesiology 48:409, 1978
89. Brown WU Jr, Bell GC, Alper MH: Acidosis, local anesthetics, and the newborn. Obstet Gynecol 48:27, 1976
90. Finster M: Toxicity of local anesthetics in the fetus and newborn. Bull NY Acad Med 52:222, 1976

91. Caldwell J, Moffatt JR, Smith RL, et al: Determination of bupivacaine in human fetal and neonatal blood samples by quantitative single ion monitoring. Biomed Mass Spectrom 4:322, 1977
92. Kuhnert B, Kuhnert PM, Philipson EH, et al: The half-life of 2-chloroprocaine. Anesth Analg 65:273, 1986
93. Scanlon JW, Brown WU Jr, Weiss JB, et al: Neurobehavioral responses of newborn infants after maternal epidural anesthesia. Anesthesiology 40:121, 1974
94. Nyirjesy I, Hawks BL, Hebert JE, et al: Hazards of the use of paracervical block anesthesia on obstetrics. Am J Obstet Gynecol 87:231, 1963
95. Rosefsky JB, Petersiel ME: Perinatal deaths associated with mepivacaine paracervical block anesthesia in labor. N Engl J Med 278:530, 1968
96. Shnider SM, Asling JH, Holl JW, et al: Paracervical block anesthesia in obstetrics. I. Fetal complications and neonatal morbidity. Am J Obstet Gynecol 107:619, 1970
97. Teramo K, Widholm O: Studies of the effect of anaesthetics on foetus. Par 1. The effect of paracervical block with mepivacaine upon fetal acid-base values. Acta Obstet Gynecol Scand (suppl) 46-2:3, 1967
98. Morishima HO, Covino BG, Yeh M-N, et al: Bradycardia in the fetal baboon following paracervical block anesthesia. Am J Obstet Gynecol 140:775, 1981
99. Cibils LA: Response of human uterine arteries to local anesthetics. Am J Obstet Gynecol 126:202, 1976
100. Fishburne JI Jr, Griess FC Jr, Hopkinson R, et al: Responses of the gravid uterine vasculature to arterial levels of local anesthetic agents. Am J Obstet Gynecol 133:753, 1979
101. Weiss RB, Halevy S, Almonte RO, et al: Comparison of lidocaine and 2-chloroprocaine in paracervical block: clinical effects and drug concentrations in mother and child. Anesth Analg 62:168, 1983
102. Freeman DW, Arnold NI: Paracervical block with low doses of chloroprocaine—fetal and maternal effects. JAMA 231:56, 1975
103. Philipson EH, Kuhnert BR, Syracuse CB, et al: Intrapartum paracervical block anesthesia with 2-chloroprocaine. Am J Obstet Gynecol 146:16, 1983
104. Kangas-Saarela T, Jouppila R, Puolakka J, et al: The effect of bupivacaine paracervical block on the neurobehavioural responses of newborn infants. Acta Anaesthesiol Scand 32:566, 1988
105. McGowan GW: A plea for low-dosage anesthesia with paracervical and pudendal block. Trans Pacific Coast Obstet Gynecol Soc 38:38, 1970
106. Philipson EH, Kuhnert BR, Syracuse CD: Maternal, fetal, and neonatal lidocaine levels following local perineal infiltration. Am J Obstet Gynecol 149:403, 1984
107. Philipson EH, Kuhnert BR, Syracuse CD: 2-Chloroprocaine for local perineal infiltration. Am J Obstet Gynecol 157:1275, 1987
108. Merkow AJ, McGuinness GA, Erenberg A, et al: The neonatal neurobehavioral effects of bupivacaine, mepivacaine, and 2-chloroprocaine used for pudendal block. Anesthesiology 52:309, 1980
109. Abboud TK, Khoo SS, Miller F, et al: Maternal, fetal, and neonatal responses after epidural anesthesia with bupivacaine, 2-chloroprocaine, or lidocaine. Anesth Analg 61:638, 1982
110. Tronick E, Wise S, Als H, et al: Regional anesthesia and newborn behavior: effect over the first ten days of life. Pediatrics 58:94, 1976
111. Rosenblatt DB, Belsey EM, Lieberman BA, et al: The influence of maternal analgesia on neonatal behaviour. II. Epidural bupivacaine. Br J Obstet Gynaecol 88:407, 1981
112. Abboud TK, Sarkis F, Blikian A, et al: Lack of adverse neonatal neurobehavioral effects of lidocaine. Anesth Analg 62:473, 1983.
113. Abboud TK, Afrasiabi A, Sarkis F, et al: Continuous infusion epidural analgesia in parturients receiving bupivacaine, chloroprocaine, or lidocaine—maternal, fetal, and neonatal effects. Anesth Analg 63:421, 1984
114. Abboud TK, Kern S, Jacobs J, et al: The neonatal neurobehavioral effects of mepivacaine for epidural anesthesia in labor. Reg Anesth 11:143, 1986
115. Wang JK, Nauss LA, Thomas JE: Pain relief by intrathecally applied morphine in man. Anesthesiology 149, 1979
116. Bromage PR: Epidural and spinal narcotics. Semin Anesth 2:75, 1983
117. Cousins MJ, Mather LE: Intrathecal and epidural administration of opioids. Anesthesiology 61:276, 1984
118. Nordberg G, Hedner T, Mellstrand T, et al: Pharmacokinetic aspects of epidural morphine analgesia. Anesthesiology 58:545, 1983
119. Nybell-Lindahl G, Carlsson C, Ingemarsson I, et al: Maternal and fetal concentrations of morphine after epidural administration during labor. Am J Obstet Gynecol 139:20, 1981
120. Hughes SC, Rosen MA, Shnider SM, et al: Maternal and neonatal effects of epidural morphine for labor and delivery. Anesth Analg 63:319, 1984
121. Wolfe MJ, Davies GK: Analgesic action of extradural fentanyl. Br J Anaesth 52:357, 1980
122. Carrie LES, O'Sullivan GM, Seegobin R: Epidural fentanyl in labour. Anaesthesia 36:965, 1981
123. Heytens L, Cammu H, Camu F: Extradural analgesia during labour using alfentanil. Br J Anaesth 59:331, 1987
124. Writer WDR, James FM III, Wheeler AS: Double-blind comparison of morphine and bupivacaine for continuous epidural analgesia in labor. Anesthesiology 54:215, 1981
125. Cohen SE, Tan S, Albright GA, et al: Epidural fentanyl/bupivacaine mixtures for obstetric analgesia. Anesthesiology 67:403, 1987
126. Phillips G: Continuous infusion epidural analgesia in labor: the effect of adding sufentanil to 0.125% bupivacaine. Anesth Analg 67:462, 1988
127. Abboud TK, Afrasiabi A, Zhu J, et al: Epidural morphine or butorphanol augments bupivacaine analgesia during labor. Reg Anesth 14:115, 1989
128. Hunt CO, Naulty S, Malinow AM, et al: Epidural butorphanol-bupivacaine for analgesia during labor and delivery. Anesth Analg 68:323, 1989

129. Bonnardot JP, Maillet M, Colau JC, et al: Maternal and fetal concentration of morphine after intrathecal administration during labor. Br J Anaesth 54:487, 1982
130. Nordberg G, Hedner T, Mellstrand T, et al: Pharmacokinetic aspects of intrathecal morphine analgesia. Anesthesiology 60:448, 1984
131. Srinivasan T: Intrathecal morphine for obstetric analgesia. Anesthesiology 55:A298, 1981
132. Baraka A, Noueihid R, Hajj S: Intrathecal injection of morphine for obstetric analgesia. Anesthesiology 54:136, 1981
133. Leighton BL, DeSimone CA, Norris MC, et al: Intrathecal narcotics for labor revisited: the combination of fentanyl and morphine intrathecally provides rapid onset of profound, prolonged analgesia. Anesth Analg 69:122, 1989
134. Crawford JS: Intrathecal morphine in obstetrics (Letter to the editor). Anesthesiology 55:487, 191.

PAIN RELIEF AND CESAREAN DELIVERY

Cesarean delivery has increased in frequency in the United States from 5.5 percent in 1970 to 20.3 percent in 1983.[1] For cesarean delivery, subarachnoid or epidural anesthesia or general anesthesia is utilized.[2] This section reviews the effects of each anesthetic technique on the fetus and neonate.

METHODS OF PAIN RELIEF FOR CESAREAN DELIVERY

Intraspinal (Subarachnoid and Epidural) Anesthesia

Subarachnoid anesthesia and epidural anesthesia are the two most commonly administered methods of regional anesthesia for cesarean delivery. Effects on the fetus can occur as a result of altered oxygen content of the blood, a decrease in uteroplacental blood flow (resulting from maternal hypotension or prolonged uterine manipulation by the obstetrician during delivery), the effects of sedative medications, and/or the effects of the local anesthetic drugs or anesthetic technique (subarachnoid or epidural) administered.

Oxygenation. In 1982, Ramanathan et al.[3] demonstrated higher PO_2 values in the umbilical cord and maternal blood with higher maternal FIO_2 values (Table 3-11). This was done in parturients undergoing epidural anesthesia with bupivacaine. Although Apgar scores were similar in their groups, supplemental oxygen administration is recommended for all parturients undergoing intraspinal anesthesia for cesarean delivery to improve oxygen stores.

Table 3-11. Mean PO_2 Values (in mmHg) of Maternal and Umbilical Cord Blood at Various Inspired Maternal Oxygen Concentrations (FIO_2)

FIO_2	0.21	0.47	0.74	1.0
Maternal PO_2	96	232	312	423
Umbilical vein PO_2	28	36	41	47
Umbilical artery PO_2	15	19	21	25

(From Ramanathan et al.,[3] with permission.)

Hypotension. Hypotension is defined as a maternal systolic blood pressure below 100 mmHg or a fall in maternal systolic blood pressure of 30 mmHg or more. Hypotension results from maternal sympathetic nervous system blockade with the vasodilation that develops, as well as from aortocaval compression if the mother lies in the supine position. Hypotension will occur in about 80 percent of parturients receiving subarachnoid anesthesia if measures are not taken to prevent it. Methods to prevent and to treat the hypotension include left uterine displacement, intravascular volume expansion, administration of vasopressors, and placing the parturient in the Trendelenburg position. Because the sympathetic block develops faster with subarachnoid anesthesia than with epidural anesthesia, the incidence of hypotension is higher with subarachnoid anesthesia.

In 1982, Corke et al.[4] looked at blood gas values and neurobehavioral scores (ENNS performed at 2 to 4 hours and at 24 hours after birth) in neonates whose mothers received subarachnoid anesthesia. In one group (18 neonates) the mothers had hypotension for less than 2 minutes; in the other group (13 neonates) the mothers remained normotensive. They noted that a short period of hypotension (less than 2 minutes) is associated with more maternal and neonatal acidosis; however, the neurobehavioral performance of the neonates appears unaffected.

In 1982, Datta et al.[5] looked at the blood gas values of neonates and their mothers who were given subarachnoid anesthesia after hydration with 1,500 ml of 5 percent dextrose in lactated Ringer's solution and placed at a 15 degree left uterine tilt. They evaluated three groups: group A (22 parturients) did not develop hypotension and received no vasopressors; group B (18 parturients) developed hypotension and were rapidly treated with ephedrine; and group C (20 parturients) had any decrease in systolic blood pressure as an indication for ephedrine (aggressive management). Although the parturients in group C had a fall in systolic blood pressure, they did not develop hypotension as defined above. The induction to delivery (I–D) and uterine incision to delivery (UI–D) intervals were similar among the three groups. Infants in group B had lower 1-minute Apgar scores and lower average pH values of the umbilical artery and vein when compared to groups A and C (no hypotension). Lower Apgar scores and poorer blood gas values developed when maternal hypotension occurred.

In 1988, Ramanathan et al.[6] compared three groups of patients given epidural anesthesia. Group 1 (53 parturients) did not develop hypotension; Groups 2 (37 parturients) and 3 (37 parturients) did develop hypotension. Hypotension was treated in group 2 with 5-mg boluses of ephedrine and in group 3 with 100-μg boluses of phenylephrine to maintain a systolic blood pressure above 100 mmHg. There was no difference in 1- and 5-minute Apgar scores or in blood gas values. In addition, no differences were noted in umbilical cord glucose, lactate, or pyruvate values among the three groups.

Because oxygen delivery to the fetus depends on adequate blood pressure, aggressive treatment of any fall in systolic blood pressure (i.e., more crystalloid, vasopressors, more left uterine displacement, and use of the Trendelenberg position) appears important if prophylactic methods fail. Most anesthesiologists would favor ephedrine over phenylephrine as a vasopressor since ephedrine is associated with a higher maternal cardiac output.

Uterine Manipulation. In 1981, Datta et al.[7] looked at parturients who underwent subarachnoid anesthesia with tetracaine for cesarean delivery. They noted that in the absence of hypotension, a prolonged UI–D interval of more than three minutes was associated with an increase in neonatal acidosis and depressed Apgar scores when compared to neonates whose maternal UI–D interval was less than 3 minutes.

Sedation. In 1977, Rolbin et al.[8] compared two groups of patients undergoing cesarean delivery under epidural anesthesia. One group was given up to 10 mg of diazepam prior to delivery; the other group received no diazepam. They found no differences in Apgar scores (7 to 10), although the 1-minute scores demonstrated a decrease in muscle tone in the diazepam group. No differences existed in umbilical cord blood gas values. The neurobehavioral scores (ENNS) showed a decrease in muscle tone at 4 hours of age in the diazepam-treated group, but by 24 hours of age no differences were seen.

Subarachnoid Anesthesia. Subarachnoid anesthesia can affect the fetus by a direct mechanism (local anesthetic blood concentration) or by an indirect mechanism (altered uteroplacental blood flow), as discussed above.

In 1984, Chantigian et al.[9] compared tetracaine with dextrose (group I, 10 patients) with tetracaine and procaine (group II, 11 patients) for elective cesarean delivery. All parturients received 1,500 to 2,000 ml of lactated Ringer's solution, had left uterine displacement, and received oxygen by face mask. Ephedrine was used (as suggested by Datta et al.[5]) in eight patients in each group, as their blood pressure fell 10 mmHg or more. Hypotension (systolic blood pressure less than 100 mmHg) occurred in two patients in group I and three patients in group II. The hypotension was rapidly treated with administration of more fluid and ephedrine. The I–D and UI–D intervals were similar. Apgar scores and umbilical blood gas values were similar between the groups.

In 1984, Santos et al.[10] looked at bupivacaine 7.5 to 10 mg in 22 patients undergoing elective cesarean delivery. Their patients received 1,500 ml of lactated Ringer's solution and ephedrine 50 mg intramuscularly 15 minutes before the anesthetic was injected, and were positioned with left uterine displacement and a 10 degree head-down tilt. Only 2 of the 22 patients (4.5 percent) developed hypotension, which was easily treated with more ephedrine. Apgar scores and umbilical blood gas values were normal.

In 1986, Kuhnert et al.[11] measured plasma lidocaine levels in maternal blood and neonatal umbilical cord blood in 10 elective cesarean deliveries. The mothers received subarachnoid anesthesia with lidocaine in doses of 60 to 100 mg. The mean plasma lidocaine level in the maternal vein was 0.65 μg/ml, in the umbilical vein was 0.20 μg/ml, and in the umbilical artery was 0.08 μg/ml. These plasma levels are much lower than the toxic level of lidocaine, which is thought to be 3 μg/ml. The only depressed neonates (one with a 1-minute Apgar score of <7, and two with cord pHs of less than 7.25) occurred in mothers who developed hypotension and were treated with ephedrine. They also detected lidocaine and its metabolites in the urine for more than 36 hours in some of the neonates.

In 1987, in a similar study, Kuhnert et al.[12] measured plasma bupivacaine levels in six elective cesarean deliveries. The mothers received subarachnoid anesthesia with bupivacaine in doses of 7.5 to 8.5 mg. The mean plasma bupivacaine level in the maternal vein was 59 ng/ml, in the umbilical vein was 20 ng/ml, and in the umbilical artery was 14 ng/ml. These plasma levels were also much lower than the toxic levels. None of the neonates was depressed as assessed by Apgar score or cord pHs. The neonates excreted bupivacaine and its metabolites in their urine for more than 36 hours.

In the last few years, a small amount of a narcotic has been added to the local anesthetic (bupivacaine) at the time of subarachnoid injection to increase intraoperative anesthesia and to provide postoperative analgesia. In two studies in which morphine (0.1 to 0.25 mg) was added[13,14] and in one study in which fentanyl (2.5 to 50 μg/ml), was added[15] Apgar scores, umbilical cord blood gas values, and neurobehavioral evaluations were normal in the neonates.

Thus, the direct effects of the subarachnoid administration of local anesthetics appear to be small. However, hypotension or a prolonged uterine manipulation may indirectly affect the fetus. Different anesthetic drugs may differ in the speed and frequency of hypotension produced. Few comparative studies exist. The common anesthetic drugs used are lidocaine with dextrose, tetracaine with dextrose or procaine, and bupivacaine with dextrose. Recently, small amounts of a narcotic, morphine or fentanyl, have been added to the local anesthetic with no significant effects on the neonate.

The maternal administration of oxygen to increase maternal and fetal PO_2, the prevention or rapid treatment of hypotension, and a UI–D interval of less than 3 minutes are recommended.

Epidural Anesthesia. Epidural anesthesia can also affect the fetus by either a direct mechanism (local anesthetic blood concentration) or an indirect mechanism (altered uteroplacental blood flow). Most studies evaluate parturients who are undergoing an elective cesarean delivery at term and, therefore, are not in labor. This eliminates the effects of labor on the fetus when evaluating epidural anesthesia.

A common belief is that the neurobehavioral examinations will reveal alterations attributable to drug effect more frequently in cesarean-delivered babies whose mothers received epidural anesthesia than in those born vaginally under epidural anesthesia because of the higher dose of local anesthetic used during a cesarean delivery. This may not be true because the time the local anesthetic has to pass the placenta may be shorter; elective cesarean-delivered babies are delivered within minutes after the local anesthetic is injected, whereas vaginally delivered babies may be exposed to the local anesthetic for several hours. Thus, the total amount of drug transferred may be less in neonates delivered by cesarean even though the peak maternal level may be greater. Further work is needed to clarify this possibility.

In 1977, Lund et al.[16] evaluated etidocaine for cesarean delivery. All 40 neonates assessed by the neurobehavioral scores (ENNS) at 2 to 4 hours of age were normal.

In 1980, Datta et al.[17] compared 3 percent chloroprocaine (16 + 1 ml) with 0.75 percent bupivacaine (17 + 1 ml) and 1 percent etidocaine (22 + 1 ml). The mean umbilical vein level of bupivacaine was 0.12 μg/ml and of etidocaine was 0.15 μg/ml. One- and 5-minute Apgar scores, blood gas values, and the neurobehavioral scores (ENNS) performed at 2 to 4 hours after birth demonstrated no significant differences.

In 1980, James et al.[18] compared 3 percent chloroprocaine (23 + 2 ml) with 0.5 percent bupivacaine (26 + 2 ml); they also demonstrated no significant differences in time to sustained respiration, 5-minute Apgar scores, and blood gas values.

In 1983, Abboud et al.[19] compared 3 percent chloroprocaine (21.5 ml), 2 percent lidocaine (21.5 ml), 2 percent lidocaine with epinephrine 1:200,000 (20 ml), and 0.75 percent bupivacaine (17 ml). Umbilical vein levels were 2.74 ng/ml for chloroprocaine, 1.43 μg/ml for lidocaine without epinephrine, 1.15 μg/ml for lidocaine with epinephrine, and 0.21 μg/ml for bupivacaine. One- and 5-minute Apgar scores, blood gas values, and neurobehavioral scores (ENNS) at 2 and 24 hours after birth demonstrated no significant differences.

In 1984, Kileff et al.[20] compared 2 percent lidocaine (29 + 5 ml) with 0.5 percent bupivacaine (29 + 6 ml). Mean umbilical vein levels were 1.82 μg/ml for lidocaine and 0.27 μg/ml for bupivacaine. No differences were found in Apgar scores, blood gas values, or neurobehavioral scores (ENNS) performed at 4 and 24 hours of age, except for a higher score for the sucking response in the lidocaine-treated group at 24 hours. It is interesting to note that several of the women in the lidocaine-treated group had some evidence of elevated levels of local anesthetic as suggested by central nervous system (CNS) symptoms of dizziness or diaphoresis. No women in the bupivacaine group had CNS symptoms suggestive of a high local anesthetic level.

In 1986, Gaffud et al.[21] compared 0.5 percent bupivacaine (10 parturients) to 0.5 percent bupivacaine with fentanyl 100 μg (10 parturients) for epidural anesthesia for elective cesarean delivery. They noted better analgesia in the fentanyl group and no difference in Apgar scores among the neonates. The average umbilical artery concentration of fentanyl was 0.8 ng/ml, a low level not associated with neonatal depression.

In 1988, Preston et al.[22] compared 2 percent lidocaine with epinephrine (15 parturients) to 2 percent lidocaine with epinephrine plus fentanyl 1 μg/kg (15 parturients) for epidural anesthesia for nonemergent cesarean delivery. They also noted better analgesia when fentanyl was added. Apgar scores, umbilical blood gas values, and neurobehavioral scores (NACS) were not different between the groups. Plasma umbilical artery fentanyl concentrations in their study were below 0.1 ng/ml in all samples.

Of the eight currently available local anesthetics for epidural use, three (chloroprocaine, lidocaine, and bupivacaine) are commonly used for epidural anesthesia for cesarean delivery. These three drugs appear to have minimal effects on neonatal behavior, provided adequate uteroplacental perfusion is maintained. The addition of a small amount of narcotic epidurally appears to increase analgesia with no significant neonatal effects. As with subarachnoid anesthesia, maternal administration of oxygen to increase maternal and fetal PO_2, the prevention or rapid treatment of hypotension, and a UI–D interval of less than 3 minutes is recommended.

If needed, administration of a small amount of diazepam intravenously can help alleviate some of the maternal anxiety while producing minimal effects on the neonate.

Etidocaine, although safe, is rarely used today because of its marked maternal motor block.

General Anesthesia

Many variables, including drugs, affect the fetus/and neonate during general anesthesia for cesarean delivery. This section reviews several of these variables.

Preoperative Considerations. The parturient should be placed on the operating table with the uterus displaced to the left to decrease the deleterious effects of aortocaval compression. In 1972, Crawford et al.[23] demonstrated better Apgar scores, less neonatal acidosis, and less hypercarbia in those whose mothers were operated upon in the right lateral position compared to parturients who were operated upon supine. This difference was more apparent when the UI–D interval was prolonged. In 1977, Buley et al.[24] further noted better neonatal results when the parturients were in the left lateral position compared to the right lateral position.

All parturients receive supplemental oxygen before induction. In 1974, Archer et al.[25] demonstrated that after preinduction oxygenation, 1 minute of apnea will decrease maternal PO_2 from 473 to 334 mmHg and will increase PCO_2 from 31 to 40 mmHg. This study confirmed the increase in oxygen consumption at term and emphasized the need for acute oxygenation before and prompt reoxygenation and ventilation after endotracheal intubation.

Although the importance of acute oxygenation is established, the traditional technique of giving 100 percent oxygen for 3 to 5 minutes has been questioned. In 1981, Gold et al.[26] compared a group of nonpregnant patients who had 5 minutes of acute oxygenation with a similar group who took four deep breaths of oxygen and found similar oxygen levels. In 1985, Norris et al.[27] found similar results in parturients undergoing elective cesarean delivery.

Induction of anesthesia is performed after the parturient's abdomen is prepared and draped. This decreases the I–D interval and may decrease the total amount of drugs that reach the fetus. It also allows for adequate acute oxygenation and denitrogenation of the parturient.

Induction Agents. Although many drugs have been used to induce general anesthesia for cesarean delivery, thiopental is today the most frequently used drug, with ketamine second. Because thiopental is the standard, many drugs are compared to it.

Thiobarbiturates. Clinical research on the effects of thiobarbiturates includes both thiopental (Pentothal), introduced in 1934, and thiamylal (Surital), introduced in 1952. They are commonly grouped together, as there are no significant clinical differences between these drugs.[28]

For the parturient, the mean dose and standard deviation of thiopental needed to induce sleep is 3.5 ± 0.5 mg/kg pregnant body weight (PBW).[29] For the nonpregnant young woman, the dose of thiopental is 5.4 ± 0.6 mg/kg.[30] The lower dose needed to induce sleep in the parturient may be related to the lower serum albumin levels in the parturient (75 percent of normal; thiobarbiturates are bound predominantly to albumin)[31] or to the lower concentration of the drug needed to anesthetize the parturient due to the hormonal effects of pregnancy.

Thiamylal and thiopental rapidly cross the placenta, with levels detected within 45 seconds of induction and peak fetal blood levels occurring 1.5 to 3 minutes after induction.[32,33] The concentration then rapidly decreases.[31,34] Although the thiobarbiturates cross the placenta rapidly, the neonate does not lose consciousness when the mother loses consciousness after the induction of anesthesia (with low doses of barbiturates). Several factors may explain why the fetal brain appears to be protected from the maternal dose. These factors include a rapid decline in maternal and fetal blood levels due to the rapid distribution of drug,[31,32] uptake of the drug by the fetal liver as the drug passes from the placenta into the fetal circulation[35] (although this has been challenged[36]), progressive dilution of the drug in the fetal circulation due to shunting, and the higher relative water content of the fetal brain.[37]

At an induction dose of 4 mg/kg PBW of thiobarbiturate followed by succinylcholine, endotracheal intubation, and 100 percent oxygen, 91 percent of neonates had a 1-minute Apgar score of 7 to 10, whereas at an 8-mg/kg dose only 57 percent have a score of 7 to 10.[32]

Thus, because the fetal outcome as measured by the Apgar score does not appear to be affected and anesthesia is reliably induced in the parturient at this dose, 4 mg/kg PBW is the most commonly used dose for induction today. In addition, delivery should not be delayed in an attempt to allow redistribution to occur, as the fetal brain appears to be exposed only to a small concentration of drug as compared with the exposure sustained by the maternal brain.

Oxybarbiturates. Methohexital (Brevital), introduced in 1954, is 2.5 times as potent as thiopental.[38] Because it has a shorter half-life as compared with thiopental, its use has been suggested for obstetrics. In 1962, Sliom et al.[39] compared methohexital 100 mg with thiopental 250 mg, followed by succinylcholine, endotracheal intubation, and maintenance with 70 percent nitrous oxide in oxygen. They found no significant difference in time to sustained respirations or 1-minute Apgar scores between the two groups. In 1974, Holdcroft et al.[40] compared two doses of methohexital (1.0 to 1.4 mg/kg). Although they found no significant difference in the umbilical cord pH, PO_2, or PCO_2, a marked difference in Apgar scores existed. Fifty percent of the neonates in the 1.4-mg/kg group had Apgar scores of ≤ 4, whereas only 7 percent of the neonates in the 1.0-mg/kg group scored ≤ 4. (*Note:* These studies were performed more than 15 years ago with the parturients in the supine position and utilizing 70 percent nitrous oxide in oxygen.)

Nonbarbiturates. Diazepam (Valium), introduced in 1961, has an adult half-life of 15 to 25 hours and a neonatal half-life of 25 to 100 hours.[41] Induction of anesthesia with diazepam is associated with a delay of about 1 minute until sleep is induced and may require a dose in excess of 0.8 mg/kg.[42] In 1974, Stovner et al.[43] compared diazepam 20 mg with thiopental 200 mg as induction agents followed by succinylcholine, endotracheal intubation, and 60 percent nitrous oxide with 40 percent oxygen. The recall and dream rate was 35 percent in the thiopental group and 12 percent in the diazepam group. There were no significant differences in the 1-minute Apgar score or clinical appearance of the neonates in the postnatal period between the two groups. Perhaps the short I–D interval (3 to 6 minutes) permitted only a small amount of the drug to cross the placenta.

Midazolam (Versed) is a fast-acting but short-duration benzodiazepine.

In 1987, Bland et al.[44] compared midazolam 0.2 mg/kg and thiopental 3.5 mg/kg as induction agents for elective cesarean delivery. After induction and endotracheal intubation, anesthesia was maintained with 50 percent nitrous oxide in oxygen and 0.5 percent halothane. Maternal and umbilical cord blood gas values were similar. Apgar minus color scores were low (below 5) in 5 of 26 neonates in the midazolam group and 1 of 26 neonates in the thiopental group. Neurobehavioral scores (ENNS) were similar between the groups. They believed midazolam was less suitable than thiopental for induction of general anesthesia for cesarean delivery.

In 1989, Ravlo et al.[45] compared midazolam 0.3 mg/kg to thiopental 4 mg/kg thiopental as induction agents for elective cesarean delivery. After induction and endotracheal intubation, anesthesia was maintained with 67 percent nitrous oxide in oxygen. Apgar scores were similar between the groups. Neurobehavioral scores (ENNS) were similar between the groups except for general body tone and arm recoil, which were inferior with midazolam in the first 2 hours after delivery. They believed midazolam to be as safe as thiopental for induction of general anesthesia for cesarean delivery.

Ketamine (Ketalar, Ketaject), introduced in 1965, is a parenteral anesthetic that produces intense analgesia and a dissociative state regarded as sleep. In 1977, Ellingson et al.[46] demonstrated rapid placental transfer of ketamine with peak levels found between 1 and 2 minutes.

When used alone for vaginal delivery in a dose of 2 mg/kg or more, ketamine produces unpleasant dreams in more than 50 percent of parturients[47] as well as neonatal depression.[48] When used at a lower dose of about 1 mg/kg, ketamine produces an incidence of unpleasant dreams similar to that seen with thiopental 3 to 4 mg/kg (when these induction agents were combined with succinycholine, endotracheal intubation, 60 percent nitrous oxide, 40 percent oxygen, fentanyl, and/or diazepam after delivery) (i.e., less than 16 percent).[49,50]

In 1973, Peltz et al.[50] compared ketamine 1 mg/kg to thiopental 3 mg/kg followed by succinylcholine, endotracheal intubation, and 60 percent nitrous oxide with 40 percent oxygen. Anesthesia was reliably induced with the 1-mg/kg dose. No difference in Apgar scores was seen.

In 1985, Berstein et al.[51] compared ketamine 1 mg/kg and thiopental 4 mg/kg as induction agents for elective cesarean delivery. Anesthesia was maintained after endotracheal intubation with 50 percent nitrous oxide and 50 percent oxygen. They found no difference in Apgar scores or blood gas values between the two groups of neonates.

Neurobehavioral studies comparing ketamine with thiopental are few. In one study that compared thiopental–nitrous oxide and oxygen with ketamine–nitrous oxide, and oxygen for vaginal delivery, infants whose mothers received ketamine scored better on the ENNS than infants whose mothers received thiopental.[52]

Etomidate (Amidate) is an imidazole compound that was introduced clinically in 1973. Induction of anesthesia is rapid (1 circulation time) and is associated with cardiovascular stability in healthy patients[53] and in patients with cardiac disease. A dose of etomidate 0.3 mg/kg is equivalent to thiopental 4 mg/kg. Two side effects, pain on injection and myoclonus, have been noted to occur.[54] In 1977, a new formulation was introduced that decreased the incidence of pain on injection from 30 percent to 4 percent. The incidence of myoclonus was unchanged at 18 percent.[55]

In 1979, Downing et al.[56] compared etomidate 0.3 mg/kg to thiopental 3.5 mg/kg as induction agents for elective cesarean delivery. After induction and endotracheal intubation, anesthesia was maintained with 50 percent nitrous oxide in oxygen and 0.5 to 0.8 percent enflurane. Umbilical vein and artery blood gas analyses showed similar PO_2, PCO_2, hydrogen ion content, and umbilical artery base deficits. Umbilical vein base deficits were -6.5 in the etomidate group and -4.7 in the thiopental group, a statistically significant difference. The 1-, 2-, and 5-minute Apgar scores were similar. These investigators believed the neonates in the etomidate groups were clinically superior to those in the thiopental group. This was reflected in the time to spontaneous respiration, which was 1.5 seconds in the etomidate group and 4.4 seconds in the thiopental group ($0.05 < P < 0.10$).

In 1980, Ionescu et al.[57] compared etomidate 0.2 mg/kg and thiopental 3 to 4 mg/kg. After induction and endotracheal intubation, anesthesia was maintained with nitrous oxide and oxygen. They found fewer hemodynamic changes in the etomidate group. Blood gas results were similar in the two groups.

In 1989, Dailland et al.[58] looked at propofol (Diprivan), introduced in 1983, as an induction agent for elective cesarean delivery. All patients were induced with 2.5 mg/kg. In phase 1 (10 patients), anesthesia was maintained with 0.25 to 0.5 percent halothane and 50 percent nitrous oxide in oxygen. In phase 2 (11 patients), anesthesia was maintained with a constant infusion of propofol (5 mg/kg h) and 50 percent nitrous oxide in oxygen. Propofol crossed the placenta and achieved UV/MV blood ratios of approximately 0.75. Apgar scores were > 7 in 18 neonates at 1 minute, in 20 neonates at 5 minutes, and in all 21 neonates at 10 minutes. Blood gas values and neurobehavioral scores (NACS) were comparable to neonates delivered under other established methods of anesthesia. They did note a 40 percent incidence of awareness in phase 1 parturients and a 9 percent incidence in phase 2 parturients. Thus, at these low doses, propofol seems acceptable from the standpoint of neonatal well-being.

Neuromuscular Relaxants. Neuromuscular relaxants are used to facilitate endotracheal intubation and to obtain abdominal relaxation for cesarean delivery. Initially placental transfer was thought to be absent because while the mothers were relaxed their neonates were not.[59–61] This was related to the low lipid solubility of the drugs and high degree of ionization. However, with improved assays, placental transfer has been demonstrated, but is usually clinically insignificant. Placental transfer has been noted for the short-acting agent, succinylcholine[62,63]; for the intermediate-acting agents, atracurium[64] and vecuronium[65,66]; and for the long-acting agents, d-tubocurarine,[34,67–69] metocurine,[70] gallamine[34] and pancuronium.[65,71–75]

The dose of neuromuscular drug needed to cause relaxation of the neonate is extremely high. Kvisselgaard et al.[63] used 200 to 500-mg doses of succinylcholine to determine placental transmission. They were unable to detect succinylcholine until a dose of 300 mg was administered. All neonates had normal Apgar scores and showed no signs of muscle weakness.

Under some abnormal conditions in which a large gradient between the mother and the fetus exists, the neonate can be clinically paralyzed.

Baraka et al.[62] reported the administration of succinylcholine to a mother with homozygote-atypical serum cholinesterase whose neonate was also homozygote-atypical for serum cholinesterase (dibucaine numbers were below 30 for each). Ventilatory support was needed for the mother for 2 ½ hours, and for 6 hours for the neonate.

Older et al.[69] reported a case of a woman in status epilepticus who received 245 mg of d-tubocurarine over 16 hours. Her 28-week neonate made no effort to breathe until edrophonium was given.

Inhalation Agents.

Oxygen. Maternal arterial oxygen tension during cesarean delivery is an important determinant of fetal oxygenation and the clinical condition of the neonate at birth.[76–78] In 1970, Baraka[76] varied the inspiratory oxygen concentrations and looked at both maternal and fetal (umbilical vein) PO_2. Anesthesia was induced with thiopental, followed by succinylcholine and endotracheal intubation. The maintenance anesthetic was different in each of four groups. Group 1 had 20 percent oxygen and 80 percent nitrous oxide, group 2 had 33.3 percent oxygen and 66.7 percent nitrous oxide, group 3 had 50 percent oxygen and 50 percent nitrous oxide, and group 4 had 0.5 percent halothane in 100 percent oxygen.

Table 3-12. Maternal and Fetal Oxygenation

Group	Oxygen Concentration (%)	Maternal PO_2 (mmHg)	Fetal Umbilical Vein PO_2 (mmHg)
1	20	78–100	20–26
2	33	115–157	28–35
3	50	200–300	38–65
4	100	440–500	43–65

(From Baraka,[76] with permission.)

Results are shown in Table 3-12. Thus, increasing the maternal inspired oxygen concentration from 20 to 50 percent increased maternal and fetal PO_2. Increasing the maternal oxygen concentration from 50 to 100 percent increased maternal but not fetal PO_2.

Nitrous Oxide. In 1970, Marx et al.[79] demonstrated rapid placental transfer of nitrous oxide during parturition. The maternal nitrous oxide level rose rapidly in the first 4 minutes of anesthesia. After 4 minutes, the increase in maternal nitrous oxide was small. The UV/MA ratio was 0.8 after 2 minutes of anesthesia. The UA/UV ratio rose progressively with increased duration of anesthesia from 0.6 at 2 to 4 minutes to 0.9 after 15 to 19 minutes of anesthesia. After an induction to delivery interval of 15 to 19 minutes, further increase in the nitrous oxide level is small. Thus, nitrous oxide is rapidly taken up by the mother, rapidly crosses the placenta, and is rapidly taken up by the fetus.

In 1977, Palahniuk et al.,[80] and in 1978, Shnider et al.,[81] looked at uterine blood flow in pregnant ewes with the administration of nitrous oxide and oxygen. They noted a drop in uterine blood flow of 10 to 20 percent from control values. This may be related to an elevation of plasma catecholamines that may occur with light levels of anesthesia and the uterine artery vasoconstriction that may result.

Neonatal depression at birth may result from the anesthetic effect of nitrous oxide, diffusion hypoxia as the nitrous oxide is excreted by the neonate, and/or a decrease in oxygen delivery to the fetus in utero as a result of elevated catecholamines. Thus, oxygen should be available for the neonate and used especially when administration of nitrous oxide has been prolonged.[82]

Because of its narcotic-like effects, some anesthesiologists decreased the level of nitrous oxide from 70 to 50 percent and found less narcosis of the neonate. Maternal awareness rose from about 5 to 20 percent. With the addition of a small amount of a volatile agent, maternal awareness approaches zero when the nitrous oxide concentration is reduced to 50 percent.

Volatile Agents. After induction of anesthesia, maintenance of the anesthetic state is required. Oxygen with the addition of nitrous oxide does not always provide adequate anesthesia. The addition of a small amount of volatile agents (halothane, enflurane, or isoflurane) permits the use of a higher oxygen concentration (i.e., 50 percent oxygen with 50 percent nitrous oxide) and, at the same time, decreases the incidence of maternal intraoperative recall toward zero.[83–86] Because volatile agents cause a dose-related decrease in uterine contactility, it has been claimed that they might also cause an increase in postpartum hemorrhage. However, no increased blood loss has been demonstrated with a low dose [½ to ⅔ minimal alveolar concentrations (MAC)] of halothane,[84–86] enflurane[83,86] or isoflurane[86] when used during cesarean delivery.

In 1978, Shnider et al.[81] looked at uterine blood flow in pregnant ewes with the administration of 50 percent nitrous oxide, and oxygen, as noted above, and also with the addition of 0.5 percent halothane or 1 percent enflurane. With nitrous oxide alone, uterine blood flow fell 10 to 15 percent from control values. However, with the addition of halothane, uterine blood flow was increased about 20 percent over control, and with enflurane, increased about 5 percent over control. The addition of the volatile agent may have decreased the level of plasma catecholamines and decreased the uterine artery vasoconstriction that may result from nitrous oxide alone.

In 1983, Warren et al.,[86] using the standard anesthetic induction consisting of preinduction oxygenation for 3 minutes followed by thiopental and succinylcholine, endotracheal intubation, and ventilation with a tidal volume of 10 ml/kg PBW at a rate of 10 breaths/min, compared four maintenance groups: 50 percent oxygen–50 percent nitrous oxide alone, and 50 percent oxygen–50 percent nitrous oxide combined with 0.5 percent halothane, with 0.75 percent isoflurane and with 1.0 percent enflurane. The recall rate was 17 percent in the 50 percent oxygen–50 percent nitrous oxide group. None of the patients with the added volatile agent had recall. Blood loss was similar in all groups. No differences were noted in I–D and UI–D intervals, 1- and 5-minute Apgar scores, maternal and fetal blood gas values, lactate values, or the neurobehavioral scores (ENNS) at 2 to 4 hours.

Ventilation. In 1983, Burger et al.[87] compared controlled maternal ventilation under general anesthesia at tidal volumes of 8 ml/kg, 9 ml/kg, and 10 ml/kg PBW and at a respiratory rate of 10 breaths/min. They found no differences in Apgar scores or fetal oxygenation but did find less fetal acidosis in the 10-ml/kg group. This group also showed more normal maternal PCO_2 values. Thus, 10 ml/kg PBW at 10 breaths/min is the suggested maternal minute ventilation.

Timing of Delivery. In evaluating the effect of anesthesia on neonatal outcome, two time intervals are commonly evaluated: the I–D interval and the UI–D interval.[2] Recent investigations have demonstrated that the UI–D interval is equally as important as the I–D interval. When the UI–D interval is greater than 3 minutes, a greater proportion of neonates will demonstrate depressed Apgar scores and will have more acidosis than those delivered with UI–D intervals of less than 3 minutes.[7]

Comparison of Anesthetic Techniques

In 1982, Zagorzycki et al.[88] compared general anesthesia with epidural anesthesia for repeat cesarean delivery (195 patients). They found no difference in 1- and 5-minute Apgar scores between the groups. In addition, they did not see any significant differences in Apgar scores when the I–D interval was prolonged (at least 15 minutes).

In 1983, Fisher et al.[89] compared epidural anesthesia with general anesthesia for elective cesarean delivery. They compared Apgar scores, acid-base values, and respiratory function (tidal volume, respiratory rate, minute ventilation, and inspiratory and expiratory times) and found no significant differences except for slightly better umbilical artery blood gas values (PO_2, pH, and PCO_2) in the general anesthesia group.

In a retrospective study, Ong et al.[90] in 1989 looked at 3,940 cesarean deliveries performed between 1975 and 1983 to determine the effect of anesthetic technique on neonatal outcome. They found several factors related to a low 1-minute Apgar score ($\leq$ 4). These factors included primiparity, grand multiparity, antepartum disease, complicated labor, fetal distress, low birthweight, low gestational age, use of narcotics in labor, breech presentation, nonelective cesarean delivery, and general anesthesia. They further subdivided the cesarean deliveries into three groups: elective, urgent, and emergent. For elective cesarean deliveries the choice of anesthesia was made by the patient and anesthesiologist. For urgent cesarean deliveries a slight delay for regional anesthesia was acceptable. For emergent cesarean deliveries regional anesthesia was used only when it was already established. In each group, they noted lower 1-minute Apgar scores in the general anesthesia group. At 5 minutes, a marked improvement occurred in the Apgar scores, suggesting transient neonatal depression. At 5 minutes, there was no significant difference in the Apgar scores between neonates delivered using general anesthesia and regional anesthesia for the elective cesarean deliveries. However, in the urgent and emergent cesarean deliveries, the neonates were better after regional anesthesia. There was no difference in neonatal mortality in the three groups.

If neonates are depressed at delivery, attention should be directed to each of three areas: anesthesia, surgery, and the fetal condition prior to delivery. For intraspinal anesthesia, one needs to consider the use of sedative drugs before delivery, and a decrease in uterine blood flow as a consequence of maternal hypotension or of poor patient positioning (supine position).[91] With general anesthesia, too light an anesthetic may decrease uterine blood flow because of elevated plasma catecholamines, and too deep an anesthetic may depress the fetus directly. Surgical considerations include the potential for a difficult delivery with prolonged uterine manipulation to cause a decrease in uteroplacental perfusion or for an anterior placenta to result in neonatal blood loss. With regard to the fetus, intrauterine distress before delivery or congenital abnormalities may be underlying factors causing neonatal depression.

SPECIAL SITUATIONS

The above discussion relates primarily to elective cesarean deliveries. Individualization, especially with maternal, obstetric, or medical conditions, may require a change in technique. A few brief comments are listed below.

Fetal Distress

Whenever fetal distress develops, steps should be taken immediately to increase oxygen delivery to the fetus while preparations are made for rapid delivery. These steps include oxygen administration, more left uterine displacement, use of ephedrine to raise maternal blood pressure (if hypotension exists), more intravenous fluid (if indicated), and the discontinuation of an oxytocin infusion (if one is administered). Recently, the administration of intravenous or subcutaneous terbutaline has been suggested to help decrease uterine tone and increase uterine blood flow.[92–94]

In 1984, Marx et al.[95] compared general anesthesia (71 anesthetics) with regional anesthesia (33 spinal anesthetics, 22 extension of established labor epidural anesthetics). The choice of anesthetic was made by the mother unless medical or obstetric abnormalities (such as coagulopathy or prolapsed cord) dictated otherwise. They noted similar umbilical vein and artery blood gas and pH values between the general and regional anesthetic groups. In addition, the 1-minute Apgar scores were better following regional anesthesia. (*Editor's note:* I will use subarachnoid anesthesia after consultation with the obstetrician in selected circumstances when an emergent delivery is required.)

For general anesthesia in the presence of fetal distress, ketamine may be a better choice for induction over thiopental. With fetal distress (i.e., in the acidotic fetal sheep model), a low dose of ketamine (2 mg/kg) preserves fetal blood pressure and cerebral blood flow better than thiopental (6 mg/kg). Higher doses of ketamine (4 mg/kg) or thiopental (10 mg/kg) were associated with a marked reduction in fetal blood pressure and fetal cerebral blood flow.[96] The clinical significance of this requires further study.

The choice of volatile agent may be important in the asphyxiated fetus. In the pregnant ewe model, Palahniuk et al., in 1980,[97] demonstrated a marked decrease in fetal cerebral blood flow when halothane-oxygen anesthesia was administered to asphyxiated ewes, whereas Baker et al.,[98] in 1990, demonstrated a maintenance of cerebral oxygen delivery when isoflurane-oxygen was administered to asphyxiated ewes. A comparison study of anesthetic agents may prove to be of clinical significance.

If an epidural anesthetic has been established for labor and fetal distress develops, chloroprocaine may be the drug of choice to make the block higher and more dense. Chloroprocaine has a faster onset than lidocaine or bupivacaine. In addition, with fetal distress and the associated fetal acidosis that develops, amide local anesthetics may become trapped on the fetal side of the placenta and may lead to excessively high blood levels. With chloroprocaine, fetal blood levels remain clinically insignificant; this may be related to the rapid maternal and fetal metabolism of chloroprocaine.[99] (*Editor's note:* With the reported higher incidence of back pain when large volumes of chloroprocaine are required, I have found alkalinized lidocaine provides a similar onset of surgical anesthesia. Since delivery is rapid, I have not observed any untoward neonatal effects.)

Hypovolemia

In a parturient whose intravascular volume is reduced (e.g., with bleeding as seen in placenta previa, placenta abruption, and uterine rupture), general anesthesia may prove safer for the neonate because placental perfusion is better preserved. Because of the better cardiovascular stability that ketamine gives in the hypovolemic patient, ketamine is preferred to thiopental.[51]

Pregnancy-Induced Hypertension

The choice of anesthetic technique in patients with pregnancy-induced hypertension must be carefully considered, as hypovolemia, coagulopathies, and decreased renal function may be present.

If coagulation studies are relatively normal, regional anesthesia may be performed. Epidural anesthesia may be safer than subarachnoid anesthesia, as the level of anesthesia can be more gradually established as the intravascular volume is expanded. This may give better control of blood pressure, allowing placental perfusion to be better maintained.

If general anesthesia is chosen, precautions should be made to blunt the hypertensive response to intubation. Because of the cardiovascular stimulation that occurs with ketamine, it is not recommended as an induction agent for general anesthesia in these parturients.[46] Thiopental is more commonly used.

REFERENCES

1. Notzon FC, Placek PJ, Taffel SM: Comparisons of national cesarean-section rates. New Engl J Med 316:386, 1987
2. Datta S, Alper MH: Anesthesia for cesarean section. Anesthesiology 53:142, 1980
3. Ramanathan S, Gandhi S, Arismendy J, et al: Oxygen transfer from mother to fetus during cesarean section under epidural anesthesia. Anesth Analg 61:576, 1982
4. Corke BC, Datta S, Ostheimer GW, et al: Spinal anesthesia for caesarean section—the influence of hypotension on neonatal outcome. Anaesth 37:658, 1982
5. Datta S, Alper MH, Ostheimer GW, et al: Method of ephedrine administration and nausea and hypotension during spinal anesthesia for cesarean section. Anesthesiology 56:68, 1982
6. Ramanathan S, Grant GJ: Vasopressor therapy for hypotension due to epidural anesthesia for cesarean section. Acta Anaesthesiol Scand 32:559, 1988
7. Datta S, Ostheimer GW, Weiss JB, et al: Neonatal effect of prolonged anesthetic induction for cesarean section. Obstet Gynecol 58:331, 1981
8. Rolbin SH, Wright RG, Shnider SM, et al: Diazepam during cesarean section—effects on neonatal Apgar scores, acid-base status, neurobehavioral assessment and maternal and fetal plasma norepinephrine levels. Abstracts of Scientific Papers, No. 449. Annual Meeting, American Society of Anesthesiologists, Chicago, 1977
9. Chantigian RC, Datta S, Burger GA, et al: Anesthesia for cesarean delivery utilizing spinal anesthesia—tetracaine versus tetracaine and procaine. Reg Anesth 9:195, 1984
10. Santos A, Pedersen H, Finster M, et al: Hyperbaric bupivacaine for spinal anesthesia in cesarean section. Anesth Analg 63:1009, 1984
11. Kuhnert BR, Philipson EH, Pimental R, et al: Lidocaine disposition in mother, fetus, and neonate after spinal anesthesia. Anesth Analg 65:139, 1986
12. Kuhnert BR, Zuspan KJ, Kuhnert PM, et al: Bupivacaine disposition in mother, fetus, and neonate after spinal anesthesia. Anesth Analg 66:407, 1987
13. Abboud TK, Dror A, Mosaad P, et al: Mini-dose intrathecal morphine for the relief of post-cesarean section pain: safety, efficacy, and ventilatory responses to carbon dioxide. Anesth Analg 67:137, 1988
14. Abouleish E, Rawal N, Fallon K, et al: Combined intrathecal morphine and bupivacaine for cesarean section. Anesth Analg 67:370, 1988

15. Hunt CO, Naulty JS, Bader AM, et al: Perioperative analgesia with subarachnoid fentanyl-bupivacaine for cesarean delivery. Anesthesiology 71:535, 1989
16. Lund PC, Cwik JC, Gannon RT, et al: Etidocaine for caesarean section—effects on mother and baby. Br J Anaesth 49:457, 1977
17. Datta S, Corke BC, Alper MH, et al: Epidural anesthesia for cesarean section: a comparison of bupivacaine, chloroprocaine, and etidocaine. Anesthesiology 52:48, 1980
18. James FM III, Dewan DM, Floyd HM, et al: Chloroprocaine vs. bupivacaine for lumbar epidural analgesia for elective cesarean section. Anesthesiology 52:488, 1980
19. Abboud TK, Kim KC, Noueihed R, et al: Epidural bupivacaine, chloroprocaine, or lidocaine for cesarean section—maternal and neonatal effects. Anesth Analg 62:914, 1983
20. Kileff ME, James FM III, Dewan DM, et al: Neonatal neurobehavioral responses after epidural anesthesia for cesarean section using lidocaine and bupivacaine. Anesth Analg 63:413, 1984
21. Gaffud MP, Bansal P, Lawton C, et al: Surgical analgesia for cesarean delivery with epidural bupivacaine and fentanyl. Anesthesiology 65:331, 1986
22. Preston PG, Rosen MA, Hughes SC, et al: Epidural anesthesia with fentanyl and lidocaine for cesarean section: maternal effects and neonatal outcome. Anesthesiology 68:938, 1988
23. Crawford JS, Burton M, Davies P: Time and lateral tilt at cesarean section. Br J Anaesth 44:477, 1972
24. Buley RJR, Downing JW, Brock-Utne JG, et al: Right versus left lateral tilt for cesarean section. Br J Anaesth 49:1009, 1977
25. Archer GW Jr, Marx GF: Arterial oxygen tension during apnoea in parturient women. Br J Anaesth 46:358, 1974
26. Gold MI, Duarte I, Muravchick S: Arterial oxygenation in conscious patients after 5 minutes and after 30 seconds of oxygen breathing. Anesth Analg 60:313, 1981
27. Norris MC, Dewan DM: Preoxygenation for cesarean section—a comparison of two techniques. Anesthesiology 62:827, 1985
28. Tovell RM, Anderson CC, Sadove MS, et al: A comparative clinical and statistical study of thiopental and thiamylal in human anesthesia. Anesthesiology 16:910, 1955
29. Christensen JH, Andreasen F, Jansen JA: Pharmacokinetics of thiopental in caesarean section. Acta Anaesth Scand 25:174, 1981
30. Christensen JH, Andreasen F, Jansen JA: Pharmacokinetics of thiopentone in a group of young women and a group of young men. Br J Anaesth 52:913, 1980
31. Morgan DJ, Blackman GL, Paull JD, et al: Pharmacokinetics and plasma binding of thiopental. II. Studies at cesarean section. Anesthesiology 54:474, 1981
32. Kosaka Y, Takahashi T, Mark LC: Intravenous thiobarbiturate anesthesia for cesarean section. Anesthesiology 31:489, 1969
33. McKechnie FB, Converse JG: Placental transmission of thiopental. Am J Obstet Gynecol 70:639, 1955
34. Crawford JS, Kane PO, Gardiner JE: Some aspects of obstetric anesthesia. Br J Anaesth 28:146, 1956
35. Finster M, Morishima HO, Mark LC, et al: Tissue thiopental concentrations in the fetus and newborn. Anesthesiology 36:155, 1972
36. Woods WA, Stanski DR, Curtis J, et al: The role of the fetal liver in the distribution of thiopental from mother to fetus. Anesthesiology 57:A390, 1982
37. Flowers CE Jr: The placental transmission of barbiturates and thiobarbiturates and their pharmacological action on the mother and the infant. Am J Obstet Gynecol 78:730, 1959
38. Egbert LD, Oech SR, Eckenhoff JE: Comparison of the recovery from methohexital and thiopental anesthesia in man. Surg Gynecol Obstet 109:427, 1959
39. Sliom CM, Frankel L, Holbrook RA: A comparison between methohexitone and thiopentone as induction agents for caesarean section anesthesia. Br J Anaesth 34:316, 1962
40. Holdcroft A, Robinson MJ, Gordon H, et al: Comparison of effect of two induction doses of methohexitone on infants delivered by elective caesarean section. Br Med J 2:472, 1974
41. Wood M, Wood AJJ: Drugs and Anesthesia—Pharmacology for Anesthesiologists. Williams & Wilkins, Baltimore, 1982
42. Brown SS, Dundee JW: Clinical studies of induction agents. XXV. diazepam. Br J Anaesth 40:108, 1968
43. Stovner J, Vangen O: Diazepam compared to thiopentone as induction agent for caesarean sections. Acta Anaesth Scand 18:264, 1974
44. Bland BAR, Lawes EG, Duncan PW, et al: Comparison of midazolam and thiopental for rapid sequence anesthetic induction for elective cesarean section. Anesth Analg 66:1165, 1987
45. Ravlo O, Carl P, Crawford ME, et al: A randomized comparison between midazolam and thiopental for elective cesarean section anesthesia. II. Neonates. Anesth Analg 68:234, 1989
46. Ellingson A, Haram K, Sagen N, et al: Transplacental passage of ketamine after intravenous administration. Acta Anaesth Scand 21:41, 1977
47. Ellingson A, Haram K, Sagen N: Ketamine and diazepam as anesthesia for forceps delivery. A comparative study. Acta Anaesth Scand 21:37, 1977
48. Janeczko GF, El-Etr AA, Younes S: Low-dose ketamine anesthesia for obstetrical delivery. Anesth Analg 53:828, 1974
49. Dich-Nielsen J, Holasek J: Ketamine as induction agent for caesarean section. Acta Anaesthesiol Scand 26:139, 1982
50. Peltz B, Sinclair DM: Induction agents for caesarean section—a comparison of thiopentone and ketamine. Anaesthesia 28:37, 1973
51. Bernstein K, Gisselsson L, Jacobsson L, et al: Influence of two different anaesthetic agents on the newborn and the correlation between foetal oxygenation and induction-delivery time in elective caesarean section. Acta Anesthesiol Scand 29:157, 1985
52. Hodgkinson R, Marx GF, Kim SS, et al: Neonatal neurobehavioral tests following vaginal delivery under ketamine,

thiopental, and extradural anesthesia. Anesth Analg 56:548, 1977
53. Gooding JM, Corssen G: Etomidate: an ultrashort-acting nonbarbiturate agent for anesthesia induction. Anesth Analg 55:286, 1976
54. Fragen RJ, Caldwell N, Brunner EA: Clinical use of etomidate for anesthesia induction: a preliminary report. Anesth Analg 55:730, 1976
55. Hendry JGB, Miller BM, Lees NW: Etomidate in a new solvent. A clinical evaluation. Anaesthesia 32:996, 1977
56. Downing JW, Buley RJF, Brock-Utne JG, et al: Etomidate for induction of anaesthesia at caesarean section: comparison with thiopentone. Br J Anaesth 51:135, 1979
57. Ionescu T, Besse TC, Smalhout B: Etomidate during caesarean section, general anaesthesia in obstetrics. Seventh World Congress of Anaesthesiologists, Hamburg, West Germany. International Congress Series, No. 533, 17:318, Excerpta Medica Amsterdam, 1980
58. Dailland P, Cockshott ID, Lirzin JD, et al: Intravenous propofol during cesarean section: placental transfer, concentrations in breast milk, and neonatal effects. A preliminary study. Anesthesiology 71:827, 1989
59. Cohen EN, Paulson WJ, Wall J, et al: Thiopental, curare, and nitrous oxide anesthesia for cesarean section with studies on placental transmission. Surg Gynecol Obstet 97:456, 1953
60. Gray TC: d-Tubocurarine in caesarean section. Br Med J 1:444, 1947
61. Whitacre RJ, Fisher AJ: Curare in cesarean section. Anesth Analg 27:164, 1948
62. Baraka A, Haroun S, Bassili M, et al: Response of the newborn to succinylcholine injection in homozygotic atypical mothers. Anesthesiology 43:115, 1975
63. Kvisselgaard N, Moya F: Investigation of placental thresholds to succinylcholine. Anesthesiology 22:7, 1961
64. Flynn PJ, Frank M, Hughes R: Use of atracurium in caesarean section. Br J Anaesth 56:599, 1984
65. Dailey PA, Fisher DM, Shnider SM, et al: Pharmacokinetics, placental transfer, and neonatal effects of vecuronium and pancuronium administered during cesarean section. Anesthesiology 60:569, 1984
66. Demetriou M, Depoix JP, Diakite B, et al: Placental transfer of ORG NC 45 in women undergoing caesarean section. Br J Anaesth 54:643, 1982
67. Cohen EN: Thiopental-curare-nitrous oxide anesthesia for cesarean section 1950–1960. Anesth Analg 41:122, 1962
68. Finster M, Poppers PJ, Horowitz PE, et al: Placental transer of d-tubocurarine. Abstracts of Scientific Papers, Annual Meeting, American Society of Anesthesiologists, Chicago, 1973, p. 43
69. Older PO, Harris JM: Placental transfer of tubocurarine. Case report. Br J Anaesth 40:459, 1968
70. Kivalo I, Saarikoski S: Placental transfer of 14C-dimethylcurarine during caesarean section. Br J Anaesth 48:239, 1976
71. Abouleish E, Wingard LB Jr, De La Vega S, et al: Pancuronium in caesarean section and its placental transfer. Br J Anaesth 52:531, 1980
72. Booth PN, Watson MJ, McLeod K: Pancuronium and the placental barrier. Anaesthesia 32:320, 1977
73. Duvaldestin P, Demetriou M, Henzel D, et al: The placental transfer of pancuronium and its pharmacokinetics during caesarean section. Acta Anaesthesiol Scand 22:327, 1978
74. Heaney GAH: Pancuronium in maternal and fetal serum. Br J Anaesth 46:282, 1974
75. Speirs I, Sim AW: The placental transfer of pancuronium bromide. Br J Anaesth 44:370, 1972
76. Baraka A: Correlation between maternal and foetal pO_2 and pCO_2 during caesarean section. Br J Anaesth 42:434, 1970
77. Marx GF, Mateo CV: Effects of different oxygen concentrations during general anaesthesia for elective caesarean section. Can Anaesth Soc J 18:587, 1971
78. Rorke MJ, Davey DA, Du Toit HJ: Foetal oxygenation during caesarean section. Anaesthesia 23:585, 1968
79. Marx GF, Joshi CW, Orkin LR: Placental transmission of nitrous oxide. Anesthesiology 32:429, 1970
80. Palahniuk RJ, Cumming M: Foetal deterioration following thiopentone—nitrous oxide anaesthesia in the pregnant ewe. Can Anaesth Soc J 24:361, 1977
81. Shnider SM, Wright RG, Levinson G, et al: Plasma norepinephrine and uterine blood flow changes during endotracheal intubation and general anesthesia in the pregnant ewe. Abstracts of Scientific Papers, Annual Meeting, American Society of Anesthesiologists, Chicago, 1978, p.115
82. Mankowitz E, Brock-Utne JG, Downing JW: Nitrous oxide elimination by the newborn. Anaesthesia 36:1014, 1981
83. Coleman AJ, Downing JW: Enflurane anesthesia for cesarean section. Anesthesiology 43:354, 1975
84. Galbert MW, Gardner AE: Use of halothane in a balanced technic for cesarean section. Anesth Analg 51:701, 1972
85. Moir DD: Anaesthesia for caesarean section—an evaluation of a method using low concentrations of halothane and 50 per cent oxygen. Br J Anaesth 42:136, 1970
86. Warren TM, Datta S, Ostheimer GW, et al: Comparison of the maternal and neonatal effects of halothane, enflurane, and isoflurane for cesarean delivery. Anesth Analg 62:516, 1983
87. Burger GA, Datta S, Chantigian RC, et al: Optimal ventilation in general anesthesia for cesarean delivery. Anesthesiology 59:A420, 1983
88. Zagorzycki MT, Brinkman III CR: The effect of general and epidural anesthesia upon neonatal Apgar scores in repeat cesarean section. Surg Gynecol Obstet 155:641, 1982
89. Fisher JT, Mortola JP, Smith B, et al: Neonatal pattern of breathing following cesarean section. Epidural versus general anesthesia. Anesthesiology 59:385, 1983
90. Ong BY, Cohen MM, Palahniuk RJ: Anesthesia for cesarean section—effects on neonates. Anesth Analg 68:270, 1989
91. Goodlin RC: Aortocaval compression during cesarean section. A cause of newborn depression. Obstet Gynecol 37:702, 1971
92. Burke MS, Porreco RP, Day D, et al: Intrauterine resuscitation with tocolysis an alternate month clinical trial. J Perinatal 9:296, 1989

93. Mendez-Bauer C, Shekarloo A, Cook V et al: Treatment of acute intrapartum fetal distress by β_2-sympathomimetics. Am J Obstet Gynecol 156:638, 1987
94. Shekarloo A, Mendez-Bauer C, Cook V, et al: Terbutaline (intravenous bolus) for the treatment of acute intrapartum fetal distress. Am J Obstet Gynecol 160:615, 1989
95. Marx GF, Luykx WM, Cohen S: Fetal-neonatal status following caesarean section for fetal distress. Br J Anaesth 56:1009, 1984
96. Pickering BG, Palahniuk RJ, Cote J, et al: Cerebral vascular responses to ketamine and thiopentone during foetal acidosis. Can Anaesth Soc J 29:463, 1982
97. Palahniuk RJ, Doig GA, Johnson GN, et al: Maternal halothane anesthesia reduces cerebral blood flow in the acidotic sheep fetus. Anesth Analg 59:35, 1980
98. Baker BW, Hughes SC, Shnider SM, et al: Maternal anesthesia and the stressed fetus: effects of isoflurane on the asphyxiated fetal lamb. Anesthesiology 72:65, 1990
99. Philipson EH, Kuhnert BR, Syracuse CD: Fetal acidosis, 2-chloroprocaine, and epidural anesthesia for cesarean section. Am J Obstet Gynecol 151:322, 1985

PATIENT-CONTROLLED ANALGESIA FOR LABOR PAIN

Patient-controlled analgesia (PCA) is a modality that may have some useful applications during labor. Various techniques (inhalational, intravenous, and epidural) have been used, and the concept of PCA during labor is still evolving.

The technique of inhalational analgesia for labor bears some special consideration.[1] Although now largely of historical interest, inhalational analgesia was actually the first example of a self-administered (i.e., patient-controlled) modality. Virtually all inhaled agents (ether, trichloroethylene, cyclopropane, chloroform, nitrous oxide, halothane, enflurane, isoflurane, and methoxyflurane), have been advocated although only nitrous oxide is used with any regularity today. A predetermined mixture of nitrous oxide and oxygen (Entonox) is rarely used in this country but enjoys greater popularity in Great Britain. The concept underlying the inhalational technique is similar regardless of which agent is used. Some sort of device (mouthpiece, inhaler, face mask, or demand valve) is given to the patient, who is instructed to take several rapid breaths at the onset of a contraction. Self-administration of the agent ends when analgesia is obtained (which is often simply because the contraction has ended) or when maternal drowsiness causes inability to use the device. Inhalational analgesia is not a panacea. Excessive maternal drowsiness is clearly a problem. Some mothers are amnestic for the birth of the baby. In addition, the propensity of parturients toward regurgitation and aspiration of gastric contents if general anesthesia ensues without a secured airway has largely contributed to the decline in popularity of this modality. At the Brigham and Women's Hospital, inhalational analgesia during labor has not been used in over two decades.

Patient-controlled analgesia (PCA) with intravenous opioids during labor is a new and exciting development. Although first described for labor pain by Scott in 1964,[2] the technique has not gained widespread acceptance in labor units despite the fact that opioid analgesia is by far the most common type of pain relief offered to laboring women. However, the recent blossoming of PCA as a postsurgical analgesic modality has resurrected the interest in PCA for labor pain.

Why has PCA been slow to appear in labor units? The reason is multifactorial. One of the advantages of postsurgical PCA is that the already harried surgical ward nurse will not be bothered by numerous demands for intramuscular analgesics from as many as 20 (or more!) patients. In contrast, labor nurses rarely care for more than one or two patients at a time. Hence, the inconvenience of opioid injections is minimized. One may postulate that the process of assembling the pump and infusion apparatus is a deterrent, but this has certainly not deterred the use of PCA in the surgical ward, where personnel are even more scarce than in labor and delivery units. A further objection may be the concern of obstetricians that excessive narcotic administration, particularly during the second stage of labor, may cause neonatal respiratory depression. This is a valid concern that bears further consideration, although preliminary studies have so far failed to document any neonatal compromise.[3–5]

One must remember that although PCA is an improved method for administering systemic opioids, the ultimate result is still opioid-induced analgesia. Complete abolition of sensation (i.e., anesthesia) will not be obtained. Thus, this modality will not, and is not, designed to replace epidural anesthesia. Those patients who desire complete pain relief or who do not cope well with even moderate pain would not be suitable candidates for narcotic anesthesia either by bolus or PCA. However, for the subset of patients who do not desire epidural analgesia or in institutions where regional anesthesia for childbirth is unavailable, PCA offers several advantages over intermittent dosing with opioids.

First, the ability to control one's analgesic administration provides a psychological benefit. The anxiety and stress associated with childbirth are considerable, and the physical as well as emotional "trespasses" imposed upon patients during labor can be overwhelming. Returning some degree of control back to the patient is often a much-appreciated gesture.

Second, single or intermittent doses of intravenous or intramuscular opioids are usually administered during the early stages of labor. During the later stages of labor, obstetricians are often reluctant to readminister intravenous or intramuscular opioids as high peak maternal plasma levels are readily reflected in the neonate.[6] So as labor progresses and pain intensity increases, the plasma level of opioid fades. It is in the later stages of labor that patients most need a therapeutic plasma level of opioid, and such a level is only rarely obtained with a single- or intermittent-dose technique. The ability of PCA to maintain a therapeutic plasma level of opioid while avoiding high peak levels means that the analgesic regimen will still be effective during the more painful later stages of labor. In fact, the theory behind such a dosing regimen is alluded to in a major obstetric textbook: "In general, a small dose given more frequently is preferable to a larger one administered less often. Then, if delivery occurs during the next hour or so after injection, the infant is less likely to be depressed by the medication.[6]

Several investigators have recently evaluated PCA for labor analgesia.[3–5] The technique originally described by Scott[2] utilized meperidine, which to this day remains the most commonly used narcotic analgesic in obstetrics. However, two recent studies have evaluated nalbuphine via PCA for labor analgesia.[3,4] Nalbuphine[7] is a mixed agonist–antagonist opioid that is appealing for use in laboring women. As a k-receptor agonist, it has minimal psychomimetic effects. The incidence of gastrointestinal side effects is lower as compared to pure opioid agonists. In addition, a ceiling effect for respiratory depression will theoretically enhance the safety margin of this drug when maternal safety or placental transfer to the neonate is a concern.[8]

See chapter 7 for a discussion of patient-controlled epidural anesthesia.

References

1. Bonica JJ: Principles and Practice of Obstetric Analgesia and Anesthesia. FA Davis, Philadelphia 1972
2. Scott JS: Obstetric analgesia: A consideration of labor pain on a patient-controlled technique for its relief with meperidine. Am J Obstet Gynecol 106:959, 1970
3. Podlas J, Breland BD: Patient-controlled analgesia with nalbuphine during labor. Obstet Gynecol 70:202, 1987
4. Frank M, McAteer EJ, Cattermole R, et al: Nalbuphine for obstetric analgesia. A comparison of nalbuphine with pethidine for pain relief in labour when administered by patient-controlled analgesia. Anesthesia 42:697, 1987
5. Robinson JO, Rosen M, Evans JM, et al: Self-administered intravenous and intramuscular pethidine. A controlled trial in labour. Anaesthesia 35:763, 1980
6. Pritchard JA, Macdonald PC, Grant NF (eds): William's Obstetrics. 17th Ed. Appleton-Century-Crofts, East Norwalk, CT, 1985
7. Erick JK, Heel RC: Nalbuphine. A preliminary review of its pharmacological properties and therapeutic efficacy. Drugs 26:191, 1983
8. Wilson SJ, Erick JK, Balkon J: Pharmacokinetics of nalbuphine during parturition. Am J Obstet Gynecol 155:340, 1986

PHARMACOLOGY OF LOCAL ANESTHETICS

CHEMICAL STRUCTURE

Most chemical compounds that possess local anesthetic activity are made up of an aromatic portion, an intermediate chain, and an amine portion (Table 3-13). These agents can be chemically subdivided into two groups (Table 3-13). *Aminoesters* have an ester link between the aromatic portion and the intermediate chain. Examples include procaine, chloroprocaine, and tetracaine. *Aminoamides* have an amide link between the aromatic portion and the intermediate chain. Examples include lidocaine, mepivacaine, prilocaine, bupivacaine, and etidocaine.

Aminoesters and aminoamides differ in both their metabolism and their allergic potential. Aminoesters are hydrolyzed by plasma pseudocholinesterases, whereas aminoamides are enzymatically degraded in the liver. One of the metabolites of aminoester hydrolysis is para-aminobenzoic acid (PABA), which is capable of including allergic-like reactions in a small percentage of the population. Aminoamides are not metabolized to PABA, and reports of allergic reactions are extremely rare.

MECHANISM OF ACTION

Local anesthetic agents reduce pain by inhibiting neural excitation via a direct effect on the nerve cell membrane.

The Resting Neuron

The resting nerve cell membrane maintains steep ionic gradients between the extracellular fluid and the intracellular milieu. The intracellular potassium (K^+) concentration is high compared to the extracellular fluid, and the intracellular sodium (Na^+) concentration is low.

Table 3-13. Physicochemical Properties of Local Anesthetics

Agent	Chemical Configuration: Aromatic Lipophilic	Chemical Configuration: Intermediate Chain	Chemical Configuration: Amine Hydrophilic	Physicochemical Properties: Molecular Weight (base)	Physicochemical Properties: pK_a (25°C)	Physicochemical Properties: Partition Coefficient	Physicochemical Properties: % Protein Binding
Esters							
Procaine	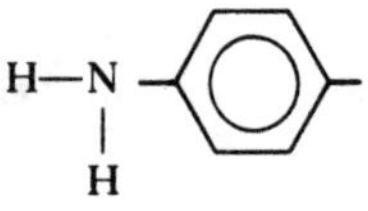	$COOCH_2CH_2$	$-N(C_2H_5)_2$	236	8.9	0.02	5.8
Tetracaine	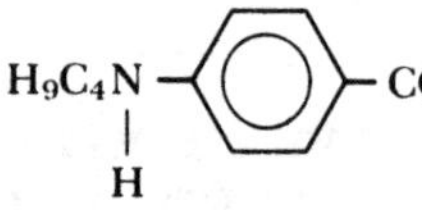	$COOCH_2CH_2$	$-N(CH_3)_2$	264	8.5	4.1	75.6
Chloroprocaine	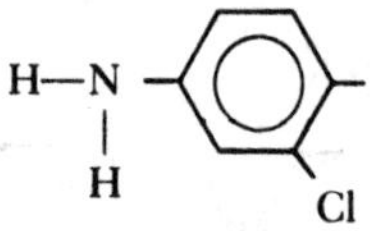	$COOCH_2CH_2$	$-N(C_2H_5)_2$	271	8.7	0.14	—
Amides							
Prilocaine	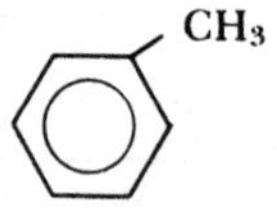	$NHCOCH(CH_3)$	$-N(H)(C_3H_7)$	220	7.9	0.9	55 approx.
Lidocaine	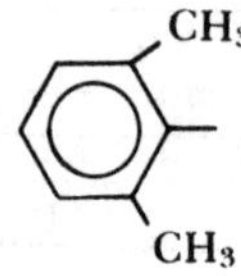	$NHCOCH_2$	$-N(C_2H_5)_2$	234	7.9	2.9	64.3
Mepivacaine		NHCO	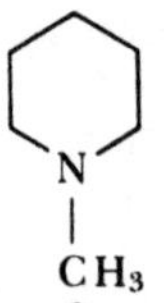	246	7.6	0.8	77.5
Bupivacaine		NHCO	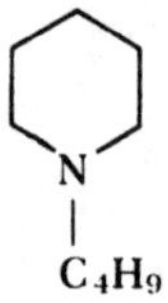	288	8.1	27.5	95.6
Etidocaine		$NHCOCH(C_2H_5)$	$-N(C_2H_5)(C_3H_7)$	276	7.7	141	94

This ionic asymmetry is due in part to the selective permeability of the cell membrane to these ions. The resting membrane is only slightly permeable to Na^+ ions, whereas it is highly permeable to K^+ ions. Furthermore, the K^+ ions, which can freely diffuse into the cell, are retained there by the negative charges on intracellular proteins.

Because the K^+ permeability (and hence conductance) is far greater than the Na^+ permeability, the resting membrane potential is largely determined by the K^+ gradient. This potential, reflecting the high intracellular concentration of potassium, is approximately −90 mV.

Depolarization-Generation of the Action Potential

With excitation, the Na^+ permeability rises and Na^+ ions enter the cell. With the rise in Na^+ gradient to the membrane potential, the membrane is depolarized eventually to the threshold or firing level, −50 to −60mV. At threshold, the Na^+ conductance rises abruptly and there is an explosive influx of Na^+ ions into the cell. The membrane potential is now largely a function of the Na^+ gradient and rises to +40 mV. This dramatic rise in the membrane potential represents the depolarization phase of the action potential.

Repolarization

At the conclusion of the depolarization phase, the Na^+ permeability again decreases and the high K^+ permeability is restored. K^+ moves out of the cell, resulting in repolarization of the membrane. The depolarization phase occupies approximately 30 percent of the entire action potential, whereas repolarization accounts for the remaining 70 percent. With return to the resting membrane potential, a very slight excess of Na^+ is present within the cell, as well as a very slight decrement of K^+. The original equilibrium is restored by the active transport of Na^+ out of the cell. This is in contrast to the flux of Na^+ into the cell during depolarization and K^+ out of the cell during repolarization; these are passive processes in which each ion moves down its concentration gradient. The energy to drive this "sodium pump" is derived from the oxidative metabolism of ATP. This pump is also believed to move K^+ from the extracellular space back into the cell.

EFFECT ON THE NERVE CELL MEMBRANE

Local-acting anesthetics do not affect the resting membrane potential or the threshold potential of nerve cells. The predominant effect of these agents is to decrease the maximum rate of rise of the action potential. As a result, threshold cannot be achieved and a propagated action potential fails to develop. Conduction is therefore blocked.

After a 15-minute exposure to a solution of 0.005 percent (0.2 mmol/L) lidocaine, the maximum rate of rise of the action potential of an isolated frog lumbar spinal ganglion decreases[1] from a control value of 190 V/s to 120 V/s. There is no significant change in the rate of repolarization. This effect of local-acting anesthetics is due to a direct effect on the cell membrane, blocking Na^+ conductance.[2] There is only a minimal decrease in K^+ conductance. Voltage clamp experiments have shown that lidocaine completely inhibits Na^+ conductance while causing only a 5 percent decrease in K^+ conductance. Tetrodotoxin, a puffer fish poison with potent local anesthetic activity, manifests a similar selective blocking effect at a concentration of 30 nmol/L.

Local-acting anesthetics are believed to act at or near the sodium channel of the nerve membrane. The specific membrane receptor differs according to the type of agent. Conventional agents, such as lidocaine and procaine, are believed to bind at receptor sites located on the inner surface of the nerve membrane. Biotoxins, such as tetrodotoxin and saxitoxin, act at sites located on the external surface of the membrane.[3] Other agents, such as benzocaine and benzyl alcohol, penetrate the nerve membrane, causing membrane expansion and a resultant decrease in the diameter of the sodium channel.[4]

ACTIVE FORM

Most of the clinically useful anesthetic preparations are available in the form of solutions of a salt. Lidocaine, for example, is usually prepared as a 0.5 to 2 percent solution of lidocaine hydrochloride. In solution, these salts exist both as uncharged molecules (B) and positively charged cations (BH^+). The ratio of B to BH^+ depends on the pH of the chemical compound and the pH of the solution:

$$pH = pK_a - \log(BH^+) \div (B)$$

Because the pK_a is constant for a given compound, the proportion of free base to charged cation depends essentially on the pH of the solution:

$$BH^+ \rightleftharpoons B + H^+$$

As the pH decreases (H^+ concentration increases) the equilibrium shifts toward the charged cationic form. As the pH increases, the equilibrium shifts toward the free base form.

Both charged and uncharged forms are involved in the process of conduction block. The base diffuses more readily through the nerve sheath and is therefore required for optimal penetration, reflected clinically in the onset of anesthesia.[5] Following diffusion through the epineurium, equilibrium recurs between B and BH^+. The charged form actually binds to the receptor site in the nerve membrane and is responsible for suppression of action potential generation, reflected clinically in the profoundness of anesthesia.

PHARMACOLOGIC BASIS

The anesthetic profile of a chemical compound depends on its lipid solubility, protein-binding capacity, pK_a, non-nervous tissue diffusibility, and intrinsic vasodilator activity (Table 3-14).

Lipid Solubility

Lipid solubility appears to be a primary determinant of intrinsic anesthetic potency. Procaine is least potent in suppressing conduction in an isolated nerve, and its partition coefficient measurements reveal its lipid solubility to be very low (less than 1). Bupivacaine, tetracaine, and etidocaine block conduction even at low concentrations, and their partition coefficient ranges from approximately 30 to 140, indicating an extremely high degree of lipid solubility. Their intrinsic anesthetic potency is about 20 times greater than that of procaine. The correlation between lipid solubility and anesthetic potency is due to the ease with which highly lipid-soluble agents can penetrate the nerve cell membrane.

Protein-Binding Capacity

The protein-binding capacity of local anesthetic agents primarily influences the duration of anesthetic action (see Table 3-14). Procaine has a short duration of action and is poorly bound to proteins. Tetracaine, bupivacaine, and etidocaine have a long duration of action and are highly bound to proteins.[6]

This correlation is also a result of the composition of the nerve membrane. Proteins account for about 10 percent of the membrane. Agents that penetrate the axolemma and attach more firmly to membrane proteins will therefore tend to have a prolonged duration of anesthetic activity.

pK_a

The pK_a of a chemical compound is the pH at which its ionized (BH^+) and unionized (B) forms are in complete equilibrium. The percentage of a local anesthetic agent present in the base form is inversely proportional to its pK_a Lidocaine, which has a pK_a of 7.74, is 35 percent nonionized at a tissue pH of 7.4. Tetracaine, which has a pK_a of 8.6, is only 5 percent unionized at a tissue pH of 7.4.

The base form, as indicated above, is primarily responsible for diffusion across the nerve sheath and thus the rate of onset of anesthesia. Both in vitro and in vivo studies confirm that drugs with a low pK_a, closer to the tissue pH, such as lidocaine, have a more rapid time of onset (Table 3-15).

Non-Nervous Tissue Diffusibility

Although in an isolated nerve the onset time is largely a function of the rate of diffusion through the epineurium, the situation in vivo is more complex, since the drug must diffuse initially through non-nervous connective tissue barriers. This rate of diffusion differs among the various drugs. Procaine and chloroprocaine both have a pK_a of 9.1 and similar onset times for conduction blockade in isolated nerves. In vivo, however, chloroprocaine has a shorter time of onset. Lidocaine and prilocaine also have the same pK_a and onset time in isolated nerve preparations, but lidocaine results in a slightly faster onset of anesthesia in vivo. The factors

Table 3-14. Relationship of Physicochemical Properties to Local Anesthetic Activity

Agent	Relative in Vivo Potency	Approximate Lipid Solubility	Duration (min)	Approximate Protein Binding (%)
Low potency/short duration				
Procaine	1	<1	60–90	5
Intermediate potency and duration				
Mepivacaine	2	1	120–240	75
Prilocaine	2	1.5	100–240	55
Lidocaine	2	4	90–200	65
High potency/long duration				
Bupivacaine	8	30	180–600	95
Tetracaine	8	80	180–600	85
Etidocaine	6	140	180–600	94

Table 3-15. Relationship of pK_a to Percentage Base Form and Time for 50 Percent Conduction Block in Isolated Nerve

Agent	Chemical Class	pK_a	% Base (at pH 7.4)	Onset (min)
Prilocaine	Aminoamide	7.7	35	2–4
Lidocaine	Aminoamide	7.7	35	2–4
Etidocaine	Aminoamide	7.7	35	2–4
Bupivacaine	Aminoamide	8.1	20	5–8
Tetracaine	Aminoester	8.6	5	10–15
Procaine	Aminoester	8.9	2	14–18

governing the rate of non-nervous tissue diffusibility have not been clearly defined.

Intrinsic Vasodilator Activity

Intrinsic vasodilator activity influences potency and duration of action in vivo. Following injection of a local anesthetic agent, some of the drug is taken up by the nerve and some is absorbed by the vascular system. The degree of vascular absorption is related to the blood flow through the area where the drug is deposited. All local anesthetic agents, except cocaine, are vasodilators (increasing vascular absorption) but their degrees of vasodilation differ.

In vitro, the intrinsic anesthetic potency of lidocaine is greater than that of mepivacaine, although their durations of action are similar. In vivo, however, mepivacaine is of equal potency and longer duration. These differences between in vitro and in vivo results are due to the greater vasodilator ability of lidocaine, which results in greater vascular absorption and a diminished availability for nerve blocks.

Structural Correlations

Within the aminoester series, the addition of a butyl group to the aromatic end of procaine produces tetracaine, a drug with greater lipid solubility and protein-binding and hence with greater intrinsic potency and a longer duration of action. Within the aminoamide series, the addition of a butyl group to the amine end of mepivacaine produces bupivacaine, a drug with greater lipid solubility and protein-binding and also greater potency and a longer duration of action. Substitution of a propyl for an ethyl group at the amine end of lidocaine, plus the addition of an ethyl group to the α-carbon in the intermediate chain yields etidocaine. This drug is more lipid soluble and more highly protein bound and therefore of greater potency and longer duration.

Classification

On the basis of differences in anesthetic potency and duration of action, it is possible to classify the clinically useful injectable local anesthetic compounds into three categories (Table 3-14). Group I includes agents of low anesthetic potency and short duration of action, such as procaine and chloroprocaine. Group II agents are those of intermediate anesthetic potency and duration of action, including lidocaine, mepivacaine, and prilocaine. Group III agents have high anesthetic potency and duration of action, such as tetracaine, bupivacaine and etidocaine.

THE PHYSIOLOGIC DISTRIBUTION

The potential toxicity of local anesthetic agents is largely determined by their vascular absorption, tissue distribution, metabolism, and excretion.

Absorption

Absorption depends on the site of injection, the dosage, the addition of a vasoconstrictor agent, and the specific agent employed.

Site of Injection. A comparison of the blood level profile of local anesthetic agents following various types of obstetric regional anesthetic techniques reveals that the most rapid rate of absorption occurs after paracervical blocks. This is followed, in order of diminishing blood levels, by administration into the caudal canal, lumbar epidural injection, and subarachnoid injection. Paracervical blocks with lidocaine 300 mg produce peak venous plasma levels of 3 to 12 μg/ml, an absorption ratio of 1 to 4 μg/ml per 100 mg lidocaine.[7] Subarachnoid administration of lidocaine 75 mg produces peak venous plasma levels of 0.2 to 0.66 μg/ml.[8]

Dosage. The blood level of local anesthetic agents is related to the total dosage of drug (mass) administered rather than the specific volume or concentration of solution employed.[9] A linear relationship tends to exist between the injected amount of drug and the peak anesthetic blood level.

In one experiment, as the total dosage of lidocaine injected into the lumbar epidural space or caudal canal was raised from 3.0 to 14.2 mg/kg, the arterial levels of lidocaine at the time of delivery increased[10] from about 0.5 μg/ml to 6μg/ml. No significant differences in lidocaine, prilocaine, and etidocaine levels have been observed following the epidural administration of these agents in varying volumes and concentrations, provided the total dosage is constant. For example, 20 ml of 3 percent prilocaine (600 mg) and 30 ml of 2 percent prilocaine (also 600 mg) were found to produce equivalent peak venous plasma levels of approximately 4.0 μg/ml following epidural administration to nonpregnant patients.[10]

Addition of a Vasoconstrictor Agent. Incorporation of vasoconstrictor agents in local anesthetic solutions decreases the rate of absorption of certain agents. The addition of 5 μg/ml of epinephrine (1:200,000) reduces the peak blood levels of lidocaine and mepivacaine by approximately 30 percent, regardless of the site of administration.[6] Epinephrine decreases the peak blood levels of prilocaine, bupivacaine, and etidocaine when they are administered as peripheral nerve blocks, but has little effect on their absorption following lumbar epidural administration.[9,11] Phenylephrine and norepinephrine can also reduce local anesthetic absorption, but not as effectively as epinephrine.

Specific Anesthetic Agent. Lidocaine is absorbed more rapidly than prilocaine,[12] probably because of prilocaine's tendency to produce less vasodilation. Bupivacaine is absorbed more rapidly than etidocaine, probably due in part to etidocaine's greater lipid solubility and enhanced uptake by peripheral fat.

Tissue Distribution

Local anesthetic agents distribute throughout the total body water. An initial rapid disappearance from the blood (the α phase) is due to uptake by rapidly equilibrating tissues (i.e., tissues with a high vascular perfusion).[13] A second, slower disappearance (the β phase) reflects distribution to slowly perfused tissues as well as metabolism and excretion of the drug. Prilocaine disappears more rapidly than lidocaine or mepivacaine.[14] Similarly, the α and β half-lives of etidocaine are significantly shorter than those of bupivacaine.[15]

Although all tissues take up local anesthetic agents, the highest concentrations are found in the more highly perfused organs, such as the lungs and kidneys. The greatest percentage of an injected dose distributes to the skeletal muscle because of the large mass of this tissue in the body. All local anesthetic drugs employed for obstetric anesthesia diffuse across the placenta and can be found in fetal tissues. The rate of placental diffusion is related to the degree of plasma protein binding in maternal blood (Table 3-16).[16]

Table 3-16. Relationship between Plasma Protein-Binding Capacity and Umbilical Vein/Maternal Vein (UV/MV) Ratio of Various Local Anesthetic Agents

Agent	Protein-Binding Capacity (%)	UV/MV Ratio
Prilocaine	55	1.0–1.18
Lidocaine	64	0.52–0.69
Mepivacaine	77	0.69–0.71
Bipivacaine	95	0.31–0.44
Etidocaine	94	0.14–0.35

Prilocaine has the lowest degree of plasma protein binding and the highest umbilical vein/maternal vein (UV/MV) ratio. Bupivacaine and etidocaine are highly bound to plasma proteins and have the lowest UV/MV ratios. Nevertheless, the fetal uptake of highly protein-bound agents, such as bupivacaine and etidocaine, has been found to be similar to that of less protein-bound drugs, such as lidocaine (Finster and Morishima, personal communication). This phenomenon is probably a result of the greater lipid solubility of bupivacaine and etidocaine, which favors tissue uptake. These data clearly suggest little difference in the potential fetal toxicity of the various amide agents.

Chloroprocaine, an ester agent, is rapidly hydrolyzed in maternal plasma, and little unchanged drug diffuses across the placenta. Chloroprocaine thus possesses the least potential systemic toxicity to mother and fetus and is employed for epidural obstetric anesthesia.

Metabolism and Excretion

The aminoesters are hydrolyzed in the plasma by plasma cholinesterases. Chloroprocaine is hydrolyzed at 4.7 μmol/ml/h, procaine at 1.1 μmol/L, and tetracaine at 0.3 μmol/L, respectively.[17] Less than 2 percent of procaine is excreted unchanged, whereas approximately 90 percent of PABA, its primary metabolite, appears unchanged in the urine. Only 33 percent of diethylaminoethanol, the other major metabolite of procaine, is excreted in the urine unchanged.

The aminoamides are primarily enzymatically degraded in the liver. Their metabolism is more complex than that of the ester drugs, and has not been fully elucidated. Prilocaine undergoes the most rapid rate of hepatic metabolism. Lidocaine, mepivacaine, and etidocaine are intermediate, and bupivacaine is metabolized most slowly. Some degradation occurs outside the liver, as indicated by the formation of certain metabolites following the incubation of prilocaine with kidney slices. The metabolism of lidocaine has been the most extensively studied. It undergoes oxidative de-ethylation to monoethylglycinexylidide and is then hydrolyzed to hydroxyxylidide.[18]

Less than 5 percent of each amide drug is excreted

unchanged into the urine. The major portion of an injected dose appears in the form of various metabolites. For example, 73 percent of lidocaine can be accounted for in the urine as hydroxyxylidine.[19] The renal clearance of amide agents is inversely related to their protein-binding capacity. Prilocaine has a lower protein-binding capacity than lidocaine and a higher clearance value. Renal clearance is also inversely proportional to the urine pH, suggesting urinary excretion by nonionic diffusion.[20]

SYSTEMIC TOXICITY

Central Nervous System Toxicity

Local anesthetic agents readily cross the blood–brain barrier, and toxic levels can produce signs and symptoms of central nervous system (CNS) excitation followed by CNS depression. Initial symptoms of toxicity consist of lightheadedness and dizziness, followed by auditory and visual disturbances, such as tinnitus and difficulty in focusing. Drowsiness, disorientation, and a temporary period of unconsciousness may also occur. Slurred speech, shivering, muscle twitching, and tremors of the face and extremities appear to be the immediate precursors of a generalized convulsive state.

A further increase in the dosage results in CNS depression: a cessation of convulsive activity, respiratory arrest, and a flattening of the brain wave pattern. This progression of symptoms is due to the inhibition of cerebral cortical neurons. An initial selective blockade of inhibitory cortical neurons and synapses allows facilitory fibers to function unopposed, leading to convulsions. Further increases in dosage depress facilitory pathways as well, causing a generalized state of CNS depression.

Local anesthetic toxicity is usually due either to an unintentional rapid intravenous injection or to extravascular administration of an excessive dosage.[21] CNS toxicity following rapid intravenous administration is related to the intrinsic anesthetic potency of the agent. Bupivacaine, tetracaine, and etidocaine are the most potent anesthetics and are most liable to cause CNS convulsive activity. CNS symptoms appear at venous blood levels of 1.5 to 4 μg/ml. Procaine, the least potent local anesthetic, is least toxic following rapid intravenous administration. CNS symptoms occur at blood levels of 20 μg/ml. Lidocaine, mepivacaine, and prilocaine are intermediate in potency and convulsive activity. CNS effects appear at blood levels of 5 to 10 μg/ml.

The toxicity of local anesthetic agents administered extravascularly depends on the rate of absorption, tissue distribution, and metabolism. Although prilocaine and lidocaine have similar potency and rapid intravenous toxicity, prilocaine is approximately 60 percent less toxic following subcutaneous administration because of its rapid hydrolysis in the plasma.

Other factors, such as the patient's acid-base status, also influence local anesthetic toxicity. There is an inverse relationship between the PCO_2 level and the convulsive threshold of local anesthetic agents. When the PCO_2 in cats is elevated from 25 to 40 mmHg to 65 to 81 mmHg, the convulsive threshold of procaine decreases[22] from approximately 35 mg/kg to 15 mg/kg.

Cardiovascular Toxicity

Local anesthetic agents can produce profound cardiovascular changes by a direct cardiac and peripheral vascular action and, indirectly, by conduction blockade of autonomic nerve fibers. Lidocaine can serve as a prototype for the pattern of cardiovascular toxicity of all local anesthetic agents. At concentrations of 5 to 10 μg/ml, it may prolong conduction through various portions of the heart (increased P-R interval and QRS duration), increase the diastolic threshold, and decrease automaticity (sinus bradycardia). Lethal concentrations produce asystole.

Lidocaine dosages and blood levels considered nontoxic (2 to 5 μg/ml) cause no alterations in myocardial contractility, diastolic volume, intraventricular pressure, and cardiac output.[23] Blood levels of 5 to 10 μg/ml decrease myocardial contractility, increase diastolic volume, decrease intraventricular pressure, and decrease cardiac output. At these levels, the drug also reduces the peripheral vascular resistance by a direct relaxant effect on the smooth muscle of peripheral arterioles. These combined effects can cause profound hypotension and circulatory collapse. The dosages of local anesthetic agents employed for most regional procedures do not produce blood levels associated with a cardiodepressant effect, and cardiovascular toxicity usually results only from unintentional rapid intravenous injection or administration of an excessive dosage. Recent studies suggest that the more potent agents, such as bupivacaine, may be more cardiotoxic, particularly in obstetric patients, than the less potent agents, such as lidocaine. This enhanced cardiac toxicity of bupivacaine appears related to the production of ventricular arrhythmias by this agent following rapid intravenous injection of large doses. Lidocaine appears to be devoid of arrhythmogenic activity.[24]

The regional anesthetic procedure itself may cause cardiovascular changes. Lumbar epidural and spinal anesthesia are frequently associated with a fall in systemic blood pressure.[25] The hypotension following epidural anesthesia is correlated with the level of anesthesia, the dosage of the agent, the addition of a vasoconstrictor, and blood volume.[26] Subarachnoid blocks that extend to the T5, level decrease stroke volume, cardiac output, and peripheral vascular resistance solely as a result of sympathetic nerve blockade. Anesthetic levels extending to the T1 or higher lead to a decrease in the mean arterial blood pressure because of a reduction of total peripheral resistance and a block of the cardioaccelerator fibers. Analgesia to T4 or below, however, does not produce a significant change in blood pressure, peripheral resistance, or cardiac output.

Allergy

True allergic reactions to local anesthetic agents are rare. Ester derivatives of PABA, such as procaine and tetracaine, are associated with most reported allergic phenomena. Reports of allergic reactions to aminoamide agents are extremely rare. Multiple-dose vials of some amide agents contain methylparaben, a preservative, which may cause cutaneous allergic-type reactions.[27]

Maternal–Fetal Toxicity

The relative susceptibility of mother and fetus to local anesthetic agent toxicity has been investigated in pregnant sheep.[28] In adult sheep, signs of CNS toxicity occur when blood levels of 5 to 10 μg/ml of lidocaine are attained. Infusion of lidocaine to newborn lambs results in convulsive episodes at arterial lidocaine levels of 10 to 20 μg/ml, whereas levels of 40 μg/ml are required in fetal sheep. The newborn lamb and the fetal sheep may therefore be somewhat more tolerant to the convulsive effects of local anesthetic agents. In the nonacidotic, nonasphyxiated baboon fetus, convulsions occur[14] at lidocaine levels of 10 to 20 μg/ml. Acidosis and asphyxia markedly increase fetal sensitivity, and convulsions occur at lidocaine levels of 4 to 7 μg/ml.

In pregnant sheep, cardiovascular toxicity—manifested by a transient increase in arterial pressure and heart rate—occurs at lidocaine levels that cause convulsions. Infusion of lidocaine into the fetus results initially in a bradycardia, and subsequently in an increase in fetal heart rate. The fetal bradycardia, observed in humans and sheep at relatively low fetal anesthetic levels, does not appear to be related to a direct anesthetic action on the heart. Present data suggest it is probably a result of a reduction in uterine blood flow.

Local Tissue Toxicity

Local anesthetic agents can act as tissue irritants. Histologic changes in skeletal muscle have been observed with most local anesthetic agents. In general, the more potent agents, such as bupivacaine and etidocaine, cause the most muscle damage. The effect is reversible; regeneration begins rapidly and is usually complete within 2 weeks.

In vitro and in vivo animal studies have shown that neural tissue is resistant to the potential irritant effect of local anesthetic agents. However, several cases of prolonged sensory-motor deficits have been reported following the unintentional subarachnoid injection of large volumes of chloroprocaine.[29,30] Isolated nerve and intact animal studies indicate that the neurotoxicity of chloroprocaine solutions is related to the low pH and presence of sodium bisulfite. Chloroprocaine itself does not appear to be neurotoxic. Recently, sodium bisulfite has been replaced by EDTA as an antioxidant in solutions of chloroprocaine.[31]

REFERENCES

1. Aceves J, Machne X: The action of calcium and of local anesthetics on nerve cells, and their interaction during excitation. J Pharmacol Exp Ther 140:138, 1963
2. Hille B: Common mode of action of three agents that decrease the transient change in sodium permeability in nerves. Nature 210:1220, 1966
3. Ritchie JM: Mechanism of action of local anesthetic agents and biotoxins. Br J Anaesth (Suppl) 47:191, 1975
4. Ritchie JM, Ritchie B, Greengard P: The effect of the nerve sheath on the action of local anesthetics. J Pharmacol Exp Ther 150:160, 1965
5. Ritchie JM, Ritchie B, Greengard P: The active structure of local anesthetics. J Pharmacol Exp Ther 150:152, 1965
6. Covino BG, Vassallo HG: Local Anesthetics: Mechanisms of Action and Clinical Use. Grune & Stratton, New York, 1976
7. Evans JA, Chastain GM, Phillips JM: The use of local anesthetic agents in obstetrics. South Med J 62:519, 1969
8. Giasi RM, D'Agostino E, Covino BG: Absorption of lidocaine following subarachnoid and epidural administration. Anesth Analg 58:360, 1979
9. Scott DB, Jebson PJR, Braid DP, et al: Factors affecting plasma levels of lignocaine and prilocaine. Br J Anaesth 44:1040, 1972
10. Shnider SM, Way EL: Plasma levels of lidocaine (Xylocaine) in mother and newborn following obstetrical conduction anesthesia. Anesthesiology 29:251, 1968
11. Lund PC, Bush DF, Covino BG: Determinants of etidocaine concentration in the blood. Anesthesiology 42:497, 1975
12. Akerman B, Astrom A, Ross S, et al: Studies on the absorption, distribution and metabolism of labelled prilocaine and lidocaine in some animal species. Acta Pharmacol Toxicol (Kbh) 24:389, 1966
13. Dhuner K-G, Lewis DH: Effect of local anesthetics and vasoconstrictors upon regional blood flow. Acta Anesth Scand (Suppl) 23:347, 1966
14. Lund PC, Covino BG: Distribution of local anesthetics in

man following peridural anesthesia. J Clin Pharmacol 7:324, 1967
15. Tucker GT, Mather LE: Pharmacokinetics of local anaesthetic agents. Br J Anaesth (Suppl) 47:213, 1975
16. Covino BG: Comparative clinical pharmacology of local anesthetic agents. Anesthesiology 35:158, 1971
17. Foldes FF, Davidson GM, Duncalf D, et al: The intravenous toxicity of local anesthetic agents in man. Clin Pharmacol Ther 6:328, 1965
18. Keenaghan JB, Boyes RN: The tissue distribution, metabolism and excretion of lidocaine in rats, guinea pigs, dogs and man. J Pharmacol Exp Ther 180:454, 1972
19. Truant AP, Takman B: Differential physical-chemical and neuropharmacologic properties of local anesthetic agents. Anesth Analg 38:478, 1959
20. Erilsson E, Granberg P-O: Studies on the renal excretion of Citanest and Xylocaine. Acta Anesth Scand (Suppl) 16:79, 1965
21. Covino BG, Marx GF, Finster M, Zsigmond EK: Prolonged sensory/motor deficits following inadvertent spinal anesthesia. Anesth Analg 59:399, 1980
22. Englesson S: The influence of acid-base changes on central nervous system toxicity of local anesthetic agents. Doctoral Thesis, University of Uppsala, Sweden, 1973
23. Collinsworth KA, Kalman SM, Harrison DC: The clinical pharmacology of lidocaine as an antiarrhythmic drug. Circulation 50:1217, 1974
24. Reiz S, Nath S: Cardiotoxicity of local anaesthetic agents. Br J Anaesth 38:736, 1986
25. Ward RJ, Bonica JJ, Freund FG, et al: Epidural and subarachnoid anesthesia: cardiovascular and respiratory effects. JAMA 191:275, 1965
26. Stanton-Hicks M: Cardiovascular effects of extradural anesthesia. Br J Anaesth (Suppl) 47:253, 1975
27. Aldrete JA, Johnson DA: Evaluation of intracutaneous testing for investigation of allergy to local anesthetic agents. Anesth Analg 49:173, 1970
28. Morishima HO, Pedersen H, Finster M, et al: Toxicity of lidocaine in the adult, newborn and fetal sheep. Anesthesiology 55:57, 1981
29. Ravindran R, Bond VK, Taseh MD, et al: Prolonged neural blockade following regional analgesia with 2-chloroprocaine. Anesth Analg 39:447, 1980
30. Reisner LS, Hochman BN, Plumer MH: Persistent neurologic deficit and adhesive arachnoiditis following intrathecal 2-chloroprocaine injection. Anesth Analg 59:452, 1980
31. Gissen AJ, Datta S, Lambert D: The chloroprocaine controversy. II. Is chloroprocaine neurotoxic? Reg Anesth 9:133, 1984

ALKALINIZATION OF LOCAL ANESTHETICS

Local anesthetics contain a tertiary nitrogen atom that confers the properties of a weak base on these drugs. In the clinical setting, manipulation of the solution to increase the pH will enhance the rate of diffusion across the nerve sheath and nerve membrane and hasten the onset of a regional block. With a focus on epidural administration, this section outlines the application of pH adjustment of commercially supplied local anesthetic solutions to the anesthetic management of the obstetric patient.

PHARMACOLOGY

The tertiary nitrogen atom of the local anesthetic molecule can bind a proton to yield a charged form.[1] The tendency to bind a proton is determined by the pK_a of the individual agent and the acidity or alkalinity (pH) of the solution. At equilibrium, when the solution pH equals the pK_a of the molecule, the concentrations of charged and uncharged local anesthetic forms are equal. Thus half of the molecules are charged ions, and the remainder are neutral.

When the solution pH is less than the pK_a of a particular drug, the extra acidity shifts the equilibrium concentrations to favor the protonated molecule, which thus becomes charged. Conversely, at a pH more alkaline than the pK_a, the uncharged, nonprotonated form predominates. Thus manipulation of the pH can influence the charge on large fractions of local anesthetic molecules in a solution.

Although it is likely that the protonated, charged molecules of the local anesthetic are the active form inside the target sodium channel, the local anesthetic must pass hydrophobic lipid barriers to reach the site of action. Neutral molecules traverse these barriers more readily than do charged molecules. Consequently, the increased fraction of neutral local anesthetic molecules at alkaline pH favors access to the target proteins.

Commercially available local anesthetic preparations are generally acidic solutions.[2] Acid pH promotes solubility of several of the agents that are prone to precipitate as pH approaches neutral (7.0). Acid pH also promotes stability of adjuvants such as epinephrine. The measured pH's of commercially available local anesthetic solutions commonly used in the practice of obstetric anesthesia are listed in Table 3-17. It can be noted that the pH's of commercially available local anesthetic solutions are substantially below the pK_a's. For a theoretical molecule with a pK_a of 8.0, Table 3-18 indicates the relative proportions of neutral (B) and charged (HB^+) forms for a range of solution pH's. Because pH is alogarithmic scale, a change of pH from 4 to 7 is associated with a thousand-fold increase in the proportion of neutral molecules.

Alkalinization of local anesthetic solutions is practically achieved in the clinical setting by the addition of sodium

Table 3-17. pK_a and pH of Commercially Available Anesthetic Solutions

Agent	Concentration	pK_a[a]	pH[b]
Chloroprocaine	2%	9.1	3.40 ± .02
	3%		3.38 ± .02
Lidocaine	1%	7.9	6.40 ± .07
	1% + epi[c]		4.30 ± .05
	1.0% + epi[d]		6.42 ± .06
	1.5%		6.38 ± .06
	1.5% + epi[c]		4.28 ± .06
	1.5% + epi[d]		6.39 ± .06
	2.0%		6.43 ± .06
	2.0% + epi[c]		4.10 ± .10
	2.0% + epi[d]		6.40 ± .07
Bupivacaine	0.25%	8.1	5.58 ± .02
	0.5%		5.35 ± .03
	0.5% + epi[c]		4.14 ± .02
	0.5% + epi[d]		4.97 ± .11
	0.75%		5.49 ± .06
	0.75% + epi[c]		4.15 ± .01
	0.75% + epi[d]		5.43 ± .02

[a] Data from Carpenter and Mackey.[1]
[b] Data from Peterfreund et al.[2]
[c] Commercially added epinephrine 1:200,000.
[d] Freshly added epinephrine 1:200,000.

Table 3-18. pH Dependence of the B/HB⁺ Ratio[a]

pH	B/HB^+
4	1/10,000
5	1/1,000
6	1/100
7	1/10
8	1/1

[a] The dissociation relationship for a weak base is defined as $pH = pK_a + \log_{10}([B]/[HB^+])$, where B represents the free base and HB^+ indicates the protonated form of the molecule. Data show the ratio of nonprotonated to protonated molecules at the specified pH for a theoretical drug with a pK_a of 8.

OBSTETRIC ANESTHESIA IMPLICATIONS

Epidural Anesthesia for Labor

Rapid onset of epidural anesthesia for the laboring patient may be practically provided by administering bicarbonate. Bicarbonate solutions of 4 or 8.4 percent may be used.[2] Unfortunately, precipitation of the local anesthetic limits the degree of alkalinization possible with some solutions. Of the drugs commonly employed in obstetric epidural anesthesia, chloroprocaine, lidocaine, and bupivacaine, only the first two agents remain in solution for reasonable durations at physiologic pH. Bupivacaine precipitates rapidly with small additions of alkalinizing agent. Table 3-19 lists guidelines for alkalinization of chloroprocaine, lidocaine, and bupivacaine solutions with commercially available preparations of sodium bicarbonate. Although preparations of lidocaine and chloroprocaine might be alkalinized to a solution pH greater than 7.4, dilution of the drug by the requisite addition of large volumes of the readily available sodium bicarbonate preparations might limit utility. Moreover, potential toxic effects of large quantities of alkali administered near neural structures must be considered if alkalinization above the physiologic range is contemplated. Sources of alkali to pH adjust solutions include other chemicals such as tromethamine. However, the nature of the particular agent used to adjust the pH of the local anesthetic influences the behavior of the observed block.[3] It has thus been suggested that carbon dioxide generated by the addition of sodium bicarbonate to the local anesthetic may have intrinsic direct or indirect anesthetic action.

Table 3-19. Suggested Alkalinization Doses and pH Achieved of Commercially Available Anesthetic Solutions[a]

Agent	Concentration	HCO_3^-, ml/ 20 ml Agent	pH after HCO_3^-
Chloroprocaine	2%	4.0	7.51
	3%	4.0	7.43
Lidocaine	1%	4.0	7.43
	1% + epi[b]	4.0	7.21
	1.0% + epi[c]	4.0	7.37
	1.5%	4.0	7.31
	1.5% + epi[b]	4.0	7.16
	1.5% + epi[c]	4.0	7.35
	2.0%	4.0	7.24
	2.0% + epi[b]	4.0	7.08
	2.0% + epi[b]	4.0	7.08
	2.0% + epi[c]	4.0	7.26
Bupivacaine	0.25%	0.10	6.97
	0.5%	0.05	6.62
	0.5% + epi[b]	0.30	6.37
	0.5% + epi[c]	0.05	6.78
	0.75%	0.05	6.56
	0.75% + epi[b]	0.30	6.32
	0.75% + epi[c]	0.05	6.58

[a] Data compiled for 4 percent sodium bicarbonate (w/v) (0.48 mEq/ml). One-half of this volume dose (approximately the same milliequivalents) of sodium bicarbonate, 8.4% (w/v) (1.0 mEq/ml) may be substituted. No precipitation observed after 1 hour at room temperature with sodium bicarbonate added in these doses.
[b] Commercially added epinephrine 1:200,000.
[c] Freshly added epinephrine 1:200,000.
(Adapted from Peterfreund et al.,[2] with permission.)

large doses of a concentrated drug (i.e., 2 percent lidocaine with epinephrine) or by adjusting the pH of more dilute solutions. A disadvantage of large-dose administration is the potential for profound sensory, motor, and autonomic blockade of extended duration, although pain is quickly diminished. Administration of an alkalinized solution of dilute local anesthetic such as 1 or 1.5 percent lidocaine can hasten the onset of an anesthetic block. After administration of sufficient volume to ensure adequate dermatomal spread, pain relief with limited motor block can be quickly achieved. At the Brigham and Women's Hospital we provide long-term anesthesia by intermittent bolus or continuous infusion of bupivacaine with or without opioids.

A small test dose of alkalinized local anesthetic may also help to ensure correct epidural placement.

Epidural Anesthesia for Surgical Procedures

For the patient requiring a surgical procedure such as cesarean delivery, forceps extraction, repair of lacerations, or episiotomy, provision of an epidural block sufficiently dense for surgery may be expedited by pH adjustment of a local anesthetic. The combination of a high dose of local anesthetic with pH adjustment has potential value in settings where a labor epidural must be urgently "converted" to a surgical anesthetic for abdominal or forceps delivery. Useful combinations include alkalinized 3 percent chloroprocaine and alkalinized 2 percent lidocaine with epinephrine.

Anesthetic Implications

Concurrent with a hastened onset of anesthesia, alkalinized epidural local anesthetics potentially cause more precipitous hemodynamic changes.[4] This potential disadvantage of pH adjustment mandates adequate preparation, including good intravenous access, intravascular volume expansion, attention to patient positioning, and vigilant monitoring. Treatment of hypotension includes increased volume infusion, patient positioning to ensure adequate displacement of the uterus from the major vessels, and administration of ephedrine and oxygen if indicated.

Clinical Utility

Because of the susceptibility to precipitation, alkalinization of bupivacaine is less useful than lidocaine or chloroprocaine. Although the theoretical basis of pH adjustment of local anesthetic solutions is accepted, controversy exists as to the clinical utility of alkalinization.[5–9] Although differences in measured onset of blocks may achieve statistical significance for alkalinized solutions compared to controls for some blocks in some studies, these reported differences are sometimes small and thus are of questionable practical value. Further controlled clinical trials are needed to clarify the importance of alkalinization to clinical practice. However, our clinical experience indicates that in appropriate settings, alkalinization of local anesthetics with sodium bicarbonate provides the anesthesiologist with useful management options.

REFERENCES

1. Carpenter RT, Mackey DC: Local anesthetics. p. 371. In: Barash PG, Cullen BF, Stoelting RK (eds): Clinical Anesthesia. JB Lippincott, Philadelphia, 1989
2. Peterfreund RA, Datta S, Ostheimer GW: pH adjustment of local anesthetic solutions with sodium bicarbonate: laboratory evaluation of alkalinization and precipitation. Reg Anesth 14 (6):265, 1989
3. Ackerman WE, Juneja MM, Denson DD, et al: The effect of pH and pCO_2 on epidural analgesia with 2% 2-chloroprocaine. Anesth Analg 68:593, 1989
4. Parnass SM, Curran MJ, Becker GL: Incidence of hypotension associated with epidural anesthesia using alkalinized and nonalkalinized lidocaine for cesarean section, Anesth Analg 66:1148, 1987
5. Glosten B, Dailey PA, Preston PG, et al: pH-adjusted 2-chloroprocaine for epidural anesthesia in patients undergoing postpartum tubal ligation. Anesthesiology 68:948, 1988
6. McMorland, GH, Douglas MJ, Jeffery WK, et al: Effect of pH adjustment of bupivacaine on onset and duration of epidural analgesia in parturients. Can Anaesth Soc J 33:537, 1986
7. DiFazio CA, Carron H, Grosslight KR, et al: Comparison of pH-adjusted lidocaine solutions for epidural anesthesia. Anesth Analg 65:760, 1986
8. Hilgier M: Alkalinization of bupivacaine for brachial plexus block. Reg Anesth 10:59, 1985
9. Bedder MD, Kozody R, Craig DB: Comparison of bupivacaine and alkalinized bupivacaine in brachial plexus anesthesia. Anesth Analg 67:48, 1988

TOXICITY OF LOCAL ANESTHETICS

The local anesthetic toxicity resulting from unintentional intravenous injection or accumulation during a regional anesthetic procedure is of major concern to the anesthesiologist. Lalli and Amaranath reviewed 53 deaths associated with local anesthetics from 1971 to 1978.[1] The majority of deaths resulted from unintentional intravenous injections in obstetrics, a setting in which epidural anesthesia with a potent long-acting local anesthetic such as bupivacaine is utilized extensively. Although one may find recommendations providing maximum safe dosages of local anesthetics, appropriate clinical judgment must be used in the specific case because many factors will modify local anesthetic toxicity. For example, site of injection, patient age, clinical status of the patient, and concomitant medications will tend to affect the absorption and physiologic disposition of local anesthetics, and so influence their potential toxicity.

THE PARTURIENT

The preponderance of local anesthetic toxicity seen in the parturient has classically been attributed to the physiologic changes of pregnancy, which include increased cardiac output, increased blood volume, aortocaval compression, decreased functional residual capacity, increased oxygen consumption, and reduced plasma proteins. These alterations increase the volume of distribution, alter the metabolic state, and reduce the cardiopulmonary reserve of the parturient. However, numerous animal studies also suggest that parturients are at greater risk because of increased tissue sensitivity to local anesthetic toxicity. The mean dosages of bupivacaine that induce seizures and circulatory collapse are significantly lower in pregnant sheep than in their nonpregnant controls.[2] Conduction block in isolated nerves and cardiac tissue is achieved at lower concentrations of local anesthetics.[3] Experimental evidence suggests that this may be due to the elevated progesterone levels found in pregnancy. Of even greater clinical import is that whereas neural tissue appears to be more sensitive to all local anesthetics, the increased cardiac sensitivity of pregnant animals is specific to bupivacaine.[4,5]

Several additional factors increase the potential for local anesthetic toxicity. Pregnancy predisposes to the hypoglycemic state, and this may aggravate bupivacaine cardiac toxicity.[6] There is the theoretical concern that the pregnant patient has a relative plasma cholinesterase deficiency and, therefore, may be more sensitive to ester anesthetics. Pregnant patients are more likely to be hypomagnesemic, and this will aggravate local anesthetic toxicity by disrupting the sodium-potassium exchange pump. Lastly, venous engorgement increases the risk of an unintentional intravenous injection, especially during epidural anesthesia.

Based on reports of cardiac toxicity associated with the use of bupivacaine in pregnant patients, the Food and Drug Administration recommended that the 0.75 percent concentration of bupivacaine not be employed in obstetrics. Provided that the volume is not increased, reducing the concentration of bupivacaine decreases the total dose administered, thereby limiting the potential for toxicity.

THE FETUS

Anesthetic management of the parturient actually entails care of two patients. Observations of a significant incidence of fetal bradycardia following regional blocks with bupivacaine triggered concern that the fetus may be more sensitive to local anesthetics.[7] They can affect the fetus in three ways. Loss of sympathetic tone will decrease maternal blood pressure and cardiac output, thereby reducing placental perfusion. Local anesthetics may directly vasoconstrict the placental vessels. Lastly, local anesthetics can cross the placenta and act on fetal cardiac and neural tissue directly. Preliminary studies suggest that fetal sheep are less able to respond to a hypoxic stress with appropriate sympathetic responses when exposed to "nontoxic" plasma levels of bupivacaine.[8]

The presence of persistent fetal bradycardia must be presumed to represent fetal acidosis until proven otherwise by fetal scalp pH. In this setting, the anesthesiologist should consider using chloroprocaine rather than an amide-type local anesthetic. Because chloroprocaine is an ester, it will be rapidly metabolized by plasma cholinesterase before crossing the placenta. This minimizes the risk of ion trapping of protonated local anesthetics in the acidotic fetus. Once in the fetal circulation, local anesthetics are more likely to depress cardiac function, especially under acidotic conditions.

Despite the evidence of increased sensitivity of parturients and fetuses to local anesthetics, regional anesthesia has tremendous benefit in this population. Furthermore, unrelieved pain, such as that experienced by the laboring patient, correlates with elevated catecholamines and other stress markers that may reduce placental perfusion directly.

CENTRAL NERVOUS SYSTEM TOXICITY

Systemic toxicity of local anesthetics is usually first manifested by central nervous system (CNS) signs and symptoms. Neurologic symptoms include incoherent speech, restlessness, nervousness, lightheadedness, and dizziness. Some patients report a metallic taste, blurred vision, or tinnitus. Higher blood levels can lead to tremors and convulsions. Local anesthetics affect the CNS in a two-stage fashion. Within the limbic system, local anesthetics depress inhibitory neurons first, allowing unopposed action of facilatory neurons. This excitatory state resembles temporal lobe epilepsy and may culminate in generalized convulsions. Higher local anesthetic levels lead to global CNS depression and ultimately an isoelectric electroencephalogram.

The relative potential for CNS toxicity of the various agents is directly related to their relative potency as local anesthetics. For example, intravenously administered procaine produces convulsions in animals at a dose of approximately 35 mg/kg, whereas tetracaine and bupivacaine cause seizures at doses of approximately 5 mg/kg. Thus, tetracaine and bupivacaine, which are eight times more potent as local anesthetics, are seven times more toxic than procaine in terms of inducing seizure activity. Therefore, little difference exists between the therapeutic index of these agents if one considers the comparative dosages required for effective surgical anesthesia and the dose that will cause convulsions.

DIRECT TISSUE TOXICITY

Chloroprocaine has been associated with prolonged spinal nerve injury when unintentionally administered into the subarachnoid space. In isolated nerve preparations, the neurologic toxicity appeared to be due to the preservative sodium bisulfite in the setting of a low pH.[9] Bisulfite has subsequently been eliminated from commercially available chloroprocaine with no apparent loss in potency.

However, recent reports have linked chloroprocaine with both severe backache and localized muscle soreness. The alkalotic nature of the local anesthetic solution may cause direct tissue trauma. Another postulated mechanism is that alterations in intracellular calcium levels may cause derangement of neural function, inducing painful muscle fasciculations that may affect the patient well into the postoperative period. Judicious use is still advised, employing chloroprocaine only when the benefit to a distressed fetus outweighs the potential harm to the mother.

CARDIOVASCULAR TOXICITY

Direct Cardiac Effects

At higher serum levels, local anesthetics may depress the cardiovascular system by decreasing heart rate, reducing myocardial contractility, provoking ventricular arrhythmias, and causing profound vasodilation. The combination of myocardial depression and peripheral vasodilation can lead to cardiovascular collapse that is quite resistant to resuscitative efforts.

Two early signs of local anesthetic cardiac toxicity are bradycardia and P-R interval lengthening, resulting from inhibition of both impulse generation within the SA node, and conduction from the SA node down to the ventricular muscle.[10–12] Bupivacaine is more likely to produce asystole than lidocaine, especially in an acidotic or hypoxic milieu.[10] Furthermore, the highly lipid-soluble, protein-bound local anesthetics, such as bupivacaine and etidocaine, will induce ventricular arrhythmias, both through direct effects on ventricular muscle[13–19] and also indirectly, through a mechanism involving the CNS.[20–22]

Local anesthetics will depress myocardial contractility in a dose-dependent manner.[10,23] As local anesthetic concentration increases, myocardial contractility decreases. Furthermore, local anesthetics exert a negative inotropic effect that is more profound at low heart rates. Therefore, any agent that also causes bradycardia will decrease contractility even further.

Bupivacaine and etidocaine appear to be relatively more cardiotoxic than the less-potent agents such as lidocaine. This is quantified by the CC/CNS ratio, which is the serum concentration that induces cardiovascular collapse divided by that which produces seizures; it is narrower for the potent local anesthetics. One possible explanation arises from a theoretical model of local anesthetic–sodium channel interactions described by Clarkson and Hondeghem.[18] They concluded that lidocaine avidly binds to sodium channels but readily dissociates (fast in-fast out), whereas bupivacaine binds more tightly to sodium channels (fast in-slow out). According to this fast in-slow out theory, bupivacaine is more likely to accumulate in cardiac tissue, thereby increasing toxicity.

Peripheral Vascular Effects

The effect of local anesthetics on vascular smooth muscle is also concentration dependent, but demonstrates a biphasic character. For example, lidocaine in low concentrations increases vascular tone, but in high concentrations causes vasodilatation.[24] Bupivacaine also demonstrates a biphasic effect, although its vasodilator activity is not as pronounced as that of lidocaine. Most local anesthetics will cause vasodilatation in humans at toxic serum levels, thereby decreasing venous return and cardiac output. Significant hemodynamic compromise can result.

PREVENTION OF LOCAL ANESTHETIC TOXICITY

In light of the potential for serious sequel of systemic local anesthetic toxicity, one must focus on the prevention of an adverse reaction. Careful consideration of patient characteristics, sound preparation, appropriate monitoring, and attention to technique will help ensure a good outcome (Figure 3-11).

Patient Characteristics

There are many patient-specific characteristics that will affect anesthetic decisions when using local anesthetics. Of most importance are the pregnant state, the presence of coexisting disease, and concurrent medications. The physiologic changes of pregnancy and the parturient's increased sensitivity to local anesthetics have been mentioned. The implication is that local anesthetic toxicity will be seen earlier, at lower doses, and the parturient will be less able to cope with them. Allergy to amide local anesthetics is exceedingly rare and is usually due to a reaction to added preservatives. Allergy to ester local anesthetics is less rare and is due to sensitivity to a metabolite, para-aminobenzoic acid (PABA).

There is no evidence that individuals with seizure disorders are at increased risk of local anesthetic-induced seizures. The most common cardiovascular problem in the parturient is pregnancy-induced hypertension (PIH). PIH may be marked by the presence of neurologic irritability, hypertension, intravascular volume depletion, total body edema, renal and hepatic dysfunction, and alterations of hemostasis. The physiological alterations produced by a regional anesthetic will probably be more problematic than local anesthetic toxicity per se. Local anesthetics have been safely used in patients with congenital heart disease or pregnancy-associated cardiomyopathy. However, lidocaine rather than a more cardiotoxic agent such as bupivacaine should be used in the setting of a low cardiac output or severe arrhythmias. Epidural anesthesia in patients with bifascicular block right bundle branch block and left anterior hemiblock did not produce atroventricular conduction difficulty.[25] Altered hepatic metabolism may lead to local anesthetic accumulation, and toxicity from ester anesthetics in a patient with a plasma cholinesterase deficiency was reported recently.[26]

Concurrent medications may also affect local anesthetic toxicity. For example, calcium channel blockers increase the local anesthetic cardiac toxicity resulting from exposure to bupivacaine or lidocaine in animal experiments.[27–29] Patients taking β-blockers may be more at risk from local anesthetic toxicity because local anesthetics decrease myocardial contractility more severely at low heart rates (reverse frequency dependence).[30] β-blocking agents can alter amide local anesthetic metabolism by reducing hepatic and splanchnic blood flow. Furthermore, a significant amount of local anesthetic is removed from the circulation by passage through the lungs. A preliminary report notes that propranolol may decrease the clearance of bupivacaine in the pulmonary circuit.

Combined regional/general anesthesia is being used with increasing frequency as studies credit it with reductions in thromboembolic phenomena,[31] pulmonary dysfunction,[32,33] and better postoperative pain control.[34] The net effect of general anesthesia on local anesthetic toxicity is not clear. General anesthesia reduces hepatic blood flow, thereby decreasing local anesthetic elimination. In prolonged operative procedures, patients often become hypothermic, further depressing enzymatic function. Hypothermia of 35°C has been found to augment increases in QRS duration induced by bupivacaine.[35] General anesthesia reduces the central, adrenergically mediated reflexes that help to maintain vascular tone and cardiac contractility in the awake patient exposed to toxic serum levels of local anesthetics.

Preparation and Monitoring

Maximizing the margin of safety begins with optimal patient preparation. Oxygen via face mask or nasal prongs provides a well-oxygenated patient should catastrophe ensue. Ideally, the patient should be NPO to minimize the risk of aspiration. The gastrointestinal changes associated with pregnancy include decreased lower esophageal sphincter tone, increased gastric volume and acidity, and decreased gastric emptying. A nonparticulate antacid should be given prior to the establishment of any anesthetic. Metoclopramide has been advocated to enhance gastric emptying and decrease the incidence of nausea. Intravascular volume should be sufficiently expanded to accommodate any decrease in vascular tone, as sole reliance on sympathomimetics may decrease uterine perfusion. Should they be needed, both ephedrine and neosynephrine appear to be safely tolerated by both mother and fetus when titrated carefully to effect.

Resuscitation equipment to manage changes in ventilatory and cardiac status must be immediately available. Continuous monitoring of maternal neurologic and cardiac function should provide early warning of elevated blood levels of a local anesthetic, enabling more timely intervention. Continuous assessment of the well-being of the fetus must include fetal heart rate monitoring any time an anesthetic is administered. It is not widely appreciated that tetanic uterine contraction may be an early sign of maternal local anesthetic toxicity, which may be seen prior to overt neurologic or cardiac toxicity.

The importance of communicating with an awake patient cannot be overemphasized. Sedation should be

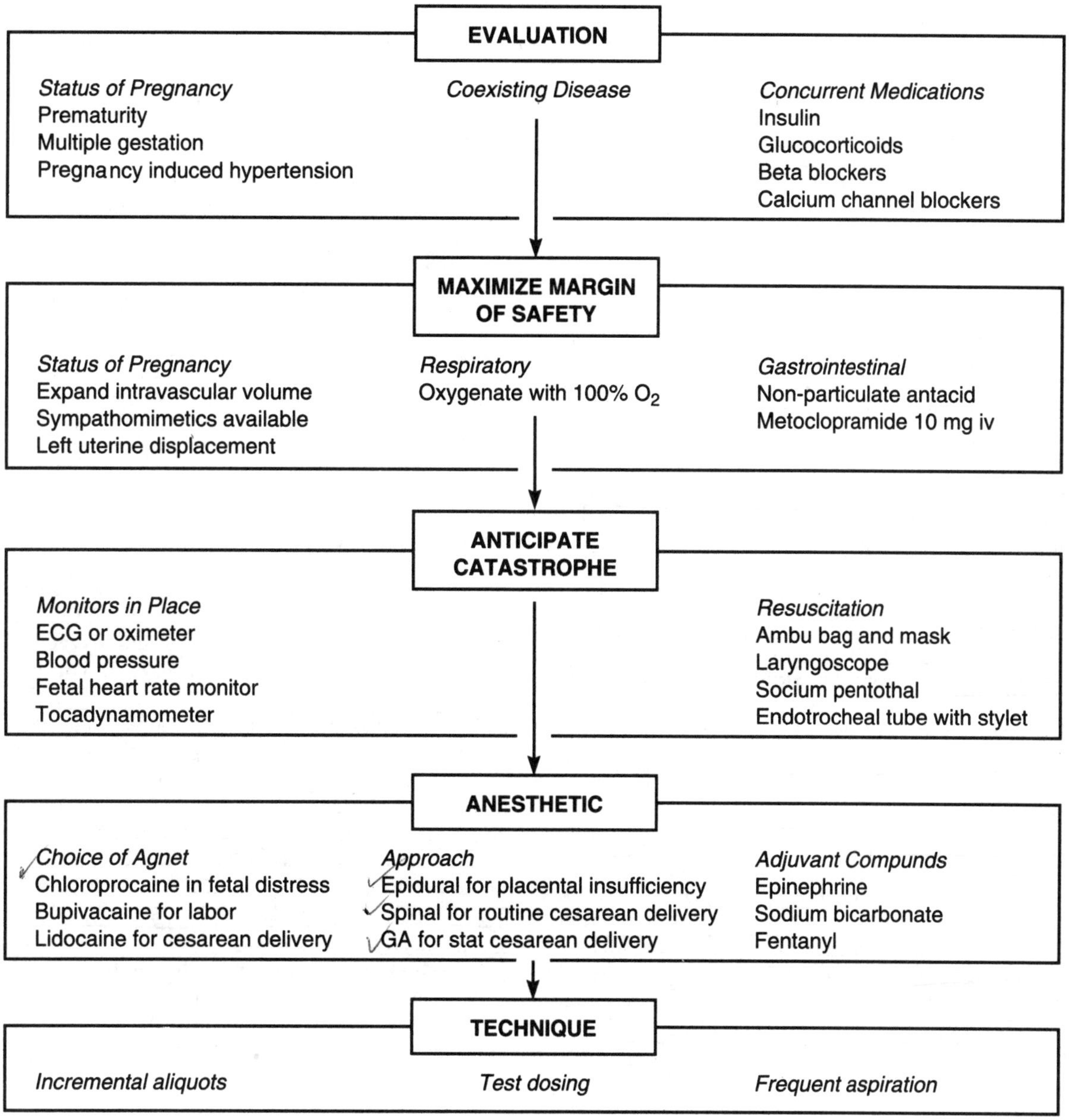

Fig. 3-11. Prevention of local anesthetic toxicity.

considered only after delivery, if possible, and the level of anesthesia adequately assessed. A recent study reviewing deaths occurring in conjunction with spinal anesthetics concluded that oversedation was a strong contributing factor in many cases, presumably because of respiratory acidosis and hypercarbia.[36]

Anesthetic Technique

Careful attention to anesthetic procedure is imperative in the choice of agents, technique, use of adjuvant compounds, and dosing. The use of bupivacaine in the cardiovascularly compromised patient should be carefully considered. Chloroprocaine is the most appropriate agent in the patient in whom the possibility of fetal distress is being entertained. If a patient is hemodynamically fragile, a case can be made in favor of epidural rather than spinal anesthesia, as the more gradual onset of an epidural anesthetic allows time for compensatory cardiovascular changes. In such a situation, the addition of bicarbonate or epinephrine has little utility, as they will hasten onset and cause unwanted peripheral vascular effects, respectively.

The rationale for test dosing is to confirm appropriate placement of a needle or catheter prior to injecting the total dose of local anesthetic. In the case of epidural anesthesia, the two sites to avoid are the subarachnoid and intravascular spaces. The addition of epinephrine has most often been advocated but whether it should be added depends on the clinical circumstance. In the laboring patient, epinephrine may reduce placental blood flow.[37] In some instances, the epinephrine effect is not specific enough to be useful given the wide variations in heart rate. The use of epinephrine is potentially hazardous in the patient with PIH. The necessity of a test dose may be obviated by the use of small fractionated dosing. If the anesthetic is injected in the wrong place, this error will be detected before the total dose is given. One caveat is that although small aliquots of both lidocaine and chloroprocaine may first present with neurologic symptoms after intravascular injection, low concentrations of bupivacaine may not. Bupivacaine, appropriately used, is a valuable tool in obstetric anesthesia.[39,40] The controversy of what constitutes an effective test dose continues, with recent reports advocating the use of small quantities of air, fentanyl, and ephedrine because of either higher sensitivity or specificity in relation to epinephrine.

The minimal concentration and total dose necessary must always be used. Frequent aspiration will help detect intravascular placement of your needle or catheter but a negative aspiration does not rule it out as the vein may collapse under the negative pressure. Inability to obtain effective pain relief should alert one to the possibility of intravascular placement of an epidural catheter. The use of continuous infusion techniques should include all the above careful considerations and demands an established plan of patient monitoring.

TREATMENT OF LOCAL ANESTHETIC TOXICITY

Management of systemic local anesthetic toxicity begins with a high degree of vigilance, close attention to the airway, supporting the circulation, and treating ventricular arrhythmias. The first signs of systemic local anesthetic toxicity usually are CNS changes. Most seizures caused by local anesthetics are self limiting, unless a massive intravenous overdose is given. Acidosis can occur very rapidly in a convulsing patient. Maintaining a normal acid–base status is critical. Respiratory acidosis will lower the seizure threshold and decrease protein binding of local anesthetics, increasing free drug levels and, therefore, toxicity.[11,41]

Secure an Airway

Initial therapy involves appropriate airway management. A patient airway must be secured and the patient adequately ventilated with 100 percent oxygen. The possibility of aspiration should always be considered. The patient should be intubated if adequate mask ventilation cannot be achieved. In the operating room or where assistance in airway management is readily available, succinylcholine may be used. In other situations, thiopental or diazepam may halt the seizures and allow one person to manage the airway. If seizure activity persists, therapy with an appropriate CNS depressant should be utilized. Thiopental (50 to 100 mg), diazepam (5 to 10 mg), or midazolam (2 to 5 mg) should control seizure activity and associated masseter contractions. (Midazolam appears to be less effective than diazepam in this regard). However, diazepam may be a double-edged sword in this setting, as it may complicate treatment of local anesthetic cardiac toxicity by aggravating hemodynamic instability.

Support the Circulation

Deteriorations in hemodynamic status must be treated aggressively. Hypotension due to local anesthetic cardiac toxicity is best treated with a sympathomimetic agent such as epinephrine, which will increase cardiac contractility as well as produce peripheral vasoconstriction. Bradycardia should be treated with atropine. The anesthesiologist must be aware of the potential for aortocaval compression or obstruction at all times. Partial vena caval obstruction can greatly increase mortality after bupivacaine-precipitated cardiovascular collapse. Resuscitation of dogs given a toxic dose of local anesthetics was prolonged by a factor of 10 when the inferior vena cava was occluded.[42] Left uterine displacement is a simple maneuver that will aid venous return. Elevation of the legs will also increase venous return. In extremis, a cesarean delivery may be able to reverse intractible hemodynamic deterioration. Clinical support for this aggressive approach is provided by a case in which a cesarean delivery during a cardiac arrest following toxic reaction led to successful resuscitation of both mother and fetus.[43]

Aggressive treatment transcends basis cardiopulmonary resuscitation. Closed-chest compressions are grossly inadequate in maintaining adequate circulation during cardiac arrest for any extended period of time. Local anesthetic cardiac toxicity may not resolve quickly and more definitive interventions could be required. In a viable individual, one must consider open-chest massage or cardiopulmonary bypass. Studies by Sanders et al.[44] show improved resuscitation from cardiac arrest with open chest massage, although in a different arrest situation.

Treat Ventricular Arrhythmias

The appropriate means of treating local anesthetic-induced ventricular arrhythmias have not been well established. Ventricular tachycardia or fibrillation is probably best treated with electrical cardioversion. Animal studies suggest that bretylium and not lidocaine is more efficacious for the pharmacologic treatment of bupivacaine-induced premature ventricular contractions or ventricular tachycardia. Recently, amiodarone has also been suggested for the treatment of bupivacaine-induced arrhythmias.

REFERENCES

1. Lalli AF, Amaranath L: A critique on mortality associated with local anesthetics. Anesth Rev 9:29, 1982
2. Morishima HO, Pedersen H, Finster M, et al: Bupivacaine toxicity in pregnant and nonpregnant ewes. Anesthesiology 63:134, 1985
3. Datta S, Lambert DH, Gregus J, et al: Differential sensitivities of mammalian nerve fibers during pregnancy. Anesth Analg 62:1070, 1983
4. Moller RA, Datta S, Jox J, et al: Progesterone-induced increase in cardiac sensitivity to bupivacaine. Anesthesiology 69:A675, 1988
5. Morishima HO, Finster M, Arthur GR, Covino BG: Lidocaine toxicity in pregnant sheep. Anesthesiology 69:A672, 1988
6. Lu GP, Batiller GM, Marx GF: Hypoglycemia enhances bupivacaine cardiotoxicity in the rat. Anesthesiology 65:A191, 1986
7. Abboud TK, Khoo SS, Miller F, et al: Maternal, fetal, and neonatal responses after epidural anesthesia with bupivacaine, 2-chloroprocaine or lidocaine. Anesth Analg 61:638, 1982
8. Heavner JE: Refresher Course Lecture: Local Anesthetic Toxicity. Annual Meeting, American Society of Regional Anesthesiology, 1989
9. Gissen AJ, Datta S, Lambert D: The chloroprocaine controversy. II. Is chloroprocaine neurotoxic? Reg Anesth 9:135, 1984
10. Sage DJ, Feldman HS, Arthur GR, et al: Influence of lidocaine and bupivacaine on isolated guinea pig atria in the presence of acidosis and hypoxia. Anesth Analg 63:1, 1984
11. Wojtczak JA, Griffin RM, Pratilas V, Kaplan JA: Mechanisms of arrhythmias during intoxication in rabbits. Anesth Analg 64:A302, 1985
12. Wheeler DM, Bradley EL, Woods WT: The electrophysiologic actions of lidocaine and bupivacaine in the isolated perfused canine heart. Anesthesiology 68:201, 1985
13. DeJong RH, Gamble CA, Ronin JD: Bupivacaine causes arrhythmias in normokalemic cats. Reg Anesth 8:84, 1983
14. Kotelko DM, Shnider SM, Dailey PA, et al: Bupivacaine induced cardiac arrhythmias in sheep. Anesthesiology 60:10, 1984
15. Sage D, Feldman H, Arthur G, et al: The cardiovascular effects of convulsant doses of lidocaine and Bupivacaine in the conscious dog. Reg Anesth 10:175, 1985
16. Nath S, Haggmark S, Johansson G, Reiz S: Differential depressant and electrophysiologic cardiotoxicity of local anesthetics. Anesth Analg 65:1263, 1986
17. Moller RA, Covino BG: Cardiac electrophysiologic effects of lidocaine and bupivacaine. Anesth Analg 67:107, 1988
18. Clarkson CW, Hondeghem LM: Mechanism for bupivacaine depression of cardiac conduction. Anesthesiology 62:382, 1985
19. Kasten GW: Amide local anesthetic alterations of effective refractory period temporal dispersion. Anesthesiology 65:61, 1986
20. Heavner JE: Cardiac dysrhythmias induced by infusion of local anesthetics into the lateral cerebral ventricles of cats. Anesth Analg 65:133, 1986
21. Hockman CS, Mauck HP, Hoff EC: ECG changes resulting from cerebral stimulation. Am Heart J 71:695, 1967
22. Thomas RD, Behbehani MM, Coyle DE, Denson DD: Cardiovascular toxicity of local anesthetics. Anesth Analg 65:444, 1986
23. Lynch C: Depression of myocardial contractility in vitro by bupivacaine, etidocaine, and lidocaine. Anesth Analg 65:551, 1986
24. Johns RA, DiFazio CA, Longnecker DE: Lidocaine constricts or dilates rat arterioles in a dose dependent manner. Anesthesiology 61:A204, 1984
25. Coriat P, Harari A, Ducardonet A, et al: The risk of advanced heart block during extradural anaesthesia in

patients with right bundle branch block and left anterior hemiblock. Br J Anaesth 53:545, 1981
26. Smith AR, Hur D, Resano F: Grand mal seizures after 2-chloroprocaine epidural anesthesia in a patient with plasma cholinersterase deficiency. Anesth Analg 66:677, 1987
27. Howie MB, Candler E, Mortimer W, et al: Does Nifedipine enhance the cardiovascular toxicity of bupivacaine? Anesthesiology 63:A225, 1985
28. Tallman RD, Rosenblatt RM, Weaver JM, Wang Y: Verapamil increases the toxicity of local anesthetics. J Clin Pharmacol 28:317, 1988
29. Edouard A, Froideuaux R, Berdeaux A, et al: Bupivacaine accentuates the cardiovascular depressant effect of verapamil in conscious dogs. Eur J Anesthesiol 4:249, 1987
30. Timour Q, Freqsz M, Betrix L, et al: Drug interactions and intraventricular conduction disorders induced by bupivacaine. Anesthesiology 69:A867, 1988
31. Thorburn J, Louden JR, Vallance R: Spinal and general anaesthesia in total hip replacement: frequency of deep vein thrombosis. Br J Anaesth 52:1117, 1980
32. Modig J, Borg T, Karlstrom G, et al: Thromboembolism after total hip replacement: role of epidural and general anesthesia. Anesth Anesth 62:174, 1983
33. Shulman M, Sandler AN, Bradley JW, et al: Post thoracotomy pain and pulmonary function following epidural and systemic morphine. Anesthesiology 61:569, 1984
34. Rawal N, Sjöstrand U, Christoffersson E, et al: Comparison of intramuscular and epidural morphine for postoperative analgesia in the grossly obese: influence on postoperative ambulation and pulmonary function Anesth Analg 63:583, 1984
35. Freysz M, Timour Q, Mazze RI, et al: Potentiation by mild hypothermia of ventricular conduction disturbances and reentrant arrhythmias induced by bupivacaine in dogs. Anesthesiology 70:799, 1989
36. Caplan RA, Ward RJ, Posner K, Cheney FW: Unexpected cardiac arrest during spinal anesthesia. Anesthesiology 68:5, 1988
37. Hood JDD, Dewan DM, James FM: Maternal and fetal effects of epinephrine in gravid ewes. Anesthesiology 64:610, 1986
38. Cartwright PD, McCarroll SM, Antzaka C: Maternal heart rate change with a plain epidural test dose. Anesthesiology 65:226, 1986
39. Albright GA, Jouppila R, Hollmen AI, et al: Epinephrine does not alter human intervillous blood flow. Anesthesiology 54:131, 1981
40. Moore DC, Batra MS: Components of an effective test dose prior to epidural Anesthesia. Anesthesiology 55:693, 1981
41. Englesson S, Grevsten J: The influence of acid-base changes on central nervous system toxicity of local anesthetics agents. Acta Anaesthesiol Scand 18:88, 1974
42. Kasten GW, Martin ST: Resuscitation from bupivacaine induced cardiovascular toxicity during partial inferior vena cava occlusion. Anesth Analg 65:341, 1986
43. DePace NL, Betesh JS, Kotler MN: 'Postmortem' cesarean section with recovery of both mother and offspring. JAMA 248:971, 1982
44. Sanders AB, Kern KB, Ewy GA, et al: Resuscitation from cardiac arrest with open-chest massage. Ann Emerg Med 13:672, 1984

INTRASPINAL OPIOIDS IN THE MANAGEMENT OF OBSTETRIC PAIN

After Queen Victoria accepted chloroform during the delivery of Prince Leopold, the concept of pain relief during childbirth became more socially accepted. Opioids have been used to provide pain relief for thousands of years and a wide variety of these drugs have been employed in an attempt to provide analgesia for childbirth. However, until recently, even marginally effective pain relief for labor required relatively large parenteral doses that were often associated with maternal or fetal sedation and respiratory depression. The discovery of opioid receptors in the spinal cord presented the intriguing possibility that narcotic agonists could be locally administered to specific receptors to produce analgesia, while minimizing systemic effects. Such an approach has theoretical advantages for the pregnant patient as it might significantly reduce fetal exposure to opioids.

In 1979, Behar et al.[1] first used epidural morphine and Wang et al.[2] reported the use of subarachnoid morphine, both in the clinical setting. Studies on the effects of epidural opioids in the pregnant patient followed in rapid succession. The epidural route has been especially attractive, as the incidence of post-dural puncture headache is increased in pregnant patients and epidural local anesthetics are being used with increasing frequency for labor and delivery.

Extensive animal and human studies have not demonstrated neurotoxicity with any commercially available, preservative-free opioid agent administered via the epidural or spinal route.[3] Epidural opioids appear to exert most of their effect on receptors in the substantia gelatinosa of the spinal cord.[4] Presumably, epidurally administered opioids reach these receptors via the cerebrospinal fluid (CSF), following direct penetration of the dura, as well as by passing around nerve root sleeves.[5] Opioids given via the epidural space also diffuse into the systemic circulation with resultant measurable blood concentrations comparable to levels seen with intramuscular parenteral administration. The rate at which these processes occur depends on the physicochemical properties of the opioid (e.g., the rate is directly proportional to lipid solubility and inversely proportional to molecular weight).[3]

Clinically, opioids can be classified as lipid insoluble (e.g., morphine), which tend to have a delayed onset of action and long duration of effect, or lipid soluble (e.g., fentanyl), which tend to have a shorter onset time but shorter duration of effect. The clinical epidural:spinal ratio (i.e., the dose of opioid required to exert a clinical effect when given via the epidural route as compared to the subarachnoid route) is about 10:1 for morphine. Morphine is not rapidly taken up into tissue following intraspinal administration and a slow cephalad spread in the CSF can occur; this can result in delayed respiratory depression. Fentanyl, which is 600 times more lipid soluble than morphine, has a clinical epidural/spinal ratio of about 3:1. Since it is bound tightly within the central nervous system (CNS), there is minimal CSF redistribution and thus minimal risk of respiratory depression.[3] Nevertheless, when fentanyl is administered epidurally, significant plasma levels occur that can approach those observed after parenteral administration.

Nausea, vomiting, pruritus, and urinary retention are side effects that can occur with any μ-agonist given by the epidural or subarachnoid route. Often, these side effects can be managed with small intravenous doses of naloxone, which usually can be titrated to relieve the side effect without antagonizing analgesia. Butorphanol, a κ-agonist, given epidurally, causes minimal nausea and pruritus and may actually be useful epidurally in combination with μ-agonists to minimize these side effects.[6]

Clinically effective epidural doses of morphine or fentanyl result in small but detectable blood levels of opioid. Comparable doses of opioid given epidurally instead of parenterally produce more profound analgesia and are of greater duration. Thus smaller doses given less often can be used. This minimizes peak maternal plasma levels and resultant fetal exposure. The recent resurgence of interest in the subarachnoid route for opioids in labor may further reduce this fetal exposure.

ANALGESIA FOR LABOR AND DELIVERY

Spinal opioids for the management of labor pain, either alone or in combination with local anesthetics, may provide analgesia without causing motor and sympathetic block.

Subarachnoid Opioids

In 1979, Yaksh and co-workers[7] reported that subarachnoid morphine produced analgesia in pregnant rats. Early reports of subarachnoid morphine in humans for labor were enthusiastic and controversial.[8] It soon became clear that subarachnoid morphine, while useful in early labor, did not consistently provide adequate pain relief for the second stage.[9,10] Subarachnoid morphine was also associated with a high incidence of side effects, including somnolence, severe pruritus, and nausea and vomiting. However, Brookshire et al.[11] found that an intravenous infusion of naloxone could significantly reduce the side effects without inhibiting the analgesia provided by subarachnoid morphine 1 mg.

The use of subarachnoid morphine without combination with local anesthetic has found limited application for the relief of labor pain in recent years. For example, Abboud and associates[12] reported the successful use of preservative-free morphine 1 mg with 7.5 percent dextrose in a parturient with severe pulmonary hypertension, in whom pain relief without sympathetic blockade was essential.

The goal of providing labor analgesia with a single dose of subarachnoid opioid is laudable and other efforts have been made. Subarachnoid opioid administration may eventually prove to be a simple method of providing at least partial analgesia for labor in hospitals where conventional epidural coverage is unavailable or impractical. Leighton et al.[13] recently reported the use of a combination of subarachnoid morphine and fentanyl. Theoretically, the fentanyl should provide rapid onset and the morphine should provide prolonged duration of analgesia. Morphine 0.25 mg was administered with fentanyl 25 μg through a single dural puncture early in the first stage of labor. Analgesia was achieved in less than 5 minutes and lasted until delivery (3 to 3.5 h) in 60 percent of the patients. The remaining 40 percent ultimately required conventional lumbar epidural anesthesia with local anesthetics. The risk of delayed respiratory depression limits increasing the dose of subarachnoid morphine to further prolong the duration of analgesia. Perhaps a safer and more controllable approach would utilize continuous subarachnoid infusion of a highly lipid-soluble agent such as fentanyl through a subarachnoid catheter. However, until recently, only relatively large catheter (19 and 20 gauge) and needle (17 and 18 gauge) combinations were available. Dural punctures with these needles were associated with a prohibitively high rate of postdural puncture headache. In 1989, the Food and Drug Administration approved a 32-gauge polyimide catheter for continuous spinal anesthesia. This microcatheter (Microspinal, TFX Medical, Duluth, GA) will pass through the lumen of a standard 25- or 26-gauge spinal needle. We used one of these microcatheters to provide labor analgesia with subarachnoid meperidine for a patient with a history of allergy to amide and ester local anesthetics. Meperidine is apparently unique in that it has some local anesthetic as well as spinal opioid receptor activity.[14] Perineal surgery[15] and cesarean delivery[16] have been performed with subarachnoid meperidine alone.

Oyama and co-workers,[17] in 1980, reported the use of synthetic β-endorphin administered subarachnoid to women in labor. The results were amazing. Labor pain in all 14 patients disappeared completely within 3 to 4 minutes and this analgesia lasted 12 to 32 hours. Side effects were minimal and all infants appeared normal. The relatively large size (3,300 daltons) of β-endorphin limited diffusion through the dura and necessitated subarachnoid placement of the drug. Subarachnoid administration may be advantageous, however, since it risks little or no transmission to the fetus. Unfortunately, the cost of the drug is prohibitive and appropriate toxicity testing should be accomplished before further studies are done.

Although the subarachnoid route for labor analgesia is not frequently used by the clinician today, the future of this approach for relief of labor pain with subarachnoid opioids and epidural opioid-local anesthetic combinations appears bright.

Epidural Opioids

Administration of opioids via the epidural space for labor is becoming increasingly popular. The effect of epidural opioids is complicated by the need for the drug to cross the dura and by the presence of a rich venous epidural plexus that absorbs the drug and is often distended secondary to the inferior vena caval obstruction associated with pregnancy. As a consequence of these effects, the use of epidural opioids alone has generally proved to be of limited utility as a labor analgesic.[18,19] However, they are useful in combination with local anesthetics.

Morphine. As the only currently approved opioid for intraspinal use, morphine is a logical choice for combination with bupivacaine for labor anesthesia. Niv et al.[20] added epidural morphine 2 mg to 0.25 percent bupivacaine and significantly increased the duration of pain relief before reinforcement. Pruritus was the only significant side effect observed and no neonatal depression was seen. The slow onset of morphine (30 to 60 min) and relatively high incidence of side effects (pruritus, nausea, vomiting, and potential respiratory depression) will likely prevent widespread clinical acceptance of this technique.

Butorphanol. Butorphanol, a κ-agonist and weak μ-agonist–antagonist, is a commonly administered systemic opioid for labor and has been demonstrated to be quite safe. Hunt et al.[21] suggested that butorphanol 2 mg added to 0.25 percent bupivacaine 8.5 to 10 ml was the optimal dose for epidural anesthesia during labor. The duration of analgesia was significantly greater and the time to onset of analgesia significantly shorter than when no butorphanol was added. The most common maternal side effect was somnolence, which was occasionally accompanied by an altered sensorium. Care must be taken not to administer this drug to patients who are physically dependent on opioids since this agonist–antagonist drug may precipitate an acute withdrawal syndrome even when given epidurally.[22]

Nalbuphine. Nalbuphine, a κ-agonist, is now available in preservative-free solution. After appropriate testing for neurotoxicity, one can assume that nalbuphine will be administered into the epidural and subarachnoid spaces with and without local anesthetics to determine its efficacy in providing pain relief during labor and postoperatively.

Sufentanil and Alfentanil. As might be expected, epidural alfentanil and sufentanil are now being studied alone or in combination with bupivacaine during labor. Heytens et al.[23] used epidural alfentanil alone in 16 primiparous patients at an infusion rate of 30 μg/kg/h, with boluses of 30 μg/kg as needed. Excellent pain relief was rapidly obtained in early labor but analgesia was inadequate for the latter part of stage I and stage II. The Amiel-Tison Neonatal Neurologic and Adaptive Capacity (NACS) examination revealed significant hypotonia. A preliminary report[24] suggests that combining lower-dose alfentanil with bupivacaine can provide excellent pain relief for labor with no detectable neonatal depression.

Sufentanil should be attractive because of its very high lipid solubility and affinity for the μ-receptor. Van Steenberge et al.[25] and Phillips[26] showed that sufentanil in combination with bupivacaine provided prolonged pain relief, reduced the total bupivacaine dose, and gave limited motor block. However, in the epidural space, sufentanil appears to be only two to three times more potent than fentanyl, whereas systematically it is five to 10 times more potent. Therefore, unintentional intravascular injection of sufentanil 30 μg would be likely to cause respiratory depression and has recently been reported to have done so (Ostheimer GW, personal communication). Van Steenberge did find epidural sufentanil to be associated with maternal dizziness and lowered 1-minute Apgar scores, which may indicate significant systemic absorption. Sufentanil is also associated with significantly more pruritus and nausea and is more expensive then fentanyl.

Fentanyl. The most popular narcotic for use in labor is undoubtedly fentanyl. Justins et al.,[27] in 1982, added fentanyl 80 μg to 0.5 percent bupivacaine 3 ml. Since then Youngstrom et al.[28] in 1984, Skerman et al.,[29] Vella et al.,[30] and Cohen et al.[31] in 1987, and Cellano and Copogna[32] and Chestnut et al.[33] in 1988 have touted the efficacy of the combination of bupivacaine and fentanyl. Bupivacaine concentrations as low as 0.028 percent combined with fentanyl 100 μg have provided adequate pain relief for labor.

Respondents to a recent survey at the annual meeting of the Society for Obstetric Anesthesia and Perinatology indicated that 56 percent used epidural opioids for labor, with the vast majority favoring fentanyl. The solutions most popular were fentanyl 50 to 100 μg in 0.25 or 0.125 percent bupivacaine 10 ml. About 20 percent of the respondents used fentanyl in an infusion; the preferred solution was fentanyl 1 to 2 μg/ml in 0.125 percent bupivacaine, which was administered at rates of 8 to 10 ml/h.

ANALGESIA FOR CESAREAN DELIVERY AND POSTOPERATIVE PAIN RELIEF

The recommended doses of subarachnoid and epidural opioids for cesarean delivery and postoperative pain relief are listed in Table 3-20.

Table 3-20. Recommended Doses of Subarachnoid and Epidural Opioids for Cesarean Delivery and Postoperative Pain Relief

	Dose	Onset	Duration
Subarachnoid			
Morphine sulfate	0.2–0.3 mg	30–45 min	12–15 h
Fentanyl	10–20 μg	5 min	2–4 h
Epidural			
Morphine sulfate	2–3 mg/ up to 10 ml NS	45–60 min	12–18 h
Fentanyl	50–100 μg/ 10 ml NS	5 min	2–3 h
Sufentanil	25–50 μg/ 10 ml NS	3–5 min	2–4 h
Butorphanol	1–2 mg/ 10 ml NS	10–15 min	3–5 h

NS, normal saline.

Subarachnoid Opioids

Subarachnoid morphine has been used successfully in many types of surgery, including cesarean delivery. A high incidence of side effects, including life-threatening respiratory depression, can be seen if doses greater than 0.5 mg are used. Chadwick and Ready[34] concluded that subarachnoid morphine sulfate in doses of 0.3 to 0.5 mg provided similar postoperative analgesia to epidural morphine 3 to 5 mg but with greater duration and no greater side effects. Two especially interesting reports in 1988 by Abboud et al.[35] and Abouleish et al.[36] showed that morphine 0.1, 0.2, and 0.25 mg mixed with hyperbaric bupivacaine provided excellent postoperative analgesia and may cause less respiratory depression than standard subcutaneous morphine injection. Hunt et al.[37] showed that fentanyl in doses as low as 6.25 μg is also an effective subarachnoid adjunct that provides effective postoperative analgesia for 3 to 4 hours.

Epidural Opioids

Epidural morphine, fentanyl, and butorphanol have been studied for cesarean delivery. Hughes[38] reported 1,700 consecutive patients who had received epidural morphine with excellent long-lasting postoperative analgesia. Four patients were noted to have respiratory depression, two required treatment with naloxone, and one was seriously acidotic. The issue of monitoring patients after intraspinal morphine is controversial (see Monitoring of the Obstetric Patient Receiving Intraspinal Opioids, below).

Fentanyl is the most popular opioid for epidural use in cesarean delivery. Fentanyl appears to be very safe, with 50 μg giving pain relief lasting approximately 2 to 3 hours.[39] Fentanyl 50 μg should be diluted in at least 10 ml of preservative free normal saline (or local anesthetic) for fastest onset and longest duration.[40] Epidural fentanyl augments intraoperative anesthesia with epidural bupivacaine[41] or lidocaine[42] and may reduce the incidence of peripartum shivering.[43] Thus it is advantageous to give the epidural fentanyl once the epidural block has been established and prior to delivery. An additional dose of fentanyl 50 μg in normal saline 10 ml can be given postoperatively just prior to removal of the epidural catheter to provide several hours of analgesia after the resolution of the local anesthetic block.

While the effects of epidural lidocaine and bupivacaine[41,42] are additive with epidural fentanyl, chloroprocaine is antagonistic. Malinow et al.[44] found no clinically significant period of fentanyl analgesia after 3 percent chloroprocaine was administered epidurally for cesarean delivery. The low pH of chloroprocaine

(3.3 to 3.5) or some secondary metabolite may be responsible for this interaction.

Epidural sufentanil has also been studied in patients undergoing cesarean delivery. Doses of 30 to 50 μg diluted in preservative free normal saline 10 ml provided analgesia with onset and duration similar to fentanyl.[45] At clinically effective doses, it is associated with a greater incidence of nausea and pruritus than fentanyl.[37] Interestingly, in epidural doses of 50 μg or greater, sufentanil can abolish shivering and effect maternal temperature control in a dose-dependent fashion.[42,44–47]

Epidural sufentanil appears to offer little advantage over fentanyl in the setting of cesarean delivery and it presents significantly greater risk. Should the epidural catheter become intravascular, a dose of 30 to 50 μg could precipitate respiratory depression or chest wall rigidity.

Epidural butorphanol, in doses of 1 to 2 mg,[21] has also been studied in patients following cesarean delivery. It has an onset of 15 to 20 minutes and a duration of 3 to 4 hours. It has not been associated with pruritus or significant respiratory depression. Naulty et al.[6] reported on the uses of an epidural butorphanol–fentanyl combination to minimize side effects of fentanyl. Epidural butorphanol can produce some maternal sedation and may affect the fetal heart rate, producing a sinusoidal-type pattern. No evidence of fetal distress has been detected by scalp capillary block pH monitoring. It may be most useful for postoperative analgesia after the fetus is delivered.

FETAL TOXICITY AND INTRASPINAL OPIOIDS

The considerable advantages of intraspinal opioids must always be weighed against the possibility of fetal depression. Drugs administered to the mother are transported rapidly to the uterus and the concentrations of free drug available to cross the placenta will depend on the agent, total dose, route of administration, lipid solubility, pK_a, maternal pH, protein binding, metabolism, and excretion.[3] All commercially available narcotics have low molecular weights and readily cross the placenta by diffusion.[48]

Although there is an extensive literature concerning maternal effects of intraspinal morphine, evaluation of the infant has most often been confined to Apgar scores or the occurrence of apnea. Subtle effects of drugs on the neonate require subtle neurobehavioral tests. However, most investigators would agree that the risk of neonatal depression with epidural morphine appears to increase with higher doses and shorter interval between dosing and delivery time because of higher maternal blood levels of morphine.[49] The prolonged onset, the high incidence of maternal side effects, and the risk of delayed respiratory depression have limited the use of epidural morphine in laboring patients.

Fentanyl has an impressive safety record. Neonatal depression has only been reported with very high repeated epidural doses. When administered by the epidural route, fentanyl produces peak plasma levels similar to those produced by the same dose given intramuscularly. Gaffud et al.[41] administered fentanyl 100 μg epidurally approximately 20 minutes before cesarean delivery. Theoretically this should produce near maximal fetal exposure. They found that epidural fentanyl 100 μg resulted in an average umbilical artery concentration of 0.8 ng/ml. This is below the concentration implicated in respiratory depression of the neonate.[50] In another study, the optimal dose of epidural fentanyl in the parturient was determined to be 50 μg[40] in normal saline 10 ml, which should minimize fetal exposure and possible depression.

Phillips[26] has compiled much of the data regarding the use of epidural sufentanil. Undetectable levels in maternal venous and umbilical cord blood are consistent with very high lipid solubility of this drug. Overall, 156 parturients received sufentanil with only one study reporting a decrease in the mean Apgar scores. Unfortunately, neurobehavioral testing of the neonate has not been reported.

While the published evaluations are few, alfentanil has been associated with neonatal depression. Heytens et al.[23] continuously infused epidural alfentanil alone and stopped at the onset of the second stage of labor. Although Apgar scores and umbilical blood gas values were normal, the NACS showed significant depression of active and passive tone. Again, subtle effects require subtle evaluations. More recent work using much lower doses of alfentanil may be promising.[51]

Butorphanol in epidural doses of 1 to 2 mg is not usually associated with respiratory depression. Thus far, neonatal depression has not been seen. However, butorphanol given via epidural or other parenteral routes may be associated with a low amplitude–high frequency sinusoidal-like fetal heart rate pattern.[52] This pattern usually resolves spontaneously and is usually associated with normal fetal scalp capillary blood pH.

REFERENCES

1. Behar M, Magora F, Olshwang D, Davidson JT: Epidural morphine in treatment of pain. Lancet 1:527, 1979
2. Wang JK, Nauss LE, Thomas JE: Pain relief by intrathecally applied morphine in man. Anesthesiology 50:149, 1979
3. Cousins MJ, Mather LE: Intrathecal and epidural administration of opioids. Anesthesiology 61:276, 1984

4. Calvillo O, Henry JL, Neuman RS: Effects of morphine and naloxone on dorsal horn neurons in the cat. Can J Physiol Pharmacol 52:1207, 1974
5. Ketahata LM, Kosaka Y, Taub A: Lamina-specific suppression of dorsal horn unit activity by morphine sulfate. Anesthesiology 41:39, 1974
6. Naulty JS, Labove P, Datta S, et al: Epidural butorphanol/fentanyl for post-cesarean delivery analgesia. Anesthesiology 67:A463, 1987
7. Yaksh TL, Wilson RP, Kaiko RF, Intrussi CE: Analgesia produced by a spinal action of morphine and effects upon parturition in the rat. Anesthesiology 51:386, 1979
8. Alper MH: Intrathecal morphine; a new method of obstetric analgesia? Anesthesiology 51:378, 1979
9. Scott PV, Bowen FE, Cartwright P, et al: Intrathecal morphine as sole analgesic during labour. Br Med J 281:351, 1980
10. Baracca A, Noueihed R, Najj S: Intrathecal injection of morphine for obstetric analgesia. Anesthesiology 54:136, 1981
11. Brookshire GL, Shnider SM, Abboud TK, et al: Effects of naloxone on the mother and neonate after intrathecal morphine for labor analgesia. Anesthesiology 59:A417, 1983
12. Abboud TK, Raya J, Noueihed R, Daniel J: Intrathecal morphine for relief of labor pain in a parturient with severe pulmonary hypertension. Anesthesiology 59:477, 1983
13. Leighton BL, DeSimone CA, Norris MC, Ben-David B: Intrathecal narcotics revisited: the combination of fentanyl and morphine intrathecally provides rapid onset of profound, prolonged analgesia. Anesth Analg 69:122, 1989
14. Famewo CE, Naguiob M: Spinal anaesthesia with meperidine as the sole agent. Can Anaesth Soc J 32:533, 1985
15. Acalouschi I, Ene V, Lorinezi E, Nicholaus F: Saddle block with pethidine for perineal operations. Br J Anaesth 58:1012, 1986
16. Talafre ML, Jacquinot P, Legagneux F, et al: Intrathecal administration of meperidine versus tetracaine for elective cesarean section. Anesthesiology 67:A620, 1987
17. Oyama T, Matsuki A, Taneichi T, et al: Beta-endorphin in obstetric analgesia. Am J Obstet Gynecol 137:613, 1980
18. Husemeyer RP, O'Connor MC, Davenport HT: Failure of epidural morphine to relieve pain in labour. Anaesthesia 35:161, 1980
19. Writer WDR, James FM, Wheeler AS: Double blind comparison of morphine and bupivacaine for continuous epidural analgesia in labor. Anesthesiology 54:215, 1981
20. Niv D, Rudick V, Golan A, Chayen MS: Augmentation of bupivacaine analgesia by epidural morphine. Obstet Gynecol 67:206, 1986
21. Hunt CO, Naulty JS, Malinow AM, et al: Epidural butorphanol-bupivacaine for analgesia during labor and delivery. Anesth Analg 68:323, 1989
22. Weintraub SJ, Naulty JS: Acute abstinence syndrome after epidural injection of butorphanol. Anesth Analg 64:452, 1985
23. Heytens L, Cammu H, Camu F: Extradural analgesia using alfentanil. Br J Anaesth 59:331, 1987
24. Carp H, Johnson MD, Bader AM: Continuous epidural infusion of alfentanil and bupivacaine for labor and delivery. Anesthesiology 69:A687, 1988
25. Van Steenberge A, DeBroux HC, Noorduin H: Extradural bupivacaine with sufentanil for vaginal delivery: a double-blind trial. Br J Anaesth 59:1518, 1987
26. Phillips G: Continuous infusion of epidural analgesia in labor—the effect of adding sufentanil to 0.125% bupivacaine. Anesth Analg 67:462, 1988
27. Justins DM, Francis D, Houlton PG, Reynolds F: A controlled trial of extradural fentanyl in labour. Br J Anaesth 54:409, 1982
28. Youngstrom P, Sedensky M, Frankmann D, Spagnuolo S: Continuous epidural infusion of low-dose bupivacaine-fentanyl for labor analgesia. Anesthesiology 69:686, 1988
29. Skerman JH, Thompson BA, Goldstein MT, et al: Combined continuous epidural fentanyl and bupivacaine in labor: a randomised study. Anesthesiology 63:A450, 1985
30. Vella LM, Willatts DG, Knott C, et al: Epidural fentanyl in labour. Anaesthesia 40:741, 1985
31. Cohen SE, Tan S, Albright GA, Halpern J: Epidural fentanyl/bupivacaine for obstetric analgesia. Anesthesiology 67:403, 1987
32. Cellano D, Capogna G: Epidural fentanyl plus bupivacaine 0.125 per cent for labour: analgesic effects. Can J Anaesth 35:375, 1988
33. Chestnut DH, Owen CL, Bates JN, et al: Continuous infusion epidural analgesia during labor: a randomized, double-blind comparison of 0.0625% bupivacaine/0.0002% fentanyl versus 0.125% bupivacaine. Anesthesiology 68:754, 1988
34. Chadwick HS, Ready LB: Intrathecal and epidural morphine sulfate for post cesarean analgesia. Anesthesiology 68:925, 1988
35. Abboud TK, Dror A, Mosaad P, et al: Mini-dose intrathecal morphine for the relief of postcesarean section pain. Anesth Analg 67:370, 1988
36. Abouleish E, Rawal N, Fallon K, Hernandez D: Combined morphine and bupivacaine for cesarean section. Anesth Analg 67:370, 1988
37. Hunt CO, Naulty JS, Bader AM, et al: Perioperative analgesia with subarachnoid fentanyl-bupivacaine. Anesthesiology 67:A621, 1987
38. Hughes SC: Intraspinal narcotics in obstetrics. Clin Perinatol 1:167, 1982
39. Naulty JS, Datta S, Ostheimer GW, et al: Epidural fentanyl for postcesarean delivery pain management. Anesthesiology 63:694, 1985
40. Birnbach DJ, Johnson MD, Arcario T, et al: Effect of diluent volume on analgesia produced by epidural fentanyl. Anesth Analg 68:808, 1989
41. Gaffud MP, Bansal P, Lawton C, et al: Surgical analgesia for cesarean delivery with epidural bupivacaine and fentanyl. Anesthesiology 65:331, 1986
42. Preston PG, Rosen MA, Hughes SC, et al: Epidural anesthesia with fentanyl and lidocaine for cesarean section: Maternal effects and neonatal outcome. Anesthesiology 68:938, 1988

43. Matthews NC: Epidural fentanyl for shaking in obstetrics. Anaesthesia 43:783, 1988
44. Malinow A, et al: Choice of local anesthetics affects postcesarean epidural fentanyl analgesia. Reg Anesth 15:141, 1988
45. Tan S, Cohen SE, White PF: Sufentanil for analgesia after cesarean section: intravenous versus epidural administration. Anesth Analg 65:S158, 1986
46. Rosen MA, Dailey PA, Hughes SC, et al: Epidural sufentanil for postoperative analgesia after cesarean section. Anesthesiology 68:448, 1988
47. Sevarino FB, Johnson MD, Lema MJ, et al: The effect of epidural sufentanil on shivering and body temperature in the parturient. Anesth Analg 68:530, 1989
48. Hug CC: Pharmacokinetics of new synthetic narcotic analgesics. p. 52. In Estafanous FG (ed): Opioids in Anesthesia. Butterworths, Boston, 1984
49. Nybell-Lindahl G, Carisson C, Ingemarsson I, et al: Maternal and fetal concentrations of morphine after epidural administration during labor. Am J Obstet Gynecol 139:20, 1981
50. Milon D, Bentue-Ferrer D, Noury D, et al: Anesthesie peridurale pour cesarienne par association bupivacaine-fentanyl. Ann Fr Anesth Reanim 2:273, 1983
51. Ray NL, Datta S, Johnson MD: Continuous infusion of epidural bupivacaine with fentanyl or alfentanil. SOAP Abstracts, 1989
52. Hutjis CG, Meis PJ: Sinusoidal fetal heart rate pattern associated with butorphanol administration. Obstet Gynecol 67:377, 1986

FETAL AND NEONATAL EFFECTS OF INTRASPINAL OPIOIDS

Epidural and subarachnoid opioids have several potential advantages when used for obstetric analgesia.[1] When administered alone, there is no sympathetic block. Hypotension, a frequent problem when local anesthetics are used, is avoided. Motor block is also absent. The motor block experienced with local anesthetics may be distressing to the parturient and may decrease her expulsive efforts during the second stage of labor. However, opioids are rarely administered alone for labor and delivery as analgesia is often inadequate. To overcome this problem, administration of combinations of local anesthetics with opioids has become standard practice. These combinations administered epidurally for labor analgesia result in improved pain relief, reduced local anesthesia requirements, and less motor block. For cesarean delivery, both epidural and subarachnoid administration of narcotic with local anesthetic provide improved intraoperative anesthesia and postoperative analgesia.

Despite these advantages, the exposure of the fetus to opioids should be considered. The desire to avoid fetal exposure to opioids was one of the motivating forces behind the introduction of intraspinal anesthesia into obstetrics.

PLACENTAL TRANSFER OF DRUGS

Maternally administered drugs are rapidly transported to the uterus, which receives approximately 10 percent of the cardiac output. The concentration of free drug available to cross the placenta will depend on the total dose and route of administration as well as the pK_a of the drug and maternal pH, protein binding, metabolism, and excretion.[2] Drugs cross the placenta by passive diffusion according to Fick's law, which states that the rate of diffusion is proportional to the concentration gradient, that is, to the change in concentration per unit length in the direction of diffusion. Diffusion is enhanced by a high uterine artery concentration of a drug that has a low molecular weight and is lipid soluble, nonionized, and minimally protein bound. The concentration of free drug in the umbilical artery will depend on the concentration of drug entering the fetal circulation via the umbilical vein and other factors, including fetal pH, protein binding, tissue uptake, metabolism and excretion. All opioids have low molecular weights and readily cross the placenta (Table 3-21). Differences in placental transfer can be anticipated from the differences in the physiochemical properties of the different drugs.

EPIDURAL OPIOIDS

Morphine

Morphine has been one of the most extensively studied opioids. In postsurgical patients, Weddel and Ritter examined epidural morphine in clinically administered doses of 5 or 10 mg per 70 kg of body weight.[3] The serum levels they reported, 28.0 ± 20.6 ng/ml after 5 mg and 49.7 ± 35.6 ng/ml after 10 mg, closely correlated to those following similar doses of intramuscular morphine. Peak concentrations were found between 15 and 30 minutes. Wide variation from patient to patient was noted. Youngstrom et al. examined plasma concentrations of morphine following epidural injection (4 mg) and intramuscular morphine injection (4 mg) in postcesarean patients.[4] Their peak plasma levels following epidural administration were 12.5 ng/ml, approximately half that seen after intramuscular injection, 24.8 ng/ml. The difference between their levels and those of Weddel and Ritter may reflect the small number of patients

Table 3-21. Physicochemical Factors Affecting the Disposition of Opioid Analgesics

	Molecular Weight	pK_a	Percent Non-ionized at pH 7.40	Free Fraction in Human Plasma at pH 7.4	Octanol-Water Partition Coefficient (apparent at pH 7.4)
Morphine	285	7.9	23	70	1.4
Meperidine	247	8.5	7.4	30	39
Fentanyl	336	8.4	8.5	16	816
Alfentanil	417	6.5	89	7.9	89
Sufentanil	386	8.0	20	7.5	1727

(From Hug CC Jr: Pharmacokinetics of new synthetic narcotic analgesics. p. 52. In Estafanous FG (ed): Opioids in Anesthesia. Butterworth, Boston, 1984, with permission.)

studied, differences in sample times, or altered hemodynamics in the pregnant patient.

Only two studies directly examined the placental transfer of morphine to the fetus. First, Craft et al. examined maternal and fetal effects of epidural morphine 5 mg in the chronically instrumented sheep.[5] This study of 10 pregnant ewes documented stable maternal cardiovascular status. Intrauterine pressures were unaffected and uterine blood flow was maintained except for a small decrease at 120 minutes. Even more encouraging were the very low fetal femoral artery morphine levels. It would be tempting to conclude that placental transfer is minimal, however, extrapolation of animal data to humans can be misleading. Nybell-Lindahl et al. examined the plasma concentration of morphine in maternal and cord blood following administration of epidural morphine 4 to 6 mg.[6] The morphine concentrations were almost identical and the greatest concentrations were found with the shortest injection to delivery times. One of the infants experienced respiratory depression at birth and periods of apnea during the first 16 minutes of life.

Neonatal assessment after exposure to epidural morphine has been limited. Husemeyer et al. examined 10 neonates whose mothers were given epidural morphine 2 mg and commented only on the neonatal time to sustained respiration, which occurred within 1 minute in all infants.[7] Booker et al. reported no neonatal central nervous system or cardiovascular depression following epidural morphine 2.5 or 4 mg administered to 25 parturients.[8] Crawford studied eight patients receiving epidural morphine 2 to 6 mg and reported Apgar scores of 8 at 1 and 5 minutes in all infants.[9] Niv et al. compared the combination of 0.25 percent bupivacaine with morphine (2 mg) to plain 0.25 percent bupivacaine and found improved maternal analgesia without neonatal depression as assessed by the Apgar score.[10] However, all of these studies assessed only the vital functions of the neonate.

Subtle effects of drugs require neurologic and neurobehavioral examinations. Writer et al. evaluated infants whose mothers received epidural morphine 2 to 8 mg (mean, 3.25 mg).[11] They found no alterations of the fetal heart rate (FHR) tracing. There was no evidence of neonatal depression as reflected by the Apgar score or umbilical cord gas data. However, at 2 to 6 hours, six infants had "borderline" Early Neonatal Neurobehavioral Scale (ENNS) examinations, which were then normal at 20 to 26 hours. Hughes et al. compared patients given 0.5 percent bupivacaine to those given morphine[12] 2, 5, or 7.5 mg. They found no alterations in the FHR tracing and no neonatal depression as evidenced by normal Apgar scores, cord blood gas analysis and Neurological and Adaptive Capacity Scores (NACS). Although the neurobehavioral assessments were encouraging, the use of the NACS has been questioned because of its abbreviated nature and reliance on the evaluation of motor tone.

In these studies, 131 patients received epidural morphine (Table 3-22). Morphine by itself provided ineffective analgesia and required the subsequent use of a local anesthetic, usually bupivacaine. One infant had evidence of respiratory depression attributed to the narcotic and six infants had neurobehavioral depression when examined using the ENNS. The influence of the local anesthetic was considered to be negligible.

The risk of neonatal depression by epidural morphine appears to be greatest with high doses and when the injection to delivery (I-D) interval is short. The long latency of epidural morphine, the high incidence of maternal side effects and fear of delayed maternal respiratory depression have limited its use in laboring patients.

Meperidine

Husemeyer et al. examined pregnant patients given epidural, intramuscular, or intravenous meperidine.[13] They found similar plasma levels with intravenous and

Table 3-22. Fetal and Neonatal Effects of Epidural Morphine

Investigator	Dose	Patients No.	Reported Effects
Nybell-Lindhal et al.[6a]	4–6 mg	20	One infant had respiratory depression at birth and periods of apnea for the first 16 min
Husemeyer et al.[7a]	2 mg	10	All infants had sustained respiration within 1 minute of delivery
Booker et al.[8a]	2.5 mg or 4 mg	25	No central nervous system or cardiovascular depression
Crawford[9a]	2–6 mg	8	All infants had Apgar scores of 8 at 1 and 5 min
Niv et al.[10a]	2 mg	30	No depression of Apgar scores
Writer et al.[11b]	2–8 mg (× 3.25)	8	No alteration of FHR tracing Apgar scores. Umbilical cord blood gas data similar to control group six infants with "borderline" ENNS at 2 to 6 h, all normal at 20 to 26 h
Hughes et al[12a]	2 mg 5 mg 7.5 mg	9 10 11	No alteration of FHR tracing No depression of Aggar scores, NACS, umbilical cord blood gas data (control group (n = 10) received 0.5% bupivacaine)

[a] Received supplemental bupivacaine.
[b] Received supplemental chloroprocaine.

epidural administration. The umbilical cord plasma meperidine concentrations were similar to the maternal venous samples that were collected at delivery (Fig. 3-12). Infants were considered depressed if the 1-minute Apgar score was <7 or there were any signs of impaired respiration in the first 5 minutes. A total of six infants were depressed, three of whose mothers received epidural meperidine. The highest incidence of neonatal depression was seen when the drug was administered between 2 and 3 hours before delivery. Neonatal depression was not correlated with umbilical cord meperidine concentration and the investigators postulated that me-

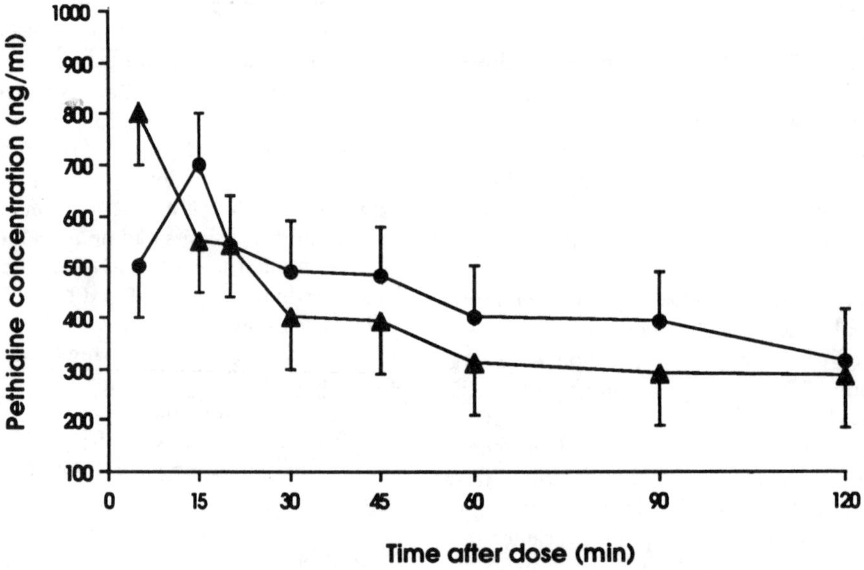

Fig. 3-12. Comparison of mean (± SD) plasma pethidine (meperidine) concentrations after intravenous (▲) and epidural (●) administration of pethidine 100 mg to patients in labor. (From Husemeyer et al.,[13] with permission.)

tabolites of meperidine may have caused the depression of the infants.

As would be expected, Skjoldebrand et al. found much lower plasma concentrations when lower doses of meperidine, 25 mg, were administered epidurally.[14] They also documented a close correlation between maternal and umbilical plasma concentrations. Two of 19 infants had 1-minute Apgar scores of <7 and one of these infants had a 5-minute Apgar score of <7.

Several reports including those by Perriss and Baraka et al. documented the lack of changes on the FHR tracing with epidural meperidine.[15–17] Baraka et al. also evaluated Apgar scores, which were all ≥8 at 5 minutes, and ENNS scores, which were normal. Hammonds et al. did report borderline ENNS scores but they were not different from those whose mothers received 0.125 percent bupivacaine.[18]

In these studies, a total of 89 patients received epidural meperidine, with three infants experiencing respiratory depression (Table 3-23). These mothers had been given the highest dose of meperidine 100 mg.[13] Two infants had low Apgar scores. These infants were delivered by forceps for "threatening asphyxia."[14] It was the opinion of most of the investigators that epidural meperidine should be administered only once and early in the course of labor to minimize the risk of neonatal depression from the cumulative effects of meperidine and its metabolites.

Fentanyl

A potential advantage of epidural fentanyl is the very low plasma concentrations produced by this form of administration. Plasma levels of fentanyl were reported by Wolfe and Davies in 1980 in parturients who received epidural fentanyl 100 μg following cesarean delivery.[19] Only one of four patients had a detectable fentanyl level. However, rapid placental transfer of fentanyl has been confirmed in animal studies with rabbits and sheep.[20–22]

Carrie et al. reported the efficacy of epidural administration of fentanyl 150–200 μg, often as repeated doses in laboring parturients.[23] Umbilical artery levels were much lower than maternal levels measured 30 minutes after administration. Unfortunately, maternal levels at delivery and I–D intervals were not reported. Neonatal evaluation was limited to the Apgar scores at 1 minute, which were 7 to 10 in all infants except one. This infant had an Apgar score of 3 and required intubation, oxygen, and naloxone. The plasma fentanyl level was 0.25 ng/ml. However, the investigators noted that other infants had similar levels and did not experience respiratory depression.

Maternal venous plasma concentrations of fentanyl following epidural or intramuscular administration of fentanyl 100 μg at the same time as the epidural test dose of bupivacaine were examined by Justins et al.[24] Although there was wide interindividual variation, the peak plasma concentrations were higher in the first 10 minutes with the epidural administration (Fig. 3-13). The peak plasma concentrations occurred at 5 to 10 minutes following epidural administration, whereas in the intramuscular group, the plasma levels were still rising at 20 minutes. Unfortunately, plasma levels were measured only for the first 20 minutes. No neonatal respiratory depression was found with these doses.

Youngstrom et al. examined maternal venous and

Table 3-23. Fetal and Neonatal Effects of Epidural Meperidine

Investigator	Dose	Patients No.	Reported Effects
Husemeyer et al.[13]	100 mg	10	Three infants had respiratory depression
Skjoldebrand et al.[14a]	25 mg	19	Two infants had Apgar scores <7 at 1 min, one infant scored <7 at 5 min
Perriss et al.[16]	25–100 mg	12	No effect on the FHR tracing
Perriss et al.[15]	50 mg	20	No effect on the FHR tracing
Baraka et al.[17a]	100 mg	13	No changes in FHR variability, one transient late deceleration All Apgar scores ≥7 at 1 min, ≥8 at 5 min All infants had normal ENNS (compared to 0.25% bupivacaine group)
Hammonds et al.[18]	25 mg	15	No differences in ENNS, borderline scores in both groups (compared to 0.125% bupivacaine group)

[a] Subsequently received 0.25 percent bupivacaine.

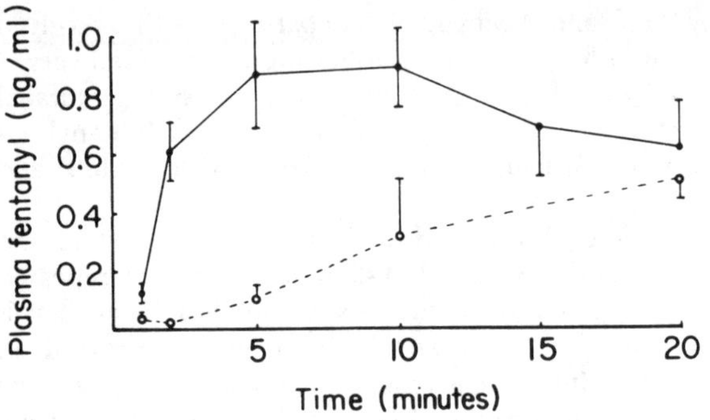

Fig. 3-13. Mean plasma concentrations of fentanyl after epidural fentanyl (-●-) and intramuscular fentanyl (-○-). Vertical bars represent standard errors. The differences between groups are significant at 1 and 10 minutes ($P<0.05$) and at 2 and 5 minutes ($P<0.001$). (From Justins et al.,[24] with permission.)

umbilical venous fentanyl concentrations in patients who received as their initial epidural injection fentanyl 150 μg either alone or with 0.125 percent bupivacaine.[25] The highest maternal concentrations were found with the shortest I–D interval (Table 3-24). Fentanyl was not detected in any of the umbilical samples. Median Apgar scores were 9 at 1 and 5 minutes in both groups. Umbilical venous pH's were within normal limits.

Similarly, low concentrations of fentanyl in maternal blood were found by Skerman et al.[26] They examined fentanyl combined with bupivacaine administered as a continuous infusion. An initial level was established with 0.25 percent bupivacaine with fentanyl 5 μg/ml. Twenty minutes later 0.125 percent bupivacaine with fentanyl 2.5 μg/ml was infused at 10 ml/h. They noted an increase in maternal plasma concentration as the duration of infusion increased, although exact values were not reported. Umbilical cord blood revealed undetectable fentanyl levels. There was no evidence of neonatal depression and Apgar scores were normal. Continuous epidural infusions have also been studied by Chestnut et al.[27] They found no difference in Apgar scores or umbilical cord blood gas data when 0.0625 percent bupivacaine with fentanyl 2 μg/ml was compared to 0.125 percent bupivacaine.

Several other studies of epidural fentanyl have confirmed the lack of adverse effects on the neonate. Vella et al. reported no neonatal depression with fentanyl administered as an epidural bolus (80 μg) or as an infusion to produce similar plasma levels.[28] Gaffud et al. found no difference in Apgar scores when parturients received either 0.5 percent bupivacaine alone or with fentanyl 100 μg for cesarean delivery.[29] Preston et al. compared two groups of patients who received 2 percent lidocaine epidurally for cesarean delivery with or without fentanyl (1 μg/kg).[30] There were no differences between groups in Apgar scores or neurobehavioral examinations (NACS). Fentanyl was detected in only one umbilical venous sample (0.24 ng/ml).

Cohen et al. have extensively evaluated the neonate.[31] They investigated four groups. Three groups received 0.025% bupivacaine with fentanyl 0, 50, or 100 μg. The fourth group received 0.068 percent bupivacaine and fentanyl 100 μg. There were several incidences of fetal bradycardia resembling one another. The only difference found was in the time to sustained respiration, which was longest in the control group. One neonate in the control group required mask ventilation. There was no difference in the incidence of low Apgar scores or low NACS. Umbilical blood gas analyses were within the normal range.

Capogna et al. also evaluated two groups of neonates whose mothers received bupivacaine with or without fentanyl 100 μg.[32] There were 13 control parturients and 29 who received fentanyl. All Apgar scores were >7 at 1 and 5 minutes. Neonates were also evaluated with the ENNS. The fentanyl group infants were noted to have more vigorous truncal tone and placing. By 24 hours, there were no differences between groups. Further, no effect was noted on the lability of state, which reflects the neonate's ability to maintain control of his reactions to environmental stimuli. The capacity to habituate, a measure of pharmacologic depression, was similar in both groups.

In these studies, fentanyl was administered to 286 parturients with only one case of neonatal depression (Table 3-25). Fentanyl appears to be the safest narcotic to administer epidurally. There are very low maternal

Table 3-24. Plasma Concentrations after Epidural Fentanyl, 150 μg

I–D Interval (h)	Patients No.	Maternal Conc. (ng/ml)	Cord Conc. (ng/ml)
0–1	1	0.65 <0.10[a]	
1–2	7	0.41 ± 0.18[b]	<0.10[a]
2–3	6	0.26 (0.06)	<0.10[a]
3–4	6	0.15 (0.03)	<0.10[a]
4–5	3	0.13 (0.04)	<0.10[a]
5–6	4	0.11 (0.05)	<0.10[a]
>6	7	<0.10[a]	

[a] Limit of detection 0.10 ng/ml with ± 10 percent precision at levels of 0.5 ng/ml.
[b] Mean ± standard deviation.
(Modifed from Youngstrom et al.[25] with permission.)

Table 3-25. Fetal and Neonatal Effects of Epidural Fentanyl

Investigator	Dose	Patients No.	Reported Effects
Carrie et al.[23a]	150–200 μg 15 repeated doses	38	One infant with 1-min Apgar score of 3 requiring resuscitation
Justins et al.[24]	100 μg	18	Mean Apgar score of 8 at 1 min, 9.3 at 5 min (no difference from IM fentanyl groups)
Justins et al.[24]	80 μg	35	No change in FHR tracing Mean Apgar score of 7.9 ± 0.2 at 1 min, 9.4 ± 0.3 at 5 min (no difference from control group (n = 33)
Youngstrom et al.[25]	150 mg	21(alone) 21(w/0.125% bupiv)	Median Apgar score of 9 at 1 and 5 min Umbilical vein pH 7.32 (no difference from control group (n = 23)
Skerman et al.[26]	2.5 μg/ml	25	No neonatal depression No difference in Apgar score from control group (n = 25)
Vella et al.[28]	80 μg	20	Mean Apgar score of 7.6 at 1 min, 9.2 at 5 min
	vs. IV infusion	20	Mean Apgar score of 7.2 at 1 min, 9.2 at 5 min
Gaffud et al.[29]	100 μg	10	Mean Apgar score of 7.9 at 1 min, 9 at 5 min
Cohen et al.[31]	50 μg 100 μg	22 39	Similar frequency of bradycardia, low Apgar scores, low NACS
Capogna et al.[32]	100 μg	29	Apgar score >7 at 1 and 5 min At 2 h, truncal tone and placing were more vigorous in fentanyl group (control group n = 13)
Chestnut et al.[27]	2 μg/ml	41	No difference in Apgar scores or umbilical blood gas data from control group (n = 39)
Preston et al.[30]	1 μg/kg	15	No difference in Apgar scores or NACS from control group (n = 15)

[a] These patients did not receive supplemental bupivacaine.

plasma levels and very little placental transfer. However, there does appear to be evidence of maternal accumulation of drug from Skerman's infusion study.[26] Neonatal depression has been found only with high repeated doses.

Sufentanil

Little et al. examined the addition of a very small dose of sufentanil, 5 μg, to an initial dose of 0.25 percent bupivacaine compared to 0.25 percent bupivacaine alone.[33] There were no differences between groups in Apgar scores or NACS. Sufentanil levels were at or below the limits of detectability in maternal venous samples collected 2 minutes after the initial dose and at the time of delivery as well as in the cord blood.

Van Steenberge et al. examined three groups of patients who received an initial epidural injection of 10 ml of 0.125 percent bupivacaine with 10 ml epinephrine combined with sufentanil 15 μg, 7.5 μg, or 0 μg.[34] The 1-minute Apgar sores were lower in the sufentanil 15 μg group with a mean of 7.9 ± 1.3 versus 8.8 ± 1.3 ($P < .005$) in the control group. At 5 minutes, there were no differences between the groups.

Phillips has reported the use of sufentanil (combined with bupivacaine) as an initial bolus (1 μg/ml), intermittent boluses (1, 10, 20, or 30 μg), and continuous infusions (sufentanil 2 μg/ml).[35–37] Compared to controls, he reported no differences in Apgar scores and no respiratory depression in the first 3 hours. Despite administering sufentanil 40 to 151 μg, plasma levels were undetectable in maternal venous and umbilical cord blood. Similarly, low levels (less than 0.1 mg/ml) have been reported by Steinberg et al. when up to 50

Table 3-26. Neonatal Effects of Epidural Sufentanil

Investigator	Study Group	Reported Effects
Little et al.[33]	0.25% bupiv + 5 μg sufentanil (n = 8) vs. 0.25% bupiv (n = 6)	No difference in Apgar score or NACS Undetectable sufentanil group, equal at 5 min
Van Steenberge et al.[34]	15 μg sufentanil + 12.5 mg bupiv + 12.5 μg epi (n = 37) vs. 7.5 μg sufentanil + 12.5 mg bupiv + 12.5 μg epi (n = 36) vs. 12.5 mg bupiv + 12.5 μg epi (n = 34)	Apgar scores significantly lower at 1 min in 15-μg sufentanil group, equal at 5 min

μg of sufentanil was added to their initial dose of bupivacaine.[38]

Unfortunately, few studies have evaluated the neonate with neurobehavioral examinations (Tables 3-26 and 3-27). Capogna et al., using both the ENNS and NACS, did find a reduced adaptive capacity at 1 hour in infants whose mothers received sufentanil 50 μg with the initial dose of bupivacaine.[39] There were no differences from control at 4 hours. When sufentanil 80 μg was used, mild hypotension, poor primary reflexes, and reduced habituation was found at 1 and 4 hours. Preliminary reports with very low doses of sufentanil have not found adverse neurobehavior effects.[40,41]

Alfentanil

Heytens et al. administered epidural alfentanil as a 30-μg/kg loading dose followed by a continuous infusion of 30 μg/kg/h.[42] Top-up doses consisted of alfentanil 30 μg/kg or 0.2 percent bupivacaine 10 ml. The infusion was stopped at the beginning of the second stage of labor and no further drugs were given. The mean total dose of alfentanil was 198.9 μg/kg (range, 54.4 to 334.7 μg). Although there were no differences in Apgar scores or umbilical cord gas analyses compared to the control group whose mothers received no analgesia, the Amiel-Tison score (a neurobehavioral evaluation similar to the NACS) showed significant depression of passive and active tone (Table 3-28). This clearly demonstrates the importance of more extensive neurologic evaluations of neonates. There was a lack of correlation between the duration of second stage and the maternal venous concentration of alfentanil in this study.

Several preliminary reports with low doses of alfentanil have not shown adverse neonatal effects.[43,44] Although these results are encouraging, more extensive double-blind studies must be done before this drug can be advocated for clinical use.

Table 3-27. Neonatal Effects of Epidural Sufentanil

Initial Dose	Subsequent Doses	Neonatal Effect
3 ml 1.5% lido + 7 ml 0.25% bupiv + 1 ml saline (n = 10) or 10 μg sufentanil (n = 10) or 20 μg sufentanil (n = 10) or 30 μg sufentanil (n = 10)	Intermittent doses of 0.25% bupiv	No difference in Apgar scores
10 ml of 0.25% bupiv (n = 25) or 0.125% bupiv with 2 μg/ml sufentanil (n = 25)	Intermittent doses of assigned solution	No difference in mean Apgar scores: 1 min 8 (4–9) 5 min 9 (7–9) No respiratory depression in first 3 h
10–15 ml of 0.125% bupiv + 2 μg/ml sufentanil (n = 20)	Continuous infusion at 10 ml/hr	No difference in mean Apgar score: at 1 min 8 (6–9) at 5 min 9
or 10–15 ml of 0.25% bupiv	or 0.125% bupiv + 1 μg/ml suf or 0.125% bupiv	No respiratory depression in first 3 h Undetectable sufentanil levels

(Data from Phillips.[35–37])

Table 3-28. NACS in Neonates following Maternal Epidural Administration of Alfentanil

	Control Group	Alfentanil Group
Passive tone (max. 8)	7.31 ± 0.20	6.07 ± 0.25[a]
Active tone (max. 10)	7.63 ± 0.20	5.75 ± 0.52[b]
Primary reflexes (max. 6)	5.50 ± 0.13	5.07 ± 0.18
General assessment (max. 6)	5.63 ± 0.15	5.87 ± 0.13
Total score (max. 30)	26.06 ± 0.34	22.92 ± 0.68[a]

[a] $P < 0.005$.
[b] $P < 0.001$.
(Modified from Heytens et al.,[42] with permission.)

Butorphanol

Butorphanol is a strong κ- and weak μ-receptor agonist-antagonist not associated with respiratory depression and, combined with bupivacaine, has also been evaluated for labor analgesia.[45] Parturients received butorphanol 0, 1, 2, or 3 mg with their initial dose of 0.25 percent bupivacaine. Detectable fetal effects were found in the butorphanol 3 mg group. Four of six fetuses developed low amplitude sinusoidal-like FHR patterns which began around 10 minutes after drug injection and resolved spontaneously over 25 minutes (Fig. 3-14). Fetal scalp capillary pH samples obtained from one fetus were 7.35 and 7.31. There were no differences between groups in Apgar scores which were ≥7 at 1 minute and ≥9 at 5 minutes. Umbilical blood gas data were within normal range for all neonates. The ENNS results were similar in all groups. The NACS results have also been evaluated following maternal administration of epidural butorphanol 1 and 2 mg.[46] No differences from the control group were noted.

SUBARACHNOID OPIOIDS

Morphine

Scott et al. were among the first to investigate subarachnoid morphine for the relief of labor pain.[47] In their pilot study, morphine 1.5 mg was administered. One infant was delivered by emergency cesarean delivery because of bradycardia and late decelerations. Three infants had Apgar scores of 6 at 1 minute and all were ≥8 at 5 minutes. One infant required intubation and naloxone.

Shortly thereafter, Chauvin et al. examined plasma concentrations of subarachnoid morphine injection in surgical patients. Even when administered in large doses, 0.2 mg/kg, lower plasma levels resulted than with epidural or intramuscular administration of the same dose.[48] When small doses of morphine (0.02 mg/kg) were administered, the greatest plasma concentration was 13 μg/ml at 1 hour.[49] The method used by Chauvin measured both morphine and its metabolites.

Using a similar radioimmunoassay but separating morphine from its metabolites, Bonnardot et al. measured plasma concentrations of morphine obtained at delivery from maternal vein and umbilical cord blood.[50] All mothers received subarachnoid morphine 1 to 1.75 mg. All plasma concentrations measured less than 6 ng/ml. As the I–D interval increased, maternal concentrations tended to decrease, whereas neonatal concentrations increased (Fig. 3-15). Twenty-two infants had Apgar scores of ≥ 9 at 5 minutes. Three scores of 8, 7, and 5 were attributed to umbilical cord compression.

Baraka et al. administered subarachnoid morphine 1 or 2 mg to 20 laboring patients.[51] In 19 cases the FHR pattern was normal with no loss of variability. These neonates also cried immediately at birth. Apgar scores at 1 minute ranged from 7 to 9 and at 5 minutes ranged from 8 to 10. One patient who received morphine 2 mg had a prolonged labor. The FHR tracing demonstrated bradycardia. The 1-minute Apgar was 5 and the 5-minute score was 7. The neonates were evaluated within 24 hours using the ENNS and were all considered normal.

In 1984, Abboud et al. studied subarachnoid morphine 0.5 and 1 mg for labor analgesia.[52] She observed no effect on the FHR tracing. All 30 infants had sustained respiration by 90 seconds. The 1-minute Apgar was depressed in six infants. By 5 minutes all infants scored ≥ 7, NACS results at 15 minutes were less than 35 (35 to 40 being normal) in eight infants but, by 24 hours, all were normal. The maternal doses of morphine were not specified for the depressed infants.

In an attempt to decrease the incidence of maternal side effects of subarachnoid morphine 1 mg, Dailey et al. administered intravenous naloxone as a 0.4-mg bolus followed by a 0.4- to 0.6-mg/h infusion.[53] Twenty-three patients received naloxone and 17 served as controls. In both groups the FHR and variability were not changed by the morphine or naloxone. One infant in the naloxone group did not have sustained respirations within 90 seconds. Three infants in each group had 1-minute Apgar scores < 7 although all were ≥ 7 at 5 minutes. A similar incidence of low scores on the NACS was found at 15 minutes. All NACS results were between 35 and 40 at 24 hours. The only significant difference between the groups was in the umbilical arterial gas analyses. The naloxone group had higher pH and PO_2 values.

In these studies, 127 patients received subarachnoid morphine (Table 3-29). All five of these studies demonstrated fetal depression as evidenced by low 1-minute Apgar and 15-minute NACS scores. However, by 5

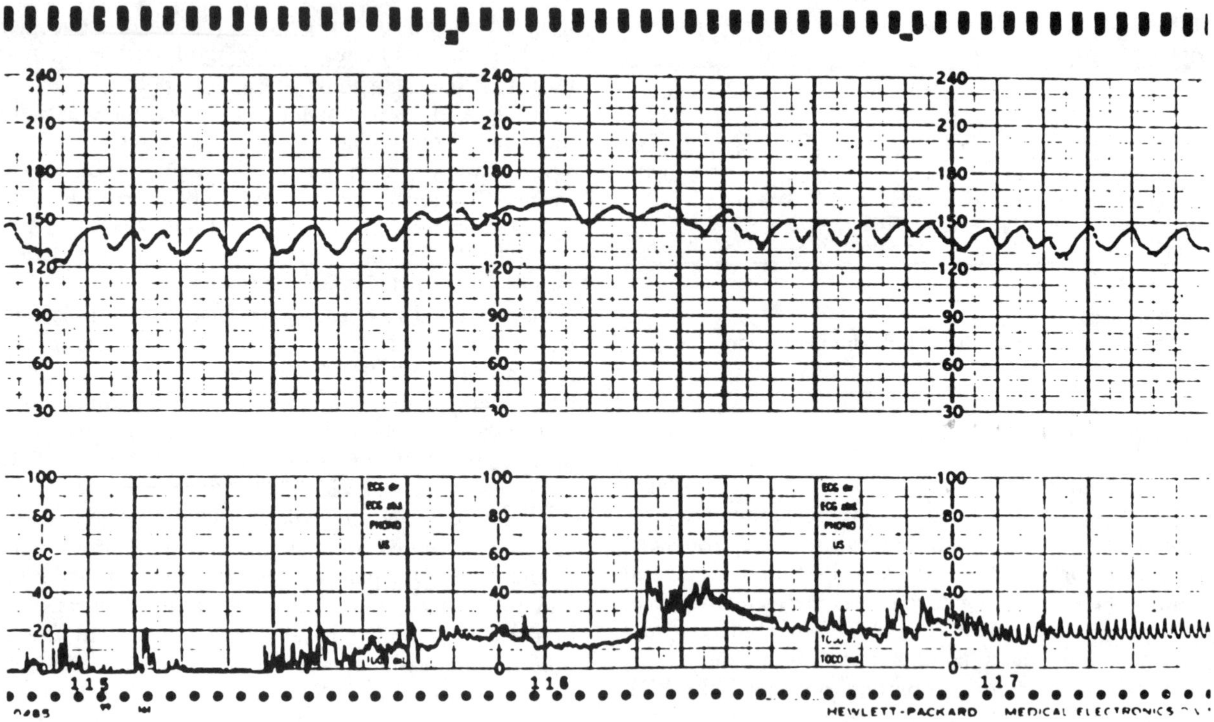

Fig. 3-14. A transient sinusoidal FHR tracing developing within 10 minutes of maternal epidural administration of butorphanol 3 mg.

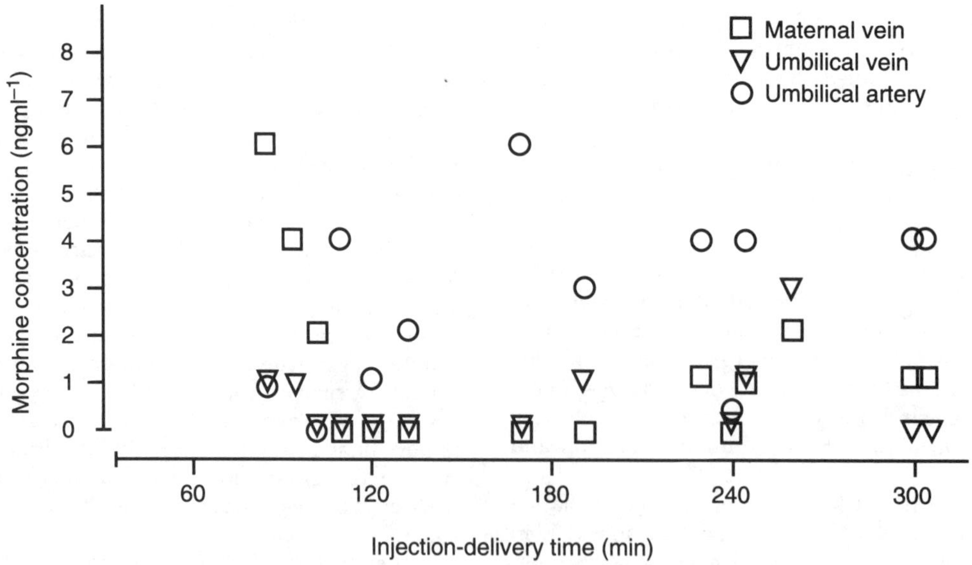

Fig. 3-15. Maternal and fetal concentrations (radioimmunoassay) after intrathecal administration of morphine hydrochloride 0.8 mg/ml. The ratio of maternal:fetal plasma concentrations of morphine were reversed with I–D times, maximum rates being equal to or less than 6 ng/ml. (From Bonnardot et al.,[50] with permission.)

Table 3-29. Fetal and Neonatal Effects of Subarachnoid Morphine for Labor and Delivery

Investigator	Dose	No. Patients	Reported Effects
Scott et al.	1.5 mg	12	One fetus had bradycardia and late decelerations
Bonnardot et al.[47]	1–1.75 mg	25	No neonatal respiratory depression Three had low Apgar scores All plasma concentrations in mother and neonate <6 mg/ml
Baraka et al.[51]	1 or 2 mg	20	One fetus had bradycardia Apgar scores: 7–9 (one 5), at 1 min 8–10 (one 7) at 5 min ENNS all normal
Abboud et al.[52]	0.5 or 1 mg	30	No effect on FHR tracing All had sustained respirations by 90 sec Apgar scores: 24 ≥7 at 1 min 30 ≥7 at 5 min Umbilical cord blood gases within normal range NACS: 21 ≥35 at 15 min All ≥35 at 24 h
Dailey et al.[53]	1 mg	40	No changes of FHR tracing One infant with respiratory depression Three 1-min Apgar scores >7, all >7 at 5 min Three low NACS at 15 min, all normal by 24 h

minutes all Apgar scores were ⩾ 7. By 24 hours, the neurobehavioral scores were normal. Bonnardo et al. attributed the low Apgar scores in their study to cord compression. The depressed infant in the Baraka et al. study was attributed to a prolonged labor. Abboud et al. suggested that forceps or cesarean delivery may have caused the early neonatal depression in their study. It should be noted that there are no data for patients not receiving analgesia, a problem shared by all investigators. Furthermore, most of these patients required additional anesthesic for the delivery; local perineal infiltration, pudendal block, or epidural block was administered, and may also have influenced neonatal outcome.

A more promising use of subarachnoid morphine is the combination of very small doses with hyperbaric bupivacaine for improved intraoperative and postoperative pain relief. Abboud et al. administered morphine 0.1 or 0.25 mg mixed with hyperbaric bupivacaine.[54] There were no differences between groups in Apgar scores. At 1 minute, one infant in each morphine group and two in the control group had a score of ⩽ 6. At 5 minutes, all scored ⩾ 7. All umbilical vein and artery pH and PO_2 values were within normal limits. NACS results were not different for any test items. Abouleish et al. also has reported good Apgar scores and umbilical cord gas data when morphine 0.2 mg was added to hyperbaric bupivacaine[55] (Table 3-30).

Table 3-30. Neonatal Effects of Subarachnoid Morphine-Bupivacaine for Cesarean Delivery

Investigator	Dose	No. Patients	Reported Effects
Abboud et al.[54]	0.25 mg 0.10 mg 0 mg	11 10 12	No differences in incidence of low 1-min Apgar scores All 5-min Apgar scores ≥7 Umbilical blood gas data within normal range
Abouleish et al.[55]	0.2 mg 0	17 17	Apgar scores: 1 min ≥7 5 min ≥8 All umbilical blood gas data within normal range

Fentanyl

The combination of hyperbaric bupivacaine with fentanyl in doses of 0, 2.5, 5, 6.25, 12.5, 25, 37.5 and 50 μg has also been evaluated.[56] All neonates except one had Apgar scores at 1 and 5 minutes of ≥ 7. There was one depressed infant whose mother received fentanyl 12.5 μg. This mother was hypotensive prior to delivery despite administration of intravenous fluids and ephedrine. All infants had umbilical blood gas analyses within normal limits. There were no differences in ENNS results between groups on days 1 and 3.

Meperidine

In a recent case report, subarachnoid administration of meperidine provided adequate pain relief during labor and for cesarean delivery because of its local anesthetic-like properties.[56]

REFERENCES

1. Kanto J, Erkkola R: Epidural and intrathecal opiates in obstetrics. Int J Clin Pharmacol Therap Toxicol 22:316, 1984
2. Mirkin BL, Singh S: Placental transfer of pharmacologically active molecules. In Perinatal Pharmacology and Therapeutics. Academic Press, Orlando, FL, 1978
3. Weddel SJ, Ritter RR: Serum levels following epidural administration of morphine and correlation with relief of postsurgical pain. Anesthesiology 54:210, 1981
4. Youngstrom PC, Cowan RI, Sutheimer C, et al: Pain relief and plasma concentrations from epidural and intramuscular morphine in post-cesarean patients. Anesthesiology 57:404, 1982
5. Craft JB, Bolan JC, Coaldrake LA, et al: The maternal and fetal cardiovascular effects of epidural morphine in the sheep model. Am J Obstet Gynecol 142:835, 1982
6. Nybell-Lindahl G, Carisson C, Ingemarsson I, et al: Maternal and fetal concentrations of morphine after epidural administration during labor. Am J Obstet Gynecol 139:20, 1981
7. Husemeyer RP, O'Connor MC, Davenport HT: Failure of epidural morphine to relieve pain in labour. Anaesthesia 35:161, 1980
8. Booker PD, Wilkes RG, Bryson THL, Beddard J: Obstetric pain relief using epidural morphine. Anaesthesia 35:377, 1980
9. Crawford JS: Experiences with epidural morphine in obstetrics. Anaesthesia 36:207, 1981
10. Niv D, Rudick V, Golan A, et al: Augmentation of bupivacaine analgesia in labor by epidural morphine. Obstet Gynecol 67:206, 1986
11. Writer WDR, James FM, Wheeler AS: Double-blind comparison of morphine and bupivacaine for continuous epidural analgesia in labor. Anesthesiology 54:215, 1981
12. Hughes SC, Rosen MA, Shnider SM, et al: Maternal and neonatal effects of epidural morphine for labor and delivery. Anesth Analg 63:319, 1984
13. Husemeyer RP, Cummings AJ, Rosankiewicz JR, et al: A study of pethidine kinetics and analgesia in women in labour following intravenous, intramuscular and epidural administration. Br J Clin Pharmacol 13:171, 1982
14. Skjoldebrand A, Garle M, Gustafsson LL, et al: Extradural pethidine with and without adrenaline during labour: Wide variation in effect. Br J Anaesth 54:415, 1982
15. Perriss BW: Epidural pethidine in labour. A study of dose requirements. Anaesthesia 35:380, 1980
16. Perriss BW: Pain relief in labour using epidural pethidine with adrenaline. Anaesthesia 36:631, 1981
17. Baraka A, Maktabi M, Noueihid R: Epidural meperidine-bupivacaine for obstetric analgesia. Anesth Analg 61:652, 1982
18. Hammonds W, Bramwell RS, Hag CC, et al: A comparison of epidural meperidine and bupivacaine for relief of labor pain. Anesth Analg 61:187, 1982
19. Wolfe MJ, Davies GK: Analgesic action of extradural fentanyl. Br J Anaesth 52:357, 1980
20. Vella LM, Knott C, Reynolds F: Transfer of fentanyl across the rabbit placenta. Br J Anaesth 58:49, 1986
21. Craft JB, Coaldrake LA, Bolan JC, et al: Placental passage and uterine effects of fentanyl. Anesth Analg 62:94, 1983
22. Craft JB, Robinchaux AG, Kin H, et al: The maternal and fetal cardiovascular effects of epidural fentanyl in the sheep model. Am J Obstet Gynecol 148:1098, 1984
23. Carrie LES, O'Sullivan GM, Seegobin R: Epidural fentanyl in labour. Anaesthesia 36:965, 1981
24. Justins DM, Knott C, Luthman J, et al: Epidural versus intramuscular fentanyl. Analgesia and pharmacokinetics in labor. Anaesthesia 38:937, 1983
25. Youngstrom P, Eastwood D, Patel H, et al: Epidural fentanyl and bupivacaine in labor: double-blind study. Anesthesiology 61:A414, 1984
26. Skerman JH, Thompson BA, Goldstein MT, et al: Combined continuous epidural fentanyl and bupivacaine in labor: a randomized study. Anesthesiology 63:A450, 1985
27. Chestnut DH, Owen CL, Bates JN, et al: Continuous infusion epidural analgesia during labor: a randomized, double-blind comparison of 0.0625% bupivacaine/0.0002% fentanyl versus 0.125% bupivacaine. Anesthesiology 68:754, 1988
28. Vella LM, Willatts DG, Knott C, et al: Epidural fentanyl in labour. An evaluation of the systemic contribution to analgesia. Anaesthesia 40:741, 1985
29. Gaffud MP, Bansal P, Lawton C, et al: Surgical analgesia for cesarean delivery with epidural bupivacaine and fentanyl. Anesthesiology 65:331, 1986
30. Preston PG, Rosen MA, Hughes SC, et al: Epidural anesthesia with fentanyl and lidocaine for cesarean section: maternal effects and neonatal outcome. Anesthesiology 68:938, 1988
31. Cohen SE, Tan S, Albright GA, et al: Epidural fentanyl/bupivacaine mixtures for obstetric analgesia. Anesthesiology 67:403, 1987
32. Capogna G, Celleno D, McGannon P, et al: Neonatal

neurobehavior effects following maternal administration of epidural fentanyl during labor. Anesthesiology 67:A461, 1987
33. Little MS, McNitt JD, Choi JH, et al: A pilot study of low dose epidural sufentanil and bupivacaine for labor anesthesia. Anesthesiology 67:A444, 1987
34. Van Steenberge AV, Debroux HC, Noordin H: Extradural bupivacaine with sufentanil for vaginal delivery. Br J Anaesth 59:1518, 1987
35. Phillips GH: Epidural sulfentanil in labor. Anesth Analg 66:S140, 1987
36. Phillips GH: Combined epidural sufentanil and bupivacaine for labor analgesia. Reg Anesth 12:165, 1987
37. Phillips GH: Continuous infusion epidural analgesia in labor: the effect of adding sufentanil to 0.125% bupivacaine. Anesth Analg 67:462, 1988
38. Steinberg RB, Powell G, Hee X, Dunn SM: Epidural sufentanil for analgesia for labor and delivery. Reg Anesth 14:225, 1989
39. Capogna G, Celleno P, Tomassetti M: Maternal analgesia and neonatal effects of epidural sufentanil for cesarean section. Reg Anesth 14:282, 1989
40. Naulty JS, Ross R, Bergen W: Epidural sufentanil-bupivacaine for analgesia during labor and delivery. Anesthesiology 71:A842, 1989
41. Vandemeulen E, Vertommen J, Van Aken H, et al: Epidural bupivacaine with sufentanil in labor. Anesthesiology 71:A844, 1989
42. Heytens L, Cammu H, Camu F: Extradural analgesia during labor using alfentanil. Br J Anaesth 59:331, 1987
43. Carp H, Johnson MD, Bader AM, et al: Continuous epidural infusion of alfentanil and bupivacaine for labor and delivery. Anesthesiology 69:A687, 1988
44. Fernando E, Shevede K, Eddi D: A comparative study of epidural alfentanil and fentanyl for labor pain relief. Anesthesiology 71:A846, 1989
45. Hunt CO, Naulty JS, Malinow A, et al: Epidural butorphanol-bupivacaine for analgesia during labor and delivery. Anesth Analg 68:323, 1989
46. Abboud TK, Reyes A, Richardson M, et al: Epidural morphine or butorphanol augments bupivacaine analgesia during labor. Reg Anesth 14:115, 1989
47. Scott PV, Bowen FE, Cartwright P, et al: Intrathecal morphine as sole analgesia during labour. Br Med J 281:351, 1980
48. Chauvin M, Samii K, Schermann JM, et al: Plasma concentrations of morphine after I.M., extradural, and intrathecal administration. Br J Anaesth 53:911, 1981
49. Chauvin M, Samii K, Schermann JM, et al: Plasma morphine concentration after intrathecal administration of low doses of morphine. Br J Anaesth 53:1065, 1981
50. Bonnardot JP, Maillet JC, Colau JC, et al: Maternal and fetal concentration of morphine after intrathecal administration during labour. Br J Anaesth 56:1351, 1982
51. Baraka A, Noueihid R, Hajj S: Intrathecal injection of morphine for obstetric analgesia. Anesthesiology 54:136, 1981
52. Abboud TK, Shnider SM, Dailey PA, et al: Intrathecal administration of hyperbaric morphine for the relief of pain in labour. Br J Anaesth 56:1351, 1984
53. Dailey PA, Brookshire GL, Shnider SM, et al: The effects of naloxone associated with the intrathecal use of morphine in labor. Anesth Analg 64:658, 1985
54. Abboud TK, Dror A, Mosaad P, et al: Mini-dose intrathecal morphine for the relief of post-cesarean section pain: safety, efficacy, and ventilatory responses to carbon dioxide. Anesth Analg 67:137, 1988
55. Abouleish E, Rawal R, Fallon K, et al: Combined intrathecal morphine and bupivacaine for cesarean section. Anesth Analg 67:370, 1988
56. Hunt CO, Datta S, Hauch M, et al: Perioperative analgesia with subarachnoid fentanyl-bupivacaine. Anesthesiology 71:535, 1989
57. Johnson MD, Hurley RJ, Gilbutson LI, Datta S: Continuous microcatheter spinal anesthesia with subarachnoid meperidine for labor and delivery. Anesth Analg 70:658, 1990

OTHER INTRASPINAL ANALGESICS

The search for the ideal anesthetic technique for the parturient began centuries before the era of modern anesthesia. In 1818, Benjamin Rush described the essential characteristics of the ideal anesthetic for obstetrics.[1] He expressed the hope that "a medicine would be discovered which should suspend sensibility altogether and leave irritability or powers of motion unimpaired." After more than a century, the ideal anesthetic for labor analgesia has still not been found. However, recent developments in the neurophysiology and neuropharmacology of pain have led to major advances toward this goal.

PROPOSED MECHANISM OF INTRASPINAL ANALGESIA: ION CHANNELS, HYPERPOLARIZATION, AND THE INHIBITION OF NERVE CELLS

The processing of pain information begins in the dorsal horn of the spinal cord and is modulated in part by the excitation of the so-called wide dynamic response neurons.[2] Although this process is not entirely understood, the primary action of most analgesics, including opiates and adrenergic agonists, is thought to involve inhibition of activation of neural pain encoding networks by their effects on individual nerve cell ion channels. Although single nerve cells do not act independently in vivo, in vitro studies using single cells have shown that spinal analgesic agents may act to inhibit nerve cell firing by hyperpolarizing these cells as a result of increases in potassium (or chloride) ion conductance.[3]

Inhibition of nerve cells is an important modulator of nerve cell function. One example of the importance of nerve cell inhibition is the reduction in excitability of motoneurons supplying opposing muscles groups. This is brought about by the opening of chloride channels that permits chloride to enter the cell leading to hyperpolarization and inhibition of nerve cell excitation.[3] Interestingly, nerve cell hyperpolarization as a result of increased chloride ion conductance may be the mechanism underlying the spinal analgesic effects of benzodiazepines.

Another way to hyperpolarize nerve cells and thus inhibit firing is to open potassium channels, which will allow potassium ions to diffuse out of the cells. In fact, the bradycardic effects of acetylcholine binding to muscarinic receptors in the heart is the result of increased potassium ion conductance that hyperpolarizes and inhibits the cardiac pacemaker and slows the heart rate.[3]

Interestingly, the bulk of experimental evidence also suggest that hyperpolarization of nerve cells, as a result of increased potassium conductance with subsequent inhibition of firing, may explain the spinal analgesic action of many drugs, including opioids and adrenergic agonists.[3] Many of the in vitro experiments that form the basis for this conclusion were carried out by Dr. Alan North and his colleagues on small pieces of nerve tissue with the tip of a glass microelectrode positioned in the cell interior so that the membrane potential can be measured.[3] The results of such in vitro experiments demonstrate that opioids, norepinephrine, clonidine, and somatostatin produce membrane hyperpolarization and inhibition of neuronal firing. This is shown in Figure 3-16 for an enkephalin derivative.[4]

Next, experiments to confirm the mechanism of nerve cell hyperpolarization were conducted using the voltage clamp method. The results of voltage clamp experiments demonstrate that the action of opioids, clonidine, norepinephrine, and somatostatin[4] is to open ion channels in the membrane that are selectively permeable to potassium.[3] In the normal cellular environment this current is outward and leads to hyperpolarization and inhibition of cell firing. This may be the effector mechanism underlying the spinal analgesic action of these agents.[3]

However, increased potassium conductance following opiate or adrenergic agent receptor binding requires the subsequent activation of a signal transducer, known as a G-protein, that is linked to the ion channel.[3–5] This is summarized in Figure 3-17. Binding of an opioid or adrenergic agonist to its spinal cord receptor activates the associated G-protein. The G-protein then directly

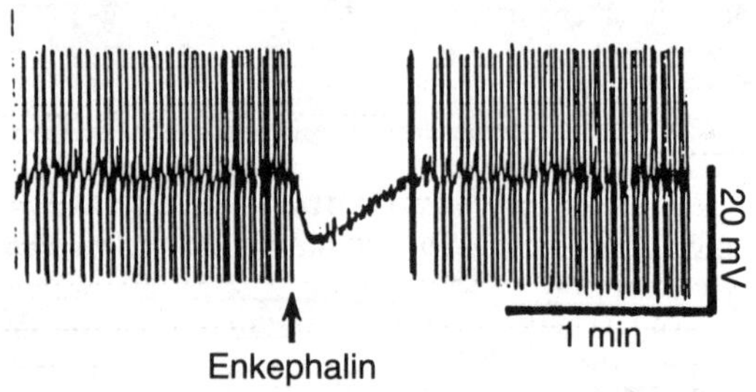

Fig. 3-16. Enkephalin inhibits nerve cell firing. An intracellular recording from a spontaneously firing locus coeruleus neurone. Enkephalin (D-Ala^2-D-leu^5-enkephalin) was applied to a pipet positioned just above the brain slice at the times indicated by the arrows. The cell hyperpolarized and the action potential discharge was transiently inhibited. (Adapted from Williams et al.,[4] with permission.)

opens a potassium channel in the membrane to produce hyperpolarization of the nerve cell and inhibition of nerve cell firing in a pain-sensitive neuron with resultant analgesia.[3–5]

The interposition of a G-protein between receptor and effector allows for further diversification of the action of the particular agonist. In fact, the same G-proteins mediating increases in potassium ion conductance by spinal analgesics may also open other ion

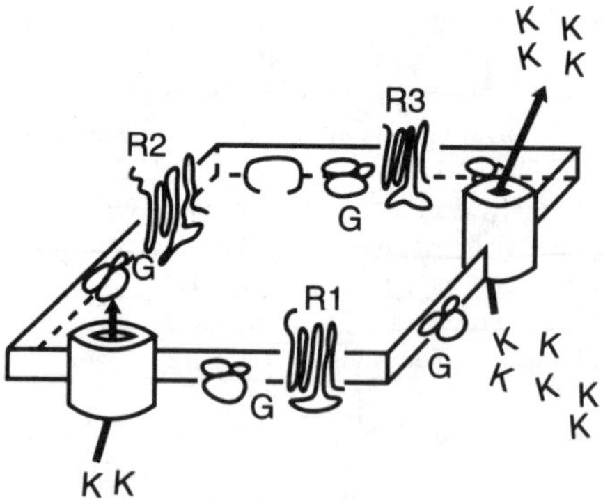

Fig. 3-17. Possible mechanism of intraspinal analgesia: A nerve cell membrane (exterior surface upward) and its associated membrane receptors and ion channels. The cellular response to intraspinal analgesic agents is initiated by binding to specific cell surface receptors (R1, R2, R3) followed by activation of a common G-protein (G). Next, the activated G-protein directly opens potassium channels (K) to produce membrane hyperpolarization, inhibition of nerve cell firing, and analgesia. R1, R2, R3, represent opioid, adrenergic agonist, or somatostatin receptors.

channels such as calcium or activate cellular enzymes such as adenylcyclase, and these effects may also be important.[3–5] Interestingly, indirect evidence suggests that the action of general anesthetics may be mediated by G-proteins.[6]

In summary, based on in vitro studies, a variety of drugs capable of producing spinal analgesia interact with their specific cell surface receptors to hyperpolarize nerve cells. Hyperpolarization of nerve cells will inhibit nerve cell firing, causing a reduction in neurotransmitter release and the production of analgesia. Opioids, adrenergic agents, and somatostatin may produce this effect by increasing potassium ion conductance, and benzodiazepines increase chloride conductance.

Understanding the basic cellular mechanisms of pain and analgesia will certainly lead to the development of more effective analgesic agents and techniques capable of producing analgesia without maternal or fetal side effects.

SPECIFIC AGENTS

Adrenergic Agonists

Recent studies in experimental animals and humans demonstrate that adrenergic agonists, including epinephrine, norepinephrine, and clonidine, are capable of producing profound analgesia following epidural or intrathecal administration.[7–9]

Despite its relatively poor selectivity for the α_2-receptor, clonidine is the only α_2-agonist currently available for clinical use in this country.[7] Epidural clonidine produces analgesia by a nonopioid mechanism and may offer advantages over other agents for labor analgesia.[8] Unlike local anesthetics, clonidine does not produce motor or sensory blockade and unlike opioids, clonidine has not been reported to produce delayed respiratory depression, nausea, pruritus, or urinary retention. In fact, a recent study in pregnant ewes demonstrated that epidural clonidine in analgesic doses did not produce significant maternal or fetal side effects.[8] Furthermore, epidural clonidine has been used to provide post-cesarean delivery analgesia in humans and was found to provide analgesia of intermediate duration with minimal maternal side effects.[9] However, under certain conditions epidural or subarachnoid clonidine may produce hypotension, bradycardia, and decreased ventilatory response to carbon dioxide.[10–12] Hemodynamic depression may limit the usefulness of clonidine in the laboring patient. However, more specific α_2-adrenergic agonists, including dexmedetomidine[7] and tizanidine,[11] may produce analgesia with fewer side effects than clonidine. Finally, α_2-agonists may act synergistically with co-administered local anesthetic or opioid to improve the quality and duration of analgesia.[7]

α_2-Adrenergic agonists appear to be promising agents for analgesia in obstetrics.

Enkephalins

Methionine-enkephalin (met-enkephalin), a rapidly metabolized, naturally occurring opioid peptide, may be an ideal intraspinal narcotic for use in obstetric anesthesia. Although met-enkephalin produces analgesia following intracerebroventricular administration,[13] preliminary studies in guinea pigs demonstrate that continuous subarachnoid infusion of met-enkephalin produces prolonged analgesia (H. Carp, unpublished observations). However, it does not produce analgesia or respiratory depression following systemic administration because of its rapid degradation by proteases contained in maternal and fetal plasma and tissues (plasma half-life, 1 minute).[13] Interestingly, following acute intravenous administration of large doses of met-enkephalin to pregnant ewes, the drug was rapidly degraded in the maternal and fetal plasma and was unable to affect the fetal lambs.[14]

Subarachnoid administration of met-enkephalin to laboring patients could produce analgesia without the risk of fetal respiratory depression, because of rapid metabolism, and without the motor weakness and hypotension associated with currently used local anesthetics. This may result in improved fetal and maternal safety as well as a lesser effect on the labor process.

In contrast to the rapid degradation of met-enkephalin, metkephamid is a synthetic peptide derivative of met-enkephalin resistant to degradation and capable of producing analgesia following subarachnoid or even systemic administration in animals and man.[15] Interestingly, studies in pregnant rates and sheep showed that metkephamid does not cross the placental barrier following maternal systemic administration of analgesic doses. Therefore, metkephamid may be an ideal analgesic agent for labor, capable of producing analgesia but unable to produce fetal depression because of an inability to cross the placental barrier.

Benzodiazepines

A number of representatives of the nonopioid, noncatecholamine drug class, including benzodiazepines, can produce intraspinal analgesia. Several studies have suggested that systemic administration of benzodiazepines may depress nociception.[16] More importantly, further studies have also shown that benzodiazepines may have profound analgesic properties following subarachnoid administration.[17–20] Lumbar subarachnoid administration of small doses of midazolam in anesthetized dogs depresses sympathetic reflexes evoked by nociceptive stimulation of the animals' hind-, but not forelimbs.[17] Furthermore, subarachnoid administration of midazolam to patients with postoperative and chronic pain produced significant analgesia.[18] In that study, relatively large doses were used and significant sedation was produced. However, a more recent study clearly showed that subarachnoid administration of small doses of midazolam produced analgesia in rats.[19] In contrast, control animals receiving intraperitoneal injections of the same dose of midazolam did not demonstrate analgesia and actually developed hyperalgesia. These investigators suggested that the analgesic effect of midazolam may stem from its action at the spinal level, whereas its sedative and hyperalgesic effects are a function of its supraspinal action.

Finally, Serrao and co-workers, using rats, investigated the effects of subarachnoid midazolam on the threshold for pain induced by brief passage of electric current between pairs of electrodes placed on the tail and the skin of the neck.[20] They concluded that subarachnoid midazolam produces segmental, spinally medicated analgesia and presented indirect evidence suggesting that midazolam may produce spinally mediated analgesia by binding to nonopioid receptors in the spinal cord (i.e., benzodiazepine receptors). In support of their idea, benzodiazepine binding sites have been demonstrated in the spinal cord and endogenous benzodiazepine-like substances have been discovered in human cerebrospinal fluid.

Membrane preparations of benzodiazepine receptors have been linked with the receptors for γ-aminobutyric acid (GABA). The benzodiazepine-GABA receptor complex consists of four elongated subunits, each of which contains a central axial chloride channel outside of which is the GABA receptor and benzodiazepine receptor.[21,22] The main function of the complex is to allosterically regulate GABA receptor-mediated gating of the chloride channels. It may be that the combination of midazolam with benzodiazepine receptors in the spinal cord potentiates the effect of GABA on the chloride channel and increases chloride ion conductance so that chloride ions enter the cell, leading to hyperpolarization and inhibition of nerve cell firing and potentiation of the analgesic effect of GABA. (This effect is analogous to the hyperpolarization of nerve cells produced by opioids and clonidine as a result of increases in potassium ion conductance.)

These experimental findings with midazolam suggest that, in addition to opioids, benzodiazepines may be capable of producing intraspinal analgesia.

Progesterone

It is becoming increasingly evident that steroid hormones, including progesterone, can act on the central nervous system to produce a variety of behavioral effects, independent of their hormonal action. In fact, the anesthetic effects of steroids may be related to their ability to potentiate GABA-mediated increases in chloride ion conductance, in a manner similar to benzodiazepines.[23]

Interestingly, the subarachnoid administration of progesterone markedly potentiates the analgesic effects of neuraxial opiates in rats (H. Carp and A. Jayaram, unpublished observations). This effect of progesterone is blocked by prior administration of picrotoxin or bicuculline, both agents that block GABA-mediated increase in chloride ion conductance.

These experimental results suggest that increased progesterone levels during pregnancy may potentiate the analgesic action of endogenous opioids secreted in response to labor pain and may help to explain the decreased analgesic requirements in these patients.

In addition to analgesic effects, increased progesterone levels may be related to the decrease in minimum alveolar concentration (MAC) for potent inhaled agents, as well as the increased sensitivity to local anesthetic blocks associated with pregnancy. In support of this, chronically administered progesterone decreases halothane MAC in rabbits.[24]

Calcitonin

Calcitonin is a polypeptide hormone initially detected in thyroid and recently found also in brain, pituitary, and cerebrospinal fluid. In addition to its effect on calcium and phosphate metabolism, prolonged analgesia in animals and humans has been reported following calcitonin administration.[25–27] Indirect evidence suggests that calcitonin-mediated analgesia may act through the serotinergic system.

Puig and colleagues reported that subarachnoid calcitonin produced profound analgesia in a study of 56 postoperative patients with minimal side effects.[25] However, further experience using subarachnoid calcitonin suggests that unacceptable side effects limit its usefulness as a spinal analgesic (M. Puig, personal communication).

Somatostatin

The nonopioid tetradecapeptide, somatostatin, was first isolated from bovine hypothalamus. The presence of somatostatin in dorsal root ganglia and small primary sensory neurons (C-afferents) suggests a possible role as a neurotransmitter or neuromodulator of pain. In fact, somatostatin has been shown to produce analgesia in experimental animals.[28] However, in some reports the analgesic action of subarachnoid somatostatin has been associated with spinal cord neurotoxicity and flaccid paralysis.[29] In humans, intracerebroventricular, subarachnoid, and epidural administration of somatostatin have been reported to produce analgesia when used to treat chronic pain without evidence of neurotoxicity.[29–31]

However, there are conflicting reports of the efficacy of epidural somatostatin in the treatment of acute postoperative pain. Chrubasik and co-workers reported effective analgesia following epidural somatostatin in eight postoperative patients[31] and further reported that epidural somatostatin produced segmental analgesia.[32] In contrast to the results obtained by Chrubasik, a more recent study by other investigators reported that epidural somatostatin failed to provide adequate analgesia after cholecystectomy in 24 patients.[33] This study also failed to demonstrate any cutaneous analgesia following somatostatin.

The role of somatostatin as an effective analgesic agent needs to be clarified by further study.

CONCLUSIONS

Recent developments in the neurophysiology and neuropharmacology of pain and analgesia will bring us closer to development of the ideal anesthetic for obstetrics through the discovery of drugs that are capable of altering neural transmission in such a way that analgesia results without motor, sensory, or sympathetic block.

After more than a century, we are moving closer to discovering the ideal analgesic for obstetrics that in 1818 Banjamin Rush hoped would be able to "suspend sensibility altogether and leave irritability or powers of motion unimpaired."[1]

REFERENCES

1. Heaton CE: The history of anesthesia and analgesia in obstetrics. J Hist Med Allied Sci 1:567, 1946
2. Watkins DE: Multiple endogenous opiate and non-opiate analgesia systems: evidence of their existence and clinical implications. Ann NY Acad Sci 467:273, 1986
3. North RA: Drug receptors and the inhibition of nerve cells. Br J Pharmacol 98:13, 1989
4. Williams JT, Egan TM, North RA: Enkephalin opens potassium channels on mammalian central neurones. Nature 299:74, 1982
5. Brown AM, Birnbaumer L: Direct G protein gating of ion channels. Am J Physiol 23:H401, 1988
6. Firestone S, Firestone LL: Anesthetic alcohols modulate membrane-bound protein kinase C function. FASEB J 2:A1381, 1988
7. Maze M, Segal IS, Bloor BC: Clonidine and other alpha-2-adrenergic agonists: strategies for rational use of these novel anesthetic agents. J Clin Anesth 1:146, 1988
8. Eisenach JC, Castro MI, Dewan DM, Rose JC: Epidural clonidine analgesia in obstetrics: sheep studies. Anesthesiology 70:51, 1989
9. Viscomi CM, Eisenach JC: Epidural clonidine for post cesarean section analgesia. Society of Obstetric Anesthesia and Perinatology (Abstracts) D24, 1989
10. Eisenach JC, Lysak SZ, Viscomi CM: Epidural clonidine analgesia following surgery: phase 1. Anesthesiology 71:640, 1989
11. Lubenow T, et al: Analgesic and hemodynamic evaluation of intrathecal clonidine and tizanidine. Anesthesiology 71:A648, 1989
12. Penon C, Ecoffey C, Cohen SE: Ventilatory effects of epidural clonidine. Anesthesiology 71:A649, 1989
13. Buscher HH, et al: Evidence for analgesic activity of enkephalin in the mouse. Nature 261:423, 1976
14. Lagamma EF, Itskovitz J, Abraham MR: Maturation of circulatory responses to methionine-enkephalin. Pediatr Res 17:162, 1983
15. Frederickson RCA, et al: Preclinical pharmacology of metkephamid (LY 127623) a met-enkephalin analogue. p. 150. In Harris LS (ed): National Institute on Drug Abuse Research Monograph, 1982
16. Boralessa H, Senior DF, Whitwam JG: Cardiovascular response to intubation. A comparative study of thiopentone and midazolam. Anaesthesia 38:623, 1983
17. Niv D, Whitwam JG, Loh L: Depression of nociceptive sympathetic reflexes by the intrathecal administration of midazolam. Br J Anaesth 55:541, 1983
18. Rigoli M: Epidural analgesia with benzodiazepines. p. 69. In Tiengo M, Cousins MJ (eds): Pharmacological Basis of Anesthesiology: Clinical Pharmacology of New Analgesics and Anesthetics. Raven Press, New York, 1983
19. Niv D, Davidovich, S, Geller E, Urca G: Analgesic and hyperalgesic effects of midaszolam: dependence on route of administration. Anesth Analg 67:1169, 1988
20. Serrao JM, Goodchild CS, Stubbs SC, Gent JP: Intrathecal midazolam and fentanyl in the rat: evidence for different spinal antinociceptive effects. Anesthesiology 70:780, 1989
21. Braesfrap C, Nielsen M: Neurotransmitters and CNS disease: anxiety. Lancet 2:1030, 1982
22. Schoefield PR, et al: Sequence and functional expression of the GABA receptor shows a ligand-gated receptor superfamily. Nature 328:221, 1987
23. Kavaliers M, Wiebe JP: Analgesic effects of the progesterone metabolite 3 α-hydroxy-5 α-pregnan-20-one and possible modes of action in mice. Brain Res 415:393, 1987
24. Datta S, Migliozzi RP, Flanagan HL, Krieger NR: Chronically administered progesterone decreases halothane requirements in rabbits. Anesth Analg 68:46, 1989
25. Bates RFI, et al: Comparison of the analgesic effects of subcutaneous and intracerebroventricular injection of calcitonin on acetic acid induced abdominal constrictions in the mouse. Br J Pharmacol 72:575, 1981

26. Miralles FS, et al: Post-operative analgesia induced by subarachnoid lidocaine plus calcitonin. Anesth Analg 66:615, 1987
27. Fraioli F, et al: Subarachnoid injection of salmon calcitonin induces analgesia in man. Eur J Pharmacol 78:381, 1982
28. Chrabasik J, et al: Somatostatin: a potent analgesic substance. Lancet 2:1208, 1984
29. Gaumann DM, Yaksh TL: Intrathecal somatostatin in rats: antinociception only in the presence of toxic effects. Anesthesiology 68:733, 1988
30. Meynadier J, Chrubasik J, Dubar M, Wunsch E: Intrathecal somatostatin in terminally ill patients. A report of two cases. Pain 23:9, 1985
31. Chrubasik J, Meynadier J, Scherpereel P, Wunsch E: The effect of epidural somatostatin on postoperative pain. Anesth Analg 64:1085, 1985
32. Carli P, Ecoffey C, Chrubasik J, et al: Spread of analgesia and ventilatory response to CO_2 following epidural somatostatin. Anesthesiology 65:Suppl. A216, 1986
33. Desborough JP, et al: Hormonal and metabolic responses to cholecystectomy: comparison of extradural somatostatin and diamorphine. Br J Anaesth 63:508, 1989

MONITORING OF THE OBSTETRIC PATIENT RECEIVING INTRASPINAL OPIOIDS

ASSOCIATED RISKS

Wang et al. and Behar et al. first reported pain relief by the injection of morphine into the subarachnoid and epidural spaces, respectively, in 1979.[1,2] Subsequently, intraspinal opioids have been extensively used with reasonable safety. The first application of intraspinal opioids was for patients in chronic pain who had become tolerant to substantial parenteral amounts of opioids. There were few reports of major respiratory depression in these early clinical reports. In contrast, patients acutely treated for postoperative pain who have not developed tolerance were at much greater risk.

What are the risks associated with the use of intraspinal opioids, and what options are available to reduce these risks? The only narcotic agent presently approved by the FDA for intraspinal use is preservative-free morphine (Astromorph, Duramorph). Morphine, the prototypical intraspinal opioid, is the least lipid soluble and the most hydrophilic of the opioids used at present. While it provides the longest duration of action, it has the slowest onset. When administered epidurally, only 0.3 percent of the total morphine dose is detectable in CSF. Much of the remainder is absorbed into the circulation and thus may cause respiratory depression. Because of low lipid and high water solubility, morphine has the greatest propensity of any opioid to sequester in CSF. Following the lumbar epidural administration of morphine, it can be detected in the cervical CSF within 30 to 60 minutes[3] and detectable levels may be present up to 24 hours. Thus, in contrast to the more lipid-soluble opioids such as fentanyl and sufentanil, morphine is more likely to reach respiratory centers in the fourth ventricle by rostral flow and cause respiratory depression.

MECHANISMS OF RESPIRATORY DEPRESSION

The hydrophilic properties of morphine, though associated with increased side effects, can be clinically useful. Diffusion of water-soluble opioids along the spinal cord may make analgesia available at areas far from the insertion site of the spinal needle or epidural catheter. However in the post-cesarean delivery patient, there is little to be gained from this effect as good pain control can be achieved with drug placed in the lumbar area. Perhaps the greatest benefit of the more water-soluble opioids is their longer duration of pain relief, especially if the anesthetic technique employs at a single administration of drug. While rostral spread in the CSF may have a beneficial effect, it can also produce an insidious second peak of respiratory depression that is variable in onset, usually seen in 8 to 12 hours although it may not occur for up to 24 hours.[4]

Opiate binding at medullary and pontine respiratory centers can reduce respiratory drive by reducing the sensitivity to increased $PaCO_2$. When the effects of intravenous and epidural morphine were compared in healthy young subjects, significantly greater depression of the slope of the ventilatory response curve to end-tidal PCO_2 and tidal volume was observed with epidural morphine. Maximum respiratory depression occurred at 30 minutes after the intravenous bolus of morphine, whereas with epidural morphine, this occurred between 3 and 22 hours and lasted up to 22 hours.[5] Of particular concern is the wide variability in the late onset of a second peak of respiratory depression. With an average onset time of 8 to 12 hours, this peak may often occur at night when supervision is minimal. It is the variable nature of secondary respiratory depression that demands our vigilance. Fentanyl, despite its high lipid solubility, has been reported to cause respiratory depression when given epidurally either by bolus[6] or infusion.[7] Although the degree of respiratory depression associated with intraspinal fentanyl is extremely low at ordinary doses as compared with morphine, fentanyl has a shorter duration of action and repeated dosing may result in an additive effect.

RISK ASSESSMENT

The risk of respiratory depression has been quantified in several studies. In a retrospective survey, Gustafsson and colleagues found severe respiratory depression in 29 of some 9,000 patients (0.3 percent) receiving intraspinal morphine.[8] The majority of these patients were elderly and there was an association with the presence of pulmonary disease. A review by Reiz and Westberg of 1,200 patients receiving epidural morphine revealed 4 patients with a respiratory rate less than 10 breaths/min. One patient exhibited marked respiratory compromise, with the onset of hypoxemia, hypercarbia, and respiratory acidosis.[9] As these studies were conducted prior to the routine use of pulse oximetry and apnea monitoring, the incidence of respiratory depression was surely underestimated. Factors that influence late onset of respiratory depression associated with intraspinal morphine include age, chronic obstructive pulmonary disease, body position, spinal level of catheter insertion, increased intrathoracic pressure, positive-pressure ventilation, use of concurrent parenteral opioids, preexisting tolerance to opioids, kyphoscoliosis, obstruction of the inferior vena cava, and baricity of the injectate.[10]

In a recent review, Ready and his colleagues treated 623 patients postoperatively with epidural morphine and 167 with intravenous patient-controlled analgesia (PCA). Patients were cared for in an ICU setting and had continuous respiratory monitoring. Four patients treated with epidural morphine developed marked respiratory depression. These were elderly, high-risk patients who had undergone prolonged operative procedures. The lowest recorded respiratory rates ranged between 8 and 12 breaths/min with $PaCO_2$ ranging from 63 to 95 mmHg. Even with an apparent adequate respiratory rate, the patients became somnolent and were not easily arousable. The lowest blood pH recorded was 7.07. Time to peak depression ranged from 2.75 to 13.5 hours. Respiratory depression was reversed with naloxone. None of the patients using PCA developed signs of respiratory depression.[11]

Cheng and Stommel studied 15 subjects receiving epidural sufentanil, an opioid whose greater lipid solubility should limit the degree of respiratory depression, and had four episodes where the oxygen saturation fell below 90 percent and, in three patients, end-tidal PCO_2 was greater than 50 mmHg.[12]

Cousins had stated that the margin of safety of epidural morphine (i.e., the difference between an effective analgesic dose and one that will cause significant respiratory depression) is about 2:1.[13] Bromage reported one patient who suffered apnea and loss of consciousness 4.5 hours after receiving hydromorphone 1 mg epidurally. This occurred in an ICU and the patient required intubation.[14] Parenteral opioids and sedative-tranquilizers can interact synergistically with intraspinal opioids, thus increasing the risk of respiratory depression. In addition, one needs to be concerned that drug administration errors may be increased in a non-ICU setting.

Little work has been reported concerning the respiratory effects of intraspinal opioids in the postpartum patient. Abboud et al. compared epidural butorphanol and morphine for post-cesarean delivery and demonstrated that the respiratory response to carbon dioxide was depressed with the use of morphine 5 mg or butorphanol 2 and 4 mg. Ventilatory depression was found to be more prolonged with morphine. Recently the use of "mini-dose" subarachnoid morphine 0.1 to 0.25 mg has been described in a few patients who had prolonged pain relief with no evidence of ventilatory depression.[15] At the Brigham and Woman's Hospital, fentanyl 10 μg is routinely given along with the usual dose of hyperbaric bupivacaine for subarachnoid anesthesia for cesarean delivery to blunt the discomfort felt with peritoneal tugging or exteriorization of the uterus. If epidural anesthesia has been chosen, fentanyl 50 μg is given in preservative-free normal saline 10 ml or local anesthetic postdelivery. Several thousand patients have been treated in this manner with no evidence of respiratory depression.

Migration of epidural catheters into both subarachnoid[16,17] and intravascular[18,19] spaces has been reported. An analysis by Dawkins suggests an incidence of unrecognized dural puncture of 0.2 percent and of intravascular puncture of 2.8 percent.[20] Injections of incorrect medications, including diazepam and hyperalimentation solution into the epidural catheter, have been reported, which emphasizes the importance of properly labeling the epidural catheter and syringes.

APPROPRIATE MONITORING SYSTEMS

What monitoring systems should be used to optimize patient safety when intraspinal opioids are used? Observation of respiratory rate and mental status by trained personnel is the optimal monitoring technique at present but such labor intensive measures are considered to be unrealistic in this time of cost containment. Even with observation of an adequate respiratory rate, tidal volume may be diminished, resulting in hypercapnea.[11] Current monitoring technology includes impedance apnea monitoring, pulse oximetry, capnography, and arterial blood gas analysis. Cheng and Stommel compared the efficacy of pulse oximetry and end-tidal CO_2 monitoring to detect respiratory depression in 15 patients given epidural sufentanil. They concluded that measurement of end-tidal CO_2 is a more sensitive indicator of respiratory depression than pulse oximetry but that pulse oximetry is a useful adjunct.[12] This study and the review by Ready et al.[11] suggested that capnography is the more sensitive monitoring system. While capnography may be a more sensitive monitor, unintubated patients naturally find a tight-fitting mask to be objectionable. When the mask is not properly fitted, capnography is not reliable. Pulse oximetry is a more practical mode of monitoring because of these constraints. Although pulse oximetry is not sensitive to increasing PCO_2 levels, the adequacy of oxygen delivery to the peripheral tissues is assured. The pulse oximeter is less expensive, and is reliable, easy to use, and readily accepted by patients. Impedance apnea monitors are simple and useful if properly adjusted to ensure a low false-positive rate; however, patient movement can often result in false alarms.

The incidence of respiratory depression (and other side effects such as pruritis, urinary retention, nausea and vomiting) can be reduced by infusions of low concentrations of naloxone (5 μg/kg/h)[21] or bolus administration of nalbuphine.[22] The antagonistic effects of these agents when used in low doses can decrease the side effects of intraspinal opioids with minimal effects on analgesia. Interesting work is being done using oral naltrexone after the use of intraspinal morphine to try to limit the incidence of respiratory depression.

Research on alternatives to morphine for intraspinal use has branched into a number of different areas. Many opioids have been tried intraspinally. Their therapeutic ratios are now being assessed. Lipid-soluble agents such as fentanyl, while less likely to cause respiratory depression, require a more frequent dosing schedule. While lofentanil and sufentanil ware more lipid soluble than fentanyl, their greater avidity for opiate receptors enables a longer duration of action. Duration of analgesia with fentanyl is about 2 to 3 hours, whereas that of sufentanil is 4 to 6 hours. However, there are indications that tighter receptor binding may make reversal of side effects more difficult.

Agonist-antagonist opioids have been studied. Epidural butorphanol has provided up to 5 hours of analgesia with minimal respiratory depression. Combinations of local anesthetics and opioids may reduce total dose requirements and side effects associated with each drug.[23] Addition of epinephrine to intraspinal opioids appears to lengthen duration of analgesia but also increase incidence of side effects.[24] The ideal opioid should produce no respiratory depression even with high doses. Most agents now in use are predominantly μ-agonists. The use of a κ-specific agent may decrease the incidence of respiratory depression.[25] Although the ideal agent has not been found, combinations of agents such as butorphanol and fentanyl hold promise in minimizing side effects and maximizing analgesia.

Oyama et al. have shown that β-endorphins can produce profound pain relief in patients with cancer[26] or labor pains.[27] Respiratory depression, nausea, vomiting, pruritus, reduced uterine contactility, or alterations in FHR were not found. Pain relief lasted up to 33 hours. Unfortunately, the cost of β-endorphins is currently prohibitive.

In summary, intraspinal opioids are a powerful new and seemingly simple technique with great potential for acute and chronic pain management but their use is associated with a small but definite risk of respiratory depression, which can occur in an unpredictable time frame. The margin of safety of epidural opioids when compared to parenteral opioids is reduced and subarachnoid catheter migration can lower this margin even more. Use of more lipid-soluble opioids such as fentanyl appears to be much safer. Small "mini-doses" of subarachnoid morphine may provide effective and safe pain relief for long periods of time but more work must be done to quantify the possible risk.

When large doses of intraspinal opioids such as morphine are used in acute postoperative situations, monitoring is absolutely necessary and should continue for 24 hours after the last dose of opioid has been given. Patients treated with continuous infusions or a repeated dosing schedule, even with the more lipid soluble fentanyl, should also be monitored. It is possible that the use of intraspinal agonist–antagonist agents may prove to be safe and not require the use of continuous monitoring but further studies are necessary to substantiate this concept. Whenever intraspinal opioids are administered a firm policy should be followed, allowing only the pain service or designated personnel to control the dosage and/or route of administration of any analgesic substance. Patients should be monitored in appropriate nursing situations with personnel aware of the side effects associated with intraspinal opioids. Apnea monitors and pulse oximetry are practical, available and essential if appropriate nursing personnel are not available. Supplemental oxygen should be used when indicated. All catheters, infusions, and syringes must be labeled, preferably with bright warning labels that are difficult to remove. There must be a constant alertness for possible subarachnoid, subdural or intravascular migration of epidural catheters. Naloxone must be kept at the bedside and resuscitative equipment must be immediately available. Safety may be enhanced by the use of appropriate naloxone or nalbuphine infusions. Intraspinal opioids have great potential for postoperative pain management but prudence requires conservative monitoring.

REFERENCES

1. Wang JK, Nauss LA, Thomas JE: Pain relief by intrathecally applied morphine in humans. Anesthesiology 50:149, 1979
2. Behar M, Olshwang D, Magora F, Davidson JT: Epidural morphine in treatment of pain. Lancet 1:527, 1979
3. Gourlay GK, Cherry DA, Cousins MJ: Cephalad migration of morphine in CSF following lumbar epidural administration in cancer patients. Pain 23:317, 1985
4. Bromage PR, Camporesi EM, Durant PAC, Nielsen CH: Rostral spread of epidural morphine. Anesthesiology 56:431, 1982
5. Camporesi EM, Nielsen CH, Bromage PR, Durant PAC: Ventilatory CO_2 sensitivity after intravenous and epidural morphine in volunteers. Anesth Analg 62:633, 1983
6. Negre I, et al: Ventilatory response to carbon dioxide after intramuscular and epidural fentanyl. Anesth Analg 66:707, 1987
7. Renaud B, et al: Continuous epidural fentanyl: ventilatory effects and plasma kinetics. Anesthesiology A234, 1985
8. Gustafsson LL, Schildt B, Jacobsen K: Adverse effects of extradural and intrathecal opiates: report of a nationwide survey in Sweden. Br J Anaesth 54:479, 1982
9. Reiz S, Westberg M: Side effects of epidural morphine. Lancet 2:203, 1980
10. Cousins MJ, Mather LE: Intrathecal and epidural administration of opioids. Anesthesiology 61:276, 1984
11. Ready LB, et al: Development of an anesthesiology based postoperative pain management service. Anesthesiology 68:100, 1988
12. Cheng EY, Stommel KA: Respiratory monitoring for postoperative patients receiving epidural opioids. Anesth Analg 67:S28, 1988
13. Cousins MJ: The experts opine. Surv Anesthesiol: 372
14. Bromage PR: The experts opine. Surv Anesthesiol: 374
15. Abboud TK, Dror A, Mosaad P, et al: Mini-dose intrathecal morphine for the relief of postcesarean section pain. Anesth Analg 67:370, 1988
16. Ravindran R, Albrecht W, McKay M: Apparent intravascular migration of epidural catheter. Anesth Analg 58:252, 1979
17. Ryan DW: Accidental intravenous injection of bupivacaine: a complication of obstetrical epidural anesthesia. Br J Anesth 45:907, 1973
18. Gilles IDS, Morgan M: Accidental total spinal with bupivacaine. Anaesthesia 28:441, 1973
19. Kim YI, Mazza NM: Massive spinal block with hemicranial palsy after a test dose of extradural analgesia. Anesthesiology 43:370, 1975
20. Dawkins CJM: An analysis of the complications of epidural and caudal block. Anesthesiology 24:554, 1969
21. Rawal N, Wattwil M: Respiratory depression following epidural morphine: an experimental and clinical study. Anesth Analg 63:8, 1984
22. Henderson SK, Cohen H: Nalbuphine augmentation of analgesia and reversal of side effects following epidural hydromorphone. Anesthesiology 65:216, 1987
23. Skerman JH, Thompson BA, Goldstein, et al: Combined continuous epidural fentanyl and bupivacaine in labor: a randomized study. Anesthesiology 63:A450, 1985
24. Klepper ID, et al: Analgesic and respiratory effects of extradural sufentanil in volunteers and the influence of adrenaline as an adjuvant. Br J Anaesth 59:1147, 1987
25. Lander CJ, et al: Analgesia and ventilatory characteristics of epidural Spiradoline—a specific kappa agonist. Presented at the International Symposium on Spinal Analgesia, Basic and Clinical Aspects. Munich, Germany, August 1987
26. Oyama T, Toshiro JIN, Yamaya R: Profound analgesic effects of beta-endorphins in man. Lancet 2:122, 1980
27. Oyama T, Matsuki A, Taheichi T, et al: Beta-endorphin in obstetric analgesia. Am J Obstet Gynecol 137:613, 1980

PERIPARTUM NAUSEA AND EMESIS

Vomiting, or emesis,[1] is a complex reflex characterized by the forceful expulsion of gastrointestinal contents through the mouth. Nausea is an unpleasant visceral sensation that may or may not be associated with vomiting. Retching is the labored rhythmic activity of the respiratory musculature that usually precedes or accompanies vomiting, but is not ordinarily accompanied by opening the mouth. The mouth opens immediately preceding the evacuation of the stomach whether vomiting is projectile or labored.

During elective cesarean delivery under either subarachnoid[2–5] or epidural[6] anesthesia, 40 to 80 percent of parturients may incur emetic symptoms despite aggressive and meticulous control of maternal hemodynamic variables. The parturient routinely receives little or no premedication prior to elective cesarean delivery to limit fetal exposure to drugs. Emetic symptoms in an unmedicated parturient occur frequently, tend to be an upsetting experience, place the parturient at risk for pulmonary aspiration of gastric contents, and often delay or interfere with surgery. In addition, retching may transiently reduce placental perfusion and adversely affect the fetus with a marginal blood supply.

PHYSIOLOGY OF THE PARTURIENT

In 1960, Bellville et al.[7] reported a three-fold increase in the incidence of postoperative nausea and/or vomiting among women, with a trend toward higher levels during the third and fourth weeks in their menstrual cycle. He speculated this resulted from elevated levels of progesterone and/or gonadotropins.[7,8] Schoeneck[9] in 1942 compared urine gonadotropin levels in parturients with and without emetic symptoms. He found them to be higher among women with emetic symptoms. The highest concentration were found during the 6th to 12th weeks of gestation, which coincides with the highest incidence of emetic symptoms during pregnancy. Cohen et al.[10] found in first-trimester parturients presenting for therapeutic abortions that 63 percent reported a history of nausea and 45 percent had a history of vomiting in early stages of pregnancy. Therefore, the parturient may be more prone to emetic symptoms secondary to the physiologic changes assciated with pregnancy. After the first trimester, the parturient should always be considered to have a full stomach because of pregnancy-induced hormonal changes and the mechanical effects of the gravid uterus. These changes trend to become clinically significant from 18 to 20 weeks of gestation[11] until 8 to 24 hours postpartum. Progesterone decreases gastrointestinal motility, enhances gastrin secretion, and decreases lower esophageal sphincter (LES) tone. By the end of the first trimester, the uterus may begin to mechanically obstruct the duodenum and divide the stomach into antral and fundal pouches. The gravid uterus displaces the pylorus upward and backward, raising intragastric pressure[12] while also rendering the physiologic LES incompetent. Collectively, these serve to delay gastric emptying, increase gastric residual volume, decrease gastric pH, and predispose the parturient to gastroesophageal reflux, regurgitation, and emetic symptoms.

GASTRIC EMPTYING

Pregnancy, labor, and opioid administration delay gastric emptying. In the parturient gastric emptying time may be increased to twice that of the nonpregnant woman.[13] Despite this, it appears that the major cause of gastric stasis during labor is the administration of opioid analgesics.[14–16] Opioids not only delay gastric emptying, but they may stimulate the chemoreceptor trigger zone (CTZ), and sensitize the vestibular apparatus to the effects of motion. Frame et al.[14] in 1984 have shown that intravenous naloxone can reverse the opioid-induced delay of gastric emptying in laboring parturients given intramuscular meperidine.

THE LOWER ESOPHAGEAL SPHINCTER

The physiologic LES is considered a major barrier that protects against spontaneous gastroesophageal reflux.[17] Symptoms of heartburn and reflux of gastric acids are common during pregnancy and are often related to LES incompetence. Pregnant women have weaker LES tone than nonpregnant women. Furthermore, parturients with heartburn tend to have lower LES tone than those without heartburn.[18] The LES incompetence associated with pregnancy appears to be related to the mechanical effects of the gravid uterus and elevated progesterone levels.[19]

Drugs administered in the peripartum period may predispose the parturient to further gastric reflux and regurgitation (Table 3-31). Atropine,[20] scopolamine, and glycopyrrolate[21] have been demonstrated to decrease LES tone. The antiemetic, promethazine (Phenergan), has significant anticholinergic properties and also reduces LES tone.[12,22] In contrast, prochlorperazine (Compazine) has minimal anticholinergic properties and, therefore, has a tendency to increase LES tone.[12] Even though droperidol does not change LES tone, it has been shown by pH probe detection 5 cm above the LES to increase the risk of regurgitation and reflux.[22] Opioid analgesics have also been reported to decrease LES tone.[23,24] Metoclopramide[12,17,18] domperidone,[17] procloperazine (Compazine), and cyclizine[12,17] are antiemetics known to increase LES tone. Metoclopramide, domperidone, and prochlorperazine are dopamine antagonists that may block adrenergic inhibitory impulses to acetylcholine at the LES, thereby potentiating its effect.[12] The mechanism behind cyclizine, a piperazine phenothiazine with marked antihistamine (H_1) properties, remains unclear.[12]

PHYSIOLOGY OF VOMITING

Vomiting Center

The vomiting center is situated in the dorsal part of the lateral reticular formation of the medulla, in the midst of cell groups governing salivation and respiration.[1] Emetic episodes may result from direct stimulation of the vomiting center. Emetic prodromata such as copious salivation, swallowing, and sweating and vasomotor activity such as pallor, tachycardia, and weakness are related to the close proximity of autonomic nuclei to the vomiting center. Sensory information regarding emesis is processed through the nucleus tractus solitarius. The motor components of vomiting are initiated by the dorsal motor nucleus of the vagus and the nucleus ambiguous. Histamine (H_1) receptors are highly concentrated in the nucleus tractus solitarius and the dorsal motor nucleus of the vagus. Muscarinic cholinergic receptors are localized in the nucleus tractus solutarius and the nucleus ambiguus.[25] Therefore, the role of antihistamines and anticholinergic medications in pre-

Table 3-31. Factors That Effect Lower Esophageal Sphincter Tone

Increase	No Change	Decrease
Antimetics	Antiemetics	Antiemetics
Metoclopramide	Droperidol	Promethazine[a]
Domperidone		
Prochlorperazine	H_2 Antagonists	Anesthetics
Cyclizine	Cimetidine	Opioids
	Ranitidine	Thiopental
Cholinergic agonists		Halothane
Bethanechol	Muscle relaxants	Enflurane
	Atracurium	
Hormones		Anticholinergics
Gastrin		Atropine
Insulin		Scopolamine
		Glycopyrrolate
Anticholinesterase		
Edrophonium		Foods
Neostigmine		Fat
		Chocolate
Muscle relaxants		Alcohol
Succinylcholine		Cigarettes
Pancuronium		
Vecuronium		Sedative-hypnotics
		Diazepam
Miscellaneous		
α-adrenergic stimulants		Vasodilators
Antacids (by raising gastric pH)		Sodium nitroprusside
		Nitroglycerin
		Ganglionic blockers
		Verapamil
		Vasopressors
		Dopamine
		Physiologic conditions
		Pregnancy
		Obesity
		Hiatal hernia

[a] Has been shown to increase gastroesophageal reflux.[19,22]
(Data from Refs. 12, 17, 18, 20–24.)

venting or treating emetic symptoms has a sound physiologic basis.

Cortical Afferents. Cortical stimuli resulting from psychogenic and/or emotional disturbances or unpleasant olfactory, visual, or gustatory stimuli may directly trigger the vomiting center. Evans[26] in 1928 described "psychic" nausea as nausea resulting from the terrifying thoughts of an overactive mind. A well-informed patient prior to regional anesthesia and a reassuring, compassionate anesthesiologist may significantly decrease the incidence of anxiety and related emetic symptoms. If the parturient is extremely anxious, mild sedation may be considered. Diazepam 0.5 to 5 mg or diphenhydramine 12.5 to 50 mg intravenously before or after the baby is delivered usually blunts anxiety and extraneous stimuli. Blunting cortical sensory afferents may ultimately decrease signals that impinge directly on the vomiting center. This may help to minimize the incidence of emetic symptoms in the operating room during regional anesthesia.

H1 blocker

Relative Brainstem Hypoxia: Hypotension and Arterial Hypoxemia. Hypotension and the resultant hypoxemia of the brainstem vomiting center may also trigger vomiting.[2,27,28] Hypotensive episodes with systolic blood pressures less than 80 mmHg have been significantly associated with the development of nausea and/or vomiting during subarachnoid anesthesia.[27] Ratra et al.,[28] in a 1972 prospective study of women undergoing gynecologic surgery under subarachnoid anesthesia, noted that the incidence of emetic symptoms increased almost twofold when the systolic blood pressure decreased below 80 mmHg (70.6 percent versus 37.7 percent).

These investigators also observed that the administration of supplemental oxygen therapy significantly decreased the incidence of emetic symptoms despite the presence of hypotension. This supports the theory that hypotension and the relative cerebral hypoxia or hypoxemia of the vomiting center may trigger vomiting.[26–28] During regional anesthetic techniques for cesarean delivery, Datta et al.[2] and Kang et al.[3] reported a 6.6- and 7.0-fold reduction in peripartum emetic symptoms during induction of subarachnoid anesthesia by avoiding maternal hypotension (keeping systolic blood pressure above 100 mmHg or within 10 to 20 percent of baseline) with the aggressive use of intravenous ephedrine by bolus[2] or infusion.[3]

Supplemental inspired oxygen by face mask and acute hydration with 1,000 to 1,500 ml of crystalloid for the healthy parturient undergoing epidural or subarachnoid anesthesia are essential. The higher the segmental sympathetic blockade (especially greater than T4), the greater the risk of hypotension and associated emetic symptoms.[22] The rapidity with which these changes occur influences the incidence of hypotension as well as the incidence of emetic symptoms. Postinduction left uterine displacement to avoid aortocaval compression and prompt intravenous administration of ephedrine as soon as maternal blood pressure begins to fall from baseline will effectively halt further downward trends in blood pressure.[2]

Visceral Autonomic Afferents. During obstetric surgery, reflex triggering of emetic symptoms often results when visceral or parietal peritoneum, or viscera themselves, are overzealously handled or stretched. Sympathetic innervation to the stomach (T6–T10) may be blocked with high segmental levels of subarachnoid or epidural anesthesia. This allows relatively unopposed vagal afferent impulses to predominate in the upper gastrointestinal tract. Harsh peritoneal traction, uterine exteriorization, lower uterine segment stretching, or repair by inexperienced surgeons may further increase afferent impulses over unblocked vagal segments to trigger the vomiting center.

Pederson et al.[29] observed two groups of parturients given a mean dose of hyperbaric bupivacaine of either 8.41 mg or 10.89 mg for cesarean delivery. The group receiving 25 percent more drug per centimeter of height had reduced intraoperative intravenous opioid supplementation and 2.2 times less visceral pain, which can result when inadequate extent, duration, or intensity of subarachnoid or epidural anesthesia occurs.[30] Under such circumstances, reflex visceral vagal afferents from the gastrointestinal tract or uterus can travel centrally to directly trigger the vomiting center. If emetic symptoms occur at this time, a reminder to the surgeons to gently handle the tissues may suffice. Emetic symptoms associated with visceral pain are usually brief and self-limited, often resolving as surgical stimulation diminishes. Anticholinergic medications, which have detrimental effects on the LES tone, are often impractical for therapy at this time unless given prophylactically. Furthermore, antiemetics with predominant antidopaminergic properties tend to be largely ineffective in treating emetic symptoms of visceral origin.

Visceral pain during subarachnoid anesthesia is often related to inadequate anesthesia, especially when plain local anesthetic mixtures are used.[29] During epidural anesthesia, an inadequate sacral block also predisposes the parturient to visceral pain sensations and emetic consequences. The degree of pain complaints by the patient represents the state of afferent blockade of the nociceptive fibers.[31] This can be modified by the quality and quantity of local anesthetics used during the operative procedure. The use of larger dosages of local anesthetics in the subarachnoid space provides for a more profound sensory afferent blockade. This may limit the incidence of visceral pain, as well as the incidence of viscerally mediated emetic symptoms.[27] Norris[32] demonstrated that adequate anesthesia for cesarean delivery (median level T3) could be obtained with 12 mg (1.6 ml) of hyperbaric bupivacaine regardless of patient height (4′11″ to 5′8″), weight, or body mass index.

Subarachnoid and epidural opioids act selectively on the nociceptive receptors in the dorsal horns of the spinal column, specifically in the substantia gelatinosa. Here, subarachnoid and epidural opioids modulate nociceptive input from small primary afferent nerves of the unmyelinated C and myelinated A-δ type.[33,34] Visceral nociceptive afferents can be blunted by intrathecal μ- and κ-agonists, such as morphine and fentanyl. Epidurally administered fentanyl 50 μg diluted in a total volume of at least 10 ml of preservative-free normal saline has been shown to help minimize the incidence of emetic symptoms associated with uterine manipulation.[35] The μ-receptor agonist/antagonists with κ-agonist properties (nalbuphine, butorphanol, and nalorphine) may similarly decrease visceral pain.[33]

Hunt et al. in 1989,[36] observed that hyperbaric bupivacaine plus subarachnoid fentanyl 6.25 μg allowed for complete intraoperative pain relief during cesarean delivery, when compared with plain subarachnoid bupivacaine solutions. No intravenous opioid supplementation was required in the subarachnoid bupivacaine/fentanyl group versus a 67 percent requirement in the plain bupivacaine group. Therefore, subarachnoid and epidural opioids may successfully decrease the

Table 3-32. Antiemetic Drug Potencies at Neurotransmitter Receptor Sites

Drug	Dopamine (D_2)	Muscarine Cholinergic	Histamine (H_1)
Anticholinergics			
Hyoscine	Negligible	+ + + + +	Negligible
Atropine	Negligible	+ + + + +	Negligible
Glycopyrrolate	Negligible	+ + + + +	Negligible
H_1 Antihistamines			
Promethazine	+ + + +	+ + + + +	+ + + + +
Diphenhydramine	Negligible	+ + + +	Negligible
Cyclizine	+	+ + +	+ + + + +
Phenothiazines			
Fluphenazine	+ + + + +	+ + + +	+ + + + +
Prochlorperazine	+ + + + +	+ + +	+ + + +
Chlorpromazine	+ + + + +	+ + + +	+ + + + +
Butyrophenones			
Droperidol	+ + + + +	Negligible	+
Haloperidol	+ + + + +	Negligible	+
Miscellaneous			
Metoclopramide	+ + + +	Negligible	+
Domperidone	+ + + +	Negligible	Negligible

(From Palazzo and Strunin,[38] with permission.)

incidence of intraoperative visceral pain. Interestingly, a threefold increase in the incidence of nausea was observed in the subarachnoid bupivacaine/fentanyl group compared to the plain bupivacaine group (32.6 percent versus 11.0 percent). Obviously, there are other mechanisms responsible for triggering emetic symptoms.

Chemoreceptor Trigger Zone

The chemoreceptor trigger zone (CTZ) lies bilaterally on the floor of the fourth ventricle in the medulla in close proximity to the vomiting center. Impulses from the CTZ are relayed to the vomiting center and a vomiting reflex initiated (Fig. 3-18). This CTZ is richly innervated with dopaminergic (D_2) receptors.[25] This is why dopamine antagonists such as phenothiazines, droperidol,[5,36] metoclopramide,[4,6,37,38] and domperidone[38] are efficacious antiemetics (Table 3-32). Triggers of the CTZ include circulating toxins and drugs (cytotoxic drugs, opioids, digoxin, and apomorphine), radiation therapy, metabolic disturbances (uremia, hypoglycemia, and hyperglycemia), as well as hyperemesis gravidarum.

Impulses mediating nausea and vomiting by vestibular stimulation (motion sickness) originate principally in the utricular maculae of the labyrinth. These impulses pass by way of the 8th cranial nerve to the lateral vestibular nuclei, to the uvula and nodulus of the cerebellum, then to the CTZ, and finally to the vomiting center. The lateral vestibular nucleus is innervated by muscarinic cholinergic and histamine (H_1) receptors. Therefore, motion sickness may be managed with anticholinergics (e.g., scopolamine) and/or antihistamines (H_1) such as promethazine (Phenergan),[25] or diphenhydramine. Interestingly, intramuscular ephedrine may also have antiemetic efficacy in patients prone to motion sickness. However, its mechanism remains unclear.[39]

PROPHYLAXIS AND TREATMENT OF EMETIC SYMPTOMS FOR THE PARTURIENT

Steps in prevention and treatment of emetic symptoms are outlined in Table 3-33.

Metoclopramide is an antiemetic[40,41] that is related to procainamide but virtually devoid of antiarrhythmic or local anesthetic activity. It accelerates gastric emptying by its direct effect on autonomic nuclei and sensitizes gastric smooth muscle to the effects of acetylcholine. In laboring primigravidae, Howard and Sharp in 1973[13] showed an almost threefold increase in gastric emptying after 10 mg of metoclopramide was given intramuscularly following a 750-ml test fluid meal (Fig. 3-19). He also showed that metoclopramide partly reversed the delayed gastric emptying produced by meperidine in laboring patients. Murphy et al.[42] similarly noted improved gastric emptying in parturients when given metoclopramide during labor and/or elective cesarean delivery. Wyner[11] demonstrated in first-trimester parturients that the preinduction administration of 10 mg of intravenous metoclopramide decreased gastric volume.

Metoclopramide's central antidopaminergic activity on the CTZ makes it a useful antiemetic whether given before[4] or after cesarean delivery.[6] Maternal and fetal safety has been well documented with metoclopramide.[14,43] McGarray[37] demonstrated its antiemetic efficacy for parturients in labor when given meperidine analgesia. Lussos et al.[4] reported that parturients given intravenous metoclopramide 10 mg prior to induction of bupivacaine/fentanyl subarachnoid anesthesia had a fivefold reduction in post-subarachnoid block, predelivery emetic symptoms compared to saline controls. Chestnut et al.[6] administered intravenous metoclopramide 0.15 mg/kg to parturients intraoperatively post-cesarean delivery. He observed a threefold reduction in postdelivery intraoperative nausea (12 percent versus 36 percent) and no vomiting in the metoclopramide group compared to 15 percent in the saline placebo group. All patients received epidural morphine or hydromorphone prior to closure of the fascia. Of note was the 2.5- to

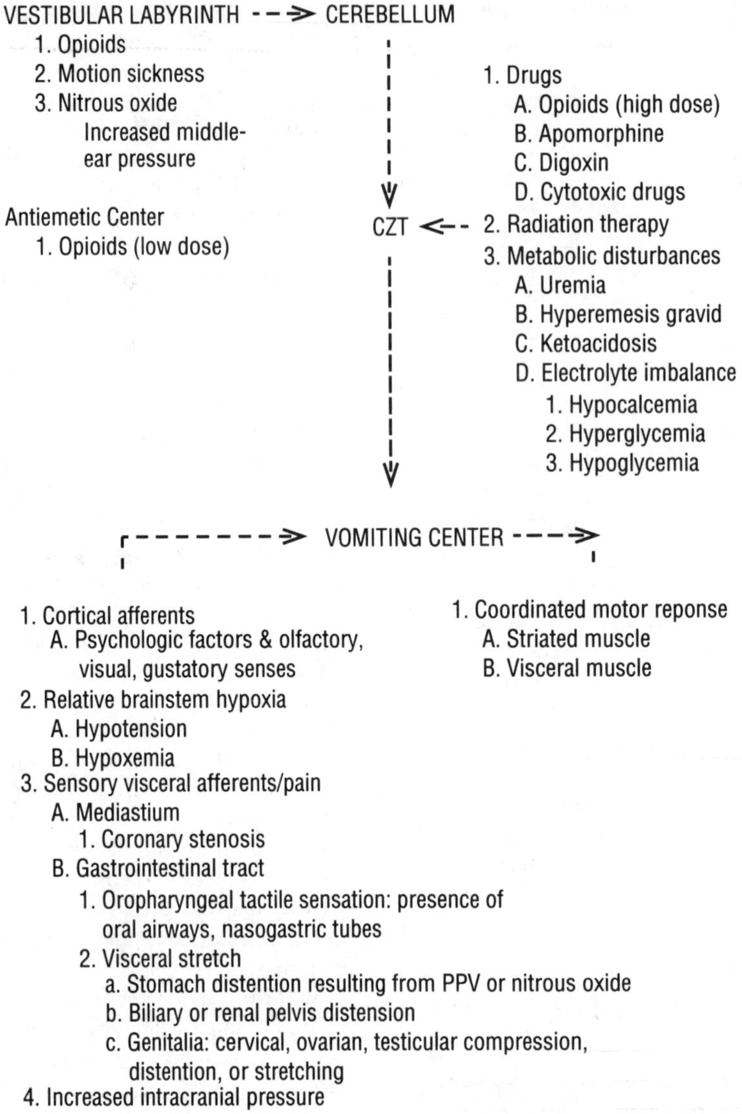

Fig. 3-18. Stimuli that cause emetic symptoms. (Data from Bellville,[8] Clarke,[53] and Palazzo and Strunin.[54])

3.0-fold reduction in emetic symptoms in the metoclopramide group during the first 4 hours postoperatively.

Adverse side effects to metoclopramide are dose related and occur infrequently in the 10- to 20-mg dose ranges used clinically.[4,41] Sedation and extrapyramidal and dystonic reactions (e.g., torticolis, oculogyric crises, and trismus) are potential adverse effects of antiemetic medications. Cohen et al.[10] reported that patients given droperidol 1.25 mg suffered from delayed awakening[10,39] and postoperative dizziness,[10] whereas patients given metoclopramide had less postoperative sedation and earlier discharge times. Patients with a history of dystonic reactions often benefit from pretreatment with diphenhydramine or avoidance of metoclopramide and droperidol altogether. The use of droperidol during subarachnoid anesthesia has been shown to have antiemetic efficacy in the parturient,[5] but may increase the risk of esophageal reflex and regurgitation.[22]

Timing of drug administration is important. Metoclo-

Table 3-33. Prophylaxis and Treatment of Emetic Symptoms for the Parturient during Obstetric Regional Anesthesia

1. Full explanation of the regional anesthetic procedure and expected sensory and motor changes to be experienced following successful block.
2. 0.3 mol/L sodium citrate 30 ml PO.
3. Acute hydration with dextrose-free crystalloid solution 1.5–2.0 L.
4. Metoclopramide 10 mg IV approximately 10–15 minutes priot to induction.
5. Oxygen 6 L PM by face mask.
6. Appropriate monitors applied: NIBP, SPO_2, ECG.
7. Post subarachnoid or epidural placement emetic symptoms: determine etiology.
   - A. Psychogenic/anxiety-related emetic symptoms
     - 1. Diphenhydramine 12.5–50 mg, diazepam 0.5–5.0 mg IV.
   - B. Relative cerebral hypoxia
     - 1. Ensure SBP >100 or 10–20% of baseline, check HR and level of blockade.
       - A. Bolus ephedrine in 10 mg IV increments as soon as sBP decreases from baseline.
       - B. Fluid bolus.
       - C. Ensure adequate left uterine displacement.
     - 2. Ensure adequate oxygenation: check SPO_2, oxygen source.
   - C. Visceral pain (usually occurs postdelivery)
     - 1. Inadequate anesthesia or excessive surgical visceral traction.
       - A. Ensure adequacy of regional block: extent, intensity, duration.
         - 1. Subarachnoid anesthesia
           - a. Begin block with higher dose of local anesthetic.
           - b. Add subarachnoid opioid to local anesthetic mixture.
           - c. Supplement with IV opioid after block is complete.
         - 2. Epidural anesthesia
           - a. Ensure adequate sacral block prior to incision.
           - b. Supplement block with epidural opioids.
           - c. Reassess sensory level: top-up local anesthetic, if indicated.
       - B. Glycopyrrolate 0.2 mg IV for persistent visceral pain.
   - D. Opioid induced
     - 1. Metoclopramide 10 mg IV q 4–6 h, or droperidol 0.625 mg IV q 6–8 h.
     - 2. Scopolamine patches.
     - 3. Low-dose naloxone 80 μg/h, nalbuphine 2–5 mg, butorphanol 1–2 mg IV.

pramide 10 mg given intravenously 5 to 10 minutes before atropine administration may counter its undesirable effects on LES tone.[44] Meperidine 1 to 2 mg/kg given intramuscularly can lower mean barrier pressure (barrier pressure = LES pressure − intragastric pressure) and LES tone, the subsequent administration of metoclopramide 10 mg has been shown to return mean barrier pressure toward baseline levels (Fig. 3-20).[23] Parturients with or without heartburn derive beneficial augmentation of LES tone and, therefore, increased barrier pressure when given metoclopramide.[12,18,19] This effect appears most pronounced in patients with greater intrinsic LES tone.[12]

Patients given epidural opioids (especially morphine) may develop emetic symptoms within 1 hour or up to 4 to 10 hours after administration. Early emetic symptoms may be related to the systemic absorption of opioids from the epidural space, analogous to intramuscular opioid administration. Delayed emetic symptoms reflect diffusion of epidural opioids into the cerebrospinal fluid and rostral spread to the brainstem.[45] The μ-opioid receptor agonists appear to mediate the supraspinal emetic response at the CTZ or the vestibular apparatus. Reported incidences of emetic symptoms with subarachnoid opioids range from 20 to 50 percent, whereas epidurally administered opioids range from 20 to 30 percent.[34]

Abouleish[46] observed a fivefold increase in nausea postoperatively in parturients given subarachnoid morphine 0.2 mg. Leicht et al.[47] observed a 20 percent incidence of postoperative emetic symptoms after cesarean delivery in parturients given epidural morphine 5 mg. Abboud et al.[48] demonstrated an 8.5-fold reduction in postoperative emetic symptoms (1.1 percent versus 9.3 percent) when butorphanol 2 to 4 mg was compared to epidural morphine 5 mg for postcesarean delivery pain relief.

Harrison et al.[49] and Eisenach et al.[50] both prospec-

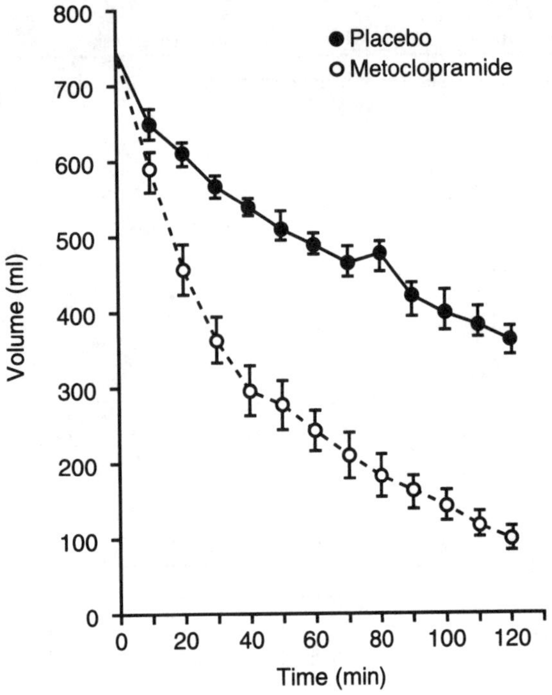

Fig. 3-19. Mean gastric volumes after a 750-ml fluid test meal remaining in laboring parturients given either metoclopramide or placebo. (From Howard and Sharp,[13] with permission.)

tively found the greatest overall quality of postcesarean analgesia with epidural morphine 5 mg when compared to patient-controlled analgesia morphine, and intramuscular morphine. Both failed to observe any statistically significant difference in the incidence of emetic symptoms between the three groups postoperatively. Interestingly, 50 percent of patients in Eisenach's[50] epidural morphine group developed nausea, 30 percent of these patients required antiemetic therapy. Although pruritus is usually the most common complication, and late respiratory depression the most feared complication of subarachnoid or epidural opioids, perhaps emetic symptoms may leave the patient with the most lasting and unpleasant impression related to their use. Therefore, when using opioids during subarachnoid anesthesia for cesarean delivery it may be prudent to administer a preoperative antiemetic such as metoclopramide beforehand to block the CTZ.

Kotelko et al.[51] demonstrated the antiemetic efficacy of transdermal scopolmaine (TDS) patches in parturients receiving epidural morphine after cesarean delivery compared to placebo. Postoperative emetic symptoms remained in the 3 to 25 percent range during the first 24 hours postoperatively despite TDS patches. For prolonged relief of emetic symptoms postoperatively intravenous metoclopramide 10 mg every 4 to 6 hours, or scopolamine patches, a mixed agonist-antagonist (e.g., nalbuphine or butorphanol), or a long-acting oral opioid antagonist such as naltrexone may be used.

Finally, during transport to and from the operating room it is important to avoid abrupt movements, such as turning, and rapid head-up movements, which may trigger vestibular response and cause emetic symptoms.[8] This is especially true if the parturient has recently received opioid medications, as these can sensitize the vestibular apparatus. Adequate pain relief also has been shown to minimize the incidence of postoperative emetic symptoms.[52]

CONCLUSION

Peripartum emetic symptoms are multifactorial in nature. A management scheme to successfully diminish the incidence of emetic symptoms must anticipate those stimuli or events that may provoke or trigger this response. The parturient is unique in that hormonal changes during pregnancy, as well as the mechanical effects of the gravid uterus, predispose the patient to emetic symptoms. Labor itself, and opioid analgesics in particular, may compound this problem by causing gastric stasis.

The intensity, extent, and duration of the intraspinal block cannot be overemphasized in preventing intraoperative visceral pain. Adequate local anesthetic dosages combined with subarachnoid or epidural opioids may improve the quality of sensory analgesia and modulate nociceptive sensory afferent impulses to limit visceral pain. Despite their ability to decrease the incidence of visceral pain, subarachnoid and epidural opioids may increase postoperative emetic symptoms by systemic absorption or by their rostral spread to the brainstem. They may also sensitize the vestibular apparatus to the effects of motion or trigger the CTZ directly. Efforts to obtain a high, dense segmental block must be weighed against the risk of precipitating hypotension. Forethought and aggressive prophylactic ephedrine in addition to acute hydration and left uterine displacement are essential to limit the fall of blood pressure from baseline. Supplemental oxygen and pulse oximetry are essential to protect against hypoxemia.

The ideal antiemetic for the parturient undergoing a regional anesthetic for cesarean section probably does not exist, especially since the etiology of pre- or post-delivery emetic symptoms may be different and may involve different pathways in triggering either the CTZ or the vomiting center. If antiemetics are utilized, proper timing and sequence of drug administration are important. Metoclopramide, which has antiemetic properties,

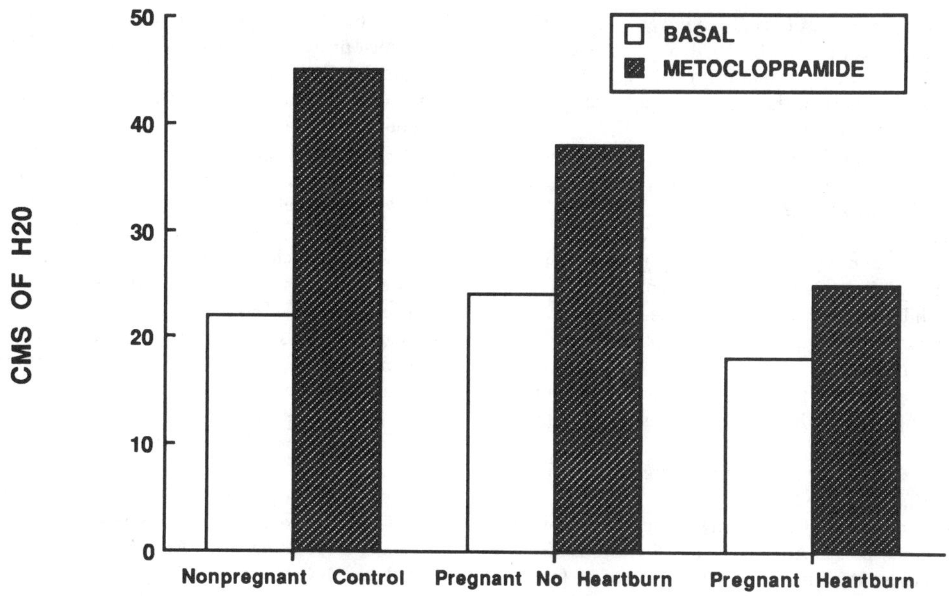

Fig. 3-20. Mean barrier pressure (LES pressure − intragastric pressure) before and after metoclopramide. (From Brock-Utne et al.,[12] with permission.)

increases LES tone and tends to reverse the gastric stasis associated with pregnancy, appears to be ideal for the parturient. Prophylactic antiemetics should be considered when the parturient describes a prior history of postoperative emetic symptoms or motion sickness, or when subarachnoid or epidural opioids are being utilized.

REFERENCES

1. Borison HL, Wang SC: Physiology and pharmacology of vomiting. Pharmacol Rev 5:193, 1953
2. Datta S, Alper MH, Ostheimer GW, Weiss JB: Methods for ephedrine administration and nausea and hypotension during spinal anesthesia for cesarean section. Anesthesiology 56:68, 1982
3. Kang YG, Abouleish E, Caritis S: Prophylactic intravenous ephedrine infusion during spinal anesthesia for cesarean section. Anesth Analg 61:839, 1982
4. Lussos SA, Bader AM, Thornhill M, Datta S: The antiemetic efficacy of prophylactic metoclopramide for cesarean delivery. Society for Obstetric Anesthesia and Perinatology; Abstracts, 1991.
5. Santos A, Datta S: Prophylactic use of droperidol for control of nausea and vomiting during spinal anesthesia for cesarean section. Anesth Analg 63:85, 1984
6. Chestnut DH, Vandewalker GE, Owen CL, et al: Administration of metoclopramide for prevention of nausea and vomiting during epidural anesthesia for elective cesarean section. Anesthesiology 66:563, 1987
7. Bellville JW, Bross IDJ, Howland WS: Post operative nausea and vomiting. IV. Factors related to post operative nausea and vomiting. Anesthesiology 21(2):186, 1960
8. Bellville JW: Post anesthetic nausea and vomiting. Anesthesiology 22(5):773, 1961
9. Shoeneck FJ: Gonadotropic hormone concentration in emesis gravidarum. Am J Obstet Gynecol 43:308, 1942
10. Cohen SE, Woods WA, Wyner J: Antiemetic efficacy of droperidol and metoclopramide. Anesthesiology 60:67, 184
11. Wyner J, Cohen SE: Gastric volume in early pregnancy: effect of metoclopramide. Anesthesiology 57:209, 1982
12. Brock-Utne JG, Dow TGB, Welman S, et al: The effect of metoclopramide on the lower oesophageal sphincter in late pregnancy. Anaesth Intens Care 6:26, 1978
13. Howard FA, Sharp DS: Effect of metoclopramide on gastric emptying during labour. Br Med J 1:446, 1973
14. Frame WT, Allison RH, Moir DD, Nimmo WS: Effect of naloxone on gastric emptying during labour. Br J Anaesth 56:263, 1984
15. Nimmo WS, Wilson J, Prescott LF: narcotic analgesics and delayed gastric emptying during labour. Lancet 1:890, 1975
16. Nimmo WS, Wilson J, Prescott LF: Further studies of gastric emptying during labour. Anaesthesia 32:100, 1977
17. Cotton BR, Smith G: The lower oesophageal sphincter and anaesthesia. Br J Anaesth 56:37, 1984
18. Hey VMF, Ostick DG: Metoclopramide and the gastro-oesophageal sphincter: a study in pregnant women with heartburn. Anaesthesia 33:462, 1978
19. Hey VMF, Ganguli PC, Skinner LD, et al: Gastro-oesophageal reflux in late pregnancy. Anaesthesia 32:372, 1977
20. Dow TGB, Cog MR, Brock-Utne JG,. et al: The effect of

atropine on the lower eosphageal sphincter in late pregnancy. Obstet Gynecol 51(4):426, 1978
21. Brock-Utne JG, Rubin J, Welman S, et al: The effect of glycopyrrolate (Robinol) on the lower oesophageal sphincter. Can Anaesth Soc J 25(2):144, 1978
22. Brock-Utne JG, Rubin J, Welman S, et al: The action of commonly used anti-emetics on the lower esophageal sphincter. Br J Anaesth 50:295, 1978
23. Hey VMF, Ostick DG, Mazumder JK, Lord WD: Pethidine, metoclopramide, and the gastroesophageal sphincter. A study in healthy volunteers. Anaesthesia 36:173, 1981
24. Hey VMF, Phillips K, Woods I: Pethidine, atropine, metoclopramide and the lower esophageal sphincter. Anaesthesia 38:650, 1983
25. Peroutka SJ, Snyder SH: Antiemetics: neurotransmitter receptor binding predicts therapeutic actions. Lancet 1:658, 1982
26. Evans CH: Possible complications with spinal anesthesia. Am J Surg 5(6):581, 1928
27. Crocker JS, Vandam LD: Concerning nausea and vomiting during spinal anesthesia. Anesthesiology 20:589, 1959
28. Ratra CK, Badola RP, Bhargava KP: A study of factors concerned in emesis during spinal anesthesia. Br J Anaesth 44:1208, 1972
29. Pedersen H, Santos AC, Steinberg ES, et al: Incidence of visceral pain during cesarean section: the effect of varying doses of spinal bupivacaine. Anesth Analg 69:46, 1989
30. Bonica JJ, Crepps W, Monk B, Bennett B: Post anesthetic nausea, retching and vomiting. Anesthesiology 19(4):532, 1958
31. Wall PD: To what would Gaston Labat be attending to today? Reg Anesth 14:261, 1989
32. Norris MC: Height, weight, and the spread of subarachnoid hyperbaric bupivacaine in the term parturient. Anesth Analg 67:555, 1988
33. Cousins MI, Mather LE: Intrathecal and epidural administration of opioids. Anesthesiology 61:276, 1984
34. Ready LB: Regional analgesia with intraspinal opioids. Ch. 95. In Bonica JJ (ed): The Management of Pain. 2nd Ed. Lea & Febiger, Philadelphia, 1990
35. Ackerman WE, Juneja MM, Colclough GW, Kaczorowski DM: Epidural fentanyl significantly decreases nausea and vomiting during uterine manipulation in awake patient undergoing cesarean section. Anesthesiology 69:A679, 1988
36. Hunt CO, Naulty S, Bader AM, et al: Perioperative analgesia with subarachnoid fentanyl-bupivacaine for cesarean delivery. Anesthesiology 71:535, 1989
37. McGarry JM: A double-blind comparison of the anti-emetic effect during labour of metoclopramide and perphenazine. Br J Anaesth 43:613, 1971
38. Palazzo MGA, Strunin L: Anaesthesia and emesis. II. Prevention and management. Can Anesth Soc J 31:407, 1984
39. Rothenberg DM, Parnass SM, Litwack K, et al: Efficacy of ephedrine in the prevention of postoperative nausea and vomiting. Anesth Analg 72:58, 1991
40. Schulze-Delrieu K: Metoclopramide. N Engl J Med 305(1):28, 1981
41. Tornetta FJ: Clinical studies with the new antiemetic, metoclopramide. Anesth Analg 48:198, 1969
42. Murphy DF, Nally B, Gardiner J, Unwin A: Effect of metoclopramide on gastric emptying before elective and emergency caesarean section. Br J Anaesth 56:1113, 1984
43. Bylsma-Howell M, Riggs KW, McMorland GH, et al: Placental transport of metoclopramide: assessment of maternal and neonatal effects. Can Anaesth Soc J 30(5):487, 1983
44. Brock-Utne JG, Rubin J, Downing JW, et al: The administration of metoclopramide with atropine. (A drug interaction effect on the gastroesophageal sphincter in man.) Anesthesia 31:1186, 1976
45. Bromage PR, Camporesi EM, Durant PAC, Neilsen CH: Non-respiratory side effects of epidural morphine. Anesth Analg 61:490, 1982
46. Abouleish E, Rawal N, Fallon K, Hernandez D: Combined intrathecal morphine and bupivacaine for cesarean section. Anesth Analg 67:370, 1988
47. Leicht CH, Hughes SC, Dailey PA, et al: Epidural morphine sulfate for analgesia after cesarean section: a prospective report of 1000 patients. Anesthesiology 65:A366, 1986
48. Abboud TK, Moore M, Zhu J, et al: Epidural butorphanol or morphine for the relief of post-cesarean section pain: ventilatory responses to carbon dioxide. Anesth Analg 66:887, 1987
49. Harrison DM, Sinatra R, Morgese L, Chung JH: Epidural narcotic and patient-controlled analgesia for post-cesarean section pain relief. Anesthesiology 68:454, 1988
50. Eisenach JC, Grice SC, Dewan DM: Patient-controlled analgesia following cesarean section: a comparison with epidural and intramuscular narcotics. Anesthesiology 68:444, 1988
51. Kotelko DM, Rottman RL, Wright WC, et al: Transderm scop (R) decreases post-cesarean nausea and vomiting in patients receiving epidural morphine. Anesthesiology 69:A666, 1988
52. Andersen R, Krohg K: Pain as a major cause of postoperative nausea. Can Anaesth Soc J 23:366, 1976
53. Clarke RSJ: Nausea and vomiting. Br J Anaesth 56:19, 1984
54. Palazzo MGA, Strunin L: Anaesthesia and emesis. I. Etiology. Can Anaesth Soc J 31:178, 1984

PRURITUS

Epidural and subarachnoid opioids are widely utilized for anesthesia during labor and vaginal and cesarean delivery, and for postoperative pain control. While their efficacy is well documented, the associated side effects—more specifically, pruritus—are also well documented, with an incidence of 20 to 93 percent,[1] depending on the investigator and the report.

The pruritus associated with opioids is seen more commonly after epidural and subarachnoid administration than after systemic administration and is more common in pregnant women than in nonpregnant patients.[2] Interestingly, the pruritus is often localized to the face,[2,3] unlike that of systemically administered opioids, in which the itching tends to be more generalized. This facial itching has recently been linked to reactivation of oral herpes simplex virus.[4,5]

The dermatomal pattern of pruritus provides valuable information regarding its mechanism, which is far from fully understood. It appears that stimulation of opioid μ-receptors may be responsible,[6] though Ballantyne and colleagues describe several other possible mechanisms.[2] It is essential to evaluate these mechanism(s) in an effort to better antagonize, prevent, and/or treat the itching.

First, one must consider how the sensation is transmitted and then, how it differs from its close companion, pain. Both share a common neuronal pathway in the ascending spinothalamic tract and both are also generated (at least partially) by polymodal nociceptor units. It remains to be defined whether itch is a primary sensation with its own system of fibers and receptors, or whether the two sensations are carried by one fiber type with different patterns of nerve impulses.[2]

The term *pruritus* needs to be defined. It is a sensation that provokes the desire to scratch and can be aroused by a variety of mechanical, electrical, and chemical stimuli.[2]

Pruritus, in general, may be described as either "itchy skin," from which itch can be aroused more readily than from normal skin, or "spontaneous itch," which occurs without any external stimulus. Keele et al. has compared "itchy skin" to hyperalgesia and "spontaneous itch" to spontaneous pain.[7] Morphine and similar opioids are known to chemically mediate pruritus, presumably through the release of histamine. With epidural and subarachnoid opioids, the segmental distribution of pruritus has been encountered. This leads one to believe that the spinal cord itself and/or the spinal roots are a significant site of this opioid-induced itching.[2]

Ballantyne and his colleagues have developed a hypothesis to explain intraspinal opioid-induced pruritus. It is their contention that the hyperalgesia and itch that occur after intraspinal administration are manifestations of opioid-mediated facilitation of protective reflexes.

Their claim is that both pain and itch are sensations that invoke defensive, or protective, behaviors. The immediate pain of injury produces a reflex withdrawal. The tenderness associated with such pain induces rubbing, as a means of soothing. Itch, as a sensation, induces scratching, which may itself be a protective reflex. In response to injury, then, protective reflexes are enhanced, resulting in hyperalgesia and itch. Both arise after cutaneous injury and involve the damaged tissue as well as the surrounding area. The tenderness of damaged tissue dissipates, however, if not further stimulated. It is important that an equilibrium be reached between the suppression and facilitation of noxiously induced reflexes. Ballantyne et al. contend that opioids have a role in facilitating noxiously induced activity by certain mechanisms described briefly below.

Opioids have excitatory effects, facilitating hyperalgesia and itch. There are opioid receptors on primary afferent neurons in the periphery and on primary sensory ganglia. It appears that peripheral opioid receptors may mediate hyperalgesia;[8,9] when opposed, they may allow central analgesia systems to act unopposed and thus potentiate analgesia.[8]

It has also been demonstrated in animals that subarachnoid injection of high doses of morphine can result in a scratch syndrome, or *hyperalgesia* syndrome.[10] In humans, both hyperalgesia and itch can occur after subarachnoid administration of opioids, in a segmental distribution with respect to injection site.[11,12] In view of this distribution, it seems likely that the process is most likely localized to the spinal cord or dorsal roots.[2]

The following mechanisms of this excitation have been postulated. First, activation of peripheral opioid receptors may produce itching, as hypothesized by Van der Kooy,[9] but this mechanism remains conjectural.

Itching may occur because certain afferent fibers with a moderating influence are suppressed, leaving only unopposed excitatory activity in other fibers.[2] High concentrations of drug—here, opioid—are required to block conduction of these fibers,[13] posing some problem when explaining the itch produced by small amounts of intraspinal opioid.

Ballantyne and his colleagues also proposed that the opioid, once introduced into the cerebrospinal fluid (CSF), may reach distinct sites within the cord and then facilitate noxiously induced activity. They used morphine, with its poor lipid solubility and its often-produced facial itching, as an example, and claimed that penetration to the ventral side of the spinal cord appears to predominate, at least in the cervical region.

Finally, they suggest that opioid antagonism of the inhibitory transmitter, glycine, may be responsible for the pruritus effected by opioids, and also indicate that metabolites of opioids (e.g., morphine 3-glucoronide) may induce and/or potentiate hyperalgesia and itch.[10]

TREATMENT

Treatment of the pruritus induced by intraspinal opioids, as well as by systemic administration such as patient-controlled analgesia (PCA), is variable in its efficacy.

In some reports, intravenous morphine (PCA) produces less pruritus than epidural morphine,[14,15] but if patients do experience pruritus with PCA, it is often helpful to decrease the demand dose (e.g., morphine 1 mg) or modify the lockout interval (e.g., morphine every 5 minutes) to decrease the pruritus. Changing from one opioid to another may be prudent in some cases. Antihistamines such as hydroxyzine or diphenhydramine are also useful.[3]

Various agents have been administered for the prevention and treatment of the pruritus and other side effects associated with subarachnoid and epidural narcotics. Rosen found that epidural sufentanil may result in a decreased incidence of pruritus compared to morphine.[16] A continuous infusion of naloxone 0.4 to 0.6 mg/h can significantly decrease pruritus while maintaining analgesia following subarachnoid administration of morphine.[17] The facial pruritus experienced by some patients can be treated with naloxone, but there remains an increased risk (about 15 percent) of oral reactivation of herpes simplex virus after epidural morphine in obstetric patients with a positive history of herpes labialis.[4,5] Naltrexone (5 mg) has been found to diminish both the frequency and severity of pruritus, nausea, and vomiting after epidural morphine 5 mg with no diminution of the quality or duration of analgesia.[18] Similarly, 6 mg has been found to be an effective oral prophylactic against the pruritus and vomiting associated with subarachnoid morphine, but it tends to decrease the duration of analgesia.[19]

Other agents with varying efficacy include nalbuphine, administered intravenously (2.5 mg) to prevent pruritus induced by epidural fentanyl.[20] Buprenorphine 0.6 mg/50 ml total was used as a replacement for morphine in an epidural infusion with 0.125 percent bupivacaine in a patient who complained of severe, unremitting pruritus, and the buprenorphine mixture allowed for excellent analgesia while sustaining rapid and complete relief from pruritus.[21] Most recently the mixed agonist–antagonist butorphanol (3 mg) has been combined with epidural opioids (morphine 4 mg) to effectively decrease the occurrence of pruritus and nausea without significantly increasing respiratory depression or sedation, and without adversely affecting duration of analgesia.[1]

REFERENCES

1. Lawhorn CD, McNitt JD, Fibuch EE, et al: Epidural morphine with butorphanol for postoperative analgesia after cesarean delivery. Anesth Analg 72:53, 1991
2. Ballantyne JC, Loach AB, Carr DB: Itching after epidural and spinal opiates Pain 33:149, 1988
3. Bonica JJ: The Management of Pain. Lea & Febiger, Philadelphia, 1990, p. 1977
4. Crone LL, Conly JM, Storgard C, et al: Herpes labialis in parturients receiving epidural morphine following cesarean section. Anesthesiology 73:208, 1990
5. Gierarts R, Navalgund A, Vaes L, et al: Increased incidence of itching and herpes simplex in patients given epidural morphine after cesarean section. Anesth Analg 66:1321, 1987
6. Martin WR: Clinical evidence for different narcotic receptors and relevance for the clinician. Ann Emerg Med 15:1026, 1986
7. Keele CA, Armstrong D: Substances Producing Pain and Itch. Edward Arnold, London, 1964
8. Van der Kooy D, Nagy JI: Hyperalgesia mediated by peripheral opiate receptors in the rat. Behav Brain Res 17:203, 1985
9. Van der Kooy D: Hyperalgesic functions of peripheral opiate receptors. In: DD Kelly (ed): Stress-Induced Analgesia. Ann NY Acad Sci 467:154, 1986
10. Yaksh TL, Harty GJ, Onofrio BM: High doses of spinal morphine produce a nonopiate receptor-mediated hyperesthesia: clinical and theoretic implications. Anesthesiology 64:590, 1986
11. Bromage PR, Camporesi EM, Durant PAC, Nielsen CH: Rostral spread of epidural morphine. Anesthesiology 56:431, 1982
12. Bromage PR, Camporesi EH, Durant PAC, Nielsen CH: Non-respiratory side effects of epidural morphine. Anesth Analg 61:490, 1982
13. Staiman A, Seeman P: The impulse-blocking concentrations of anesthetics, alcohols, anticonvulsants, barbiturates and narcotics on phrenic and sciatic nerves. Can J Physiol Pharmacol 52:535, 1974
14. Harrison DM, Sinatra R, Morgese L, Chung JH: Epidural narcotic and patient-controlled analgesia for post-cesarean section pain relief. Anesthesiology 68:454, 1988
15. Eisenach JC, Grice SC, Dewan DM: Patient-controlled analgesia following cesarean section: a comparison with epidural and intramuscular narcotics. Anesthesiology 68:444, 1988
16. Rosen MA, Dailey PA, Hughes SC, et al: Epidural sufentanil for postoperative analgesia after cesarean section. Anesthesia 68:448, 1988
17. Dailey PA, Bookshire GL, Shnider SM, et al: The effects of naloxone associated with the intrathecal use of morphine in labor. Anesth Analg 64:658, 1985
18. Cullen M, Altstatt AH, Kwon NJ, et al: Naltrexone reversal of the side effects of epidural morphine. Anesthesiology 69:A336, 1988
19. Abboud TK, Lee K, Chai M, et al: Prophylactic oral naltrexone with intrathecal morphine for cesarean section: effects on adverse reactions and analgesia. Anesthesiology 71:A836, 1989
20. Davies GG, From R: A blinded study using nalbuphine for prevention of pruritus induced by epidural fentanyl. Anesthesia 69:763, 1988
21. Keaveny JP, Harper NJN: Treatment of epidural morphine-induced pruritus with buprenorphine (letter). Anaesthesia 44:691, 1989

URINARY RETENTION

The etiology of urinary retention, a common complication of delivery, can be difficult to determine. Changes in the lower urinary system that occur toward the end of gestation include increased bladder capacity and a loss of bladder tone.[1] Consequently, urinary dysfunction may occur irrespective of the method of delivery or type of anesthesia.

EFFECT OF LABOR AND DELIVERY

The most common causes of urinary dysfunction after delivery among patients who have not received a regional anesthetic were thought to be a loss of desire to micturate and pain secondary to perineal tears, sutures, and bruising.[2] Early studies by Bennetts and Judd using cystoscopic and cystometric measurements reported a hypotonic postpartum bladder in 86 percent of patients, a finding that was supported by similar results of a study by Youssef in 1965.[3,4] More recently, Kerr-Wilson et al. in 1984 found normal urodynamic measurements at 48 hours and again at 4 weeks after delivery. The method of delivery, infant weight, and episiotomy did not result in a hypotonic postpartum bladder in several studies.[5] The authors attribute these discrepancies to changes in the management of labor and the puerperium, including more frequent use of oxytocin stimulation and cesarean delivery which shorten labor. Also, patients were catheterized 4 to 6 hours after delivery, whereas, in previous studies, patients were observed for 8 hours or longer prior to catheterization if no discomfort or bladder distension occurred.[5]

EFFECT OF ANALGESIA AND ANESTHESIA

More controversial is the effect of analgesia on the postpartum bladder. Bennetts and Judd reported that antepartum analgesia did not account for their findings of bladder hypotonicity. However, 81 percent of their patients received scopolamine, which causes bladder relaxation through its anticholinergic effects.[3,5]

Epidural anesthesia for labor and delivery has become increasingly popular as this technique provides excellent pain relief and minimal motor block. By suppressing afferent sensory impulses from the bladder and inhibiting the reflex mechanism for micturition, epidural anesthesia may delay normal voiding.[6] Even a single episode of overdistension of the bladder may produce urethrovesicle dysfunction due to irreversible damage to the detrussor muscle.[7] Increased residual volume and urinary retention are known side effects of epidural anesthesia. Weil et al. report a significant difference in residual volume and maximum cystometric capacities from the second to the fifth days postpartum between those patients who received epidural anesthesia and those who did not. They conclude that bladder distension during or after labor with an epidural anesthetic rather than the epidural block itself may be responsible for these results since the anesthetic effect of an epidural anesthetic lasts less than 24 hours.[8]

When evaluating patients receiving epidural anesthesia for vaginal or elective cesarean delivery, both bladder compliance and maximum cystometric capacity were significantly lower in the parturients following spontaneous vaginal delivery with and without epidural anesthesia. Factors thought to be contributory include the following: (1) active labor and obstetric trauma were avoided; (2) a urinary catheter was left in place postoperatively for 12 hours, thus avoiding bladder distension; and (3) an "irritable" state of the detrussor muscle and bladder contributed to a reduction in voluntary capacity.[8]

EFFECT OF INTRASPINAL OPIOIDS

The addition of opioid to the local anesthetic in epidural anesthesia has become increasingly popular for pain relief during labor. Studies specific to urinary retention in this patient population receiving epidural narcotics are lacking. However, an incidence of urinary dysfunction varying from 39 to 95 percent following epidural morphine in general surgical patients has been reported.[9,10] It must be remembered that urinary retention is also a known side effect of systemic opioid administration.

Rawal et al. report consistent, predictable relaxation of the detrussor muscle and increased bladder capacity leading to urinary retention for 14 to 16 hours following epidural morphine regardless of dose among groups receiving epidural morphine 2 mg, 4 mg, and 10 mg. The degree of detrussor relaxation was more marked after higher doses, whereas the duration, the increase in maximum bladder capacity, and duration of urinary retention were not dose related.[11] The effects of different opioids on urinary retention have yet to be studied.

A possible mechanism of urinary retention in patients receiving epidural or subarachnoid morphine is that the morphine travels rostrally in the cerebrospinal fluid to the supraspinal structures at the level of the pons, where it causes an inhibitory effect on the primary micturition center. However, the time needed for this cephalad spread of morphine is believed to be longer than the 15 to 30 minutes it takes for epidural morphine to cause bladder relaxation. Therefore, a spinal site of action through autonomic inhibition of sacral parasympathetic outflow has been suggested. The possible presence of opiate receptors in the urinary bladder able to cause this direct effect on bladder relaxation is another possible explanation.[11]

TREATMENT

Attempts at treating urinary retention following epidural narcotics have included administration of the synthetic cholinergic agonist drug, bethanechol, and the opioid antagonist, naloxone. Subcutaneous injection of bethanechol 5 mg had been recommended as initial therapy, however, intravenous naloxone 0.4 mg to 0.8 mg has been more reliable in initiating micturition.[11–13]

Current recommendations for patient care during and following epidural and subarachnoid anesthesia include frequent checks to determine if bladder distension is occurring. If attempts at spontaneous voiding are unsuccessful, catheterization is necessary. In addition, all patients after cesarean delivery should have urinary bladder catheters for 12 to 24 hours postoperatively.

REFERENCES

1. Muellner SR: Physiological bladder changes during pregnancy and the puerperium. J Urol 41:691, 1938
2. Grove LH: Backache, headache and bladder dysfunction after delivery. Br J Anaesth 45:1147, 1973
3. Bennetts FA, Judd GE: Studies of the post-partum bladder. Am J Obstet Gynecol 42:419, 1941
4. Youssef AF: Cystometric studies in gynecology and obstetrics. Obstet Gynecol 8:818, 1956
5. Kerr-Wilson RHJ, Thompson SW, et al: Effect of labor on the postpartum bladder. Obstet Gynecol 64:1, 1984
6. Katz J, Aidinis SJ: Complications of spinal and epidural anesthesia. J Bone Joint Surg 62A:1219, 1980
7. Hinman F: Post-operative overdistension of the bladder. Surg Gynecol Obstet 142:901, 1976
8. Weil A, et al: Effect of lumbar epidural analgesia on lower urinary tract function in the immediate post-partum period. Br J Obstet Gynaecol 90:428, 1983
9. Torda TA, Pubus DA: Clinical experience with epidural morphine. Anesth Intens Care 9:129, 1981
10. Lanz E, Theiss D, Riess W, Sommer V: Epidural morphine for postoperative analgesia: a double-blind study. Anesth Analg 61:236, 1982
11. Rawal N, Möllefors K, Alexlsson K, et al: An experimental study of urodynamic effects of epidural morphine and of halaxone reversal. Anesth Analg 62:641, 1983
12. Cousins MJ, Mather LE: Intrathecal and epidural administration of opioids. Anesthesiology 61:276, 1984
13. Bromage PR, Camporesi EM, Durant PAC, Nielsen CH: Non-respiratory side effects of epidural morphine. Anesth Analg 61:490, 1982

4

Nonpharmacologic Pain Relief

PREPARED CHILDBIRTH

The pregnant woman has many concerns during her pregnancy. These concerns are diverse, but can be divided into four areas: (1) the health of the baby; (2) how the mother's health is affecting the baby, how the pregnancy is affecting the mother's health, and what can be done to prevent or resolve problems (e.g., treatment of illness, nausea and vomiting, weight gain); (3) how the baby will affect family life (e.g., bring the family closer together); and (4) what delivery will be like (e.g., how long will it last, how much will it hurt, and what can be done about the pain.

As an anesthesiologist, one must recognize and address these maternal concerns as well as appreciate the physiologic changes of pregnancy. One often needs to respond to the mother's concern about the effect and safety of "anesthesia" with regard to the baby's health (e.g., "How will anesthesia affect my baby? Is it safe?"). Maternal safety during labor and delivery must be ensured; maternal comfort must be addressed; consideration of the father's role during pregnancy, labor, and delivery must also be recognized. The mother is often more relaxed during labor when a supportive husband or "significant other" is near.

One must appreciate that the mother's concerns about her pregnancy, including labor and delivery, have often been discussed with family members, friends, nurses, and her obstetrician. She may have read several books and magazines. Unfortunately, the information she obtains may not always be accurate.

Since women wish to be better prepared before they go into labor, they often attend prepared childbirth classes. The evolution and philosophy of these classes, as well as their content merits our review.

EVOLUTION OF PREPARED CHILDBIRTH

Back in the early 1930s, Grantly Dick-Read popularized the concept that women can deliver without pain medication.[1] He emphasized that the normal healthy patient has no pain, and since childbirth is *normal,* it should be painless. Some women feel pain and anxiety because they have been conditioned by society to perceive the process of childbirth as frightening. Dick-Read advocated the idea of educating women as to what happens during pregnancy and childbirth to decrease this anxiety and fear of the unknown. He strongly advised against the use of any analgesics during childbirth because "they are unnecessary." He thought that analgesics should not even be mentioned; doing so would suggest that childbirth may sometimes be associated with pain and thus analgesics might be needed. He also taught exercises that can help the parturient relax, since tension aggravates pain. Thus, the properly prepared patient can have a natural, drug-free, painless delivery once the fear-tension-pain cycle is interrupted and countered by education.

In the late 1940s, I. Z. Velvovski, a Russian neuropsychiatrist, began to teach a method of pain relief for childbirth that later became known as the psychoprophylaxis method.[1,2] This method was brought to France by the obstetrician, Ferdinand Lamaze, and later spread throughout Europe and North America. Although childbirth is described as being painful, with proper education and conditioning through exercises, the sensations felt would not be interpreted as unpleasant.

In 1975, Frederick Leboyer, a French obstetrician, introduced the concept of a gentle delivery in a dark and quiet environment.[3–5] After delivery, the neonate is immediately placed on the mother's abdomen, and the pulsations of the umbilical cord are allowed to stop before the cord is cut. Leboyer stated, "To sever the umbilicus when the child has scarcely left the mother's womb is an act of cruelty whose ill-effects are immeasurable."[4] The newborn then is calmed with a warm bath "to ensure that this separation is not a shock but a joy." This type of delivery is designed to prevent the baby from crying. Leboyer believes that the baby's cry signifies pain and suffering, which occurs from the trauma of delivery and is made worse by bright lights, rapid cutting of the cord, and drying the baby before the mother handles her baby. There is no *scientific* evidence to support his hypothesis.

The prepared childbirth classes of today have evolved from the classes taught by people like Dick-Read and Lamaze, who stressed the importance of an awake and cooperative mother. Although the initial emphasis was on delivery without any pain medications, today's classes have acknowledged that labor can be painful,[6] and include a discussion of medications that, if used judiciously, could assist in making childbirth both pleasant and safe. The education provided by these classes has helped millions of women make the transition to motherhood more pleasant and satisfying.

METHOD

Prepared childbirth classes, usually taught during the second half of pregnancy, consist of approximately 5 to 10 sessions. Each session is commonly divided into three parts. The first part consists of a lecture, and includes topics such as the fertilization process, anatomy, changes in maternal physiology, what happens during labor and delivery, what pain medications (intravenous, intramuscular, and regional) are available, and how to care for the newborn. Other topics not related to the pregnancy, but useful, include where to park the car, how to get admitted to the hospital, what to bring to the hospital, and a tour of the labor and delivery suite. In the last session, a film of a normal delivery is often shown. The second part of the sessions is devoted to questions and answers that help tailor the classes to the needs of the future parents. The last part of the sessions is devoted to exercises. These exercises include general conditioning exercises designed to keep the mother in good physical condition and breathing exercises designed to serve as a distraction during the labor and delivery process by helping the mother cope during the pain of contractions.

ADVANTAGES

1. The main advantage of prepared childbirth is a better educated and prepared mother and "significant other." Being more knowledgeable about the birth process will, it is hoped, lead to less apprehension and more cooperation during labor and delivery.[1,3] (For example, the mother can learn that pain medication given in appropriate amounts at the proper time can produce effective analgesia and be safe for her and their neonate.)
2. Lower pain scores are reported.[1,6–8]
3. Although there are no significant differences in length of labor, frequency of fetal distress, mean Apgar scores, or type of neonatal problems between prepared parturients and parturients who do not attend childbirth classes, a few reports show labor to be shorter and conditions to be better for the newborn when the parturient has attended childbirth classes.[1,8]
4. The risk of maternal aspiration of gastric contents is minimized in an awake parturient because the maternal airway reflexes are maintained.
5. Parturients who attended childbirth classes have a lower incidence of forceps deliveries compared to women who deliver under regional anesthesia.[8] This may be the result of greater motivation to expel the fetus, which may be due to increased sensation leading to the generation of greater "pushing" force, or because women view forceps as not being safe for their baby. The use of low or outlet forceps has not been shown to be harmful and may be beneficial in some circumstances.[1,3] Another possible reason for the decreased use of low forceps is that application of forceps without anesthesia is usually quite uncomfortable.[1]
6. With less systemic medication and less maternal sedation, bonding between the mother and the newborn is easier. A Leboyer delivery may have a favorable effect on bonding. It also reminds one to keep extraneous noises to a minimum to make the time of delivery more pleasant for the new family.[3–5]

DISADVANTAGES

1. One reason that many women take prepared childbirth classes is to avoid the use of all analgesics. This is an unreasonable expectation.[1,7] Only 10 to 20 percent of women who are "prepared" avoid all analgesics. An additional 30 to 50 percent of women who attended prepared childbirth classes use a small dose of analgesic. The remaining women use analgesics in total doses that are similar to those of women who have not attended prepared childbirth classes.[1]

   A point often made in favor of prepared "drug-free" delivery is that the woman is awake and is therefore cooperative. However, not all women who are awake and *in pain* are cooperative! One must recognize that regional anesthesia can provide awake, pain-free conditions for delivery, can provide a more pleasant experience, and can allow better conditions for bonding.[3]
2. Although the breathing techniques taught are useful in helping the mother through the contractions, excessive hyperventilation can be harmful. In a study by Saling and Ligdas,[9] the average PCO_2 in laboring women is 25.3 ± 8.0 mmHg, with about 7 percent having PCO_2 levels below 15 mmHg. With marked hyperventilation, fetal acidosis may develop. If excessive maternal hyperventilation occurs, fetal PO_2 may decrease as well.[10,11]
3. Although most prepared childbirth educators give accurate information, some educators may distort information to the point of producing more harm than good.[12] The following statements, which may have some truth under certain circumstances, have created some difficult situations:
   (a) "If pain medications are needed, you have failed. Your baby will be exposed to unnecessary and dangerous drugs."
   (b) "If you can make it to 8 cm dilation, then you do not need or have time for an epidural or a spinal for delivery; you can 'gut it out.'"
   (c) "Do not let the doctors and nurses force you into an unnecessary cesarean delivery; you can do it naturally."
   (d) "You should not have general anesthesia for your cesarean delivery because the drugs will depress your baby."
   (e) "You should not have spinal anesthesia for your cesarean delivery because it lowers your blood pressure."
   (f) "You should not have epidural anesthesia for your cesarean delivery because it doesn't give you a good block and you can have a 'window.'"
4. The Leboyer delivery can create problems for the mother and the neonate. When educated with the Leboyer philosophy, the mother may suffer psychological trauma if she hears her baby cry more than a few times, as she may believe her baby is suffering.[3] This type of delivery may delay evaluation and possible resuscitation of the neonate, especially if delivery occurs in a labor room, where resuscitation equipment may not be readily available. Failure to dry the infant and subsequently bathing him can cause significant neonatal hypothermia as a result of exposure to the cool environment of the delivery room and bath water with an uncontrolled temperature. If a bath is used, its temperature should be in the neutral thermal range (98 to 100°F) and should be continuously monitored. The practice of bathing the infant immediately has been discontinued in many delivery suites and has been replaced by more appropriate physiologic practices. This includes placing the baby on a baby blanket on the mother's abdomen immediately after delivery with the umbilical cord intact, if possible, drying the baby, and then placing the baby on the mother's warm and dry abdomen and covering the baby with a dry, warm cotton blanket. Here the mother again becomes an incubator, the baby is kept warm, and bonding can begin immediately. This technique was developed by Gerard W. Ostheimer and the obstetricians at the Boston Hospital for Women, who, after observing significant neonatal hypothermia with the original Leboyer approach, modified the technique.

REFERENCES

1. Bonica JJ: Principles and Practice of Obstetric Analgesia and Anesthesia. FA Davis, Philadelphia, 1967, p. 762
2. Lamaze F: Painless Childbirth—Psychoprophylactic Method. Pocket Books, New York, 1972
3. Abouleish E: Pain Control in Obstetrics. JB Lippincott, Philadelphia, 1977, p. 365
4. Nelson NM, Enkin MW, Saigal S, et al: A randomized clinical trial of the Leboyer approach to childbirth. N Engl J Med 302:655, 1980
5. Saigal S, Nelson NM, Bennett KJ, et al: Observations on the behavioral state of newborn infants during the first hour of life—a comparison of infants delivered by the Leboyer and conventional methods. Am J Obstet Gynecol 139:715, 1981
6. Melzack R: The myth of painless childbirth (the John J. Bonica lecture). Pain 19:321, 1984
7. Melzack R, Taenzer P, Feldman P, et al: Labour is still painful after prepared childbirth training. Can Med Assoc J 125:357, 1981

8. Scott JR, Rose NB: Effect of psychoprophylaxis (Lamaze preparation) on labor and delivery in primiparas. N Engl J Med 294:1205, 1976
9. Saling E, Ligdas P: The effect on the fetus of maternal hyperventilation during labor. J Obstet Gynaecol Br Commonw 76:877, 1969
10. Levinson G, Shnider SM, deLorimier AA, et al: Effects of maternal hyperventilation on uterine blood flow and fetal oxygenation and acid-base status. Anesthesiology 40:340, 1974
11. Motoyama EK, Rivard G, Acheson F, et al: Adverse effect of maternal hyperventilation on the foetus. Lancet 1:286, 1966
12. Stewart DE: Psychiatric symptoms following attempted natural childbirth. Can Med Assoc J 127:713, 1982

HYPNOSIS

Hypnosis (*hypnos*, sleep) can produce analgesia and amnesia during labor and delivery for some selected patients.[1–5]

The technique of hypnosis has been used for many centuries. Its origin is lost in antiquity. The term was coined in 1843 by James Braid, who recognized that suggestion was the basis of hypnosis.[1,2,4,6]

The subject who is hypnotized appears to be asleep. Her eyes are closed, and she appears very relaxed. In actuality, she is not asleep, but very much awake and deeply concentrating. Her eyes are closed to assist in concentration and relaxation. This state of deep concentration is called a *trance*. Once the trance state is achieved, the subject becomes highly responsive to suggestions. Suggestions are the key to hypnosis, because through them the subject can select the sensory input she wishes to obtain.[1,2,4–8]

In obstetrics, the woman who is hypnotized enters a relaxed, deeply concentrating state in which pleasurable sensations are suggested and reinforced and unpleasant sensations are transformed to more tolerable or pleasurable thoughts. For example, contractions are not pain, they are tenseness of the abdomen; bearing down is felt as pressure.[4]

The ability to reach the degree of concentration needed for labor and delivery requires a lot of time, a minimum of several training sessions, and a skilled hypnotist.[1,2,4,6] The sessions are held either in private or in groups, depending on the situation.

Those involved in the care of a patient who is hypnotized should keep in mind that she is deeply concentrating.[2] Thus, care must be taken to keep noise to a minimum and to administer sedatives and tranquilizers judiciously, as they may make her ability to concentrate more difficult.[8]

REFERENCES

1. Abouleish E: Pain Control in Obstetrics. JB Lippincott, Philadelphia, 1977, p. 365
2. Bonica JJ: Principles and Practice of Obstetric Analgesia and Anesthesia. FA Davis, Philadelphia, 1967
3. Bonica JJ: Obstetric Analgesia and Anesthesia. World Federation of Societies of Anesthesiologists, Amsterdam, 1980
4. Kroger WS: Clinical and Experimental Hypnosis. 2nd Ed. JB Lippincott, Philadelphia, 1977
5. Martin J: Hypnosis gains legitimacy, respect, in diverse clinical specialties. JAMA 249:319, 1983
6. Collins VJ: Principles of Anesthesiology. 2nd Ed. Lea & Febiger, Philadelphia, 1976
7. Cousins MJ, Bridenbaugh PO: Neural Blockade in Clinical Anesthesia and Management of Pain. JB Lippincott, Philadelphia, 1980
8. Gutsche B: Maternal analgesia and anesthesia for vaginal delivery. Refresher Course in Anesthesiology 6:67, 1978

ACUPUNCTURE

In traditional Chinese medicine, acupuncture is well established as a method for relieving pain and providing surgical anesthesia. At the present time, 10 percent of all surgical procedures in China are performed under acupuncture analgesia/anesthesia.[1]

Until recently, acupuncture had gained little acceptance in the West. Interestingly, acupuncture was known and accepted by William Osler, who touted it as the preferred treatment for acute lumbago in his medical writings. With the first organized visit of American physicians to China in 1970, acupuncture has enjoyed increasing interest in America, if not ultimate acceptance.

MECHANISM OF ACTION

The mechanism of action of analgesia is not known. Three theories have been proposed. According to the traditional meridian theory,[2–4] all organs are linked by 12 coupled and 2 midline meridians. A vital life force or energy called *Ch'i* flows through the body along meridians. If the balance of energy is upset, disease or pain results. The manipulation of needles at precise points along the meridians results in a restoration of energy balance, thereby causing analgesia or relief of symptoms.

The second hypothesis involves Melzack and Wall's

gate theory of pain.[5] Acupuncture needles stimulate large myelinated Aβ nerve fibers that "close the gate" to impulses carried by Aδ and C fibers. This is basically the same analgesic mechanism as proposed for transcutaneous electrical nerve stimulation (TENS).[6]

The third theory is neurohumoral and involves release of endorphins by acupuncture.[4,7,8] Modulation of endorphins and monoamine receptors (norepinephrine and serotonin) has been demonstrated during electroacupuncture stimulation. The effects of acupuncture have been shown to be reversible by naloxone.[8]

Cortical electrophysiologic recordings (electroencephalograms, somatosensory-evoked potentials, and cognitive-evoked potentials) have recently been made during acupuncture-induced anesthesia for removal of thyroid tumors.[9] Intraoperative recordings were unchanged as compared to preoperative recordings. The investigators hypothesized that acupuncture may primarily affect a subcortical area(s), with the endorphin system regulating the subjective appreciation of pain.[9]

ANALGESIA FOR LABOR AND DELIVERY

The use of acupuncture for labor and delivery is a recent development because Oriental women by tradition have not used acupuncture for delivery.[8] With the potential to greatly reduce or eliminate the administration of drugs to laboring women, acupuncture would appear to be an exciting alternative or adjunct to traditional analgesic modalities. Unfortunately, acupuncture, either by electrical[10] or mechanical[11] stimulation of the needles, fails to provide adequate analgesia. When 21 volunteer parturients were treated by a trained Chinese acupuncturist, 19 regarded the technique as ineffective for labor analgesia. Sixteen patients required alternative methods of analgesia.[11] Similar results were obtained in other studies using electroacupuncture.[10] No complications were noted in the mother or neonate in either study. Acupuncture did not affect maternal blood pressure, Apgar score, or the frequency or intensity of uterine contractions.

Acupuncture has also been used for cesarean delivery.[12] Ear points were used in conjunction with classical meridian acupuncture points. Interestingly, an analgesic effect of 24-hour duration was obtained in 8 of 14 (57 percent) of the study patients.

From these studies it appears that acupuncture for labor and delivery provides incomplete, unpredictable, and inconsistent analgesia. All studies suffered from the enrollment of small numbers of patients. Acupuncture can probably be used in conjunction with low doses of opioids or local anesthe… but further studies are n…

INDUCTIO…

Traditional Chinese teac… of certain acupuncture poi… uterine contractions, prem… abortion. Indeed, with the p… …gal climate, most American acupuncturist… will decline treatment of pregnant women (with the possible exception of using carefully selected ear points).

This may be turned to possible advantage, however, by use of acupuncture as an induction agent in late pregnancy. In a study of 41 women, 78 percent achieved delivery.[13] Two other studies were equally optimistic regarding the ability of acupuncture to successfully induce labor.[14,15] Certainly, further careful research is needed prior to recommendation of acupuncture as a proven agent for the induction of labor.

REFERENCES

1. Bonica JJ: Anesthesiology in the People's Republic of China. Anesthesiology 40:175, 1974
2. Abouleish E: Pain Control in Obstetrics. JB Lippincott, Philadelphia, 1977, p. 365
3. Collins VJ: Principles of Anesthesiology. 2nd Ed. Lea & Febiger, Philadelphia, 1976
4. Cousins MJ, Bridenbaugh PO: Neural Blockade in Clinical Anesthesia and Management of Pain. JB Lippincott, Philadelphia, 1980
5. Melzack R, Wall PD: Pain mechanisms: a new theory. Science 150:971, 1965
6. Shealy C: Transcutaneous electroanalgesia. Surg Forum 23:419, 1972
7. Bonica JJ: Obstetric Analgesia and Anesthesia. World Federation of Societies of Anesthesiologists, Amsterdam, 1980
8. Mayer DJ, Price DD, Rafii A: Antagonism of acupuncture analgesia in man by the narcotic antagonist naloxone. Brain Res 121:368, 1977
9. Starr A, Abraham G, Zhu Y, et al: Electrophysiological measures during acupuncture-induced surgical analgesia. Arch Neurol 46:1010, 1989
10. Abouleish E, Depp R: Acupuncture in obstetrics. Anesth Analg 54:82, 1975
11. Wallis L, Shnider SM, Palahniuk RJ, Spivey HT: An evaluation of acupuncture analgesia in obstetrics. Anesthesiology 41:596, 1974
12. Vallette C, Niboyet JEH, Imbert-Martelet M, Roux JF: Acupuncture analgesia and cesarean section. J Reprod Med 25:108, 1980
13. Tseui JJ, Lai Y, Sharma SD: The influence of acupuncture stimulation during pregnancy: the induction and inhibition of labor. Obstet Gynecol 50:479, 1977

R, Raffi F, Biechelr M, et al: Induction du travail electroacupuncture. La Nouv Presse Med 5:151, 976

Yip SK, Pang JC, Sung ML: Induction of labor by acupuncture electrostimulation. Am J Chin Med 4:257, 1976

TRANSCUTANEOUS ELECTRICAL NERVE STIMULATION

The use of stimulation modalities for the relief of pain has received widespread attention since the publication of the work of Melzack and Wall.[1] Two years after the publication of "Pain mechanisms: a new theory,"[2] transcutaneous electrical nerve stimulation (TENS) was utilized as a screening mechanism to examine the potential usefulness of dorsal column stimulators in the treatment of chronic pain.[3] The use of TENS was noted to elicit local analgesia. Since 1967, TENS has been recognized as an adjunctive treatment modality for use in pain management.

Transcutaneous electrical nerve stimulation involves passage of an electrical current through intact skin as a means of sending a measured amount of low-voltage electric current to the peripheral nervous system. Melzack and Wall predicted that selective stimulation of larger diameter afferent nerves (Aβ fibers) within a peripheral nerve would diminish the perception of pain. They proposed that the larger-diameter, primary afferent nerve fibers inhibit nociceptive neurons located in the substantia gelatinosa of the dorsal horn of the spinal cord. These myelinated, larger-diameter, primary afferent nerves have the lowest threshold to externally provided electrical stimulation.[4] The smaller-diameter, nonmyelinated (C fibers) as well as myelinated (Aδ fibers) primary afferent nerve fibers have a significantly higher threshold for stimulation. Therefore, using a low-voltage stimulation current, the larger-diameter fibers may be selectively activated. This, in turn, provides the basis for the use of TENS.

Other theories have been proposed to explain the observed efficacy of TENS. Use of TENS may increase local concentrations of endorphins and enkephalins, thereby elevating the pain threshold. Another theory entails frequency-dependent conduction block. Stated otherwise, nociception can be blocked by adjustment of the frequency of impulse generation so that impulses are delivered before ionic channels in neurons can respond. No action potential would be generated by such neurons. Pain would not be perceived.

A specific analgesic effect for TENS has yet to be proved. However, a number of studies have given support to its use for the relief of pain in obstetrics. The effect of TENS on postoperative pain was evaluated in 18 multiparous women each having undergone elective cesarean delivery.[5] The women were randomized into TENS versus placebo groups. Attempts were made to differentiate the usefulness of TENS in alleviating different types of pain. Patients reported three major pain types: (1) constant and movement-associated incisional pain (both surface and deep), (2) uterine contraction-associated pain (afterbirth pain), and (3) visceral pain due to increased abdominal distention (gas pain). The results of this study suggested that TENS was efficacious for relief of surface incisional pain and ineffective in relieving deep visceral pain.

A study by Davies in 1982 concluded that TENS was ineffective during the first 24 hours following cesarean delivery performed under epidural as compared to general anesthesia.[6] Patients receiving general anesthesia and a functional TENS unit noted less postoperative pain and required less analgesia than a control group receiving general anesthesia and a nonfunctional placebo TENS unit. In contrast, patients who delivered under epidural anesthesia did not note any additional pain decrease with the use of a functional TENS unit versus a nonfunctional placebo unit.

The use of TENS during labor and delivery has also been investigated. TENS has distinct advantages over more invasive methods of providing analgesia, as it should have no deleterious effects on the mother of the fetus. Interference with fetal heart monitoring has been noted, however.

In a study by Stewart,[7] proximal electrodes were placed to cover the dermatomes of the posterior rami of T11–L1. The distal electrode pair was placed at the dermatomal levels of S2–S4. The frequency and amplitude of the TENS unit was adjusted as labor progressed. Initially, in the early part of the first stage, only the proximal electrodes were utilized. As labor progressed, the sacral electrodes were used in an attempt to minimize suprapubic and lower back pain.

All babies were born in satisfactory condition. No disturbance of cardiotocographic recording was noted. The results of this study concluded that TENS was most helpful during the early stages of labor. Considerable pain relief was reported by 23.5 percent of the patients on whom the TENS unit was used, whereas 55.9 percent found some pain relief. In 7.4 percent the use of the unit was found to be of such value that no other form of analgesia was needed. Although this was not a controlled study, the author concluded that TENS has a definite place in the treatment of obstetric discomfort.

TENS is a noninvasive technique that may be useful in providing analgesia for labor and incisional discomfort after cesarean delivery. It may be utilized as an adjunct to the more common analgesic methods.

REFERENCES

1. Melzack R, Wall PD: Pain mechanisms: a new theory. Science 150:971, 1965
2. Abouleish E, Depp R: Acupuncture in obstetrics. Anesth Analg 54:82, 1975
3. Shealy C: Transcutaneous electroanalgesia. Surg Forum 23:419, 1972
4. Bloedel JR, McCreery DB: Organization of peripheral and central pain pathways. Surg Neurol 4:65, 1975
5. Smith CM, Guralnick MS, Gelfand MM, Jeans ME: The effects of transcutaneous electrical nerve stimulation on post-cesarean pain. Pain 27:181, 1986
6. Davies JR: Ineffective transcutaneous nerve stimulation following epidural anesthesia. Anesthesia 37:453, 1982
7. Stewart P: Transcutaneous nerve stimulation as a method of analgesia in labour. Anaesthesia 34:361, 1979

5

Drug Interactions in Labor and Delivery

Information on drug interactions specific to pregnancy, labor, and delivery is both limited and complex. While predominant obstetric advice is aimed at minimizing the drugs to which both mother and fetus are subjected during labor and delivery, it is not uncommon for a patient with a chronic disease (such as diabetes or epilepsy) to become pregnant and have an ongoing requirement for pharmacologic therapy.

A discussion of all the possible interactions between both chronically and acutely administered agents is certainly beyond the scope of this chapter. Medications other than drugs used for pain relief that are commonly administered during labor are reviewed, and the effects of these agents on anesthetic management are described.

INTERACTIONS AMONG SYSTEMICALLY ADMINISTERED AGENTS

OXYTOCICS

Oxytocics are drugs that stimulate uterine contractions. The main clinical uses for these agents are:

1. To induce or augment labor
2. To control postpartum bleeding and uterine atony
3. To cause uterine contraction after cesarean delivery or other uterine surgery
4. To induce therapeutic abortion

Oxytocin (Pitocin)

Mechanism of Action. Oxytocin has a receptor-specific action on uterine smooth muscle that stimulates both the frequency and force of contractions.

Mode of Delivery. Administration of oxytocin is always via continuous intravenous infusion.

1. *For augmentation of labor:* 10 IU (1.0 ml) is diluted in 1,000 ml of infusate. Infusion rates vary from 1 to 10 mU/min.
2. *To minimize postpartum bleeding:* rates of 20 to 100 mU/min are used. Effects appear within 3 minutes, are maximal at about 20 minutes, and disappear within 15 to 20 minutes after discontinuing the infusion. In practical terms, 20 to 40 IU are usually added to 1,000 ml of fluid and administered to effect.

Hemodynamic Effects. Of historical interest is that prior to the introduction of purely synthetic oxytocin, purified extracts of human posterior pituitary gland were used as a source of oxytocin. These extracts possessed enough "contaminant" vasopressin to cause both an independent and an additive hypertension when administered along with sympathomimetic amines.

The doses of synthetic oxytocin administered for most obstetric purposes are not sufficient to produce marked alterations of blood pressure. However, administration of large intravenous boluses of 5 to 10 IU results in

1. A 50 percent decrease in total peripheral resistance
2. A 30 percent decrease in mean arterial pressure
3. A 30 percent increase in heart rate and
4. A 30 percent increase in cardiac output[1]

Drug Interactions

Sympathomimetic Amines. As mentioned above, the commonly administered sympathomimetic amines, ephedrine and phenylephrine, have not been associated with any incidence of malignant hypertension when used concurrently with synthetic oxytocin. When almost continuous monitoring of blood pressure (every 1 to 2 minutes) is utilized, there have been no reported cases of malignant hypertension associated with the commonly administered ephedrine doses of 5 to 10 mg or with the 40- to 80-μg doses of phenylephrine.

Inhaled Agents. Although not specifically studied, inhaled agents will augment the hypotensive effects of large (5- to 10-IU) oxytocin boluses.

Agents that Will Antagonize the Uterotonic Actions of Oxytocin. Antagonists of oxytocin include halothane, propranolol, tetracaine, quinidine, and chloroprocaine.[2]

Miscellaneous Effects. Both the natural and synthetic oxytocin preparations possess antidiuretic activity. In addition, induction with oxytocin has been associated with higher neonatal bilirubin concentrations.[3]

Ergot Derivatives: Methylergonovine (Methergine) and Ergonovine Maleate (Ergotrate)

Obstetric and Gynecologic Uses. Ergot derivatives are indicated in the management of postpartum bleeding and uterine atony and are limited only to the postpartum period. After small doses, in the nonpregnant uterus, there is an increase in force and frequency of contractions followed by a normal degree of relaxation. After larger doses, or in the pregnant uterus, these agents cause contractions to become forceful and prolonged, and resting tonus is markedly increased.

Administration. A rapid and lasting response is produced with administration of 0.2 to 0.3 mg IM. Onset of activity is within 10 minutes and increased uterine activity persists for 2 to 6 hours.

Cardiovascular Effects. Potent vasoconstriction of both arteries and veins occurs, resulting in increased peripheral resistance, decreased venous capacitance, and increased mean blood pressure.[4]

Drug Interactions. The only drug interactions reported have been with sympathomimetic amines.

1. Munson[4] demonstrated a 20 percent increase in systolic blood pressure from methergine alone and an additional 20 percent increase when either ephedrine or phenylephrine was given additionally to nonpregnant rabbits.
2. Numerous cases of malignant hypertension have been associated with the intramuscular administration of ergot alkaloids and the prophylactic intramuscular administration of either ephedrine or methoxamine. Severe hypertension is more likely to occur in patients who are already mildly hypertensive. Unintentional intravenous administration may cause severe malignant hypertension.
3. Central nervous system sequelae to hypertension associated with methylergonovine have included retinal detachment,[5] ruptured cerebral aneurysm,[6] blurred vision, dizziness,[7] and even seizures.[8]

Prostaglandins

Obstetric and Gynecologic Uses. Prostaglandins (PG), primarily $PGF_{2\alpha}$, are used in the treatment of postpartum hemorrhage and for induction of midtrimester abortion; they are currently being studied as agents for induction of labor. Treatment of uterine atony usually consists of manual uterine compression and intravenous administration of oxytocin and the intramuscular administration of methylergonovine maleate. Evaluation of the coagulation profile is also necessary because ongoing postpartum bleeding may be secondary to an underlying maternal coagulopathy.

Administration and Dosage. $PGF_{2\alpha}$ or Prostin 15M, a prostaglandin analogue, is given either intramuscularly or directly via intramyometrial injection. The efficacy of each is similar. However, before repeated doses are given it must be remembered that the postpartum uterus is a highly vascular structure with a potential for rapid drug absorption.

The average dose of each agent is 500 μg (two doses

of 250 μg), which results in an 80 to 90 percent sustained response.

Failure, or the requirement for multiple injections, is often related to chorioamnionitis or retained placental tissue.[9]

Side Effects

Cardiovascular. Increases in heart rate, mean arterial blood pressure, pulmonary artery pressure, and cardiac output without changes in peripheral vascular resistance are frequently observed.

Pulmonary. Bronchospasm, dyspnea, and pulmonary edema have been observed in patients undergoing mid-trimester abortion. Pulmonary function tests demonstrate small-airway constriction, air trapping, and reduction in maximum end-expiratory flow. Decreases in PaO_2 have also been observed and are believed to be caused by ventilation: perfusion mismatching secondary to the combined bronchoconstriction and pulmonary arteriolar constriction.[10]

MAGNESIUM SULFATE

Clinical Use. Magnesium sulfate is the most frequently used agent in the management of hypertensive disorders of pregnancy.

Pharmacodynamic Properties

1. Decreases presynaptic release of acetylcholine
2. Decreases sensitivity of postjunctional membrane to liberated acetylcholine
3. Decreases excitability of muscle cell membranes
4. Reduces uterine blood flow and contractility
5. Produces moderate vasodilation with a brief decrease in blood pressure
6. Produces central nervous system depression
7. Increases uterine blood flow and cerebral blood flow

Administration and Pharmacology

1. *Loading dose:* 20 ml of 20 percent magnesium sulfate (4 g) IV over 3 minutes. *Maintenance:* 1.0 to 1.5 g/h IV as a continuous infusion.
2. Clinical neurologic signs associated with the following plasma magnesium levels:
   (a) Normal deep tendon reflexes (DTR): 1.5 to 2.5 mEq/L
   (b) Diminished DTR: greater than 4 to 5 mEq/L
   (c) Absent DTR: greater than 10 mEq/L
   (d) Respiratory paralysis: greater than 12 to 15 mEq/L

Drug Interactions

Depolarizing Neuromuscular Relaxants. Magnesium sulfate prolongs the duration of depolarizing neuromuscular blockade and decreases the dose of succinylcholine required to facilitate tracheal intubation by 50 percent.[11]

Nondepolarizing Neuromuscular Relaxants.

1. Magnesium sulfate alone acts as a nondepolarizing relaxant, with approximately 1/1,000 the potency of d-tubocurarine.[11]
2. Magnesium potentiates activity of d-tubocurarine by a factor of 4.
3. Concurrent magnesium therapy has been shown to cause an 8-fold increase in the duration of action of vecuronium.[12]
4. Calcium administration will not predictably reverse the magnesium-enhanced neuromuscular block.

Other Maternal and Neonatal Effects. Maternal hypocalcemia resulting in complete heart block, central nervous system irritability, and tetany has been observed.[13] Neonatal effects secondary to maternal administration include flaccidity, hyporeflexia, respiratory depression, and weak or absent cry.[14] Marked potentiation of neuromuscular blockade by a combination of hypermagnesemia and aminoglycoside antibiotics has also been described in neonates.[15]

TOCOLYTIC AGENTS

Tocolytic agents are used to stop premature labor while other therapeutic measures such as steroid therapy are initiated to induce maturation of fetal lungs. They prevent the myometrial response to internal or external stimuli (e.g., β-sympathomimetics, prostaglandin inhibitors, and calcium channel blockers) and decrease stimulus input to the uterus (e.g., ethanol).

β-Sympathomimetics

Of all the agents listed above, β-sympathomimetics have become the most widely accepted form of tocolytic therapy.

Mechanism of Action. The binding of these agents to B_2 receptors activates adenylate cyclase, eventually resulting in increased calcium uptake by the sarcoplasmic reticulum. The decreased intracellular free calcium causes a shorter duration of sarcomere contraction and less frequent contractions. The net result is a decrease in strength and frequency of contractions.

Administration and Dosage

Terbutaline. Terbutaline is the most popular of the tocolytic agents and can be administered orally, intramuscularly, or subcutaneously. Tocolytic therapy often involves a combination of methods of administration.

1. Our current practice is to administer three 0.25-mg doses of terbutaline SQ over a 1-hour period. This is then followed by 5 mg PO every 4 to 6 hours.
2. Dosages are limited by excessive heart rate increases and are withheld if the maternal heart rate is greater than 120 beats per minute (bpm) or the fetal heart rate is greater than 160 bpm.
3. Oral maintenance is then provided with 5 mg every 4 to 6 hours until fetal lung maturity is established via amniocentesis and assessment of lecithin:sphingomyelin ratios or the "fetal lung maturity" assay, which utilizes the surfactant:albumin ratio. Otherwise, sufficient doses of betamethasone (celestone) are administered to help ensure fetal lung maturity.

Ritodrine

1. Initial dose: 0.1 mg/min IV for 10 to 20 minutes
2. Dosage is adjusted by increasing 0.05 mg/min every 10 minutes until contractions cease
3. Oral maintenance: 10 mg every 2 hours for 1 day, then 10 to 20 mg every 4 to 6 hours

Maternal Side Effects

1. Hyperglycemia, hyperinsulinemia and lactic acidemia may occur secondary to the systemic β-sympathomimetic effects.
2. Hypokalemia occurs secondary to enhanced insulin secretion.
3. Tachycardia and hypotension: Doses should be withheld if heart rate is greater than 120 bpm.
4. Tremor, palpitations, nervousness, headache, nausea, and vomiting have been observed.

Neonatal Side Effects

1. Fetal tachycardia occurs commonly.
2. Neonatal insulin production is increased, resulting in neonatal hypoglycemia.
3. Hypotension and hypocalcemia are observed.

Drug Interactions Resulting in Pulmonary Edema. Glucocorticoids (e.g., betamethasone) are given frequently with tocolytics to promote fetal lung maturation. There is an increased incidence of pulmonary edema with the concurrent use of β-sympathomimetics and glucocorticoids.[16] The mechanism of this interaction is unknown, but maternal factors such as fluid overload, hypokalemia, twin gestations, and sustained tachycardia greater than 140 bpm may play an active role in increasing the risk of pulmonary edema.

Calcium Antagonists

Nifedipine. Although not approved for tocolytic therapy, nifedipine has been shown to be effective in abolishing uterine activity during premature labor.[17,18] The effective dose is 10 mg PO three times a day.

Maternal Side Effects. Maternal flushing and transient increases in heart rate (10 to 15 bpm) are common but do not limit therapy.

Drug Interactions. The hypotensive effects of inhaled anesthetics will likely be enhanced by this agent secondary to the peripheral vasodilating effects. In addition, the relatively long pharmacologic effects of nifedipine could result in postpartum uterine atony and hemorrhage that would be unresponsive to oxytocic agents.

Verapamil. Verapamil is ineffective for tocolysis at pharmacologically tolerable doses.

Ethanol

Intravenous ethanol was the most popular tocolytic agent in the United States during the late 1960s and early 1970s. Ethanol provides a tocolytic action via suppression of release of oxytocin from the posterior pituitary. Blood levels of 80 to 160 mg/dl produce myometrial depression but will similarly increase the incidence of nausea, vomiting, and headaches. The loss of psychic control associated with the necessary ethanol doses may increase the incidence of gastric regurgitation and pulmonary aspiration.

Prostaglandin Synthetase Inhibitors

Indomethacin. Indomethacin has been shown in numerous clinical trials to be effective in halting premature labor. Widespread popularity has not been achieved secondary to the reported incidence of premature closure of the ductus arteriosus, resulting in pulmonary hypertension and cardiac failure in the neonate.[17]

Aspirin. Maintenance aspirin therapy has been shown to prolong the duration of pregnancy while blocking the development of hypertension in pregnancy-induced hypertension (PIH)-prone patients. Several large studies are currently being performed to evaluate the use of low-dose aspirin (60 mg/day) in the treatment of PIH.

Regional Anesthesia and Prostaglandin Synthetase Inhibitors. The question will undoubtedly arise as to whether maintenance aspirin therapy increases the associated risk of receiving regional anesthesia during labor. To date, there have been no studies that indicate an increased risk of neurologic or hematologic complications in patients receiving regional anesthesia while on aspirin or nonsteroidal anti-inflammatory drug therapy.

MISCELLANEOUS AGENTS USED SYSTEMICALLY

Trimethaphan Camsylate (Arfonad)

Pharmacology and Clinical Uses

1. Trimethaphan is a ganglionic blocker that is used in acute treatment of hypertension associated with PIH. It does not cross the placenta and can be safely administered without central intravenous access as long as frequent blood pressure monitoring is observed.
2. It is rapidly metabolized, although its administration is associated with histamine release, tachycardia, and tachyphylaxis in large doses.
3. Initial starting dose by continuous intravenous infusion is 100 μg/min. Routinely, 500 mg is mixed in 500 ml of fluid and administered to effect by drip.

Drug Interactions. Trimethaphan possesses significant interactions with both depolarizing and nondepolarizing neuromuscular relaxants.

Nondepolarizing Neuromuscular Relaxants. Trimethaphan has a direct effect at the neuromuscular junction, producing a "nondepolarizing-type block" that is only a fraction of that provided by d-tubocurarine. Prolonged block will therefore be observed with concurrent use of all nondepolarizing agents.

Depolarizing Neuromuscular Relaxants. Trimethaphan noncompetitively inhibits plasma cholinesterase, resulting in prolonged blockade by succinylcholine.[19]

Sodium Nitroprusside

Sodium nitroprusside does not inhibit succinylcholine metabolism, however, the possibility of fetal cyanide accumulation exists if prolonged use is required.

Dantrolene

Clinical Use. Dantrolene is used in the treatment of malignant hyperthermia (MH) or in prophylaxis of MH-prone patients.

Pharmacologic Properties. Dantrolene decreases the release of calcium ions from the sarcoplasmic reticulum. It causes skeletal muscle relaxation with reduction in force of contraction; this effect plateaus short of total paralysis.

Administration and Dosage

1. *For treatment of MH:* initial effective dose is 2.4 mg/kg IV.
   - (a) The initial loading dose is given at 15-minute intervals until relaxation of muscle rigor and control of tachycardia and arrhythmias is achieved.
   - (b) The maximum dose is up to 10 mg/kg body weight.
   - (c) Concomitant resuscitative measures must be carried out (see Ch. 8).
2. *Prophylaxis in MH-prone individuals:* Although currently not recommended for use in either obstetric or nonobstetric patients, an oral dose of 3.4 mg/kg is roughly equivalent to an intravenous dose of 2.4 mg/kg.

Drug Interactions

1. Verapamil is used for treatment of supraventricular tachycardias and has been proposed in the treatment of MH-induced tachycardias. In animal studies, therapeutic doses of dantrolene in conjunction with verapamil have been shown to cause severe cardiovascular depression and cardiac arrest. The mechanism is unknown and this interaction has not been reported in humans.[20]
2. Concurrent use of the neuromuscular relaxants, vecuronium and dantrolene, has been shown to cause a twofold increase in the duration of neuromuscular blockade.[21]

Antibiotics

Drug interactions with anesthetic agents involve primarily potentiation of neuromuscular blockade. Virtually all of the aminoglycoside antibiotics tested show a wide range of actions. Most of these agents have combined actions on both the nerve terminals and the cholinergic receptor. When used in the presence of nondepolarizing agents, most of these effects can be reversed with either calcium or neostigmine. There have been case reports of concomitant maternal administration of vecuronium and gentamicin resulting in postpartum respiratory depression and hypotonia of the neonate.[15]

REFERENCES

1. Weis FR Jr, Markello R, Mo B, Bechiechio P: Cardiovascular effects of oxytocin. Obstet Gynecol 46(2):211, 1975
2. Anderson WG, Miller JW: Interaction between halothane and propranolol on oxytocin-induced uterine contractions. J Pharm Exp Ther 192(2):408, 1975
3. Davies DP: Neonatal jaundice and maternal oxytocin infusion. Br Med J 2:476, 1973
4. Munson WM: The pressor effect of various vasopressor-oxytocic combinations: a laboratory study and review. Anesth Analg 44:114, 1965
5. Gombos GM, Howitt D, Shinyee C: Bilateral retinal detachment occurring in the immediate postpartum period after methylergonovine and oxytocin administration. Eye Ear Nose Throat Mo 48:45, 1969
6. Casady GN, Moore DC, Bridenbaugh DL: Postpartum hypertension after use of vasoconstrictor and oxytocic drugs. JAMA 172:1011, 1960
7. Alper MH, Datta S: Agents in obstetrics: mother, fetus, and newborn. In Smith NT, Corbascio AN (eds): Drug Interactions in Anesthesia. 2nd Ed. Lea & Febiger, Philadelphia, 1986
8. Abouleish E: Postpartum hypertension and convulsion after oxytocic drugs. Anesth Analg Curr Res 55(6):813, 1976
9. O'Leary JA: Prostaglandins and psotpartum hemorrhage. Sem in Reprod Endocrinol 3(3):247, 1985
10. Greeley WJ, Leslie JB, Reves JG: Prostaglandins and the cardiovascular system: a review and update. J Cardiothorac Anesth 1(4):331, 1987
11. Morris R, Giesecke AH: Potentiation of muscle relaxants by magnesium sulfate therapy in toxemia of pregnancy. South Med J 61:25, 1968
12. Sinatra RS, Phillip BK, Naulty SJ, Ostheimer GW: Prolonged neuromuscular blockade with vecuronium in a patient treated with magnesium sulfate. Anesth Analg 64:1220, 1985
13. Eisenbat E, Lobue C: Hypocalcemia after therapeutic use of magnesium sulfate. Arch Intern Med 136:688, 1976
14. Lipsitz PJ: The clinical and biochemical effects of excess magnesium in the newborn. Pediatrics 47:501, 1971
15. L'Hommideau CS: Potentiation of magnesium sulfate-induced neuromuscular weakness by gentamicin, tobramycin and amikacin. J Pediatr 102:629, 1983
16. Benedetti TJ, Hargrove JC, Rosene KA: Maternal pulmonary edema during preterm labor inhibition. Obstet Gynecol 59(6):33s, 1982
17. Van Kets H, Thiery M, Deran R: Perinatal hazards of chronic antenatal tocolysis with indomethacin. Prostaglandins 18:893, 1979
18. Ulmsten U, Anderson KE, Wingerup L: Treatment of premature labor with the calcium antagonist nifedipine. Arach Gynecol 229:1, 1980
19. Dale RC, Schneider ET: Respiratory paralysis during treatment of hypertension with trimethephan camsylate. Arch Intern Med 136:816, 1976
20. Lynch C, Durbin CG, Fisher NA, et al: Effects of dantrolene and verapamil on atrioventricular conduction and cardiovascular performance in dogs. Anesth Analg 65:252, 1986
21. Driessen JJ, Wuis EW, Gielen MJ: Prolonged vecuronium neuromuscular blockade in a patient receiving orally administered dantrolene. Anesthesiology 62:523, 1985

INTERACTIONS BETWEEN AGENTS ADMINISTERED IN THE EPIDURAL SPACE AND AGENTS GIVEN SYSTEMICALLY

EPIDURAL OPIOIDS

Fentanyl

Fentanyl is the most commonly administered epidural opioid at the Brigham Women's Hospital. During labor, fentanyl is administered in combination with a local anesthetic, usually bupivacaine, via continuous infusion to provide 10- to 20-μg/h doses. Epidural boluses of 25 to 100 μg with a local anesthetic during labor or 50 to 100 μg in 10 ml of preservative-free normal saline or local anesthetic for postcesarean pain relief are also administered. To date, there have been no drug interactions between epidural fentanyl and systemically administered medications noted in our practice or in the literature.

Hydromorphone (Dilaudid)

Epidural hydromorphone in a dose of 1.25 mg, in conjunction with intravenous droperidol (1.25 mg), has been shown to cause profound respiratory depression that is not responsive to naloxone but does respond to physostigmine.[1]

Acute Abstinence Syndrome

Acute abstinence syndrome is characterized by tachycardia, tachypnea, diaphoresis, hypotension, abdominal discomfort, and agitation. In humans, acute abstinence reactions have been precipitated by the intravenous or epidural administration of opioid agonist-antagonists to patients who are physiologically dependent on narcotics. Epidural administration of butorphanol[2] and buprenorphine[3] has been observed to cause acute withdrawal.

EPIDURAL LOCAL ANESTHETICS

Cimetidine

Cimetidine, an H_2-receptor antagonist, is commonly administered intravenously, intramuscularly, or orally (300 mg) to raise gastric pH as prophylaxis against aspiration pneumonitis. Cimetidine interferes with hepatic oxidative metabolism and initial distribution of amide local anesthetics. A 30 percent increase in the peak plasma level of amide local anesthetics administered by the intravenous or epidural route should be expected if the patient is receiving cimetidine.[4] No adverse effects of this transient increase in levels of local anesthetics have been noted in mothers or neonates.

Effects of Altered Plasma Cholinesterase Activity

1. Prolonged epidural block has been observed in a patient with abnormal plasma cholinesterase activity (dibucaine # = 27). This individual heterozygous for plasma cholinesterase deficiency demonstrated a 90-minute block from epidural chloroprocaine.[5]
2. Grand mal seizures have been observed in a patient with absent plasma cholinesterase activity (dibucaine # = 0) after epidural chloroprocaine.[6]
3. Although of rare concern in obstetric patients, phospholine iodide eye drops significantly affect plasma cholinesterase activity. Although the duration of local anesthesia is more dependent on the rate at which the drug is transported away from the injection site, significantly decreased cholinesterase activity can be associated with increased systemic toxicity and possibly prolonged duration of epidural block with the ester local anesthetics (e.g., chloroprocaine).[7]

REFERENCES

1. Cohen SE, Rothblatt AJ, Albright GA: Early respiratory depression with epidural narcotic and intravenous droperidol. Anesthesiology 59:559, 1983
2. Weintraub SJ, Naulty JS: Acute abstinence syndrome after epidural injection of butorphanol. Anesth Analg 64:452, 1985
3. Christensen FR, Andersen LW: Adverse reaction to extradural buprenorphine. Br J Anesth 54:476, 1982
4. Feely J, Wilkinson GR, McAllister CB, Wood AJ: Increased toxicity and reduced clearance of lidocaine by cimetidine. Ann Intern Med 96:592, 1982
5. Kuhnert BR, Philipson EH, Pimental MD, Kuhnert PM: A prolonged chloroprocaine epidural block in a postpartum patient with abnormal pseudocholinesterase. Anesthesiology 56:477, 1982
6. Smith AR, Hur D, Rosano F: Grand mal seizures after 2-chloroprocaine epidural anesthesia in a patient with plasma cholinesterase defiency. Anesth Analg 66:677, 1987
7. Brodsky JB, Campos FA: Chloroprocaine analgesia in a patient receiving echothiopate iodide eye drops. Anesthesiology 48:288, 1978

INTERACTIONS BETWEEN AGENTS ADMINISTERED WITHIN THE EPIDURAL SPACE

LOCAL ANESTHETIC–OPIOID INTERACTIONS

Chloroprocaine and Opioids

Chloroprocaine administered into the epidural space decreases the subsequent effectiveness of both fentanyl[1] and morphine[2] given via epidural injection. Epidural lidocaine and bupivacaine do not antagonize epidural opioids in the same manner. The mechanism for this antagonism is not known. In fact, fentanyl may potentiate the amide local anesthetics. Current research is underway to evaluate this phenomenon.

LOCAL ANESTHETIC–LOCAL ANESTHETIC INTERACTIONS

Chloroprocaine and Bupivacaine

Epidural chloroprocaine will decrease the effectiveness and duration of anesthesia provided by bupivacaine. Chloroprocaine will alter bupivacaine effectiveness whether bupivacaine is given concurrently or subsequent to chloroprocaine.[3] Other local anesthetics commonly used in labor and delivery have not been shown to have this interaction.

Bupivacaine and Chloroprocaine

Bupivacaine inhibits chloroprocaine hydrolysis by plasma cholinesterase. Bupivacaine administered into the epidural space will reach plasma levels sufficient to decrease chloroprocaine hydrolysis by 38 percent.[4]

REFERENCES

1. Naulty SJ, Hertwig L, Hunt CO, et al: Duration of analgesia of epidural fentanyl following cesarean delivery—effects of local anesthetic drug selection. Anesthesiology 65(3):A186, 1988
2. Kotelko DM, Thigpen JW, Shnider SM, et al: Postoperative epidural morphine analgesia after various local anesthetics. Anesthesiology 59(3):A413, 1983
3. Corke BC, Carlson CG, Dettbarn WD: The influence of 2-chloroprocaine on the subsequent analgesic potency of bupivacaine. Anesthesiology 60:25, 1984
4. Lalka D, Vicuna N, Burrow SR, et al: Bupivacaine and other amide local anesthetics inhibit the hydrolysis of chloroprocaine by human serum. Anesth Analg 57:534, 1978

6

Inhalational Techniques

INHALATIONAL ANALGESIA

DEFINITION

Inhalational analgesia is the administration of low concentrations of an inhaled anesthetic, usually by mask or mouthpiece, to provide partial pain relief during labor and vaginal delivery. The anesthetic is administered by an anesthesiologist or by the patient herself. Often, pudendal nerve block and local infiltration of the perineum at the time of delivery are used in conjunction with or as a supplement to inhalational analgesia.

FREQUENCY OF USE

A survey of 1,200 hospitals in 1986[1] reports that 6 percent of hospitals use inhalational analgesia for vaginal deliveries. However, at the Brigham and Women's Hospital, inhalational analgesia for labor has not been used in over 20 years, because of the risk of aspiration of gastric contents and the lack of therapeutic effectiveness.

MATERNAL SAFETY

Several physiologic changes in pregnancy increase the risk of anesthetic overdose and loss of protective airway reflexes in the parturient using inhalational analgesia. Functional residual capacity is decreased by 20 percent and alveolar ventilation is increased by 70 percent. Furthermore, the minimum alveolar concentration (MAC) is decreased 40 percent during pregnancy. These changes lead to rapid equilibration of alveolar and inspired anesthetic concentrations, resulting in a rapid transition from the analgesic state to the anesthetic state with an unprotected airway.

FETAL AND NEONATAL EFFECTS

Analgesic concentrations of nitrous oxide, methoxyflurane, enflurane, and isoflurane do not cause neonatal depression.[2–4] If neonatal depression does occur, ventilation with 100 percent oxygen by mask and bag should rapidly eliminate any effect from these agents.

TECHNIQUE

Thirty milliliters of a clear, soluble (nonparticulate) antacid is administered orally within 30 minutes before induction. An intravenous infusion is established and blood pressure is monitored. Nitrous oxide, enflurane, methoxyflurane, or isoflurane[5] with oxygen or a combination of nitrous oxide with a volatile agent is administered by intermittent or continuous inhalational technique. The concentration is adjusted to provide adequate analgesia while maintaining maternal consciousness. The anesthesiologist must maintain verbal contact with the patient. At any sign of overdose (confusion, drowsiness, excitation) the inspired concentration is rapidly decreased and 100 percent oxygen is administered. Local perineal infiltration and pudendal nerve block by the obstetrician provide reasonably complete perineal analgesia at the time of delivery. One hundred percent oxygen is administered for 3 to 5 minutes after termination of the inhaled agent to decrease the concentration of inhaled anesthetic in the mother.

REFERENCES

1. Gibbs CP, Krischer J, Peckham BM, et al: Obstetric anesthesia: a national survey. Anesthesiology 65:298, 1986
2. Abboud TK, Shnider SM, Wright RG, et al: Enflurane analgesia in obstetrics. Anesth Analg 60:133, 1981
3. Clark RB, Cooper JO, Brown WE, et al: The effect of methoxyflurane on the fetus. Br J Anaesth 42:286, 1970
4. Hicks JS, Shnider SM, Cohen H: Isoflurane analgesia in obstetrics. Abstracts of Scientific Papers, American Society of Anesthesiologists Annual Meeting, 1975, pp. 99–100.
5. McLeod DD, Ramayya GP, Tunstall ME: Self-administered isoflurane in labour. Anaesthesia 40:424, 1985

GENERAL ANESTHESIA

GENERAL ANESTHESIA FOR VAGINAL DELIVERY

There are few indications for general anesthesia for vaginal delivery; at the Brigham and Women's Hospital, less than 2 percent of the vaginal deliveries over the last 7 years required general anesthesia. The following list describes those situations in which general anesthesia would be appropriate:

1. Need for uterine relaxation: replacement of inverted uterus, complete breech extraction, manual extraction of a trapped placenta.
2. Acute fetal distress during second stage of labor in a patient without an epidural catheter in place.
3. When a parturient is able to deliver vaginally with adequate pain relief and it is not possible to administer regional anesthesia.

GENERAL ANESTHESIA FOR CESAREAN DELIVERY

Indications

General anesthesia is the technique of choice for cesarean delivery in the following situations: acute fetal distress, maternal hypovolemia or severe hypotension, severe anemia, coagulopathy, septicemia, acute neurologic deficit, and cardiovascular disorders in which sympathetic blockade would exacerbate the disorder. At Brigham and Women's Hospital, the percentage of cesarean deliveries under general anesthesia has decreased steadily from 24 percent in 1982–1983 to 8 percent in 1989–1990.

Agents

Preoperative Medications. Thirty milliliters of a nonparticulate antacid such as 0.3 mol/L sodium citrate or a commercial preparation such as Bicitra (sodium citrate and citric acid) is administered by mouth, preferably just prior to induction since its duration of activity is 30 to 60 minutes. Sodium citrate is preferable to a particulate antacid,[1] and will significantly raise gastric pH.[2] Adequate mixing of the antacid with liquid gastric contents is obtained by rolling the parturient from side to side.[3]

Histamine receptor antagonists such as cimetidine (Tagamet) or ranitidine (Zantac) may be administered orally the night before, and orally or intravenously 1 hour before an elective cesarean delivery.[4] One should consider using metoclopramide (Reglan) in the parturient who has recently eaten a meal. Metaclopramide promotes gastric emptying, raises lower esophageal sphincter tone, and is an antiemetic.

Routine sedatives are not given because of potential neonatal depression. Anticholinergics are not routinely administered. If an anticholinergic agent is desired, glycopyrrolate is preferred because it does not cross the placenta as readily as atropine and scopolamine and is a more effective antisialagogue.

Induction Agents

Thiopental. Thiopental rapidly crosses the placenta and reaches peak umbilical vein concentration within 1 minute of maternal administration. Using a dose of 4 mg/kg pregnant body weight (PBW), the fetal brain is not exposed to high concentrations of thiopental. Fetal hepatic extraction and dilution by blood from the fetal viscera and lower extremities keeps brain barbiturate concentration low.[5] Therefore, there is no advantage to delaying delivery to allow redistribution.

Ketamine. Ketamine is not routinely used for induction because of its psychomimetic properties. However, it is the preferred induction agent for severe asthmatic patients or severely hypovolemic/hypotensive patients. In doses not exceeding 1 mg/kg PBW there are no adverse fetal effects.[6,7]

Muscle Relaxants. Muscle relaxants are highly ionized and have low lipid solubility. Minimal placental transfer occurs when conventional doses are used.[8–12]

Succinylcholine is rapidly metabolized by maternal and fetal plasma pseudocholinesterase. Metabolism of succinylcholine is usually not prolonged in the parturient despite reduced plasma pseudocholinesterase.[13]

Nondepolarizing muscle relaxants may be preferable to succinylcholine infusion for particularly long cases (cesarean delivery complicated by fibroid uterus, adhesions, etc.). The shorter-acting relaxants, atracurium and vecuronium, are becoming popular choices over pancuronium and d-tubocurarine.

Inhaled Agents. Nitrous oxide crosses the placenta rapidly but rapid fetal tissue uptake during the first 15 to 20 minutes prevents significant neonatal depression. Minimizing the induction-to-delivery (I–D) interval is important because nitrous oxide is transferred to the fetus in a time-dependent manner.[14,15] Fifty percent nitrous oxide should not depress the fetus with an I–D interval of 15 minutes or less. Any resultant narcosis can be treated by the administration of 100 percent oxygen to the infant after delivery.[16]

The volatile agents are commonly used along with nitrous oxide for general anesthesia. Use of 0.5 percent halothane, 1.0 percent enflurane, or 0.75 percent isoflurane will prevent maternal awareness and recall plus allow for a high inspired oxygen tension without increased uterine bleeding or neonatal depression.[17]

Table 6-1. Technique of General Anesthesia for Cesarean Delivery

1. Insert a large-diameter (14- or 16-gauge) intravenous catheter infusing crystalloid solution. Infusion tubing should contain a hand pressure pump.
2. Give 0.3 mol/L sodium citrate 30 ml orally within 30 minutes prior to induction.
3. Prepare the patient with left uterine displacement, ECG, blood pressure cuff, and pulse oximeter.
4. Administer 100 percent oxygen by face mask while surgeons prepare and drape abdomen.
5. Give thiopental 4 mg/kg PBW and succinylcholine 1.0 to 1.5 mg/kg PBW.
6. Apply cricoid pressure from beginning of loss of consciousness to inflation of the cuff of the endotracheal tube.
7. Administer 50 percent nitrous oxide and 50 percent oxygen, with 0.5 percent halothane, 1.0 percent enflurane, or 0.75 percent isoflurane until delivery.
8. Give succinylcholine 0.1 percent infusion as needed for relaxation.
9. Discontinue volatile agent at delivery. Give 60 to 70 percent nitrous oxide with 30 to 40 percent oxygen, intravenous narcotic, and benzodiazepine as needed.
10. Give oxytocin 20 U/L of crystalloid.
11. Empty stomach with a large-bore suction catheter before extubation.
12. Extubate when the parturient is awake and following commands.

Technique

The operating room in the delivery suite should always be ready for a general anesthetic. The anesthesia machine is checked at regular intervals and has a breathing circuit, bag, and mask connected and ready for use. A suction apparatus should be ready with a tonsil-tip suction device in place. Endotracheal tubes must be ready with stylets in place and cuffs checked. Larger tubes (6.5, 7.0, and 7.5 mm ID [inside diameter]) should be immediately available, and smaller tubes (5.0, 5.5, and 6.0 mm ID) should be available in the anesthetic cart. A short-handled laryngoscope is preferable, as the parturient may have large engorged breasts that may interfere with laryngoscopy using a standard handle (see Ch. 1). Thiopental and succinylcholine should be ready in labelled and dated syringes. A rolled blanket or other device for left uterine displacement must be available for placement under the parturient's right hip.

Thirty milliliters of a non-particulate antacid is administered orally within 30 minutes prior induction, if possible (Table 6-1). A large-diameter intravenous catheter is inserted into a peripheral arm vein and lactated Ringer's or normal saline solution infused. A hand pressure pump in the infusion tubing is helpful if large amounts of fluid need to be infused rapidly.

Upon arrival in the operating room, a wedge is placed under the right hip to ensure left uterine displacement. The patient is acutely oxygenated and, thus, denitrogenated with 100 percent oxygen by face mask while ECG, blood pressure monitoring, and pulse oximetry arc initiated. Four maximally deep inspirations over 30 seconds are adequate if time does not permit a longer period of oxygenation.[18] If an automatic blood pressure cuff is used, a manual cuff should be available as a backup measure in case of failure. The surgeons prepare the skin, drape the patient, and are ready to begin surgery before induction of general anesthesia in order to minimize the time from induction of anesthesia to delivery of the infant.

The use of a small dose of nondepolarizing neuromuscular blocker before the administration of succinylcholine is controversial. We believe that it should not be given for three reasons. First, the parturient does not fasciculate intensely and does not have significant muscle pain. Second, in nonpregnant patients with fasciculations, the rise in lower esophageal sphincter pressure is greater than the rise in intragastric pressure.[19] There is no evidence that fasciculations preferentially increase intragastric pressure more than lower esophageal sphincter pressure in the parturient. Third, it may make endotracheal intubation more difficult. Therefore, if this technique is used, the dose of succinylcholine to facilitate endotracheal intubation should be increased by 30 to 50 percent.

Induction of anesthesia is accomplished with thiopental 4 mg/kg PBW followed rapidly by succinylcholine 1.0 to 1.5 mg/kg PBW. Cricoid pressure is applied as soon as the patient begins to lose consciousness, a few seconds after the thiopental injection, and it is not removed until the cuff is inflated, the lungs are auscultated to demonstrate proper placement of the endotracheal tube, and the capnograph demonstrates CO_2 production by the lungs. Earlier application of cricoid pressure may cause the patient to cough or vomit. Positive-pressure ventilation is absolutely contraindicated. Laryngoscopy is performed when facial fasciculations decrease, the jaw is relaxed, or the peripheral nerve stimulator indicates complete inhibition of twitch. A cuffed endotracheal tube, usually 6.5 to 7.0 mm internal diameter, is inserted under direct vision and the cuff is inflated. Auscultation for bilateral breath sounds and capnography are employed to confirm proper endotracheal tube placement[20] and the surgeons are notified to begin surgery. If the patient is hypovolemic and hypotensive, ketamine 1 mg/kg PBW may be used for induction.

Anesthesia is maintained with at least 50 percent oxygen. A low concentration of a volatile agent (0.5 percent halothane, 1.0 percent enflurane, or 0.75 percent isoflurane) is used to provide amnesia. Ventilation is controlled using a tidal volume of 10 ml/kg PBW at a rate of 10 breaths/min. Maternal hyperventilation can decrease fetal oxygen tension by direct uterine artery vasoconstriction, a leftward shift of the maternal oxygen-hemoglobin dissociation curve, and decreased cardiac output caused by elevated intrathoracic pressure.[21] Hypoventilation should also be avoided because it can cause fetal carbon dioxide retention and respiratory acidosis. An esophageal stethoscope is inserted for continuous auscultation of heart and breath sounds. A 0.1 percent succinylcholine infusion is used for relaxation as needed, with the guidance of a peripheral nerve stimulator. The infusion is started when neuromuscular function has returned. A large-bore suction catheter should be passed orally to decompress the stomach before extubation.

As previously mentioned, the I–D interval under general anesthesia should be minimized. The uterine incision-to-delivery time is also critically important. An interval of greater than 180 seconds during general anesthesia is associated with fetal acidosis because uteroplacental circulation is severely compromised at this time.[22]

After delivery of the infant and clamping of the umbilical cord, the nitrous oxide concentration is increased to 60 to 70 percent with 30 to 40 percent oxygen. The volatile anesthetic is discontinued. Intravenous fentanyl 50 to 100 μg, sufentanil 5 to 25 μg, or morphine 5 mg is administered, with diazepam 2.5 to 5 mg or midazolam 1 to 3 mg as necessary. In our institution, 20 U of oxytocin are added to each 1,000 ml of intravenous fluid after delivery.

At the conclusion of surgery, the patient should have full neuromuscular function as demonstrated by the nerve stimulator. She should be awake, able to follow commands, and breathing well prior to extubation. In the recovery room, the patient should receive supplemental oxygen by face mask and vital signs should be monitored at least every 5 minutes for the first 30 minutes postoperatively.

REFERENCES

1. Eyler SW, Cullen BF, Murphy ME, et al: Antacid aspiration in rabbits: a comparison of Mylanta and Bicitra. Anesth Analg 61:288, 1982
2. Roberts RB, Shirley MA: Reducing the risk of acid aspiration during cesarean section. Anesth Analg 53:859, 1974
3. Holdsworth JS, Johnson K, Mascall G, et al: Mixing antacids with stomach contents. Anaesthesia 35:641, 1980
4. Hodgkinson R, Glassenberg R, Joyce TH, et al: Comparison of cimetidine (Tagamet®) with antacid for safety and effectiveness in reducing gastric acidity before elective cesarean section. Anesthesiology 59:86, 1983
5. Finster M, Morishima HO, Mark LC, et al: Tissue thiopental concentrations in the fetus and newborn. Anesthesiology 36:155, 1972
6. Peltz B, Sinclair DM: Induction agents for caesarean section. Anaesthesia 28:37, 1973
7. Jones MM, Joyce TH, Adenwala J, Mawji F: Comparison of thiopental-nitrous oxide-halothane with ketamine-oxygen-halothane as anesthetic agents for cesarean section. Anesth Analg 64:233, 1985
8. Cohen EN, Paulsen WJ, Wall J, Elert B: Thiopental, curare, and nitrous oxide anesthesia for cesarean section with studies on placental transmission. Surg Gynecol Obstet 97:456, 1953
9. Moya F, Kvisselgaard N: The placental transmission of succinylcholine. Anesthesiology 22:1, 1961
10. Dailey PA, Fisher DM, Shnider SM, et al: Pharmacokinetics, placental transfer, and neonatal effects of vecuronium and pancuronium administered during cesarean section. Anesthesiology 60:569, 1984
11. Demetriou M, Depoix JP, Diakite B, et al: Placental transfer of Org NC45 in women undergoing caesarean section. Br J Anaesth 54:643, 1982
12. Flynn PJ, Frank M, Hughes R: Use of atracurium in caesarean section. Br J Anaesth 56:599, 1984
13. Blitt CD, Petty WC, Alberternst EE, et al: Correlation of plasma cholinesterase activity and duration of action of

succinylcholine during pregnancy. Anesth Analg 56:78, 1977
14. Marx GF, Joshi CW, Orkin LR: Placental transmission of nitrous oxide. Anesthesiology 32:429, 1970
15. Stenger VG, Blechner JN, Prytowsky H: A study of prolongation of obstetric anesthesia. Am J Obstet Gynecol 103:901, 1969
16. Mankowitz E, Brock-Utne JG, Downing JW: Nitrous oxide elimination by the newborn. Anaesthesia 36:1014, 1981
17. Warren TM, Datta S, Ostheimer GW, et al: A comparison of the maternal and neonatal effects of halothane, enflurane and isoflurane for cesarean delivery. Anesth Analg 62:516, 1983
18. Norris MC, Dewan DM: Preoxygenation for cesarean section: a comparison of two techniques. Anesthesiology 62:827, 1985
19. Smith G, Dalling R, Williams TIR: Gastro-esophageal pressure gradient changes produced by induction of anaesthesia and suxamethonium. Br J Anaesth 50:1137, 1978
20. Birmingham PK, Cheney FW, Ward RJ: Esophageal intubation: a review of detection techniques. Anesth Analg 65:886, 1986
21. Levinson G, Shnider SM, deLorimier AA, Steffenson JL: Effects of maternal hyperventilation on uterine blood flow and fetal oxygenation and acid-base status. Anesthesiology 40:340, 1974
22. Datta S, Ostheimer GW, Weiss JB, et al: Neonatal effects of prolonged anesthetic induction for cesarean section. Obstet Gynecol 58:331, 1981

THE DIFFICULT AIRWAY

Difficulty in airway management is one of the principal risks of general anesthesia for cesarean delivery. Gibbs has estimated that difficult intubations are encountered in 5 percent of obstetric general anesthetics.[1] Difficulty intubating the trachea may lead to hypoxemia, hypoventilation, and aspiration of gastric contents. The "Report on Confidential Enquiry into Maternal Deaths" in England and Wales for the years 1979 to 1981 revealed that 14 percent of deaths related to anesthesia were from anoxia and 10 percent were from aspiration events associated with difficult intubation.[2]

Three factors contribute to the complexity of airway management in obstetric anesthesia. First, altered gastrointestinal physiology during pregnancy places every parturient at risk for possible regurgitation and acid aspiration. Second, the time required for airway management and induction of general anesthesia may be critical in obstetric emergencies such as fetal distress or maternal hemorrhage. Third, airway anatomy may be altered in pregnancy. For example, patients with pregnancy-induced hypertension (PIH) may have edema of the upper airway.[3,4]

Available data do not dictate an ideal protocol for airway management in obstetric anesthesia. Therefore, each practitioner must develop his or her own approach. Relevant data have recently been reviewed[5] and are summarized below.

PREOPERATIVE EVALUATION

Although the time required for preoperative evaluation in the parturient requiring an emergent operation may be limited, complete evaluation of the airway is essential. The causes of difficult intubation have been reviewed in detail.[6] Table 6-2 lists factors proposed to predict difficult intubation. These factors were derived from experience with surgical patients but should apply to the parturient as well. Most were suggested on the basis of case reports. However, Mallampati et al. showed in a prospective study that a classification system based on the ability to preoperatively visualize the soft palate, uvula, and faucial pillars accurately predicts difficult intubation.[7]

Patients are divided into three classes:

Class 1: Faucial pillars, soft palate, and uvula can be visualized.
Class 2: Faucial pillars and soft palate can be visualized, but uvula is masked by the base of the tongue.
Class 3: Only soft palate can be visualized.

In addition to anatomic factors, the influence of physiologic changes associated with normal or complicated pregnancy must be considered. For example, upper-airway edema can be seen with PIH and perhaps with prolonged labor.[3,4] In addition, breast enlargement associated with pregnancy can interfere with insertion of the laryngoscope.[8]

Table 6-2. Anatomic Factors Proposed to Predict Difficult Intubation

Short, muscular neck with a full set of teeth
Receding lower jaw
Protruding upper or lower incisors
Poor mobility of mandible
Long, high-arched palate
Inceased alveolar–mental distance
Decreased mental–thyroid cartilage distance
Poor mobility of cervical spine (atlanto-occipital joint)
Inability to visualize soft palate, uvula, faucial pillars
Obesity

(From Malan and Johnson,[5] with permission.)

If difficult intubation is suspected, the patient should be intubated while conscious. An acceptable alternative is to perform direct laryngoscopy under topical anesthesia. If the larynx can be visualized, intubation can be performed after induction of general anesthesia. If it is not visualized, awake intubation or regional anesthesia should be used.

AWAKE INTUBATION

The patient can be intubated while conscious using topical anesthesia. Intravenous analgesia and sedation must be used judiciously because of possible neonatal effects. The method of topical anesthesia used should preserve protective airway reflexes. When carefully administered, transoral spray with 4 percent lidocaine generally provides effective anesthesia for laryngoscopy and intubation while maintaining the tracheal cough reflex.

TECHNIQUES FOR DIFFICULT INTUBATION

When possible, intubation by direct laryngoscopy is preferred because it is rapid and effective, and provides visual confirmation of placement of the endotracheal tube in the trachea. Many techniques have been suggested to facilitate this approach and have been reviewed in detail.[9] We recommend having a variety of laryngoscope blades available. In our practice, we equip each operating room with MacIntosh No. 3 and No. 4 blades, a Miller No. 3 blade, and a Datta-Briwa short handle for use in obese or large-breasted patients. Other blades are available, but have not found widespread use. Before a complex blade or technique is used on a difficult airway, facility should be gained with that technique on elective cases. Many investigators recommend the use of a malleable introducer to guide the endotracheal tube into the trachea when the larynx cannot be visualized. This introducer may be a 14 French gum elastic bougie, although newer plastic introducers are available.

A second technique for difficult intubation is blind nasal intubation. This technique is relatively contraindicated in obstetric anesthetics because it can cause bleeding, which may hamper subsequent attempts at intubation. The risk of bleeding is particularly high in the parturient because the mucous membranes become very friable in late pregnancy. A second limitation of this technique is that it may be time consuming. Compared to orotracheal intubation using direct laryngoscopy or the lighted stylet, blind nasal intubation requires more time to perform, requires more attempts, and has a lower overall success rate.[10,11]

A third approach to intubation of the parturient with a difficult airway involves the lighted stylet. This technique is easily learned. When compared to intubation by direct laryngoscopy the lighted stylet is equally as fast and requires only slightly more attempts.[12] However, these comparisons were made in patients not preselected as having difficult airways, so further evaluation is necessary before this technique can be recommended for routine use in the parturient with a difficult airway.

A very powerful method for endotracheal intubation is fiberoptic endoscopy. Although this technique can be extremely valuable, its use may be limited by three factors. First, many anesthesiologists are not sufficiently experienced with fiberoptic endoscopy to utilize it for a difficult intubation. Second, the necessary equipment is expensive and complex, and may not be available in all obstetric operating rooms. Third, the time required for intubation in the most difficult cases may be longer than is desirable in an emergent situation (up to 17 minutes).[13] Despite these limitations, in experienced hands fiberoptic endoscopy may be the most versatile technique for a difficult intubation.

A fifth approach to intubation of the difficult airway is the retrograde method.[14] Reported success rates are high, but failures do occur. In addition, the time required for intubation has not been critically evaluated. Under ideal circumstances intubation can be accomplished within 1 minute, but can require much more time. For ethical reasons, experience with retrograde intubation cannot be gained on elective cases. However, most anesthesiologists are familiar with cricothyroid puncture and with proper preparation should be capable of using the technique.

REGIONAL ANESTHESIA

The use of regional anesthesia for the patient with a difficult airway is controversial. Ideally, it avoids airway manipulation. However, complications of the regional anesthetic technique or intraoperative development of inadequate anesthesia may require emergent intubation. The utility of regional anesthesia for the patient with a difficult airway has been reviewed.[5] The use of continuous spinal anesthesia that allow the titration of drug to produce the necessary analgesia/anesthesia for delivery should be considered.

THE DIFFICULT AIRWAY AND OBSTETRIC EMERGENCIES

A difficult and controversial issue is the management of anesthesia for cesarean delivery when the mother has a difficult airway and the fetus is in distress. True fetal distress is usually managed by cesarean delivery after rapid-sequence induction of general anesthesia. However, rapid-sequence induction is contraindicated in a patient with a suspected difficult airway because it can result in an anesthetized, paralyzed patient who cannot be intubated. Therefore, even in the setting of fetal distress, time must be taken to safely perform awake laryngoscopy, awake intubation, or a regional anesthetic. Although this practice may put the fetus at risk, the bulk of medical and legal doctrine favors overlooking the fetus before putting the mother at risk. In addition, the condition of an asphyxiated fetus may worsen if the mother becomes hypoxemic or hypercarbic. If a patient is suspected of having a difficult airway, the situation should be discussed with the obstetrician and the patient early in labor. In this way the obstetrician may elect less-emergent cesarean delivery at the earliest suspicion of fetal distress, potential conflicts can be anticipated and avoided, and the patient and surgeon will not have unrealistic expectations.

REFERENCES

1. Gibbs CP: Gastric aspiration: prevention and treatment. Clin Anesthesiol 4:47, 1986
2. Turnbull AC, Tindall VR, Robson G, et al: Report on Confidential Enquiries into Maternal Deaths in England and Wales 1979–1981. Her Majesty's Stationery Office, London, 1986
3. Brock-Utne JG, Downing JW, Seedat F: Laryngeal oedema associated with preeclampsia toxemia. Anaesthesia 32:556, 1977
4. Jouppila R, Joupila P, Hollmen A: Laryngeal oedema as an obstetric anesthesia complication. Acta Anaesthesiol Scand 24:97, 1980
5. Malan TP, Johnson MD: The difficult airway in obstetric anesthesia: techniques for airway management and the role of regional anesthesia. J Clin Anesth 1:104, 1988
6. Murrin KR: Intubation procedure and causes of difficult intubation. p. 75. In Latto IP, Rosen M (eds): Difficulties in Tracheal Intubation. Balliere Tindall, London, 1985
7. Mallampati SR, Gatt SP, Gugino LD, et al: A clinical sign to predict difficult intubation: a prospective study. Can Anaesth Soc J 32:429, 1984
8. Datta S, Briwa J: Modified laryngoscope for endotracheal intubation of obese patients. Anesth Analg 60:120, 1981
9. Latto IP: Management of difficult intubation. p. 99. In Latto IP, Rosen M (eds): Difficulties in Tracheal Intubation. Balliere Tindall, London, 1985
10. Gold MI, Buechel DR: A method of blind nasal intubation for the conscious patient. Anesth Analg 39:257, 1960
11. Fox DJ, Castro T, Rastrelli AJ: Comparison of intubation techniques in the awake patient: the Flexi-lum surgical light (lightwand) versus blind nasal approach. Anesthesiology 66:69, 1987
12. Ellis DG, Jakymec A, Kaplan RM, et al: Guided orotracheal intubation in the operating room using a lighted stylet: a comparison with direct laryngoscopic technique. Anesthesiology 64:823, 1986
13. Ovasappian A, Yelich S, Dykes MHM, Brunner EE: Fiberoptic nasotracheal intubation- incidence and causes of failure. Anesth Analg 62:692, 1983
14. Dhara SS: Guided blind endotracheal intubation. Anaesthesia 34:590, 1980

FAILED INTUBATION

Failed endotracheal intubation is a principal cause of anesthesia-related maternal morbidity and mortality. In England and Wales from 1979 to 1981, 24 percent of maternal deaths related to anesthesia were directly related to difficulties with tracheal intubation.[1] The incidence of failed intubation in obstetric anesthesia is not known, but has been estimated to be approximately 1 in 300.[2] This incidence is significantly higher than that for nonpregnant patients.

The optimal approach to failed intubation is prevention. With thorough preoperative evaluation of the airway and utilization of current techniques for endotracheal intubation, the incidence of failed intubation can be minimized. However, failed endotracheal intubation after induction of general anesthesia may still occur.

Although many approaches to failed intubation in obstetrics have been proposed,[3–8] there are few objective data on which to base a protocol. However, despite these limitations, each clinician *must* formulate a plan for management of failed intubation that will help to minimize the confusion and faulty decision-making associated with an emergent, stressful situation. The plan should include an immediate assessment of the airway, alternative approaches to intubation, options for foreseeable contingencies, and specific limits for how long to persist with intubation attempts. Our approach is illustrated in Figure 6-1 and summarized below.

MANAGEMENT OF FAILED INTUBATION

If intubation fails, the lungs should be ventilated while cricoid pressure remains applied. The prompt decision to abandon the first intubation attempt and ventilate the lungs by mask is critical. Scott has argued that patients do not die from failure to intubate, they die from failure to stop trying to intubate.[10] The oxygen saturation of the parturient at term will decline very

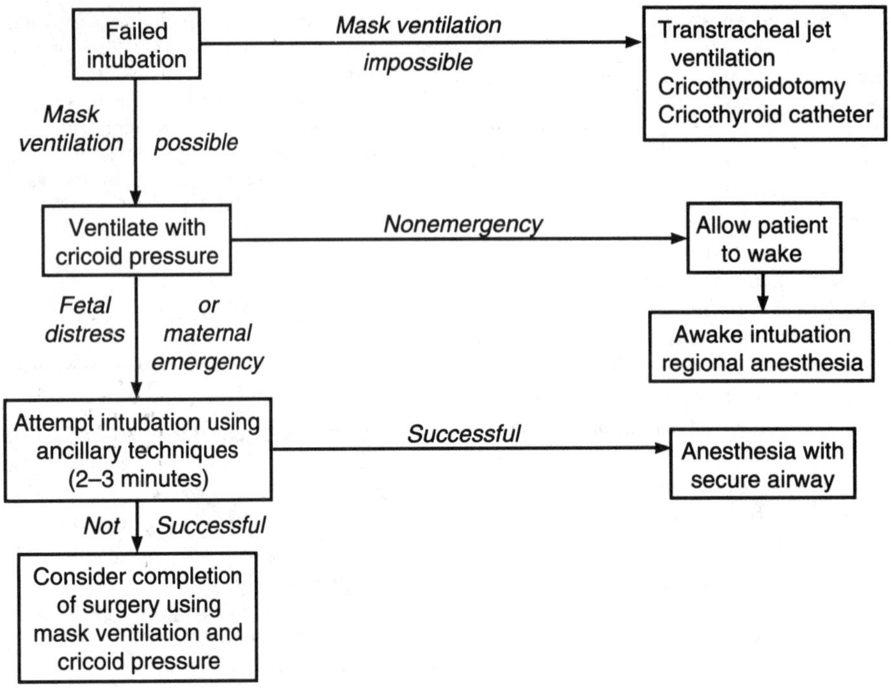

Fig. 6-1. Sample protocol for failed intubation. (Modified from Malan and Johnson,[9] with permission.)

rapidly when the patient is apneic. In addition, prolonged attempts at intubation may provoke retching, vomiting, and subsequent aspiration of gastric contents.

Subsequent attempts at intubation should be limited and well conceived in order to minimize airway trauma. Alternative methods, such as the use of the lighted stylet or fiberoptic endoscope, should be considered. Additional anesthetic or neuromuscular blocking agents should not be administered unless (1) successful intubation is considered to be certain with an additional attempt, or (2) it is elected to proceed with general anesthesia and a mask airway.

If intubation fails, one must decide whether to awaken the patient and employ an alternative anesthetic approach, such as awake intubation or regional anesthesia, or to proceed with general anesthesia and a mask airway. If the fetus does not require emergent cesarean delivery for distress, the patient should be allowed to awaken. If the fetus is at risk, the decision must be based on the clinical situation and the philosophy of the individual practitioner. Most medical and legal doctrine favors overlooking the fetus before putting the mother at risk so it is prudent to allow the patient to awaken in most cases.

Some investigators propose the use of lateral or head-down positions, laryngeal masks, esophageal obturator airways, or gastric suctioning in managing failed intubation. We do not routinely utilize these maneuvers because changes in patient position or manipulation of the pharynx and esophagus might interfere with ventilation, interfere with the competency of the lower esophageal sphincter, or stimulate vomiting or retching.

FAILURE OF INTUBATION AND VENTILATION

If the trachea cannot be intubated and the lungs cannot be ventilated via mask, two options exist: either an airway can be established by cricothyroidotomy or the lungs can be ventilated using transtracheal jet ventilation.

The utility of transtracheal jet ventilation in the management of the difficult airway has recently been reviewed.[11] This technique has been shown to provide excellent oxygenation and ventilation in experimental animals, in elective surgical patients, and in patients with complete upper airway obstruction. Using a driving pressure of 50 psi, a gas flow of 500 ml/s can be delivered through a 16-gauge catheter. This gas flow is sufficient for adequate ventilation.

Benumof and Scheller[11] have described in detail three acceptable systems for transtracheal jet ventilation. These are, in descending order of preference, a jet injector powered by regulated wall or oxygen tank pressure, a jet injector powered by unregulated wall or tank oxygen pressure and an anesthesia machine flush valve using noncompliant tubing from the fresh gas outlet. The latter system can be constructed from materials available in most operating rooms for a cost of approximately $6. Therefore, it is feasible to prepare this simple system for every obstetric operating room. Other methods proposed for transtracheal ventilation, such as using the anesthesia machine flush valve with the anesthesia circle system corrugated tubing or using the anesthesia machine reservoir bag with the circle system, do not reliably achieve adequate ventilation.

If transtracheal jet ventilation is utilized, it may be continued until the patient regains consciousness, the airway is secured by orotracheal or nasotracheal intubation, or cricothyroidotomy or tracheostomy is performed. Although transtracheal jet ventilation is a very useful technique, it does not provide protection of the airway from aspiration of gastric contents, a significant concern in the parturient.

Cricothyroidotomy is more complex and invasive than transtracheal jet ventilation, but has three potential advantages. First, insertion of a cuffed tube protects the airway from aspiration. Second, insertion of an appropriately sized tube allows tracheal suctioning. Third, there may be less likelihood of barotrauma and emphysema than with transtracheal jet ventilation. Therefore, this technique should be considered, particularly if prolonged ventilatory support is anticipated.

Although cricothyroidotomy is an invasive procedure, it is one that every anesthesiologist should be prepared to perform. Many approaches and techniques have been described. Although several adjunctive or percutaneous devices have been developed, none has found widespread use.

REFERENCES

1. Turnbull AC, Tindall VR, Robson G, et al: Report on Confidential Enquiries into Maternal Deaths in England and Wales 1979–1981. Her Majesty's Stationery Office, London, 1986
2. Morgan M: Anaesthetic contribution to maternal mortality. Br J Anaesth 59:842, 1987
3. Tunstall ME: Failed intubation drill. Anaesthesia 31:850, 1976
4. Boys JE: Failed intubation in obstetric anesthesia. Br J Anaesth 55:187, 1983
5. Campbell WI: Failed intubation in obstetric anesthesia. Br J Anaesth 55:1040, 1983
6. Sivaneswaran N, McGuiness JJ: Modified mask for failed intubation at emergency Caesarean section. Anaesth Intensive Care 12:279, 1984
7. Tunstall ME, Sheikh A: Failed intubation protocol: oxygenation without aspiration. Clin Anesthesiol 4:171, 1986
8. Rosen M: Difficult and failed intubation in obstetrics. p. 152. In Latto IP, Rosen M (eds): Dificulties in Tracheal Intubation. Balliere Tindall, London, 1985
9. Malan TP, Johnson MD: The difficult airway in obstetric anesthesia: techniques for airway management and the role of regional anesthesia. J Clin Anesth 1:104, 1988
10. Scott DB: Endotracheal intubation: friend or foe? Br Med J 292:157, 1986
11. Benumof JL, Scheller MS: The importance of transtracheal jet ventilation in the management of the difficult airway. Anesthesiology 71:769, 1989

MATERNAL ASPIRATION

By 1846, inhalational analgesia was utilized for parturition in the United States. An anesthetic morbidity/mortality treatise of the era *might* have read like this:

> ". . . and the next patient was a stout young woman of 19, in the childbirth, in whom the vapour was inhaled for four minutes whilst she delivered. From wailing, she had a fit of coughing, and was then unconscious of pain. Her vomit went to her airway, we believe, and rightly caused her pulse to fall, her hands to get cold, and complete consciousness never to return."

A scenerio 140 years later would read along these lines:

> ". . . a 20 year old full-term pregnant woman is rushed to the operating room for emergency cesarean delivery because of fetal distress. After rapid-sequence induction with thiopental and succinylcholine, the patient vomited and aspirated. She was extubated in the recovery room. Six hours later, she was found dyspneic and cyanotic on the floor, and soon thereafter, died of cardiac arrest."

The practice of obstetric anesthesia has obviously changed tremendously over the past one and one-half centuries. Something has not changed, however. Aspiration is still a killer of pregnant women.

Hall first associated the inhalation of gastric contents with obstetric patients in 1940.[1] He coined the term *chemical pneumonitis*. Mendelson went on to highlight the severe sequelae associated with gastric aspiration in 1946.[2] This unfortunate phenomenon remains a major source of anesthesia-related maternal mortality.

Pregnant patients must be considered to have a full stomach because of several factors that contribute to the retention of gastric fluid and risk of regurgitation.

INCIDENCE OF MATERNAL ASPIRATION

The documentation of incidence is erratic mainly because clinically insignificant aspirations frequently go unnoticed. If dye is placed in the stomachs of general surgical patients prior to the induction of anesthesia, the incidence of staining of the oropharynx (regurgitation) ranges from 7 to 16 percent. Of those patients with regurgitation, 8 to 16 percent have dye in their trachea.[3] We must assume that the parturient undergoing a general anesthetic lies at least within this category of risk.

The incidence of clinically significant aspiration is also unknown, mainly because only maternal *deaths* from aspiration are reported. The most recent retrospective study was done by Olsson in 1986.[4] He reviewed over 185,000 anesthetics for all types of surgical procedures and noted an incidence of aspiration of 1:2131, or 0.05 percent. Due to the enormous sample size and problems associated with documenting such events, accuracy regarding incidence will continue to be problematic.

The Confidential Enquiries into Maternal Deaths in England and Wales examined virtually all maternal deaths over a 30-year period from 1952 to 1981. While absolute maternal mortality decreased by greater than 90 percent, from 99 to 9 deaths per 100,000, no such reduction occurred in deaths from "anesthesia," the majority of which were by inhalation of gastric contents.[5–7] In fact, over this 30-year period, the percentage of true maternal anesthetic deaths increased threefold! Certainly what we are achieving is better management of high-risk obstetric cases. As such, our "figures" are telling us that we are doing a better job in some avenues, while no improvements are being made in others.

MORBIDITY AND MORTALITY

What factors affect the severity of the pneumonitis following aspiration? The initial response to the introduction of gastric material into the respiratory tree is a function of the content and character of the aspirate.[8–10] Particles of food, particularly large chunks, can lodge in bronchi and cause asphyxiation in minutes.

The acidity of the aspirate is probably the single most damaging component. Nonacid liquid has been well demonstrated to produce a mild and transient hypoxia without parenchymal damage. In such a situation, the hypoxia is a result of bronchospasm and atelectasis. Increasing acidity, either alone or with food, inflicts a severe inflammatory response resulting in tracheal mucosal and lung parenchymal injury.[11] From Teabeaut's landmark 1952 study, an inference has been made that an aspirate with a pH greater than 2.5 is relatively benign.[12] Recent animal studies contradict this. Aspiration of liquids with a pH greater than 2.5 may result in a lethal outcome.[13]

Another myth of the current literature is the notion that an aspirate volume of greater than 0.4 ml/kg is uniformly fatal.[14] This "critical volume" concept was modelled after a rhesus monkey study in which highly acidic material was instilled. More valid are the results of a study by James which suggests that "critical volume" is a function of pH.[15] In other words, for a given volume of aspirate, even though small, a lower pH will cause a higher mortality.

Partially digested food causes the worst of all possible problems. The pulmonary shunt fraction is increased and the PaO_2 falls secondary to alveolar hypoventilation.[16] Frequently, alveolar architecture is destroyed as inflammation, hemorrhage, and edema ensue.

SIGNS, SYMPTOMS, AND CLINICAL COURSE

Hypoxemia is the final common pathway after severe aspiration. The signs and symptoms are highly variable, depending on the volume and pH of the aspirated material.[17] One may or may not see gastric contents in the oral cavity. One may or may not hear bronchospasm or observe coughing. There may be tachypnea or pulmonary vasoconstriction, with associated pulmonary hypertension. Radiographic findings may occur early or as late as 12 hours postinsult. Such evidence is most often seen in the right lower lobe.

Patients sustaining a severe aspiration can be categorized into three groups by outcome.[15] One group, 10 to 15 percent, will deteriorate rapidly, with circulatory shock an early sign. Of the remaining patients, two-thirds will improve rapidly after a 1- to 4-day illness. One-third will proceed to develop a bacterial pneumonia and require antibiotic therapy. Most will eventually improve.

HOW PREGNANCY INFLUENCES RISK

The parturient is a member of the population susceptible for aspiration because of the character, quantity, and "environment" of her gastric contents. The high circulating levels of progesterone during pregnancy cause increased gastrin release, and, as a result, higher basal acid secretion rates. The parturient has a delayed gastric emptying time, also a humoral effect.[18] The gravid uterus presses upward against the stomach and poses a mechanical obstruction to the duodenum. The expanding uterus actually displaces the esophageal barrier to reflux superiorly, making the segment extra-abdominal. In addition, progesterone decreases lower-esophageal sphincter tone.[19]

There are other "risk factors" introduced iatrogenically. Parental narcotics decrease gastrointestinal motility. Increased intra-abdominal pressure encouraged during "pushing," as well as manual pressure upon the lower abdomen during delivery will serve to increase intragastric pressure.

Overlay all of these factors upon a patient for whom consciousness is impaired or ablated with anesthetics, in whom intubation may be difficult, and one must appreciate why the acid aspiration syndrome described 143 years ago continues to account for conspicuous mortality in obstetric practice.

THERAPY

Following an acute aspiration, airway management is of paramount importance. Any evident liquid or particulate matter should be immediately evacuated via suction. Placing the patient into the head-down and left-lateral posture immediately following the acute event has been recommended by some investigators. This may decrease the degree of pulmonary soilage but this has been neither proven nor is frequently practical. Copious saline lavage of the trachea and bronchi has been tried but studies demonstrating their efficacy are lacking. In fact, their action may be detrimental. Liquid gastric aspirate is distributed rapidly to the periphery of the lungs. Such washings may help disseminate the material further. Most of the instilled liquid will not reach the already disbursed gastric material.[9] One may attempt to measure the pH of the gastric aspirate as this will give an indication as to the pH of the inhaled material. Expeditious intubation, positive-pressure ventilation with supplemental oxygen, and positive end-expiratory pressure are the most critical first measures. Intravenous β_2-agonists may effectively relieve bronchospasm. While acid-injured lungs are susceptible to secondary bacterial infections, no evidence supports the prophylactic administration of antibiotics, which has been shown not to decrease the incidence of infection nor alter the outcome after aspiration of gastric fluid.[17]

The use of systemic glucocorticoids is also debatable. Some animal studies suggest a reduction in pulmonary damage if corticosteroids are given immediately following aspiration of acidic gastric material. Conversely, other data demonstrate an enhancement in the development of gram-negative pneumonia, inhibition of healing, and reduction in macrophage activity.[20]

Despite the absence of substantial evidence, it is not uncommon that an empiric dose of methylprednisolone (30 mg/kg) or dexamethasone (1 mg/kg) be given. If hypoproteinemia is present, as protein-rich edema fluid exudes across the alveolar epithelium, albumin may be administered. This approach is controversial, however, as it may exacerbate the pulmonary edema.

PROPHYLAXIS

The most significant treatment measure is *prevention*. A considerable amount of morbidity could be avoided if pregnant patients did not eat just prior to their arrival in the labor and delivery suite. This author has personally been told by "prepared childbirth" class coordinators that women *should* eat prior to coming to the hospital because "once you are there, they will not feed you." Anesthesiologist and obstetrician alike must make an impact on this misinformation through education.

One approach toward minimizing risk is by minimizing exposure to general anesthesia. This is already accomplished throughout most of the United States and Western Europe, where general anesthesia for a normal spontaneous vaginal delivery is the increasingly rare exception and not the rule.

When general anesthesia is indicated, a number of steps must be applied to either decrease the chance of aspiration or decrease the risk associated with an aspiration event.

A classic full-stomach precaution remains the technique of denitrogenation with 100 percent oxygen to provide a buffer for the apnea that ensues with induction and laryngoscopy. End-tidal nitrogen is less than 4 percent within 2.5 to 3 minutes in patients without significant pulmonary disease.[21] Recently, Norris demonstrated that four maximally deep inspirations of 100 percent oxygen over 30 seconds results in a PaO_2 on par with those after 3 minutes of 100 percent oxygen inhalation.[22]

There is an ongoing controversy as to the necessity of a pretreatment dose of a nondepolarizing muscle relaxant prior to succinylcholine administration.[23] Succinylcholine-induced muscle fasciculations produce inconsistent elevations in intragastric pressure. This rise, however, occurs concurrently with an increase in lower-esophageal sphincter pressure. Furthermore, the degree of muscle fasciculations in pregnant patients is minimal. While pretreatment with nondepolarizing muscle relaxants attenuates this response, skeletal muscle relaxation takes longer, and thus apneic time is prolonged.

Cricoid pressure is an easy and effective maneuver in preventing aspiration via passive regurgitation during induction of general anesthetic.[24,25] The pressure should not be released until the intubation is confirmed and the endotracheal tube cuff is inflated.

In 5 percent of obstetric general anesthetics, intubation is difficult.[26] If difficult intubation is anticipated, an awake laryngoscopy should be performed after satisfactory topical anesthesia. If the glottis is observed, intubation may proceed as planned following induction. However, if the glottic structures are not appreciated, and regional anesthesia is not an option, an awake intubation should be performed. If intubation warranted an awake or "rapid-sequence" protocol, an awake extubation is appropriate.[27] Extubation should only ensue once the patient regains consciousness and responds appropriately to commands. Coughing and bucking on the tube may infer that the gag reflex has returned, but it may also mean that the patient is in the excitement stage of recovery. In this stage, protective airway mechanisms may be hyperexcitable and laryngospasm is a real possibility.

The assessment of the airway, management of the failed intubation, and alternative techniques are discussed earlier in this chapter.

Antacids

There are numerous pharmacologic approaches toward minimizing the severity of maternal aspiration. Antacids remain the most reliable means of neutralizing the acidic gastric fluid.[28] Originally, particulate antacids were used, and while they were effective, if they themselves were aspirated, there was the potential for development of chronic pulmonary granulomas.[29] The alternative is a water-soluble antacid. The two most well-studied soluble antacids are 0.3 mol/L sodium citrate and Bicitra (sodium citrate and citric acid). They contain the same amount of sodium citrate and have similar neutralizing capacities, although Bicitra is slightly more acidic. Thirty milliliters of either agent, or 30 ml of water with two Alka-Seltzer Gold tablets, given prior to induction, will increase the gastric fluid pH. The patient should be rotated to her right and left following administration to allow for adequate mixing. The efficacy of the clear water-soluble antacid in raising gastric pH is immediate but there is controversy about the duration of action. Therefore, it is essential to administer the water-soluble antacid immediately prior to or within 30 minutes of induction for maximal effect.

Some recent studies suggest that if there is evidence of normal gastric motility at the time of antacid administration, the soluble antacids may pass beyond the stomach at a time when the production of gastric acid is ongoing.[30] A valid concern remains as to whether these agents are protective at the time of extubation.[31]

Histamine-2 Antagonists

Histamine has a major role in the production of hydrochloric acid by gastric parietal cells. This effect is mediated by histamine-2 (H_2) receptors. Numerous studies have evaluated this class of agents, primarily cimetidine and ranitidine, as premedicants.[32–35]

Cimetidine is the most widely studied H_2 blocker. Safety and efficacy of cimetidine prophylaxis in obstetric anesthesia has been reported by many investigators. In fact, it has been studied more in obstetric patients than in any other group. In single- or double-dose therapy, no maternal complications attributable to cimetidine have been demonstrated nor have any adverse effects been noted in infants whose mothers received cimetidine based on Apgar scores and neurobehavioral assessments.[36]

The timing of administration of H_2 blockers is important. Following oral administration, a significant effect is seen in 60 to 90 minutes, whereas following intravenous administration, efficacy is realized in 45 to 60 minutes. The delay in onset somewhat limits cimetidine's utility in an emergent situation but, if given an hour prior to induction of anesthesia, it is effective. A single 300-mg dose at bedtime results in 6 to 8 hours of significantly decreased gastric acidity and gastric juice volume. An additional 300 mg given the morning of surgery (either orally or intravenously) has resulted in an even greater increase in gastric pH.

Inhibition of drug metabolism by cimetidine is an important drug interaction.[37] Microsomal drug metabolism in the liver appears to be inhibited. Hepatic blood flow is also decreased. It is well documented that even after one or two doses, the elimination half-life of drugs such as warfarin, barbiturates, benzodiazepines, theophylline, and propranolol will be prolonged. A few reports exist relating cimetidine administration to a delay in awakening from anesthesia.[38]

Ranitidine is more potent than cimetidine and has a longer duration of action. It inhibits the hepatic mixed function oxidase system to a lesser degree.[39] A 150-mg dose the evening prior to surgery can provide gastric antisecretory effect well through the morning and a morning dose should allow for similar conditions into the extubation/recovery period.

Famotidine is a new H_2 antagonist. It can inhibit gastric acid secretion for up to 10 to 12 hours and has a faster onset of antisecretory effect (30 minutes). Studies are lacking on its use in the obstetric population.[39]

Metoclopramide

Metoclopramide possesses three characteristics that make it potentially very useful for aspiration prophylaxis:[40] (1) it is an antiemetic, (2) it increases lower-esophageal sphincter pressure, and (3) it shortens gastric emptying time. It does not directly affect gastric pH. It is equally efficacious orally or parentally, although variable blood levels are attained following oral administration secondary to a wide range in first-pass metabolism. Metoclopramide is more effective in emptying the stomach after a "light" or liquid meal than solid food. A decreased gastric volume can be demonstrated within 20 minutes of intravenous administration. The common adult dose is 10 mg IV or PO. There are isolated reports of hypotension and arrhythmias following parenteral administration. In obstetric patients, it does not appear to affect the progress of labor. Metoclopramide freely crosses the placenta although infants born to mothers who received it demonstrated no significant change in Apgar scores or neurobehavioral assessments.

Anticholinergics

In addition to histamine and gastrin, acetylcholine is an endogenous secretogogue. Anticholinergic agents have been found to inhibit gastric fluid production but only in a variable fashion. Of the anticholinergic agents available, glycopyrrolate has the most pronounced effects upon gastric secretion and pH. This class of drugs, however, has some potential drawbacks. They may decrease lower-esophageal sphincter pressure and delay gastric emptying. Practically speaking, these drugs are of limited benefit.[17]

REFERENCES

1. Hall GC: Aspiration pneumonitis as an obstetric hazard. JAMA 114:728, 1940
2. Mendelson CL: Aspiration of stomach contents into lungs during obstetric anesthesia. Am J Obstet Gynecol 53:191, 1946
3. Turndorf H, Rodis ID, Clark TS: "Silent" regurgitation during general anesthesia. Anesth Analg 53:700, 1974
4. Olsson GL, Hallen B, Hambraeys-Jonzon K: Aspiration during anaesthesia: a computer-aided study of 185,358 anaesthetics. Acta Aneasth Scand 30:84, 1986
5. Hunter AR, Moir DP: Editorial—confidential enquiry into maternal deaths. Br J Anaesth 55:267, 1983
6. Morgan M: Anaesthetic contribution to maternal mortality. Br J Anaesth 59:842, 1987
7. Rosen M: Editorial—maternal aspiration. Anaesthesia 36:145, 1981
8. LeFrock LJ, Clark TS, Davies B, Klainer AS: Aspiration pneumonia: a ten year review. Am Surg 45:305, 1979
9. Vandam LD: Aspiration of gastric contents in the operative period. N Engl J Med 273:1206, 1965
10. Gibbs CP, Schwartz KJ, Wynne JW, et al: Antacid pulmonary aspiration in the dog. Anesthesiology 51:380, 1979
11. Bynum LJ, Pierce AK: Pulmonary aspiration of gastric contents. Am Rev Resp Dis 114:1129, 1976
12. Teabeaut JR: Aspiration of gastric contents. Am J Pathol 28:51, 1952
13. Schwartz DJ, Wynne JW, Gibbs CP, et al: The pulmonary consequences of aspiration of gastric contents at pH values greater than 2.5. Am Rev Resp Dis 121:119, 1980
14. Hammelberg W, Bosomworth PP: Aspiration pneumonitis: experimental studies and clinical observations. Anesth Analg 43:669, 1964
15. James CF, Modell JH, Gibbs CP, et al: Pulmonary aspiration: effects of volume and pH in the rat. Anesth Analg 63:665, 1984
16. Wynne JW, Hood CI: Hypoxemia in the first hour after aspiration (Abstract). Chest 78:546, 1980
17. Gibbs CP: Gastric aspiration: prevention and treatment. Clin Anesth 4(1):47, 1986
18. Wyner J, Cohen SE: Gastric volume in early pregnancy. Anesthesiology 57:209, 1982
19. Ulmsten U, Sundstrom G: Esophageal manometry in pregnant and nonpregnant women. Am J Obstet Gynecol 132:260, 1978
20. Wynne JW, Reynolds JC, Hood CI, et al: Steroid therapy for pneumonitis induced in rabbits by aspiration of foodstuff. Anesthesiology 51:11, 1979
21. Hamilton WK, Eastwood DW: A study of denitrogenation with some inhalational anesthesia systems. Anesthesiology 16:861, 1955
22. Norris MC, Dewan DM: Preoxygenation for cesarean section: a comparison of two techniques. Anesthesiology 62:826, 1985
23. Miller RD, Way WC: Inhibition of succinylcholine-induced increased intragastric pressure by non-depolarizing muscle relaxants and lidocaine. Anesthesiology 34:185, 1971
24. Sellick BA: Cricoid pressure to control regurgitation of stomach contents during induction of anesthesia. Lancet ii:404, 1961
25. Sellick BA: Rupture of the oesophagus following cricoid pressure? Anaesth 37:213, 1982
26. Malinow AM, Ostheimer GW: Anesthesia for the high-risk parturient. Obstet Gynecol 69(6):951, 1987
27. Thomas JL: Awake intubation: indications, techniques, and a review of 25 patients. Anaesthesia 24:28, 1969
28. Abboud TK, Curtis J, Earl S, et al: Efficacy of clear antacid prophylaxis in obstetrics. Acta Anaesthesiol Scand 28:301, 1984
29. Eyler SW, Cullen BF, Murphy ME, Welch WD: Antacid aspiration in rabbits. Anesth Analg 61:288, 1982
30. O'Sullivan GM, Bullingham RE: Noninvasive assessment by radiotelemetry of antacid effect during labor. Anesth Analg 64:95, 1985

31. Roberts RB, Shirley MA: Reducing the risk of acid aspiration during cesarean section. Anesth Analg 53(6):859, 1974
32. Hodgkinson R, Glassenberg R, Joyce TH, et al: Comparison of cimetidine with antacid for safety and effectiveness in reducing gastric acidity before elective cesarean section. Anesthesiology 59:86, 1983
33. Howe JP, McGowan WAW, Moore J, et al: The placental transfer of cimetidine. Anaesthesia 36:371, 1981
34. Manchikanti L, Kraus JW, Edds SP: Cimetidine and related drugs in anesthesia. Anesth Analg 61(7):595, 1982
35. Stoelting RK: Gastric fluid and pH in patients receiving cimetidine. Anesth Analg 57:675, 1978
36. McGowan WAW: Safety of cimetidine in obstetric patients. J R Soc Med 72:902, 1979
37. Feely J, Wilkinson GR, Wood AJJ: Reduction of liver blood flow and propranolol metabolism by cimetidine. N Engl J Med 305(1):28, 1981
38. Lam AM, Parkin JA: Cimetidine and prolonged postoperative somnolence. Can Anaesth Soc J 28:450, 1981
39. McCammon RL: What's new in drugs that affect the gastrointestinal tract? Anesth Clin North Am 6(2):407, 1988
40. Cohen SE, Jasson J, Talafre M, et al: Does metochlopramide decrease the volume of gastric contents in patients undergoing cesarean section? Anesthesiology 61:604, 1984
41. Blysma-Howell M, McMorland GH, Rurak DW, et al: Placental transport of metochlopramide: assessment of maternal and neonatal effects. Can Anaesth Soc J 30:487, 1983

7

Regional Techniques

PAIN PATHWAYS IN PARTURITION

The pain of uterine contractions together with cervical dilation and effacement is transmitted by afferent fibers that pass to the spinal cord by way of the posterior roots of the T11 and T12 nerves and some fibers from the T10 and L1 nerves.

The pain resulting from distension of the birth canal, vulva, and perineum is conveyed by afferent fibers of the posterior roots of the S2–S4 nerves.

These pathways must be blocked in order to achieve satisfactory analgesia during labor and vaginal delivery (Fig. 7-1).

LUMBAR EPIDURAL ANESTHESIA

ANATOMY AND LANDMARKS

The spinal cord in the adult usually does not extend below the vertebral body of L2, and more often, it ends at L1 (Fig. 7-2). The dural sac, however, usually ends at the level of S1-S2. Surrounding the dural sac, delim-

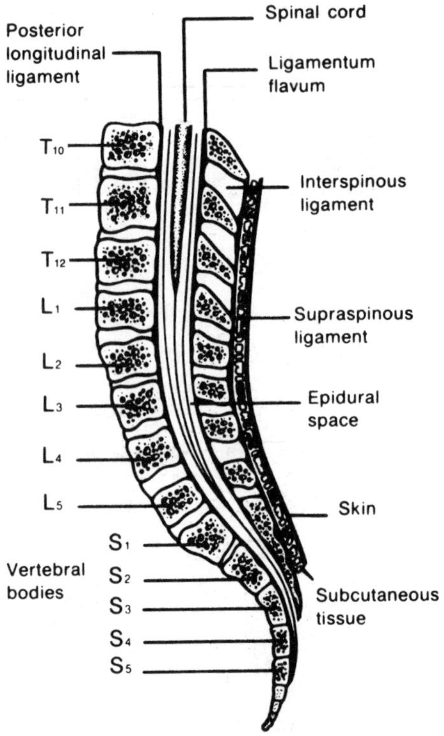

Fig. 7-2. The vertebral column.

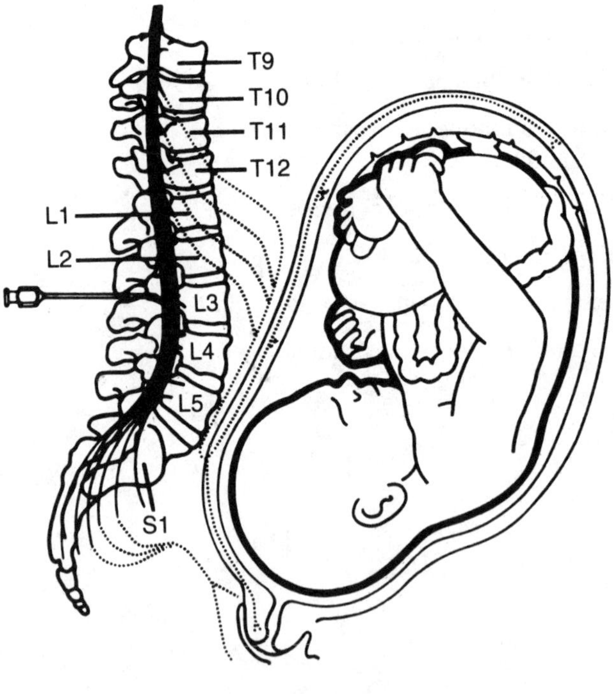

Fig. 7-1. Pain pathways during parturition.

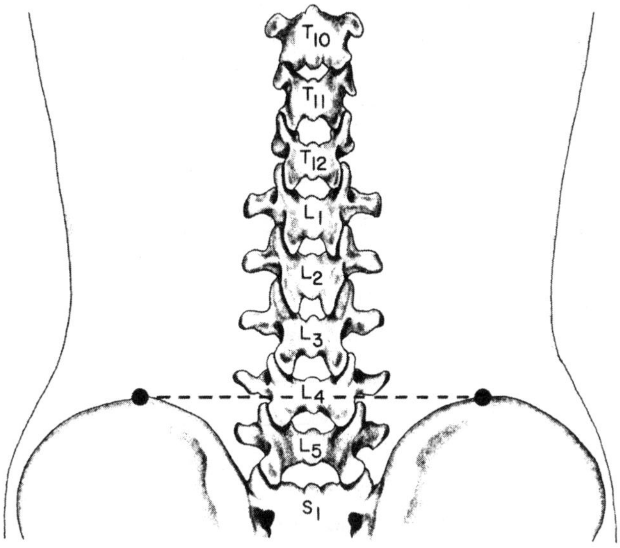

Fig. 7-3. The lumbar area. A line drawn between the right and left iliac crests crosses either the spinous process of the L4 vertebra or the L4–L5 vertebral interspace.

ited by the dura mater on one side and the periosteum of the vertebral bodies and the ligamenta flava on the other, is the epidural space, which extends from the foramen magnum superiorly to the sacral hiatus caudally. Therefore, in theory at least, epidural anesthesia may be given at any level between C1 and S5. The L2–L5 interspaces are usually chosen for obstetric epidural block.

The anatomic landmarks for epidural anesthesia are the same as for subarachnoid anesthesia: an imaginary line drawn between the right and left iliac crests crosses either the spinous process of the L4 vertebra or the L4–L5 vertebral interspace (Fig. 7-3). The selected vertebral interspace for the epidural block can be pinpointed by locating this interspace and then palpating the desired interspace in the cephalad direction.

PATIENT POSITION

The position of the patient is identical to that for subarachnoid anesthesia: either the lateral or the sitting position, although we at the Brigham and Women's Hospital prefer the right lateral position (Fig. 7-4) in order to displace the gravid uterus from the aorta and the inferior vena cava. Additionally, upon completion of the block, the parturient can be placed in the left lateral position to avoid aortocaval compression and achieve an equivalent level of anesthesia bilaterally.

MATERIALS

The following materials should be assembled when an epidural block is to be administered:

- One pair of sterile gloves
- Antibacterial solution for cleansing the skin
- One sterile cup for the antibacterial solution
- Forceps
- Sterile gauze pads
- Sterile towels for draping the field (if desired)
- One 25-gauge, 1.6- to 3.8-cm needle for skin infiltration
- One 21- or 22-gauge, 3.8-cm needle for deep infiltration (if desired)
- One 18-gauge needle to make an opening in the skin (if desired)
- One 17- to 19-gauge epidural needle with stylet (we prefer the 17-gauge Weiss modification of the Tuohy needle with the Huber tip)
- One 3-ml syringe
- One 5-ml glass syringe
- One 20-ml syringe
- One disposable epidural catheter

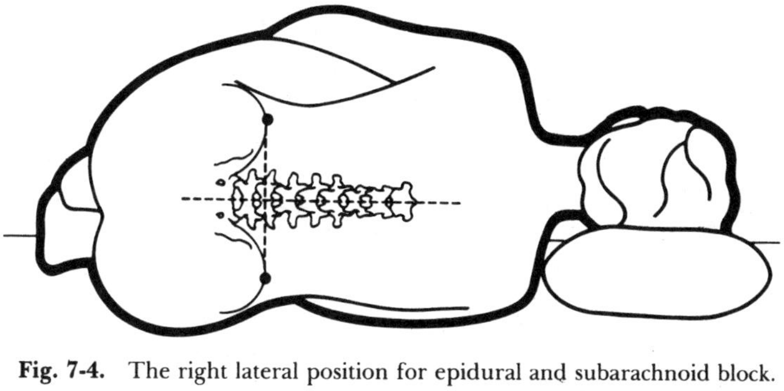

Fig. 7-4. The right lateral position for epidural and subarachnoid block.

A disposable epidural anesthetic tray usually contains all of the above items.

TECHNIQUE

Thirty milliliters of a clear antacid (0.3 mol/L sodium citrate or its equivalent) is administered before the initiation of an epidural block. No other premedication is given for vaginal delivery. For cesarean delivery, 30 ml of a clear antacid is administered (as above) and, if the patient is considered "at risk" for any reason, metaclopramide 10 mg IV and cimetidine 300 mg or ranitidine 100 mg is given intramuscularly or intravenously in the 30 to 60 minutes prior to induction of the epidural block. The technique of epidural anesthesia for the parturient is similar to that for the surgical patient except that special consideration must be given to the condition of the fetus and to the maternal physiologic changes associated with pregnancy and labor.

Although arterial blood pressure must be monitored in any patient undergoing regional anesthesia, the obstetric patient must be carefully observed for changes in blood pressure. The blood pressure is determined in the supine and lateral positions before the block is initiated to check for aortocaval compression (supine hypotensive syndrome). An automatic blood pressure monitor is useful but not mandatory. The fetal heart rate (FHR) record is reviewed. Routine electrocardiographic monitoring is optional at our institution for the initiation of an epidural block for labor of cesarean delivery unless the procedure is initiated in the operating room. However, electrocardiographic monitoring is immediately available, if desired.

The parturient selected for epidural anesthesia is acutely hydrated prior to the induction of the epidural block. A large-gauge in-dwelling plastic catheter allows the administration of 1,000 ml of warm lactated Ringer's solution or similar crystalloid solution over 10 to 20 minutes. This hydration helps to prevent the hypotension that may be caused by the sympathetic block produced by epidural anesthesia. Warm intravenous fluid diminishes pre-, intra-, and postpartum shivering experienced by the parturient. The intravenous infusion is then maintained should the patient require additional hydration or intravenous medication.

The epidural tray is opened in a sterile manner and the expiration date checked. The gloved anesthesiologist prepares the skin of the lumbar area with a bactericidal preparation, wiping off the excess solution. The field may be draped with sterile towels. The desired interspace is located. Depending on the special anatomic features of the patient and the requirements of the situation, the L2-L3, L3-L4, or L4-L5 interspace may be used. We find that the L2-L3 interspace is usually the most suitable. The selected entry point into the skin is fixed by placing two fingers on either side of the interspace selected and the skin is infiltrated with a small amount of local anesthetic. The 25-gauge needle is used to create the skin wheal. Then a small amount (about 1 to 2 ml) of local anesthetic is injected into the subcutaneous tissue and the interspinous ligament. Some anesthesiologists will insert an 18-gauge needle through the skin wheal to create a skin opening large enough to allow the epidural needle to pass through without carrying with it a plug of skin on its way to the epidural space. We do not use this technique because the subsequent release of the skin will move the hole. If one relies on the position of the skin hole, it may be very difficult to identify the epidural space. A well-fitted stylet will prevent coring of the skin.

Various types of epidural needles are available. At our institution, the winged Weiss modification of the Tuohy needle with a Huber point (Fig. 7-5A) is preferred because it can be grasped with the index finger and the thumb of both hands while it is advanced through the tissues. Resting the middle, ring, and little fingers of both hands of the anesthesiologist firmly against the patient's back gives fine control over the movement of the needle unexcelled by any other type of epidural needle. An all-purpose needle such as a 17-

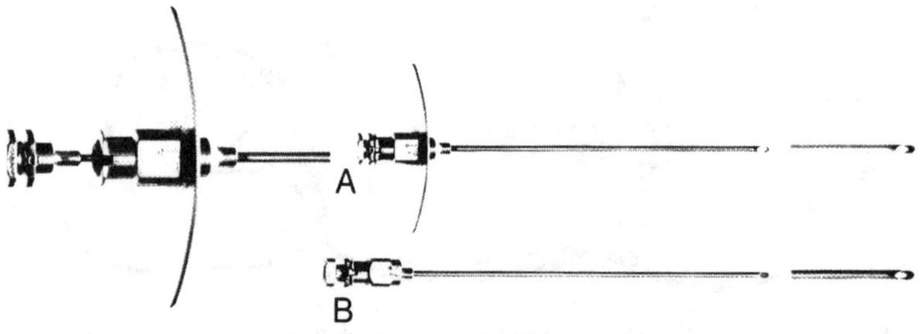

Fig. 7-5. **(A)** The winged modification of the Tuohy needle (Weiss needle). **(B)** The Tuohy needle.

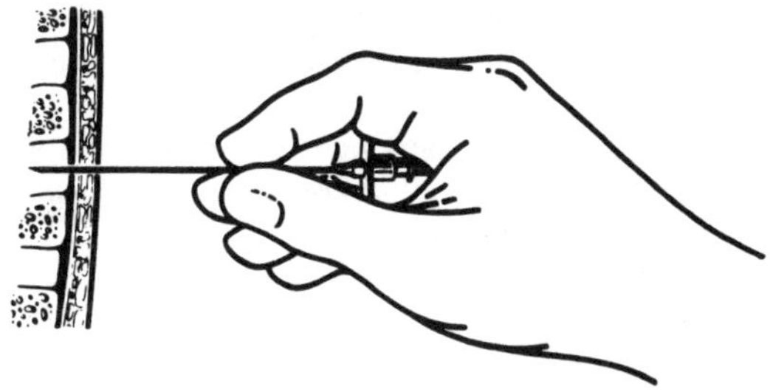

Fig. 7-6. Hand position for inserting the epidural needle.

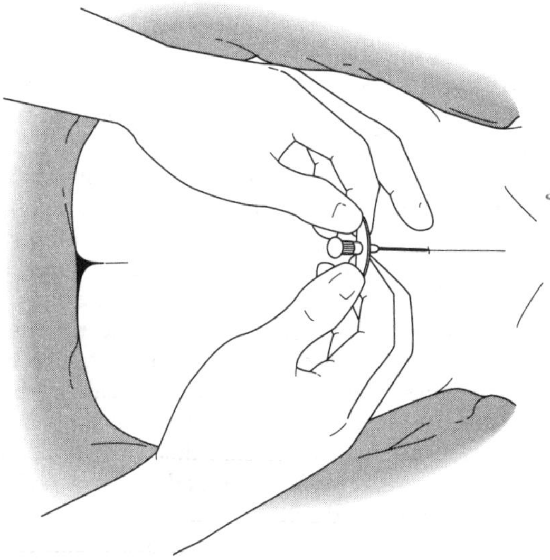

Fig. 7-7. Hand position hanging-drop technique employed when using the winged epidural needle.

to 19-gauge Tuohy needle may also be used (Fig. 7-5B).

Figure 7-2 illustrates the tissue layers and ligaments that are encountered as the needle is advanced 1.2 to 3.7 cm to a point where the tissue resistance of the interspinous ligament is felt. For this phase of the needle replacement, the shaft of the needle is held between the thumb, index, and middle fingers with the palmar aspect of the thumb resting on the head of the stylet to prevent its displacement (Fig. 7-6). We insert the needle into the interspinous ligament or ligamentum flavum with the needle bevel facing caudal or cephalad. This is done to avoid rotation of the needle once it is in the epidural space since this may result in "coring" of the dura and the production of a dural puncture.

The needle is advanced with a smooth, continuous motion. Further movement of the needle is halted when the resistance of the ligamentum flavum changes. At this point, advancing the needle only a small distance will result in its passing through the ligamentum flavum into the epidural space, which measures only 5 mm at its widest extent (in the lumbar area). The advancing needle can easily overshoot this distance, pierce the dura, and penetrate into the subarachnoid space. Therefore, it is important that the advancing movement of the epidural needle be delicately controlled.

There are two methods of identifying the epidural space. The hanging-drop method provides visual identification, whereas the loss-of-resistance method gives tactile evidence of entry.

The hanging-drop technique (Figs. 7-7 and 7-8) is based on the concept of a negative pressure within the epidural space. This method was discovered by Jantzen in 1926 and rediscovered by Heldt and Moloney in 1928. In 1930, Gutierrez used negative pressure to find

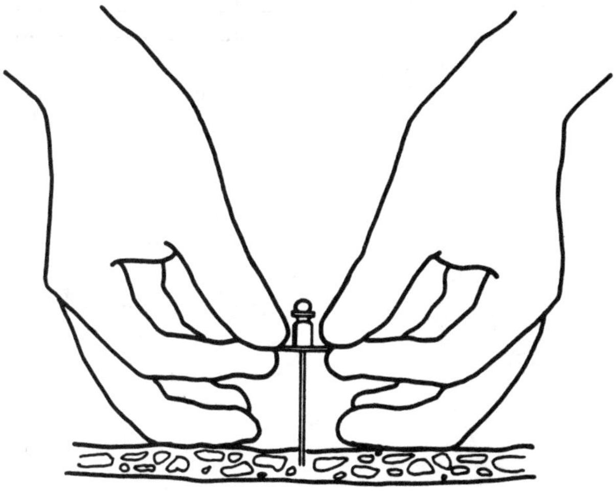

Fig. 7-8. Hand position hanging-drop technique employed when using the winged epidural needle (cross-sectional view).

the epidural space by placing a drop of saline into the hub of the advancing needle. The current technique involves placing a drop of fluid into the hub of a needle that has been inserted into the interspinous ligament or ligamentum flavum.

The wings of the needle are grasped with the thumbs and index fingers and the anesthesiologist's hands are steadied by the middle, ring, and little fingers resting on the patient's back, as shown in Figures 7-7 and 7-8.

While the drop is watched constantly, the needle is slowly and continuously advanced. As soon as the ligamentum flavum is pierced and the bevel enters the epidural space, the drop is suddenly sucked into the needle as if by a negative pressure in the epidural space. Slow and continuous movement of the needle rather than a rapid intermittent or jerky motion is essential for this technique. This sign occurs about 80 percent of the time but the reasons for it are not clear. There are four major theories:

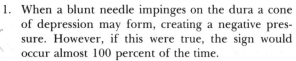

1. When a blunt needle impinges on the dura a cone of depression may form, creating a negative pressure. However, if this were true, the sign would occur almost 100 percent of the time.
2. Expansion of the thoracic cage on inspiration results in a negative pressure that may be transmitted through the paravertebral spaces and the intervertebral foraminae to the epidural space. There are no data to support this theory.
3. The epidural space may be only a potential space in the erect posture, developing only when the back is flexed and the dura mater "separates" from the ligamentum flavum. There is some evidence for this theory.
4. The pull of the abdominal viscera on the posterior thoracic and abdominal walls can cause a negative pressure, but proof of this is lacking. The negative pressure in the epidural space is probably due to a combination of the above factors.

Other mechanical devices can aid in the placement of the epidural needle and help reduce the failure rate of the visual technique.

At our institution, the hanging-drop technique is used with the Weiss needle, and there is additional confirmation of the position by using the loss-of-resistance technique with air and/or fluid.

The loss-of-resistance technique (Fig. 7-9), in which the anesthesiologist's thumb exerts continuous positive pressure on the end of the piston of a glass syringe containing air or preservative-free saline, depends on the sudden loss of resistance as the advancing needle point leaves the ligamentum flavum and enters the epidural space. This method was introduced by Sicard and Forestier in 1921 and was used to administer anesthesia for surgical procedures by Pages in the same year. Its success rate is greater than 90 percent if the dura is not entered. This technique is usually associated with Dogliotti, who popularized its use.

The needle is advanced to the level of the interspinous ligament or ligamentum flavium. The stylet is removed from the epidural needle and a small (5- or 10-ml) glass syringe filled with air or sterile saline solution is attached. The right-handed anesthesiologist holds the epidural needle firmly between the index finger and the thumb of the left hand, as illustrated in Figure 7-9. The back of the left hand rests firmly against the patient's back. This steadies the left hand so that it has fine control over the advancement of the needle. The right hand controls the syringe; with the body of the syringe between the right index and the middle finger, the thumb applies hard, *steady* pressure to the plunger of the syringe while the left hand slowly advances the epidural needle through the tissues. None of the syringe contents will be expelled as long as the point of the needle is in the interspinous ligament or the ligamentum flavum. However, as soon as these structures are pierced and the needle enters the epidural space, this resistance suddenly disappears and the entire content of the syringe is suddenly discharged. The movement of the

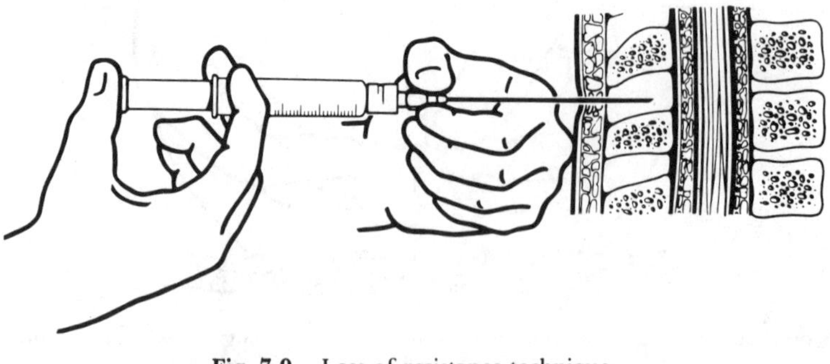

Fig. 7-9. Loss-of-resistance technique.

epidural needle is halted immediately by the counteractions of the left hand.

We prefer the hanging drop technique with the winged epidural needle over the loss-of-resistance technique because it allows better perception of the changes in tissue resistance as the needle is advanced. As their skills improve, anesthesiologists "know" the epidural space is being entered without any movement of the hanging drop. If the loss-of-resistance technique is chosen it is recommended that fluid rather than air be used because of air's compressibility and the high incidence of false-positive results when air is used.

Regardless of which technique is used, it is advisable to perform tests to confirm that the needle is in the epidural space. The first test involves aspiration with a small (5-ml) glass syringe attached to the needle. If the aspiration test yields a bloody return, it is probable that one of the veins of the epidural plexus has been punctured. To avoid intravascular injection of the relatively large amount of local anesthetic needed for an epidural block, another interspace should be chosen and the procedure repeated. If the aspiration test results in the return of cerebrospinal fluid (CSF), another interspace should be chosen for a repeat attempt to place the needle in the epidural space. Because of this potential problem, we prefer the L2-L3 interspace. If there is a dural perforation, one can move caudad and away from the initial hole by one or two interspaces. Although it may occur, we have not seen a subarachnoid block results from an epidural block performed after the puncture of the dura at another interspace. In a surgical setting, if the dura has been punctured, it may be feasible to continue the procedure as a subarachnoid anesthetic at the same interspace. However, subarachnoid anesthesia is not performed during the first stage of labor.

The next confirmatory test to ensure that the needle is in the epidural space involves either the injection of 4 to 5 cc of air or the slow injection of 3 ml of normal saline or anesthetic solution as a test dose. If air is used, a small (5-ml), empty, and dry glass syringe is attached to the epidural needle and the plunger positioned at the 4- to 5-ml mark. The air is then briskly injected into the epidural space. Pressure on the plunger is released immediately after the discharge of the total air volume. Ease of injection of the air and failure of the plunger to move back more than to the 0.5- to 1.0-ml mark usually indicate that the needle point is in the epidural space. If there is resistance to the air injection or if there is significant return of air into the syringe, then the bevel of the needle may still be located in subcutaneous tissue, interspinous ligament, or the ligamentum flavum. A *dry* glass syringe is utilized for this confirmatory test because a wet glass syringe without liquid contents in the barrel will become sticky and make interpretation difficult. In addition, the glass syringes in disposable epidural trays are made to be used *dry*.

If normal saline or local anesthetic is used as a confirmatory test, we incorporate a small (0.2-cc) air bubble into the solution. Compression of the bubble on injection indicates the tip of the epidural needle is still in the ligamentum flavum and not the epidural space, which is a *potential* space. Absence of bubble compression and smooth injection of the solution indicates injection into the epidural space. We also use this technique when identifying the epidural space with the loss-of-resistance technique employing normal saline.

Injecting a small amount (3 ml) of local anesthetic solution should not result in any major anesthetic effect if the needle is in the epidural space. However, if the dura mater has been pierced and the local anesthetic is injected into the subarachnoid space, extensive sensory and motor block may be noted. Three minutes are allowed for any sensory anesthetic effect to appear.

Table 7-1. Local Anesthetics and Suggested Dosages for Single-Dose Epidural Block for Vaginal Delivery

Local Anesthetic[a]	Dosage[b] (ml)	Dosage[b] (mg)	Clinical Onset of Action (min)	Duration of Action (min)
Bupivacaine 0.25–0.5%	8–20	20–100	3–5	60–180
2-Chloroprocaine 2.0–3.0%	8–20	160–600	3–5	40–60
Lidocaine 1.0–2.0%[c]	8–20	80–400	3–5	60–90
Mepivacaine 1.0–2.0%	8–20	80–400	3–5	60–90

[a] Without epinephrine.

[b] Dosage range depending on patient's height; total milligram dosage of the local anesthetic should not exceed manufacturer's recommendations.

[c] With or without epinephrine 1:200,000.

Table 7-2. Local Anesthetics and Suggested Dosages for Single-Dose Epidural Block for Cesarean Delivery

Local Anesthetic[a]	Dosage[b] (ml)	Dosage[b] (mg)	Clinical Onset of Action (min)	Duration of Action (min)
Bupivacaine 0.5%	20–30	100–150	3–5	90–180
Chloroprocaine 3%	12–20	360–600	3–5	40–60
Etidocaine 1.0–1.5%[c,d]	12–20	120–300	3–5	60–90
Lidocaine 2.0%[c]	12–20	240–400	3–5	60–90
Mepivacaine 2.0%	12–20	240–400	3–5	60–90

[a] Without epinephrine.
[b] Dosage range depending on patient's height; total milligram dosage of the local anesthetic should not exceed manufacturer's recommendations.
[c] With or without epinephrine 1:200,000.
[d] Etidocaine 1.5% is only manufactured with epinephrine 1:200,000.

If these tests indicate that the needle is in the epidural space, an aspiration test is performed before each of the incremental or fractional (3- to 5-ml) doses, which are injected every 60 to 90 seconds until the total dose for a single-dose epidural block has been administered. The indicated dosages have been reduced by about 25 percent from those appropriate for a similar epidural block in a surgical patient (Tables 7-1 and 7-2). After the epidural needle is withdrawn, the patient is allowed to rest in a comfortable position favoring left uterine displacement—usually a semisitting position with the right hip elevated by a wedge. We prefer to initiate an epidural block with the parturient in the right lateral position. Thus, with left uterine displacement, the dependent side will receive an adequate amount of drug. Vital signs, particularly blood pressure, and the spread of anesthesia are carefully monitored. Indications for single-dose epidural anesthetic are discussed below.

PLACING AN EPIDURAL CATHETER

The anatomic landmarks and the initial steps for placing an epidural catheter are the same as for the single-dose method of epidural block. An epidural needle must be selected that is large enough to admit the catheter for passage into the epidural space. The needle is positioned in the epidural space using the techniques described previously. Either the hanging-drop technique or the loss-of-resistance method may be used to identify the epidural space. We administer a test dose of 3 ml of local anesthetic through the needle before inserting the catheter into the epidural space.

The plastic catheter is examined for imperfections. The depth markings are noted and compared with the length of the epidural needle. The tubing may be inserted using a wire stylet to make the passage of the catheter through the needle easier. The wire stylet is withdrawn 2 to 3 cm from the tip of the catheter. The catheter is uncurled and held by the fingers of the left hand. The tip of catheter is inserted through the hub of the epidural needle by the right hand (by a right-handed anesthesiologist). As the leading point of the tubing contacts the directional bevel of the epidural needle, a sudden resistance is left. This is usually at the first mark on the epidural catheter. This resistance is gently but aggressively overcome and the tubing is advanced through the needle so that it will project 2 to 3 cm beyond the bevel of the epidural needle into the epidural space. The distance can be measured by placing the plunger of the syringe against the patient's back and noting the marking on the syringe that correlates to the centimeter mark on the catheter that is at the hub of the needle. We use the back of the plunger or piston of the syringe instead of the male end to avoid contamination of the syringe with the residual antibacterial solution, and it is preferable to use a glass syringe for the initial injection through the epidural catheter. Then the needle is removed from the tissues in the following manner: the catheter is held firmly approximately 2 to 3 cm from the hub of the needle while the "wings" or shaft and hub of the needle are held between the index and middle fingers and thumb of the other hand (Fig. 7-10). While the catheter is held in place with positive forward pressure the needle is carefully pulled out until the thumbs of the two hands meet. Forward pressure should be applied to the catheter at all times. The

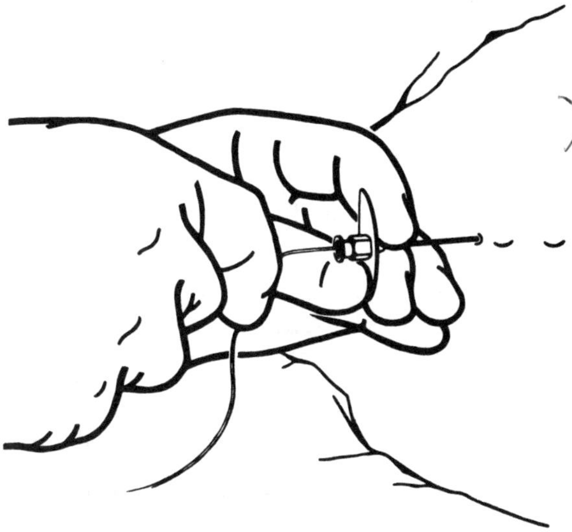

Fig. 7-10. Insertion of the epidural catheter and removal of the epidural needle over the epidural catheter.

maneuver is then repeated by grasping the tubing another 2 to 3 cm distal to the hub of the needle and repeating the same procedure. Finally, the tip of the needle will emerge from the skin. The tubing is prevented from being dislodged by applying firm pressure with the thumb and index finger of the left hand to the tubing at the point where it emerges from the skin. The needle is then moved back over the catheter. The thumb and index finger may now move some distance up the catheter and hold the catheter firmly to prevent its dislodgement while the needle and stylet are removed from the catheter by the right hand. This should always be done close to the back to avoid dislocating the catheter. Once the needle has been removed, a catheter is withdrawn the previously measured distance so that 2 to 3 cm of the catheter lies within the epidural space.

Forward repositioning of the needle is impossible once the catheter is advanced beyond the bevel. If forward repositioning is necessary, the needle and the catheter are both completely withdrawn and the procedure is repeated from the beginning. Once the catheter has advanced beyond the bevel of the epidural needle, any attempt to withdraw it can result in shearing off the catheter.

An adapter is attached to the end of the catheter, or a blunt, small-gauge needle is inserted into the tubing. Before the catheter is taped in place, an aspiration test is carefully performed to ensure that the catheter is not in the subarachnoid space or in an epidural vein. The epidural veins are thin walled; aspiration via the epidural catheter may be negative when the catheter is in an epidural vein because the aspiration has created a negative pressure that has occluded the end of the catheter with the wall of the vein. Disconnecting the syringe from a catheter adapter and holding the catheter tip *below* the level of insertion may allow blood to spontaneously appear in the lumen of the catheter as a result of venous pressure, thereby diagnosing an intravascular placement. If these tests are negative, another 3-ml test dose of local anesthetic solution is injected and the patient is observed for cardiovascular changes, sensory or motor alterations, or central nervous system toxic reaction for not less than 3 minutes. Sterile gauze pads are placed above and below the catheter as it emerges from the skin, and the catheter and pads are secured by pieces of tape. The entire catheter is then taped to the back of the patient and she is placed in a semisitting position with a wedge under the right hip to displace the uterus to the left.

If vital signs remain satisfactory and no significant anesthesia develops after this second test dose, another aspiration test is done. Fractional doses of local anesthetic (3 to 5 ml) are administered at intervals of at least 60 seconds until the full epidural dose is injected. We do not inject more than 5 ml of local anesthetic at a time. This practice translates to a maximal dose of 25 mg bupivacaine or 100 mg lidocaine in our current practice.

To obtain continuous anesthesia from T10 to S5, the first intermittent epidural dose may be the same as for the single-dose method. When the desired level of anesthesia has been achieved with the initial dose, a subsequent "top-up" dose of about two-thirds the initial dose will maintain this sensory level. Top-up doses are added as necessary. An aspiration test must be done prior to each reinforcement because perforation of the dura mater or one of the epidural veins by the catheter may have occurred since the last administration of the anesthetic. Fractional doses of local anesthetic (3 to 5 ml) are administered until the appropriate top-up dose has been given. Dosage schedules are listed in Tables 7-3 and 7-4. Alternatively, the patient may be placed on a continuous infusion of local anesthetic with or without opioid, as described subsequently in this chapter.

With the patient resting comfortably, the spread of anesthesia is checked frequently by gentle repeated pinpricks or by a cotton swab moistened with alcohol. Since the loss of pain and temperature sensation progresses simultaneously, the use of alcohol to check the spread of anesthesia may be more pleasant for the patient. Repeat pinpricks may not accurately differentiate the area of complete loss of pain sensation from that of partial sensory anesthesia. However, we still prefer the "pinprick" test. Because of the concern over blood and fluid contamination, we suggest the use of sharp plastic toothpicks to determine sensory levels.

Table 7-3. Local Anesthetics and Suggested Dosages for Continuous (Intermittent) Epidural Anesthesia for Vaginal Delivery

	Dosage[b]						
	First Dose[c]		Top-up Dose[d]		Onset of Action (min)	Duration of Action (min)	Time between Top-up Doses (min)
Local Anesthetic[a]	(ml)	(mg)	(ml)	(mg)			
Bupivacaine[e] 0.25–0.5%	8–15	20–75	6–10	15–50	3–5	60–180	Approx. 60–120
Chloroprocaine 2.0–3.0%	8–15	160–450	6–10	120–300	3–5	40–60	Approx. 45
Lidocaine 1.0–2.0%[f]	8–15	80–300	6–10	60–200	3–5	60–90	Approx. 60
Mepivacaine 1.0–2.0%	8–15	80–300	6–10	60–200	3–5	60–90	Approx. 60

[a] Without epinephrine.
[b] Total milligram dosage of the local anesthetic should not exceed manufacturer's recommendations.
[c] Dosage range depending on patient's height.
[d] The top-up dose is two-thirds of the first dose if the initial dose resulted in a satisfactory level of anesthesia and if this level is to be maintained.
[e] Some have described the use of 0.125 percent bupivacaine for vaginal delivery but we do not use this dosage for initiation of the block, just for continuous infusion.
[f] With or without epinephrine 1:200,000.

Several brands of plastic toothpicks are sharp enough to pierce olives or onions but not human skin.

PRECAUTIONS

Aspiration

Aspiration must precede the injection of local anesthetic solution in order to avoid unintentional subarachnoid injection or intravenous injection. The epidural dosage is a large multiple of that needed for subarachnoid block. Unintentional injection of such an amount of local anesthetic solution into the subarachnoid space would unavoidably result in high or total spinal block. The epidural venous plexus can be the site for an intravascular injection of a large volume of local anesthetic, which may be followed by central nervous system (CNS) excitation and convulsions. Full cardiopulmonary resuscitative equipment must be immediately available, as is customary for any regional block.

Table 7-4. Local Anesthetics and Suggested Dosages for Continuous (Intermittent) Epidural Anesthesia for Cesarean Delivery

	Dosage[b]						
	First Dose[c]		Top-up Dose[d]		Onset of Action (min)	Duration of Action (min)	Time between Top-up Doses (min)
Local Anesthetic[a]	(ml)	(mg)	(ml)	(mg)			
Bupivacaine 0.5%	20–30	100–150	8–12	40–60	3–5	90–180	Approx. 150
2-Chloroprocaine 3.0%	12–20	360–600	8–12	240–360	3–5	40–60	Approx. 45
Etidocaine 1.0%–1.5%[e,f]	12–20	120–300	8–12	80–180	3–5	60–90	Approx. 75
Lidocaine 2.0%[e]	12–20	240–400	8–12	160–240	3–5	60–90	Approx. 60
Mepivacaine 2.0%	12–20	240–400	8–12	160–240	3–5	60–90	Approx. 60

[a] Without epinephrine.
[b] Total milligram dosage of the local anesthetic should not exceed manufacturer's recommendations.
[c] Dosage range depending on patient's height.
[d] The top-up dose is two-thirds of the first dose if the initial dose resulted in a satisfactory level of anesthesia and if this level is to be maintained.
[e] With or without epinephrine 1:200,000.
[f] Etidocaine 1.5% is only manufactured with epinephrine 1:200,000.

The Test Dose

The purpose of the epidural test dose is to detect intravascular or subarachnoid injection of a local anesthetic. Moore and Batra[1] demonstrated that 3 ml of a local anesthetic with epinephrine 1:200,000 (15 μg) is an effective test dose in premedicated surgical patients. Guinard and associates[2] substantiated that:

1. A test dose containing epinephrine 10 or 15 μg is a sensitive and specific marker of intravascular injection in young, nonpregnant, healthy subjects.
2. A positive response can be reliably detected by an absolute increase in heart rate of at least 20 beats/min (bpm).
3. In the presence of acute selective or nonselective β-blockade, tachycardia is no longer a reliable sign of intravascular injection.
4. An increase in systolic blood pressure of at least 15 mmHg is a sensitive, although not entirely specific, indicator of intravascular injection of epinephrine during acute β-adrenergic blockade.

Subarachnoid injection of the local anesthetic in the test dose will produce sensory anesthesia. However, onset time of sensory block may vary from almost immediately to up to 5 or more minutes. Therefore, we believe a test dose of local anesthetic including epinephrine 15 μg should be administered on initiation of epidural anesthesia for cesarean delivery in the nonlaboring parturient as well as with any major regional anesthetic. The parturient's heart rate should be monitored continuously while the test dose is given because the increase in heart rate may occur within 25 seconds of intravascular injection and last for only 30 seconds.[2] Increases in blood pressure should occur within 2 minutes of intravenous injection. Three milliliters of 1.5 percent hyperbaric lidocaine (45 mg) with epinephrine (15 μg) is our preferred test dose to check the placement of an epidural catheter because, besides containing epinephrine as a marker for intravascular injection, it will give absolute sensory evidence of subarachnoid block within 2 minutes if placed in the subarachnoid space without worry of how high the block will go.

Leighton and Gross[3] have advocated the injection of 1 cc of air to indicate intravascular catheter placement. One theoretical concern with this technique is the possibility (albeit small) of an air embolus in the 20 percent of patients who have a probe patent foramen ovale. Other researchers have suggested the use of isoproterenol and ephedrine.

The use of a test dose for labor and vaginal delivery raises two important issues. First, what is the effect of epinephrine on labor and uterine blood flow, and second, what constitutes an adequate test dose in a laboring patient?

Matadial and Cibils[4] demonstrated a significant reduction in uterine activity when epinephrine 1:200,000 was added to local anesthetic solutions. This reduction in uterine activity is less pronounced when the epidural block is placed after labor is well established[5] The effects of epinephrine on the fetus must also be considered. Wallis et al.[6] found a decrease in uterine artery blood flow in pregnant ewes when lumbar anesthesia with chloroprocaine plus epinephrine 1:200,000 was administered. Hood et al.[7] demonstrated a significant reduction in uterine blood flow when intravenous epinephrine 5 to 20 μg was given to gravid ewes. Chestnut et al.[8] reported diminished uterine blood flow velocity in pregnant guinea pigs after intravenous epinephrine 0.2 μg/kg. Leighton et al.[9] gave 10 laboring women epinephrine 15 μg intravenously. Two FHR tracings showed signs of fetal distress. Although not statistically significant when compared to the tracings of 10 control patients who received intravenous saline, the signs of fetal distress lasted 10 to 12 minutes and were postulated by the authors to be attributed to decreased uterine blood flow.

Van Zundert et al.[10] gave bupivacaine 12.5 mg plus epinephrine 12.5 μg intravenously to laboring parturients and noted a rapid increase in maternal heart rate and a temporary increase in blood pressure along with a short-lived slowing of uterine contractions. Chestnut et al.[11] studied maternal heart rate variability during induction of epidural anesthesia in laboring women. They found increases in maternal heart rate of more than 25 bpm, lasting greater than 15 seconds in 5 of 10 laboring women during the time period of 10 minutes before to 5 minutes after epidural (not intravenous) injection of 0.5 percent bupivacaine 3 ml with epinephrine 15 μg.

At the Brigham and Women's Hospital, we do not use epinephrine in local anesthetic solutions for labor and delivery. Our maximal allowable volume of any one injection is 5 ml of any solution. Our test doses are 3 ml via the epidural needle or catheter and our maintenance injections for the intermittent dosage technique are a 3-ml test dose followed by 3 to 5 ml of local anesthetic. Alternatively, a continuous epidural infusion may be initiated. Since we frequently initiated epidural blocks during the latent phase of labor at the request of the parturient and her obstetrician, the adverse effects of epinephrine on uterine activity would become apparent, as we would be dosing a large amount of epinephrine if we gave a test dose before each injection. With our fractional or incremental injection technique, we have virtually eliminated CNS toxic reactions secondary to unintentional intravascular injection of local anesthetic during obstetric epidural anesthesia. We have seen the prodrome of a CNS reaction, but with aspiration before each incremental injection, we have avoided any sequelae. In effect, all of our injections have become test doses. With continuous epidural infusion, assessment of the parturient must be accomplished at regular intervals to monitor for unintentional subarachnoid block or intravascular migration of the epidural catheter. It must be kept in mind that negative aspiration does not rule out an intravascular or subarachnoid catheter!

Uterine Hypertonus

In our experience, the parturient may complain of increased pain with the next contraction after an intravascular injection.

Increased intravascular concentrations of local anesthetic may produce uterine hypertonus and will result in the patient perceiving more discomfort.[12] Figure 7-11 demonstrates the increase in uterine activity after an unintentional intravascular injection of approximately 50 mg of bupivacaine added to whatever circulating concentration of local anesthetic was present. In this instance, an epidural anesthetic utilizing 0.5 percent bupivacaine had been in place for several hours and involved three reinjections. At the arrow (↓), after aspiration, 5 ml of 0.5 percent bupivacaine (25 mg) was administered via an epidural catheter. After 1 minute had passed and another aspiration test was performed, another 5 ml of 0.5 percent bupivacaine (25 mg) was administered. The parturient had the prodrome of a CNS toxic reaction but no convulsion. Repeat aspiration of the epidural catheter yielded frank blood. With the next two contractions, the patient complained bitterly of pain and discomfort, which then subsided. Reinsertion of the epidural catheter was successful and satisfactory anesthesia was obtained for the remainder of the labor and delivery.

Effect on the Fetus

The pharmacologic action of the local anesthetic absorbed by the neonate during epidural anesthesia, although minimal, may be demonstrated by neurobehavioral testing. The fetal narcotization that may be seen with systemic analgesia is less likely to occur when opioids are added to the local anesthetic solutions. However, maternal hypotension with a concomitant decrease in uteroplacental perfusion producing fetal hypoxia and acidosis is possible and must be treated immediately.

Monitoring

Monitoring of vital signs is mandatory for both the mother and fetus. Maternal blood pressure must be checked frequently. If a decrease of 10 mmHg or more occurs, an immediate response is necessary. Therapy consists of an immediate change in the position of the parturient to a more pronounced left (or sometimes right) lateral position, administration of oxygen by face mask, and an increase in the intravenous infusion rate initiated by a 200- to 300-ml bolus of an appropriate intravenous crystalloid solution such as lactated Ringer's

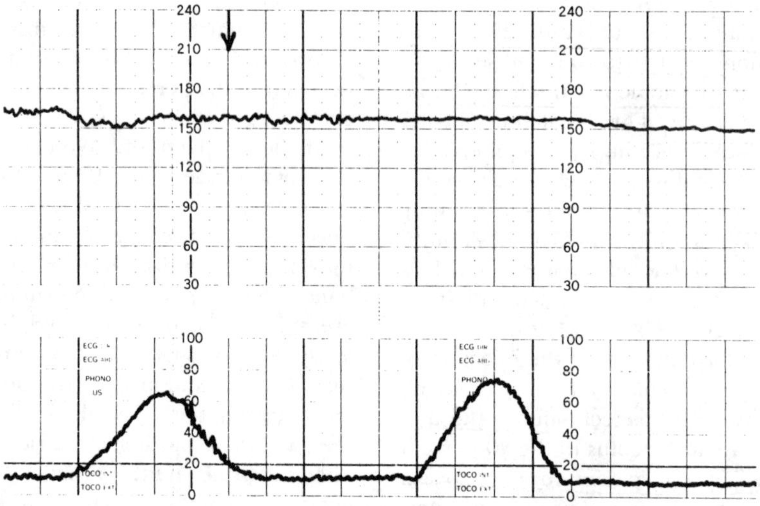

Fig. 7-11. Uterine hypertonus and decreased fetal heart rate variability after unintentional intravascular injection of local anesthetic.

solution. If these measures fail to improve the blood pressure, then ephedrine 5 to 10 mg should be injected intravenously and repeated as necessary.

COMPLICATIONS

Life-threatening complications should be rare. The unintentional accidental subarachnoid injection of a large volume of drug resulting in a total spinal block is heralded by nausea and hypotension and may progress to respiratory and cardiac arrest. Unintentional injection of a large portion of the epidural dose into an epidural vein may result in signs of CNS toxicity, including convulsions. (See discussions of unintentional injection later in this chapter.)

Other serious but rare complications include extradural hematoma at the puncture site and breakage of the needle or catheter while positioned in the epidural space.

INDICATIONS

Epidural block is very useful procedure that is of special value for the obstetric patient. It has obvious advantages for patients with pulmonary, cardiovascular, renal, or hepatic disease; diabetes; and toxemia of pregnancy (see Ch. 8).

An epidural block, providing anesthesia that extends from the level of T10 to S5 inclusively, can give total relief of pain during labor and delivery. It is therefore suitable as a single-dose technique if the anesthesiologist expects that the estimated duration of action of the local anesthetic is sufficient to cover the remaining portion of labor and delivery. The patient should be having strong contractions about 3 minutes apart, the cervix should be dilated to 5 cm or more in the multiparous patient and 6 cm or more in the primiparous patient, and the presenting part should be engaged in the pelvis.

Continuous epidural anesthesia is a more versatile technique because it extends the duration of pain relief obtainable and allows one to modify the extent and type of effect by adjusting the top-up dose of local anesthetic according to the current requirements of the patient or by using a continuous infusion of local anesthetic with or without opioid.

Pain in the first stage of labor is due primarily to the dilatation of the cervix and contractions of the uterus. It is mediated by the T11 and T12 innervation with some fibers from T10 and L1. Pain of the second and third stages of labor is perceived via S2, S3, and S4. Epidural anesthesia makes it possible to individualize the block according to the stage of labor: a segmental block may be given in the first stage, limiting the extent of anesthesia to the lower three thoracic and the upper lumbar segments. This leaves Ferguson's reflex intact and decreases both the motor block and premature relaxation of the perineum. Since flexion and internal rotation of the presenting part are not interfered with, pain relief can be offered at an earlier stage when the epidural technique is used as a segmental block or continuous infusion.

As labor progresses to the second stage, anesthesia can be extended to block the sacral innervation. A full top-up dose is given for this purpose while the patient is in the sitting position for about 5 minutes. A higher concentration of local anesthetic may be selected to achieve motor block and perineal relaxation, especially if a forceps delivery is planned or if abdominal delivery becomes necessary. However, some obstetricians prefer to have their patients pain free with a block from T10 to S5 throughout active labor and delivery.

Because of the versatility of achievable anesthetic effect and the duration of anesthesia obtainable, the continuous epidural technique is well suited for obstetric complications such as cervical dystocia or prolonged labor. Epidural anesthesia is compatible with the judicious use of intravenous oxytocin to augment and coordinate labor.

Segmental epidural block or continuous infusion can also be used for a trial of labor in patients in whom the feasibility of vaginal delivery is uncertain, such as those having had a previous cesarean delivery. If such delivery proves inadvisable, the block can be extended to T4, which makes cesarean delivery possible utilizing the existing epidural anesthetic.

In our experience, even with the epidural catheter tip placed caudad (as in our practice), the "perineal" dose for a segmental epidural block may not always provide appropriate perineal anesthesia. It may be necessary for the obstetrician to provide perineal pain relief by adding local infiltration or pudendal block.

Good nursing care is *essential* to the effective management of continuous epidural block for labor and delivery. Careful continuous monitoring of maternal vital signs, FHR, and uterine contractions is mandatory. A busy obstetric service cannot function at peak effectiveness without the cooperative interaction of the anesthesiologist, obstetrician, and labor nurse, or, in some institutions, nurse-midwives. Parturients receiving epidural anesthesia do not have to be delivered by forceps if a competent labor nurse helps the mother coordinate her "bearing down" efforts with the contractions of the uterus during the second stage of labor.

CONTRAINDICATIONS

Assuming that the anesthesiologist is experienced with the technique and treatment of possible complications, the following are relative contraindications to epidural block: the obstetrician's failure to appreciate how the epidural block may affect the management of labor, the need for immediate anesthesia, and the patient's fear of "spinal puncture." Absolute contraindications are infection at the site of the planned puncture, generalized septicemia, acute CNS disease, and blood coagulopathies.

COMPARISON WITH SUBARACHNOID BLOCK

Advantages

Epidural anesthesia offers a greater versatility of effect. For the first stage of labor, anesthesia for uterine contractions can be obtained without perineal relaxation. For the second and third stages of labor, perineal relaxation and anesthesia can result if a continuous technique is used. The onset of hypotension is slower and the degree of hypotension is less than with subarachnoid block. No post-dural puncture headache occurs.

Disadvantages

Technically, epidural anesthesia is slightly more difficult to achieve and has no definitive endpoint. The onset of anesthesia is slower than with subarachnoid block. Failure rates may be somewhat higher even for experienced anesthesiologists, however, that has not been our experience.

REFERENCES

1. Moore DC, Batra MS: The components of an effective test dose prior to epidural block. Anesthesiology 155:693, 1981
2. Guinard JP, Mulroy MF, Carpenter RL, Knopes KD: Test doses: optimal epinephrine content with and without acute beta-adrenergic blockade. Anesthesiology 73:386, 1990
3. Leighton BL, Gross JB: Air: an effective indicator of intravenously located epidural catheters. Anesthesiology 71:848, 1989
4. Matadial L, Cibils LA; The effect of epidural anesthesia on uterine activity and blood pressure. Am J Obstet Gynecol 125:846, 1976
5. Raabe N, Belfage P: Epidural analgesia in labor. IV. Influence on uterine activity and fetal heart rate. Acta Obstet Gynecol Scand 55:305, 1976
6. Wallis KL, Shnider SM, Hicks JS, et al: Epidural anesthesia in the normotensive pregnant ewe: effects on uterine blood flow and fetal acid base status. Anesthesiology 44:481, 1976
7. Hood DD, Dewan DM, James FM: Maternal and fetal effects of epinephrine in gravid ewes. Anesthesiology 64:610, 1986
8. Chestnut H, Weiner CP, Martin JG et al: Effect of intravenous epinephrine on uterine artery blood flow velocity in the pregnant guinea pig. Anesthesiology 65:633, 1986
9. Leighton BL, Norris MC, Sosis M, et al: Limitations of epinephrine as a marker of intravascular injection in laboring women. Anesthesiology 66:688, 1987
10. Van Zundert A, Vaes L, Soetens M, et al: Every dose given in epidural analgesia for vaginal delivery can be a test dose. Anesthesiology 67:436, 1987
11. Chestnut DH, Owen CL, Brown, et al: Does labor affect the variability of maternal heart rate during induction of epidural anesthesia? Anesthesiology 68:622, 1988
12. Morishima HO, Covino BG, Yeh M, et al: Bradycardia in the fetal baboon following paracervical block anesthesia. Am J Obstet Gynecol 140:775, 1981

CONTINUOUS EPIDURAL INFUSION

Epidural anesthesia for labor can be provided via a continuous-infusion technique. A low concentration of local anesthetic can be administered alone or in combination with a low dose of opioid, resulting in excellent labor anesthesia with minimal motor block.

MATERIALS

The following is a list of materials necessary for administering continuous epidural anesthesia:

Epidural tray (see the previous section for the contents of the epidural tray)
Bupivacaine 0.25 to 0.5 percent
0.9 percent sodium chloride solution in a 50-ml bag
Infusion pump and tubing
Three-way stopcock

TECHNIQUE

The epidural catheter is inserted as described in the previous section. A bilateral T10 sensory level is established with 0.25 percent bupivacaine with or without an opioid (such as fentanyl 25 to 50 μg). Fifty milliliters of 0.25 to 0.5 percent bupivacaine is added to the 50 ml of sodium chloride 0.9 percent solution in the bag. The solution will contain 100 ml of 0.125 or 0.25 percent bupivacaine. To this mixture is added fentanyl 100 to 200 μg. The resulting solution will contain 100 ml of 0.125 or 0.25 percent bupivacaine with fentanyl 1 to 2 μg/ml. The administration tubing is connected to the bag containing the local anesthetic–opioid solution and flushed well to release air bubbles. On the distal end of the tubing a three-way stopcock is attached to provide access for direct injection. The pump and anesthetic solution must be clearly labeled and any intravenous administration sites on the tubing covered with tape to prevent unintentional injections at these sites. Once all connections are secure and following an aspiration check of the epidural catheter the infusion may be started. The usual rate of infusion is 8 to 12 ml/h.

PRECAUTIONS

On an hourly basis, the blood pressure, sensory level, and adequacy of anesthesia must be assessed and recorded on the anesthetic record. Occasionally, reinforcement may be necessary. The infusion rate may be adjusted up or down depending on the dermatomal level, but it should not exceed 15 ml/h. Reinforcement by incremental injection may be necessary to correct an unequal block or to test for catheter position. It must be kept in mind that *any* injection is *always* preceded by aspiration. Anesthesia may be reinforced using 0.25 percent bupivacaine or 1.5 percent lidocaine with or without alkalinization and with or without epinephrine 1:200,000.

The possibility of migration or unintentional placement in an epidural vein or in the subarachnoid space must be considered. A test dose of 1.5 percent lidocaine 3 to 5 ml with epinephrine 1:200,000 (15 to 25 μg) should identify the unintentional placement of the epidural catheter in an epidural vein. If unintentional subarachnoid placement of the epidural catheter is a possibility, *hyperbaric* 1.5 percent lidocaine (Astra) with or without epinephrine 2 ml should be injected. If epinephrine is used, it must be freshly added and at least 15 μg administered if unintentional placement in an epidural vein is to be ruled out at the same time. (See the discussions of unintentional injection in this chapter.)

Each hour the catheter must be aspirated to monitor for possible migration of the catheter into an epidural vein or into the subarachnoid space. The aspiration check should be recorded. The motor strength of the parturient, which can be monitored by checking her ability to lift her legs, should be assessed hourly. The patient should be maintained in the lateral position throughout labor to prevent aortocaval compression. Additionally, the patient should turn from side to side every hour to avoid the development of a one-sided block.

For vaginal delivery, a dose to provide perineal anesthesia may be necessary. This should be administered incrementally and with the patient in the head-up or sitting position. For a routine vaginal delivery, 1.5 percent lidocaine 10 ml (with or without alkalinization) or 2 to 3 percent chloroprocaine 10 to 15 ml should suffice. However, a larger dose may be necessary for forceps delivery.

COMPLICATIONS

Asymmetric Sensory Block

If the patient lies continuously on one side, the level of sensory block may become asymmetric. This problem may be corrected by turning the patient to the other side and administering 0.25 percent bupivacaine or 1.5 percent lidocaine 5 to 10 ml. The patient should be encouraged to turn from side to side each hour.

Diminishing Anesthesia

Progressive diminution of sensory block and loss of analgesia may be due to a number of factors:

1. Pump malfunction or tubing disconnection
2. Inadequate rate of infusion
3. Migration of the catheter out of the epidural space
4. Migration of the catheter into an epidural vein

Differential diagnosis consists of rechecking the infusion set-up and then testing to determine where the catheter is positioned. If the block cannot be re-established or if aspiration and testing indicates intravascular migration of the catheter tip, then the catheter must be withdrawn. Depending on the clinical setting, either another catheter may be placed or alternative anesthesia may be initiated. At the usual infusion rates, bupivacaine will not produce symptoms of intravascular injection. The only clue may be diminished anesthesia.

Dense Motor Block

Patients given a continuous infusion of 0.125 to 0.25 percent bupivacaine usually exhibit mild motor block of the lower extremities. If progressively denser motor block resembling subarachnoid block ensues, then the catheter must be carefully aspirated to rule out subarachnoid migration. Suspicion of subarachnoid migration after testing mandates withdrawal of the catheter and replacement at another interspace if indicated.

Patchy Block

If a spotty or patchy block occurs, one should attempt to solidify the block by determining catheter placement and then injecting 0.25 to 0.5 percent bupivacaine or 1.5 percent lidocaine 3 to 5 ml with or without alkalinization. Fentanyl 50 μg diluted in 10 ml of preservative-free normal saline may be given incrementally via the epidural catheter as a one-time bolus. If the block remains patchy, then the catheter should be replaced.

Need for Surgical Anesthesia

If a patient requires an acute change in the character of the block for operative delivery, simply increasing the infusion rate is totally inadequate to effect the change required in the level of anesthesia. The patient must be disconnected from the infusion pump, catheter placement checked, and the anesthetic topped-up with 0.5 percent bupivacaine, 1.5 to 2 percent lidocaine with or without epinephrine, or 3 percent chloroprocaine to the desired level of anesthesia.

Inadequate Perineal Anesthesia

Often a continuous infusion of 0.125 percent bupivacaine with opioid does not provide adequate perineal analgesia. At the time of delivery, the patient may require an additional bolus of 1.5 percent lidocaine with or without alkalinization or 3 percent chloroprocaine to provide sufficient analgesia for episiotomy or forceps delivery. The patient should be placed in the head-up or sitting position prior to administering the top-up dose. Maintaining the patient in the head-up position during the second stage of labor also promotes the achievement of a more complete perineal block from the continuous infusion.

PATIENT-CONTROLLED EPIDURAL ANESTHESIA

Patient-controlled analgesia (PCA) is commonly assumed to signify the intermittent administration of intravenous opioids without physician or nursing supervision. However, "patient control" is really a conceptual framework for analgesic administration and not strictly related to opioids, the intravenous route, or intermittent mode of administration. Recent studies suggest that analgesia under patient control may be effective when given via the sublingual,[1] transbuccal,[2] subcutaneous,[3] and epidural routes.[4–7] Furthermore, the mode of administration of PCA is not restricted to intermittent boluses (*demand dosing*), but includes *constant-rate infusion plus demand dosing* (a background infusion rate is determined by a physician and may be supplemented by patient demand), and even *infusion-based PCA* (demands are granted as infusions whose rates are adjusted over time by microprocessor control).[8]

Studies of patient-controlled epidural analgesia (PCEA) as an analgesic technique have used either opioids[6,7] or bupivacaine,[4,5] alone[4,6,7] or in combination,[5] by demand dosing[4,6,7] or continuous infusion plus demand dosing.[5] As compared to intravenous PCA or continuous epidural infusion (CEI) with opioid alone,[6] PCEA appears to be "dose sparing" in nonobstetric postoperative populations. Patients using demand-dose PCEA used significantly less opioid for postoperative pain relief.[6,7]

Naturally, for a laboring population, the desired total exposure to local anesthetic and/or opioid should be as low as possible. In a randomized, single-blind, placebo-controlled study using 0.125 percent bupivacaine via demand-dose PCEA and fixed-rate CEI, Gambling et al. were able to demonstrate a significant reduction in bupivacaine use with PCEA (11.2 mg/h versus 15.2 mg/h).[4] Anesthesia was comparable in both groups. Unfortunately, due to study design, these investigators made no distinction between anesthesia and anesthetic consumption during the first and second stages of labor.

Using the constant-rate infusion plus the demand-dose mode, Lysak et al.[5] compared physician-adjusted CEI with bupivacaine (closely titrated to maintain a T10 sensory level) with three solutions administered by PCEA. The solutions contained mixtures of 0.125 percent bupivacaine alone; bupivacaine 0.125 percent with fentanyl 1 μg/ml; and 0.125 percent bupivacaine, fentanyl 1 μg/ml, and epinephrine 1:400,000. Unlike the previous study, PCEA with bupivacaine alone did not decrease total local anesthetic utilization or hourly infusion requirements for labor. Addition of fentanyl or fentanyl plus epinephrine did decrease hourly local anesthetic use (though not total dosage necessary for vaginal delivery). Use of epinephrine-containing solutions was associated with dense motor blockade. These investigators concluded that while safe and effective for labor anesthesia, PCEA did not improve anesthesia or significantly reduce anesthetic requirements as compared to CEI.

These investigators are to be applauded for their pioneering efforts. A number of questions regarding the technique of PCEA still need investigation, however.

Patient control works via a negative-feedback loop.[9] As the patient experiences pain, local anesthetic is self-administered, thereby decreasing the immediate need for further local anesthetics. Thus, the optimal local anesthetic and/or opioid for PCEA should be of fast onset, thus avoiding transient inappropriately increased patient demands. Similarly, the optimal agent should be of intermediate duration. Agents of short analgesic duration could promote a high rate of patient demand and subsequent "exhaustion" of the patient with the anesthetic process. Agents of long duration could accumulate and eventually promote toxicity or untoward side effects. The optimal local anesthetic or opioid (or combination) for use with PCEA has yet to be elucidated.

With respect to local anesthetics, the volume:concentration relations of the demand (bolus) dose need to be investigated, as well as the influence of the duration of the lockout interval on local anesthetic and/or opioid analgesic efficacy and toxicity.

When using the constant-infusion plus demand-dose mode, how much local anesthetic should be supplied by infusion? As the amount of local anesthetic supplied by infusion increases, the technique becomes less under "patient control" than "physician control." Indeed, in the study by Lysak et al.[5] the constant-rate infusion of the PCEA study groups delivered 50 percent of the hourly dose received by the CEI group. This may explain the inability to distinguish between PCEA and CEI study groups with respect to local anesthetic requirements for labor.

PCEA represents an avenue for provision of excellent pain relief for labor with the potential for utilization of lower amounts of local anesthetic agents. However, no further comment can be made on its applicability until several of the aforementioned problems with methodology have been addressed.

REFERENCES

1. Shah MV, Jones DI, Rosen M: "Patient-demand" postoperative analgesia with buprenorphine. Comparison between sublingual and I.M. administration. Br J Anaesth 58:508, 1986
2. Bell MD, Murray GR, Mishra P, et al: Buccal morphine—a new role for analgesia? Lancet 1:71, 1985
3. Urguhart ML, Klapp K, White PF: Patient-controlled analgesia: a comparison of intravenous versus subcutaneous hydromorphine. Anesthesiology 69:428, 1988
4. Gambling DR, Yu P, McMorland GH, Palmer L: A comparative study of patient controlled epidural analgesia (PCEA) and continuous infusion epidural analgesia (CIEA) during labour. Can J Anaesth 35:249, 1988
5. Lysak SZ, Eisenach JC, Dobson II CE: Patient-controlled epidural analgesia during labor: a comparison of three solutions with a continuous infusion control. Anesthesiology 72:44, 1990
6. Marlowe S, Engstrom R, White PF: Epidural patient-controlled analgesia (PCA): an alternative to continuous epidural infusions. Pain 37:97, 1989
7. Sjöström S, Hartvig D, Tamsen A: Patient-controlled analgesia with extradural morphine or pethidine. Br J Anaesth 60:358, 1988
8. Hill HF, Mackie AM, Jacobson RC: Infusion-based patient-controlled analgesia systems. p. 214. In Ferrante FM, Ostheimer GW, Covino BG (eds): Patient-Controlled Analgesia. Blackwell Scientific Publications, Boston, 1990
9. White PF: Patient-controlled analgesia: delivery systems. p. 70. In Ferrante FM, Ostheimer GW, Covino BG (eds): Patient-Controlled Analgesia. Blackwell Scientific Publications, Boston, 1990

CAUDAL ANESTHESIA

ANATOMY AND LANDMARKS

The caudal space is the most distal extension of the epidural space, delimited by the periosteum covering the first four fused sacral vertebrae and the sacrococcygeal ligament crossing the unfused fifth sacral vertebra.

Caudal block is performed by injecting local anesthetic solution through the sacral hiatus into the caudal canal.

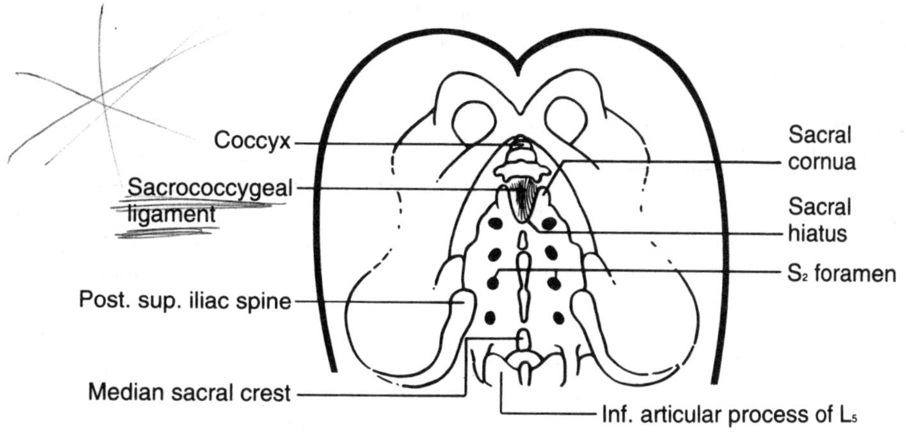

Fig. 7-12. Landmarks for caudal anesthesia.

Developmentally, the sacral hiatus is formed because the spinous process of the S5 vertebra usually fails to fuse. The two unfused parts of the spinous process can be palpated as the two sacral cornua, which constitute an important landmark for caudal block. The sacral hiatus between the sacral cornua is covered by the flat sacrococcygeal ligament (Fig. 7-12), which is pierced by the caudal needle. If the cornua cannot be identified, the end of the coccyx is located. It can be assumed that the hiatus lies approximately 5 cm cephalad to this point.

In adults, the dural sac extends to about the level of S2, or 1.5 cm caudad to a line drawn between the left and right posterior superior iliac spines. Therefore, the caudal needle should not be advanced beyond this level. The caudal canal contains the cauda equina in addition to the epidural venous plexus and the loose areolar tissue generally present in the epidural space.

The hemodynamic changes consistent with term pregnancy produce an engorgement of the venous plexus that reduces the capacity of the epidural space, including the epidural space of the caudal canal. This fact must be kept in mind because the extent of the caudal anesthesia is largely determined by the volume of the local anesthetic injected. Although, theoretically, the level of anesthesia may be extended much higher, in practice it is used for procedures at or below the level of T10.

PATIENT POSITION

For the obstetric patient, either the lateral Sims position or the modified Bowie knee-chest position may be suitable. In the latter, the patient may be positioned prone and flexed, with a pillow folded under the abdomen so as to raise the sacrum and make the parturient more comfortable. This position makes the sacral cornua more prominent and the sacral hiatus easier to identify. The Sims position is most commonly used.

MATERIALS

When a patient is scheduled for single-dose caudal block, the following materials are needed:

One pair of sterile gloves
Antibacterial solution for cleansing the skin
One sterile cup for the antibacterial solution
Forceps
Sterile gauze pads
Sterile towels for draping the field
One 25-gauge, 1.6- to 3.8-cm needle for skin infiltration
One 21- or 22-gauge, 3.8-cm needle for deep infiltration (if desired)
One 18-gauge needle to make an opening in the skin (if desired)
One 19-gauge, 7.6-cm caudal needle with stylet or one 19-gauge, 3.8-cm short-beveled needle
One 3-ml syringe
One 5-ml glass syringe
One 20-ml syringe
One disposable caudal catheter

A disposable caudal anesthetic tray usually contains all of the above items.

TECHNIQUE

Thirty milliliters of a clear antacid (0.3 mol/L sodium citrate or its equivalent) is administered before the initiation of a caudal block. No other premedication is given for vaginal delivery. The technique of caudal anesthesia for the parturient is similar to that for the surgical patient except that special consideration must be given to the condition of the fetus and to the maternal physiologic changes associated with pregnancy and labor.

Arterial blood pressure must be monitored in any patient undergoing regional anesthesia but the obstetric patient is carefully observed for changes. The blood pressure is determined in the supine and lateral positions before the block is initiated to check for aortocaval compression (supine hypotensive syndrome). An automatic blood pressure monitor is useful but not mandatory. The fetal heart rate (FHR) record is reviewed. Routine electrocardiographic monitoring is optional in our institution for the initiation of a caudal block for labor. However, an electrocardiograph is immediately available.

The obstetric patient selected for caudal anesthesia is acutely hydrated prior to the induction of the caudal block. A large indwelling plastic catheter allows the administration of 1,000 ml of warm lactated Ringer's solution or similar crystalloid solution over 10 to 20 minutes. This hydration helps to prevent the hypotension that may be caused by the sympathetic block that occurs with caudal anesthesia. Warm intravenous fluid diminishes pre-, intra-, and postpartum shivering experienced by the parturient. The intravenous infusion is then maintained should the patient require additional hydration or intravenous medication.

The caudal tray is opened in a sterile manner and the expiration date checked. The gloved anesthesiologist prepares the skin of the lumbosacral area with a bactericidal preparation, wiping off the excess solution. The field may be draped with sterile towels.

To create anesthesia at the puncture site for the caudal block, the skin overlying the sacral hiatus (the area between the sacral cornua) is infiltrated with local anesthetic solution using a 25-gauge needle. A 21- or 22-gauge, 3.8-cm needle may be used to infiltrate the deeper tissues at the entry point for the caudal needle, the subcutaneous tissues over and around the sacral hiatus, and the periosteum of the sacral cornua. A large-bore (18-gauge) needle may be used to create a small opening in the skin overlying the sacral hiatus. We do not use this step because subsequent release of the skin will move the skin hole, resulting in difficult insertion of the caudal needle.

A 19-gauge, 7.6-cm caudal needle may be used for this block. The relationship of the notching in the hub to the bevel of the needle is noted. The caudal needle is inserted into the preformed skin opening, if used, with the stylet locked in place and with the bevel turned up. The needle is controlled with the right hand. the shaft is firmly held between the thumb and the middle finger. Pressure is exerted by the index finger on the head of the stylet (Fig. 7-13). The initial entry angle for the caudal needle is 70 to 80 degrees. The needle is advanced to the level of the sacrum. The needle must not be forced against the bone; instead, it is slightly withdrawn, the entry angle reduced by a few degrees, and the needle then advanced to the level of the sacrococcygeal ligament. Depending on the body type of the patient, the resistance of the sacrococcygeal ligament is met at a depth approximately 0.5 to 3.8 cm. At this point, the bevel of the caudal needle is turned ventrally and a shallow entry angle is chosen (Fig. 7-14). In the obstetric patient, and in women generally, an angle of 30 to 40 degrees is assumed. In men (mentioned here for the sake of completeness) an even shallower angle is used (about 20 degrees) because of the lesser angulation of the male sacrum.

Keeping this bearing, the needle can now be advanced

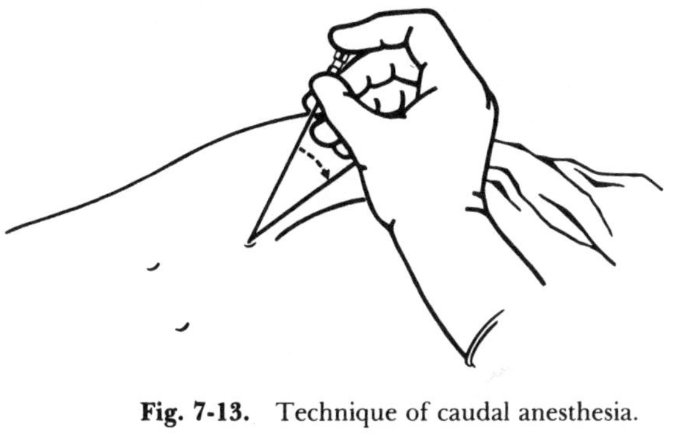

Fig. 7-13. Technique of caudal anesthesia.

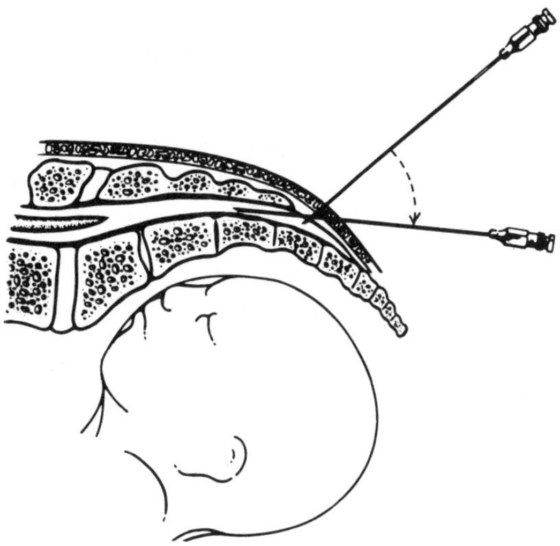

Fig. 7-14. Insertion of the needle into the caudal canal. Note the proximity of the fetus' head.

through the sacrococcygeal ligament and 2.5 to 3.8 cm into the caudal canal. The depth of the caudal needle is checked by withdrawing the stylet and holding it over the skin in approximately the same position as the inserted needle. The needle should be below the S2 level to avoid puncturing the dural sac.

Another method for avoiding the puncture of the dural sac involves using a 19-gauge, 3.8-cm short-bevel needle for the caudal injection. Although the short length of the needle may be a disadvantage in the obese patient, most patients have little subcutaneous fat overlying the sacrococcygeal ligament. The short length of the needle does not guarantee that puncture of the dural sac or an epidural blood vessel will be avoided. Aspiration tests in all four quadrants must be performed before the local anesthetic may be injected.

Any needle without a stylet, such as the 19-gauge needle recommended above, may carry a tissue plug into the caudal canal. This, however, is not of great importance unless local infection is present. The latter is a contraindication for this technique.

After the needle is placed, if the aspiration test yields cerebrospinal fluid, an alternate anesthetic technique must be chosen. A bloody return necessitates a repositioning of the caudal needle. The needle is withdrawn about 1.5 cm, the stylet is locked in place, and at least 2 minutes are allowed for the traumatized epidural veins to stop bleeding. If repeat aspiration tests after this 2-minute interval continue to produce a bloody return, the caudal approach must be abandoned in favor of another type of block. Negative results of an aspiration test are encouraging signs that the needle has been properly placed in the caudal canal. Confirmatory tests, however, must be performed to exclude the possibility of a malposition of the needle. The needle may be lodged either under the periosteal layer of the sacrum or along the dorsal surface of the sacrum, and yet give the appearance of proper positioning. Injecting 10 ml of air will identify a malpositioning along the posterior surface of the sacrum by creating crepitus in the subcutaneous tissue surrounding the tip of the needle.

A second confirmatory test must be performed to ensure that the caudal needle is positioned correctly. A small syringe is filled with 3 ml of sterile saline or local anesthetic solution and attached to the caudal needle. The solution is injected and the plunger of the syringe quickly released at the very end of the downstroke when the syringe is empty. An easy injection of the fluid without any significant (more than 0.2 ml) return into the syringe and without the appearance of tissue swelling over the sacrum suggests that the needle has been correctly placed. The syringe is detached from the caudal needle, the stylet is locked in place, and the patient's blood pressure and general condition are evaluated. After a test dose of local anesthetic is administered, no less than 3 minutes is allowed for the appearance of any anesthetic effect.

If extensive sensory or motor anesthesia is produced, it may be concluded that the dura has been punctured and that unintentional subarachnoid anesthesia has been achieved. In this case, the plans for a caudal block should be abandoned, although it is likely that the sensory block created may be useful for the obstetric procedure at hand.

If results of these tests indicate that the needle is in the caudal canal, an aspiration test is performed before administration of the local anesthetic. For a single-dose caudal block, the drug is administered in incremental or fractional (3- to 5-ml) doses injected every 60 seconds until the total dose has been given. The caudal needle is then withdrawn and the patient is placed in a comfortable semisitting position. Dosages are listed in Table 7-5.

PLACING A CAUDAL CATHETER

The technique used to position the caudal needle and to confirm its placement is the same as in the single-dose method.

As with continuous epidural techniques, it is preferable that the catheter be equipped with a wire stylet, which will make the passage of the catheter through the needle easier. The plastic catheter is examined for imperfections. The depth markings are noted and compared with the length of the caudal needle. The wire stylet is withdrawn 2 to 3 cm from the tip of the catheter. The uncurled catheter is held by the fingers of the left hand and the tip inserted into the hub of the caudal needle using the right hand (for a right-handed anesthesiologist). The catheter is advanced through the needle, which is held by the left hand, so that 2 to 4 cm projects past the bevel of the needle into the caudal space. It is important not to force the passage of the catheter as this could result in injury of a nerve root, trauma to a blood vessel, or puncture of the dura mater. The distance that the catheter is in the caudal canal can be measured by placing the plunger of the syringe against the patient's back and noting the marking on the syringe that correlates with the markings on the catheter, which is at or near the hub of the needle. The back of the plunger or piston of the syringe may be

Table 7-5. Local Anesthetics and Suggested Dosages for Single-Dose Caudal Anesthesia for Vaginal Delivery

Local Anesthetic[a]	Dosage[b] (ml)	Dosage[b] (mg)	Onset of Action (min)	Duration of Action (min)
Bupivacaine 0.25–0.5%	15–25	37.5–125	3–5	60–180
Chloroprocaine 2.0–3.0%	15–25	300–750	3–5	40–60
Lidocaine 1.0–2.0%[c]	15–25	150–500	3–5	60–90
Mepivacaine 1.0–2.0%	15–25	150–500	3–5	60–90

[a] Without epinephrine.

[b] Dosage range depending on patient's height; total milligram dosage of the local anesthetic should not exceed manufacturer's recommendations.

[c] With or without epinephrine 1:200,000.

used instead of the male end to avoid contamination of the syringe with the residual antibacterial solution if the glass syringe is to be used for the initial injection through the caudal catheter.

The needle is removed from the tissues in the following manner: the catheter is held firmly by the right hand 2 to 3 cm from the hub of the needle while the shaft and the hub of the needle are held between the index and middle fingers and thumb of the left hand. While the catheter is held in place with positive forward pressure, the needle is carefully pulled out so that the thumbs of the two hands meet. Forward pressure should be applied to the catheter at all times. The maneuver is then repeated by grasping the tubing another 2 to 3 cm distal to the hub of the needle and repeating the same procedure. Finally, the tip of the needle will emerge from the skin. The tubing is prevented from being dislodged by the application of pressure with the thumb and index finger of the left hand to the tubing at the point where it emerges from the skin. The needle is then moved back over the catheter. The thumb and index finger may now move some distance up the catheter and hold the catheter firmly to prevent its dislodgement while the needle and stylet are removed from the catheter by the right hand.

Forward repositioning of the needle is impossible once the catheter is advanced beyond the bevel. If forward repositioning is necessary, the needle and the catheter are both completely withdrawn and the procedure is repeated from the beginning. Once the catheter has advanced beyond the bevel of the caudal needle, any attempt to withdraw it can result in shearing off the catheter.

An adapter is attached to the end of the catheter or a blunt small-gauge needle is inserted into the tubing. Before the catheter is taped in place, a careful aspiration test is performed to ensure that the catheter is not in the subarachnoid space or in an epidural vein. Another test dose of 3 ml of the local anesthetic solution is injected and the patient is observed for cardiovascular changes, sensory or motor alterations, or central nervous system (CNS) toxic reaction for not less than 3 minutes. Sterile gauze pads are placed above and below the catheter as it emerges out of the skin, and the catheter and pads are secured by pieces of tape. The entire catheter is then taped to the back of the patient and the patient is placed in the left lateral position with a wedge under the right hip to displace the uterus to the left.

If vital signs remain satisfactory and no significant anesthesia develops after this second test dose, another aspiration test is done. Fractional doses of local anesthetic (3 to 5 ml) are administered with a minimum interval of at least 60 seconds until the full caudal dose is injected. We do not inject more than 5 ml of local anesthetic at a time. This translates to a maximum dosage of bupivacaine 25 mg or lidocaine 100 mg in our current practice.

To obtain continuous anesthesia from T10 to S5, the first intermittent caudal dose may be the same as in the single-dose method. When the desired level of anesthesia has been achieved with the initial dose, a subsequent "top-up" dose of about two-thirds of the initial dose will maintain this sensory level. Top-up doses are added as necessary. As aspiration test must be done prior to each reinforcement because perforation of the dura mater or of one of the epidural veins by the catheter has been reported and may have occurred since the last administration of the anesthetic. Fractional doses of local

Table 7-6. Local Anesthetics and Suggested Dosages for Continuous (Intermittent) Caudal Anesthesia for Vaginal Delivery

	Dosage[b]						
	First Dose[c]		Top-up Dose[d]		Onset of Action	Duration of Action	Time between Top-up Doses
Local Anesthetic[a]	(ml)	(mg)	(ml)	(mg)	(min)	(min)	(min)
Bupivacaine[e] 0.25–0.5%	15–25	37.5–125	8–17	20–85	3–5	60–180	Approx. 60–120
Chloroprocaine 2.0–3.0%	15–25	300–750	8–17	160–510	3–5	40–60	Approx. 45
Lidocaine 1.0–2.0%[c]	15–25	150–500	8–17	80–340	3–5	60–90	Approx. 60
Mepivacaine 1.0–2.0%	15–25	150–500	8–17	80–340	3–5	60–90	Approx. 60

[a] Without epinephrine.
[b] Total milligram dosage of the local anesthetic should not exceed manufacturer's recommendations.
[c] Dosage range depending on patient's height.
[d] The top-up dose is two-thirds of the first dose if the initial dose resulted in a satisfactory level of anesthesia and if this level is to be maintained.
[e] With or without epinephrine 1:200,000.

anesthetic (3 to 5 ml) are administered until the appropriate top-up dose has been given. Dosage schedules are listed in Table 7-6.

With the patient resting comfortably, the spread of anesthesia is checked frequently by gentle repeated pinpricks or by a cotton swab moistened with alcohol. Since the loss of pain and temperature sensation progresses simultaneously, the use of alcohol to check the spread of anesthesia may be more pleasant for the patient. Repeated pinpricks may not accurately differentiate the area of complete loss of pain sensation from that of partial sensory anesthesia. However, we still prefer the "pinprick" test. Because of the concern over blood and fluid contamination, we suggest the use of sharp plastic toothpicks to determine sensory levels. Several brands of plastic toothpicks are sharp enough to pierce olives or onions but not human skin.

PRECAUTIONS

Aspiration must precede the injection of the local anesthetic solution for two reasons: to avoid unintentional subarachnoid injection and to avoid intravenous injection. The caudal dosage is a large multiple of that needed for subarachnoid block. Unintentional injection of such an amount of local anesthetic solution into the subarachnoid space would unavoidably result in high or total spinal block. The epidural venous plexus offers a potential for an intravascular injection or a large volume of local anesthetic, which may be followed by CNS excitation and convulsions. Full cardiopulmonary resuscitative equipment must be immediately available, as is customary for any regional block. Maternal hypotension with a concomitant decrease in uteroplacental perfusion producing fetal hypoxia and acidosis is a possibility and must be treated immediately. Monitoring of vital signs is mandatory for both mother and fetus. Maternal blood pressure must be checked frequently. If a decrease of 10 mmHg or more occurs, an immediate response is necessary. Therapy consists of an immediate change in the position of the parturient to a more pronounced left (sometimes right) lateral position, oxygen by face mask, and an increase in the intravenous infusion ratio initiated by a 200- to 300-ml bolus of an appropriate intravenous crystalloid solution such as lactated Ringer's solution. If these measures fail to improve the blood pressure, ephedrine 5 to 10 mg should be injected intravenously and repeated as necessary.

It is especially important to identify the anatomic landmarks accurately in the obstetric patient. If the tip of the coccyx is mistaken for the sacrococcygeal joint, the entry point will be distal to the coccyx rather than through the sacral hiatus, and the needle may pierce the rectum and even the presenting part of the fetus. Although rare, unintentional injection of the local anesthetic into the fetal head instead of into the caudal canal has been reported. The anatomic relationship makes it obvious that this possibility is increased if caudal block is started when the fetal head is low in the pelvis.

Caudal block, along with the subarachnoid, lumbar epidural, and pudendal blocks can eliminate the reflex urge to bear down during the second stage. This may be a liability, since perineal resistance is needed for normal internal rotation to occur. To prevent the possible increased incidence of forceps deliveries, the labor nurse should monitor the patient's contractions and instruct her to "bear down" with each uterine contraction during the second stage of labor.

COMPLICATIONS

Life-threatening complications should be rare. The unintentional accidental subarachnoid injection of a large volume of drug resulting in a total spinal block is heralded by nausea and hypotension and may progress to respiratory and cardiac arrest.

Unintentional injection of a large portion of the caudal dose into an epidural vein may result in signs of CNS toxicity, including convulsions. Also, toxic blood levels of the local anesthetic can be produced even when the drug is properly deposited within the caudal space because a large volume of drug must be used. This further illustrates the need for slow, intermittent injections.

Other serious complications include extradural hematoma at the puncture site and breakage of the needle or catheter while positioned in the caudal canal.

Hypotension may arise secondary to the sympathetic block, and it occurs with greater frequency in the obstetric patient. Although the frequency and the degree of hypotension are less with caudal block than with epidural block, it does arise in a certain number of patients. The frequency varies with the level to which the caudal block is carried.

Temporary urinary retention may occur as with other blocks and with general anesthesia. The patient may have to be catheterized once or twice, after which she is usually able to void voluntarily.

INDICATIONS

The caudal block technique can be modified to fill a variety of obstetric anesthetic needs. Properly administered, it gives complete pain relief in 90 to 95 percent of obstetric patients, with the remaining 5 to 10 percent experiencing residual mild discomfort.

A caudal block up to T10 may be administered either as a single-dose technique to give anesthesia for the second and third stages of labor or by the catheter technique to manage the entire active phase of labor, including delivery. A caudal block to T6 may be used for cesarean delivery in rare instances, however, the mass (volume × concentration) of drug required is approximately twice that for lumbar epidural block of the same area and toxic blood levels could occur.

CONTRAINDICATIONS

Absolute contraindications to caudal block include infection at the puncture site involving the skin or deeper tissues (pilonidal cyst), generalized septicemia, blood coagulopathies, and active CNS disease. If sacrococcygeal deformities would make the caudal puncture technically too difficult and therefore potentially traumatic, a lumbar epidural approach may be considered as an alternative.

SUBARACHNOID ANESTHESIA

ANATOMY AND LANDMARKS

The subarachnoid space may be safely entered through one of the interspaces between L2 and L5 (see Fig. 7-2). The dural sac extends to the level of S2 and the enclosed spinal cord usually extends down to L1, rarely to L2. Therefore, a puncture below this level should not encounter the spinal cord. The puncture point for subarachnoid block is established in the following manner. After the most prominent point of the left and right posterior iliac crests is located, an imaginary line is drawn between these points. It usually crosses the L4–L5 interspace (see Fig. 7-3). This interspace and the two above it are usually chosen as points of entry for subarachnoid block. The Taylor approach utilizing the interspace of L5–S1 is rarely used in obstetric anesthesia. In the midline, the entering spinal needle (see Fig. 7-2a) traverses the skin, subcutaneous tissue, supraspinous ligament, and interspinous ligament, and then enters the ligamentum flavum which connects the laminae of vertebral arches. The needle then crosses the epidural space filled with loose areolar tissue containing the epidural venous plexus. Finally, the needle pierces the dura and the adherent arachnoid, thus entering the subarachnoid space.

PATIENT POSITION

The left or right lateral position (see Fig. 7-3) is generally the most comfortable for the parturient for vaginal delivery. Care must be taken that the line of the spinous processes of vertebrae is parallel to the table. To open up the vertebral interspaces, the patient is asked to flex her back by drawing her knees toward her chest. Her head is supported by a small pillow, and her neck should be flexed so that the chin touches the chest.

The obstetric patient usually requires a low block (T10–S5) for an uncomplicated vaginal delivery. At the Brigham and Women's Hospital, the lateral position is used for initiation of block using a hyperbaric solution.

The sitting position may also be used. The obese patient may be easier to approach in the sitting position because the line of the spinous processes is usually not obscured by the subcutaneous fat fold drooping over it. For the sitting position to be most effective for performing the subarachnoid block, the patient sits on the edge of the table with her feet resting on a stool. The neck is flexed so that the chin touches the chest. The arms should be folded across the upper abdomen, but they may rest loosely supported in the lap. A nurse or an assistant should steady the patient from the front to prevent the patient from falling if neurogenic syncope should occur.

It is best to inject the spinal anesthetic for cesarean delivery with the patient in the right lateral position. This prevents concentrating the hyperbaric local anesthetic solution on the left side of the dural sac. Such left-sided pooling of the anesthetic solution occurs when left uterine displacement by elevation of the right hip is used after initiating the spinal block with the parturient in the left lateral position. This "puddling" effect may result in an inadequate block on the right side of the patient.

MATERIALS

The following materials should be ready for use when the patient is to be given a subarachnoid block:

One pair of sterile gloves
Antibacterial solution for cleansing the skin
One sterile cup for the antibacterial solution
Forceps
Sterile gauze pads
Sterile towels for draping the field (if desired)
One 25-gauge, 1.6- to 3.8-cm needle for skin infiltration
One 21- or 22-gauge, 3.8-cm needle for preparing drugs and for deep infiltration (if desired)
One 18-gauge needle for use as an introducer

One 25-gauge Whitacre or 26-27 gauge Quincke, 8.9-cm spinal needle with stylet
One 3-ml syringe
One 5-ml glass syringe

One disposable spinal anesthetic tray usually contains all of the above items. Several small-gauge spinal needles of varying designs are available. Small-gauge needles with or without conical points have been demonstrated to reduce the incidence of post-dural puncture headache in the parturient.

TECHNIQUE

Thirty milliliters of a clear antacid (0.3 mol/L sodium citrate or its equivalent) is administered before the initiation of the block. No other premedication is given for vaginal delivery. For cesarean delivery, the patient will receive 30 ml of a clear antacid (as above) and, if considered "at risk" for any reason, will also receive intravenous metoclopramide 10 mg and intravenous or intramuscular cimetidine 300 mg or ranitidine 100 mg in the 30 to 60 minutes prior to induction of the subarachnoid block. The technique of anesthesia for the parturient is similar to that for the surgical patient except that special consideration must be given to the condition of the fetus and to the physiologic changes associated with pregnancy and labor.

Arterial blood pressure changes are noted in any patient undergoing regional anesthesia but the obstetric patient must be carefully observed for these changes. The blood pressure is determined in the supine and lateral positions before the block is initiated to check for aortocaval compression (supine hypotensive syndrome). An automatic blood pressure monitor is useful but not mandatory. The fetal heart rate (FHR) record is also reviewed. Routine electrocardiography is optional in our institution for vaginal delivery in the uncomplicated pregnancy; however, it is immediately available if needed since these deliveries are accomplished in a delivery/operating room. Electrocardiographic monitoring is mandatory for cesarean delivery.

The obstetric patient receiving subarachnoid anesthesia is acutely hydrated prior to the induction of the subarachnoid block. A large indwelling plastic catheter allows the administration of warm lactated Ringer's solution or similar crystalloid solution over 10 to 20 minutes before induction of subarachnoid block (1,000 ml for vaginal delivery and at least 1,500 ml for cesarean delivery). This hydration helps to prevent the hypotension that may be caused by the sympathetic block produced by subarachnoid anesthesia. Warm intravenous fluid diminishes pre-, intra-, and postpartum shivering experienced by the parturient. The intravenous infusion is then maintained should the patient require additional hydration or intravenous medication. In practice, approximately 1,500 to 2,000 ml of crystalloid solution is usually administered to combat the hypotension that occurs before birth during cesarean delivery. The key to the use of major regional block in obstetrics is to maintain adequate uteroplacental perfusion, which can be indirectly monitored via maternal arterial pressure. Decreased perfusion of the intervillous space can place the fetus in jeopardy.

The spinal tray is opened in a sterile manner and the expiration date checked. The gloved anesthesiologist prepares the skin of the lumbar area with a bactericidal preparation, wiping off the excess solution. The field may be draped with sterile towels. The desired interspace is located and the correct position of the patient is checked. In the lateral position, the line of the spinous processes must be parallel to the table and the surface of the back must be vertical. This will align the spinous processes in the horizontal plane. Depending on the special anatomic features of the patient, the second, third, or fourth lumbar interspace may be found most suitable.

The entry point into the skin is fixed by two fingers on either side of the interspace selected and the skin is infiltrated with a small amount of anesthesia. The 25-gauge needle is used to create the skin wheal. Then a small amount (1 to 2 ml) of local anesthetic is injected into the subcutaneous tissue and the interspinous ligament. When satisfactory analgesia of the entry point has been created, an 18-gauge needle is used as an introducer and is inserted through the skin wheal. The index and the middle fingers of the free hand straddle the interspace to fix the tissues of the underlying structures (Fig. 7-15). The introducer is used to create a passage

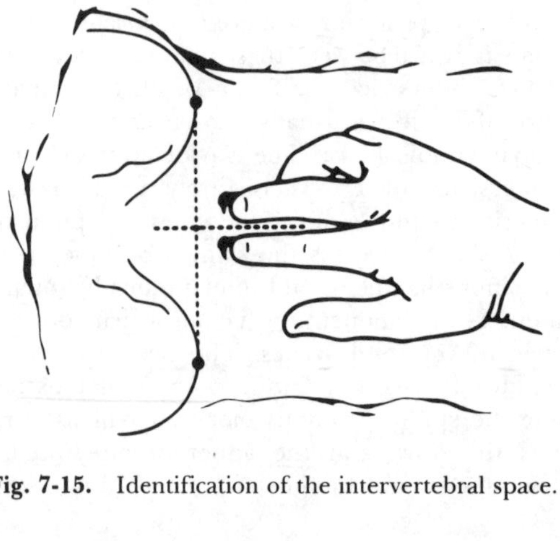

Fig. 7-15. Identification of the intervertebral space.

for the fine spinal needle and, theoretically, prevent carrying a plug of skin or fat into the subarachnoid space. However, some anesthesiologists, including the senior author, prefer not to use an introducer and will insert the spinal needle directly. If one chooses one of the conical-point needles, it may be necessary to make a hole in the skin with the introducer needle for easier insertion.

The introducer is inserted into the interspinous area maintaining this horizontal position. An improperly inserted introducer makes it impossible to point the needle in the correct direction. A small-gauge spinal needle (26- or 27-gauge Quincke or a conical-tipped needle such as the 25-gauge Whitacre needle) should be used for the procedure. The needle must first be examined for any imperfections or weaknesses. It should be noted that the bevel of the needle is on the same side as the key notch for the stylet in the hub of the needle. Once the physician is satisfied with the needle, he or she should insert it so that the bevel does not cut across the longitudinal fibers of the dura. In practice, this may not be possible. The bevel—as indicated by the key notch—should face laterally during its passage through the dura. The spinal needle is held between the thumb, index, and middle fingers and inserted through the introducer. (Fig. 7-16). The spinal needle is then slowly advanced. Its progress through the tissues is followed by noting the variations in resistance as the various structures are penetrated. First, the firm resistance of the interspinous ligament and the ligamentum flavum is felt, after which a lessening of resistance is

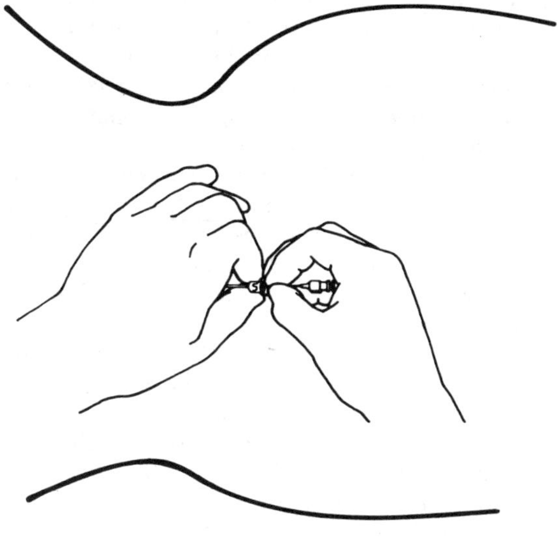

Fig. 7-16. Insertion of the spinal needle through the introducer.

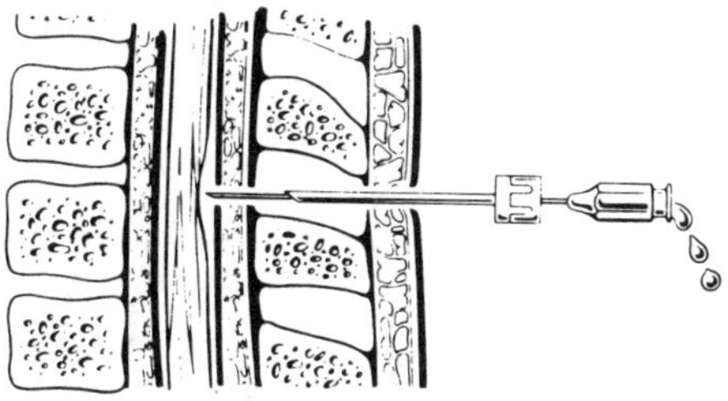

Fig. 7-17. Subarachnoid puncture and the appearance of CSF.

observed as the needle crosses the epidural space. This is followed by the characteristic "pop" (an abrupt disappearance of a last resistance) as the needle pierces the dura to enter the subarachnoid space. The anesthesiologist now may check the needle's position by withdrawing the stylet to see if cerebrospinal fluid (CSF) appears (Fig. 7-17) at the hub of the needle and by aspirating with a syringe as may not immediately appear because of the small gauge of the spinal needle.

There are several other reasons why CSF may fail to appear:

1. A nerve root or the dura may block the bevel of the needle. After withdrawing the stylet, the needle may be rotated 90 to 180 degrees in an attempt to free the bevel of the obstruction.
2. The cerebrospinal fluid pressure may be too low to push the fluid through the needle. The anesthesiologist should always confirm the needle position by achieving free flow of CSF when aspirating with a syringe.
3. A tissue plug may be blocking the bevel. This also will be dislodged by an aspiration attempt.
4. The bevel may still be in the epidural space, at least partially. Therefore, the anesthesiologist should replace the stylet in the needle and then slowly advance the needle forward. Then the above maneuvers are repeated.

If contact with bone has been made, stop. The needle must not be forced against this resistance because the needle can be bent, the lumen of the needle can be easily blocked, and the needle point can become "barbed." If it appears that the needle lumen is plugged, the needle should be removed and flushed with normal saline or local anesthetic solution. Contact with bone usually means that the vertebral lamina has been encountered. This necessitates a small change of the direction of the spinal needle. To do this effectively, the needle point is withdrawn completely into the introducer and then a fresh attempt is made at a puncture in a different direction (usually cephalad). Success is indi-

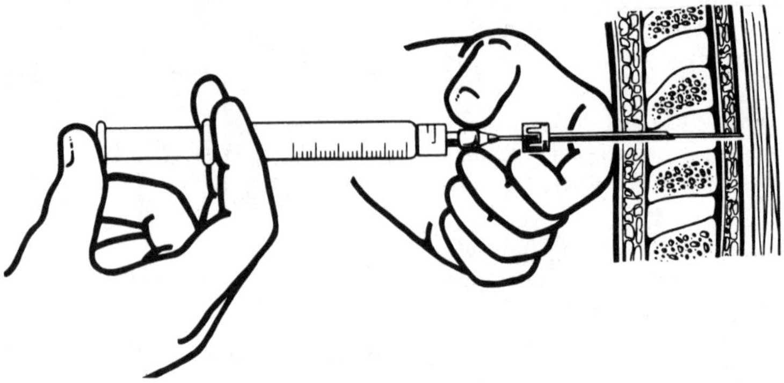

Fig. 7-18. Proper hand position during subarachnoid injection of local anesthetic.

cated by the appearance of CSF in the hub of the spinal needle. When this is achieved, the hub of the spinal needle is held firmly between the index or middle finger and the thumb of the left hand of the right-handed anesthesiologist to prevent any displacement of the needle from its proper location. The back of the anesthesiologist's hand is steadied against the patient's back (Fig. 7-18). Aspiration is performed with a syringe to ascertain free flow of cerebrospinal fluid. A syringe filled with the appropriate dose of local anesthetic solution is attached to the spinal needle.

Negative pressure is applied to the syringe to withdraw a small amount of CSF to ascertain that the proper position of the needle bevel has been maintained. Mixing of the CSF and anesthetic solution will occur during aspiration and will be visible since the local anesthetic solution will have a different baricity than CSF. Then the contents of the syringe are injected into the subarachnoid space. We prefer to aspirate and reinject a small volume (about 0.2 ml) after the local anesthetic has been injected to rule out accidental movement of the needle during the injection of the local anesthetic solution.

If aspiration is not accomplished or is difficult, we maintain the patient in position and ascertain the development of the block by testing the dependent side. If the block does not seem to be developing as expected, the spinal needle is replaced and an additional dose of anesthetic solution is administered. How much additional drug should be administered depends on the situation. The senior author administers an additional dose of 25 to 75 percent of the original volume of solution. He has not had a total spinal anesthetic using this procedure in over 25 years.

The suggested dosage of local anesthetic for the obstetric patient (Tables 7-7 and 7-8) is 30 to 50 percent lower than that given to a surgical patient. Incidentally, this dosage reduction is indicated for any patient with increased intra-abdominal pressure, including surgical patients with ascites or large intra-abdominal tumors.

Following the injection of the local anesthetic, the needle and the introducer are withdrawn and the patient is immediately placed in the supine position. Her uterus is displaced to the left by placing a wedge or a folded blanket under her right hip. Oxygen is administered by face mask at 6 to 10 L/min and the blood pressure is frequently monitored.

With the patient resting comfortably, the spread of anesthesia is checked frequently by gentle repeated pinpricks or by a cotton swab moistened with alcohol. Since the loss of pain and temperature sensation progresses simultaneously, the use of alcohol to check the spread of anesthesia may be more pleasant for the patient. Repeated pinpricks may not accurately differentiate the area of complete loss of pain sensation from that of partial sensory anesthesia. However, we still prefer the "pinprick" test. Because of the concern over blood and fluid contamination, we suggest the use of sharp toothpicks to determine sensory levels. Several brands of plastic toothpicks are sharp enough to pierce olives or onions but not human skin. The spread for the local anesthetic depends on the specific gravity relationships between the local anesthetic solution used and CSF. Normally, the specific gravity of CSF is 1.003 to 1.009.

A hyperbaric solution has a higher specific gravity than that of CSF, therefore it will move to low-lying parts of the subarachnoid space. If anesthesia of just the perineal area—the frequently used "saddle block"—is desired it is achieved by placing the patient in the sitting position as previously described.

A hypobaric solution has a specific gravity lower than CSF, therefore it will spread to higher-lying areas within the subarachnoid space. An isobaric solution, with a

Table 7-7. Local Anesthetics and Suggested Dosages for Subarachnoid Anesthesia for Vaginal Delivery

Local Anesthetic[a]	Dosage (Patient's Height) 5′	5′6″	6′0″	Onset of Action (min)	Duration of Action (min)
Lidocaine 5% in 7.5% dextrose in water (premixed)	40 mg (0.8 ml)	40–50 mg (0.8–1.0 ml)	50–60 mg (1.0–1.2 ml)	1–3	45–75
Bupivacaine 0.75% in 8.25% d/w (premixed)	7.5 mg (1.0 ml)	9.4 mg (1.25 ml)	11.3 mg (1.5 ml)	2–4	90–120
Bupivacaine 0.5% in hyperbaric solution[b]	6 mg (1.2 ml)	7 mg (1.4 ml)	8 mg (1.6 ml)	2–4	90–120
Tetracaine 1% & equal vol. 10% dextrose in water[c]	5 mg (0.5 ml) & 0.5 ml	6 mg (0.6 ml) & 0.6 ml	7 mg (0.7 ml) & 0.7 ml	3–5	120–180
Total volume	1.0 ml	1.2 ml	1.4 ml		
Tetracaine 1% & equal vol. 10% procaine/water[c]	4 mg (0.4 ml) & 40 mg (0.4 ml)	5 mg (0.5 ml) & 50 mg (0.5 ml)	6 mg (0.6 ml) & 60 mg (0.6 ml)	2–4	120–180
Total volume	0.8 ml	1.0 ml	1.2 ml		

d/w, dextrose in water.
[a] All preparations listed are hyperbaric.
[b] Not yet approved by the Food and Drug Administration.
[c] Rarely used anymore in the United States.

Table 7-8. Local Anesthetics and Suggested Dosages for Subarachnoid Anesthesia for Cesarean Delivery

Local Anesthetic[a]	Dosage (Patient's Height) 5′	5′6″	6′0″	Onset of Action (min)	DURATION ~~Onset~~ of Action (min)
Lidocaine 5% in 7.5% d/w (premixed)	60 mg (1.2 ml)	80 mg (1.6 ml)	100 m (2.0 ml)	1–3	45–75
Bupivacaine 0.75% in 8.25% d/w	9 mg (1.2 ml)	12 mg (1.6 ml)	15 mg (2.0 ml)	2–4	75–120
Bupivacaine 0.5% in hyperbaric solution[b]	8 mg (1.6 ml)	10 mg (2.0 ml)	12 mg (2.4 ml)	2–4	75–120
Tetracaine 1% & equal vol. 10% d/w[c]	7 mg (0.7 ml) & 0.7 ml	9 mg (0.9 ml) & 0.9 ml	11 mg (1.1 ml) & 1.1 ml	3–5	120–180
Total vol.	1.4 ml	1.8 ml	2.2 ml		
Tetracaine 1% & equal vol. 10% procaine/water[c]	6 mg (0.6 ml) & 60 mg (0.6 ml)	8 mg (0.8 ml) & 8 mg (0.8 ml)	10 mg (1.0 ml) & 100 mg (1.0 ml)	2–4	120–180
Total vol.	1.2 ml	1.6 ml	2.0 ml		

d/w, dextrose in water.
[a] All preparations listed are hyperbaric.
[b] Not yet approved by the Food and Drug Administration.
[c] Rarely used anymore in the United States.

specific gravity matching that of CSF, will tend to remain at the injection point. Both hypobaric and isobaric solutions are not used in single-dose subarachnoid block in obstetric anesthesia because of the lack of predictability of their spread in the subarachnoid space.

RECENT DEVELOPMENTS IN DETERMINING DOSAGE FOR SUBARACHNOID ANESTHESIA

The tables listed in this section are meant to be a guide to the appropriate dosage of hyperbaric local anesthetic for subarachnoid block for vaginal or cesarean delivery. In a recent review article, Stienstra and Green[1] reviewed the factors affecting the subarachnoid spread of local anesthetic solutions in nonpregnant patients. The following items have no clinically significant effect on the subarachnoid distribution of local anesthetics: patient weight, patient gender, barbotage, speed of injection, composition of CSF, circulation of CSF, pressure of CSF, and the presence of vasoconstrictors in the local anesthetic solution. The most important determinants for subarachnoid distribution of local anesthetic solutions are the baricity of the local anesthetic solution, the position of the patient during injection, the dosage of the local anesthetic (to some degree), and the site of injection. Less important factors (except in extreme situations) include increasing patient age, anatomic configuration of the spinal column, the direction of the spinal needle during injection, and the volume of CSF. Two controversial areas are the height of the patient and the dosage of local anesthetic (concentration × volume). Norris[2] found no difference in the spread of hyperbaric bupivacaine in term parturients regardless of age, height, or body mass index. Hartwell et al.[3] found no correlation between height, weight, or body mass index, but did find a correlation between two vertebral length measurements, C7 to the level of the iliac crest and C7 to the sacral hiatus. These investigators believed that the length of the vertebral column gave a better indication for the dose of hyperbaric local anesthetic. In practice, it has become apparent that there is a variable relationship between height of the parturient, the dose of hyperbaric local anesthetic and the ultimate level of sensory blockade. The pregnant patient is more sensitive to local anesthetics for a variety of factors that have been previously discussed (see Ch. 3). Whereas we religiously related the height of the patient to the dosage of tetracaine with glucose or procaine to produce a hyperbaric solution, such is not the situation with hyperbaric bupivacaine. Therefore, the aforementioned tables give a range and a liberal dosage scale for hyperbaric bupivacaine. We have found that the higher doses produce excellent operative anesthesia and a high level of sensory block (up to T2) that does not produce the distress in the patient that was previously seen with that level produced by hyperbaric tetracaine. Clinically, we have reached the same conclusion as Norris and Hartwell et al. that height is only a moderate determinant of the required dose of hyperbaric bupivacaine and probably only applies with the extremes of height.

There has been much controversy about the total volume of local anesthetic injected into the subarachnoid space and the subsequent production of a higher sensory level of anesthesia due to the altered hemodynamics of CSF in the parturient. Russell[4] recently investigated a range of volumes of local anesthetic with the same mass of drug and found that 15 mg of glucose-free 0.5 percent bupivacaine administered in dilutions of 3, 6, 12, or 18 ml of solution infused over 30 minutes produced the same final sensory levels when the parturient was turned supine. Therefore, volume does not appear to be a determinant of the sensory level of subarachnoid block with bupivacaine. Our own preliminary studies with isobaric (dextrose-free) bupivacaine demonstrated it to produce a variable but high block upon injection of 2 to 4 ml over a period of 1 to 2 minutes in the parturient.

Certainly the literature and our personal experience lead us to believe that the dose of hyperbaric bupivacaine is not determined by patient height nor volume of injectate. Therefore, the tables presented are to be used only as a guide that should be modified by the personal experience of the anesthesiologist. The addition of preservative-free fentanyl or morphine makes the injectate less hyperbaric but does not appear to have a significant effect on raising the final level of sensory anesthesia.

PRECAUTIONS

To ensure safety and success of subarachnoid anesthesia, several precautions should be taken.

The entry point for the needle should be below the level of L2 so as to avoid injury to the spinal cord.

The spinal needle may on occasion puncture one of the epidural vessels, resulting in a blood-tinged return of CSF at the hub of the needle. If this occurs, the anesthesiologist should wait until the return clears. If the CSF return fails to clear, an attempt should be made to repeat the block through the same or another interspace.

The vital signs must be monitored continuously, especially in the initial 20 minutes (during the fixation of the block), with close attention paid to any decrease in blood pressure. In the obstetric patient, uterine displacement and intravenous hydration will help to prevent hypotension due to aortocaval compression by the uterus and subsequent uteroplacental hypoperfusion. Oxygen administered by mask to the parturient is helpful to combat cerebral hypoxia, which will manifest itself by the appearance of nausea. Since a hyperbaric solution is used, a modified head-up position, with a pillow under the head, is advisable in order to prevent an excessive cephalad spread of the block and to make the parturient more comfortable.

COMPLICATIONS

The most common complication of subarachnoid anesthesia in obstetrics is maternal hypotension secondary to the combined effect of the decreased venous return produced by blockade of the sympathetic vascular tone and the aortocaval compression by the gravid uterus.

Should vasopressor therapy be needed, pure α-receptor-stimulating agents are usually avoided because these drugs correct the systemic blood pressure by vasoconstriction. Such an effect reduces uteroplacental perfusion and thereby compromises the fetus. However, there are exceptions to this general rule (see Ch. 3).

Ephedrine in increments of 10 mg intravenously is the best choice at present because it corrects the blood pressure predominantly by myocardial stimulation without compromising uteroplacental perfusion.

Life-threatening complications are rare and, for the most part, are due to an excessive cephalad spread of the local anesthetic causing total spinal anesthesia. This occurrence is heralded by nausea secondary to cerebral hypoxia and hypotension and can progress to respiratory and cardiac arrest. This highlights the importance of meticulous monitoring of the vital signs and the spread of anesthetic effect after the block is initiated. Standard cardiopulmonary resuscitation must be begun at once should a respiratory or a cardiac arrest occur.

Neurologic complications secondary to needle trauma are very rare but may occur if a dural puncture performed above the level of L2 results in spinal cord injury. If a paresthesia is elicited, no injection should be made. The needle should be immediately repositioned. Repeated paresthesias suggest the need to use another technique, either epidural or general anesthesia.

Minor complications include the possibility of postpartum urinary retention and postdural-puncture headache. The tendency to urinary retention is present with most types of anesthesia, including general anesthesia. The condition is temporary, and it is managed by bladder assessment and catheterization until normal bladder function resumes. Post-dural puncture headache occurs in a small percentage of patients and it is most troublesome when the patient must resume normal activity as soon as possible. Unfortunately, the parturient is in the group with the highest incidence of post-dural puncture headache (see below). The diagnosis is made by having the patient sit up or stand up. Headache commences within a few minutes and is relieved by lying down. Its incidence is diminished when the patient is acutely hydrated before the block and when small-gauge (25- to 27-gauge) needles are used. Persistent severe post-dural puncture headache not responding to hydration, bed rest, and analgesics may be treated with an epidural blood patch.

Meningitis, although rare, may result from contamination of the subarachnoid space during the initiation of subarachnoid anesthesia in the presence of septicemia, local superficial infection of the lumbar area, or contaminated equipment.

INDICATIONS

This technique provides excellent anesthesia for vaginal and cesarean delivery.

CONTRAINDICATIONS

Absolute contraindications to spinal anesthesia include infection of the meninges of the spinal cord, septicemia, local cutaneous infections at the puncture site, blood coagulopathies, and acute central nervous system disease. Proven allergy to a local anesthetic agent mandates the choice of a local anesthetic drug from a different chemical family.

In other situations, such as the presence of cardiac disease, the advantage of subarachnoid anesthesia must be weighed against potential problems arising from the cardiovascular side effects of the block.

Several deformities of the lumbosacral spine may make spinal anesthesia technically difficult and thus the potential for trauma may unacceptably high.

REFERENCES

1. Stienstra R, Greene NM: Factors affecting the subarachnoid spread of local anesthetic solutions. Reg Anesth 16:1, 1991
2. Norris MC: Patient variables and the subarachnoid spared of hyperbaric bupivacaine in the term parturient. Anesthesiology 72:478, 1990
3. Hartwell BL, Aglio LS, Hauch MA, Datta S: Vertebral column length and the spread of hyperbaric subarachnoid bupivacaine in the term parturient. Reg Anesth 16:17, 1991
4. Russell IF: Spinal anesthesia for cesarean delivery with dilute solutions of plain bupivacaine: the relationship between infused volume and spread. Reg Anesth 16:130, 1991

CONTINUOUS SUBARACHNOID ANESTHESIA

The idea of continuous subarachnoid anesthesia (CSA) was first introduced in the early 1900s by the British surgeon, Dean,[1] who used a spinal needle placed in the subarachnoid space and left in situ for reinjection. Because of technical difficulties, including needle trauma and breakage, this technique never gained popularity. It was not until 1944, with the invention of rubber ureteral catheters and their use by Tuohy,[2] that CSA began to evolve as new technological developments were made.

Bizzarri et al. were the first to use a vinyl catheter for CSA in parturients.[3] Practitioners had been using plastic and Teflon epidural catheters for many years to provide CSA[4] for surgical procedures, particularly in the geriatric population.

Administration of CSA for labor and delivery with a microcatheter (32 gauge) has been investigated by some clinicians with good results. Huckaby et al.[5] reported excellent sensory anesthesia with negligible motor block using 1 percent lidocaine. Other benefits noted in this study include the ability to achieve rapid sensory anesthesia, and to prolong its duration as required. The density and level of anesthesia could be rapidly raised if operative delivery became necessary. In addition, the danger of central nervous system or cardiac toxicity is remote because the local anesthetic is administered in small incremental doses.

The utilization of small-gauge 28- to 32-gauge catheters has caused a resurgence of interest in this technique. The incidence of post-dural puncture headache associated with CSA when large needles and catheters were used was unacceptably high for some practitioners. The nature of the procedure itself (large-gauge needle and catheter) caused the loss of clinically significant quantities of cerebrospinal fluid (CSF). Some authorities believe the presence of a catheter through the dura may potentiate further loss of CSF by a "wick" effect.

With the ongoing improvement of microcatheter technology for CSA, further investigations may demonstrate a much lower incidence of post-dural puncture headache in parturients.

ANATOMY AND LANDMARKS

Anatomy and landmarks are the same as previously discussed under Subarachnoid Anesthesia, earlier in this chapter.

PATIENT POSITION

The patient position is the same as previously discussed under Subarachnoid Anesthesia, earlier in this chapter. However, it should be noted that, for the parturient in early labor, the sitting position may sometimes be more advantageous, particularly for an obese patient, as it allows easier threading of the spinal catheter 1 to 2 cm cephalad as well as easier withdrawal of the needle without dislodgment of the catheter.

MATERIALS

The following materials should be ready for use when the patient is to be given CSA:

One pair of sterile gloves
Antibacterial solution for cleansing the skin
One sterile cup for the antibacterial solution
Forceps
Sterile gauze pads
Sterile towels for draping the field
One 25-gauge, 1.6- to 3.8-cm needle for skin infiltration
One 21- or 22-gauge, 3.8-cm needle for preparing drugs and deep infiltration (if desired)
One 18-gauge needle for use as an introducer
One 22-, 25-, or 26-gauge, 8.9-cm spinal needle with stylet
One 28- or 32-gauge microcatheter
One 3-ml syringe
One 5-ml glass syringe
Sterile gauze to protect the catheter
Tape to secure the catheter

Disposable CSA trays are commercially available that contain all of the above items.

TECHNIQUE

The technique is the same as that described for subarachnoid anesthesia earlier in this chapter, with the added steps of inserting and securing the catheter. Recently both 32-gauge catheters that can be advanced through a 25- or 26-gauge spinal needle and 28-gauge catheters that can be advanced through a 22-gauge spinal needle have become available. Most catheters have a stylet to facilitate introduction into the subarachnoid space and are marked at 1-cm intervals. Once a free flow of CSF is obtained, the catheter is advanced 1 to 2 cm into the subarachnoid space. After the introducer and spinal needle are removed, the catheter is secured in place with tape in a manner similar to an epidural catheter.

CONSIDERATIONS

The most common problem encountered when using the microcatheter is kinking of the catheter on insertion. This difficulty is due to the catheter being advanced against tissue instead of being freely passed into CSF. Hurley and Lambert[6] describe several maneuvers that may be helpful in overcoming this problem: flushing the needle with saline, rotating the needle, rotating the needle while advancing the catheter, and slowly withdrawing the needle may result in successful placement without the catheter kinking. A threading-assist adapter may also be helpful to provide lateral stabilization of the catheter within the spinal needle hub, where the catheter may flex and bend upon itself during advancement. Should all of these techniques fail, another attempt should be made at another interspace.

Following successful placement, the needle is slowly withdrawn over the catheter, the catheter is padded with gauze and then secured to the patient's back with tape, and the local anesthetic injected. Aspiration of CSF through the larger 19- or 20-gauge epidural catheter easily confirms correct subarachnoid placement, but because of the increased resistance associated with the microcatheter, aspiration may not produce CSF easily.

Some facts to be remembered when providing CSA with a microcatheter for laboring patients include the following:

1. If injection through the catheter is difficult or impossible and there is no visible evidence of occlusion, having the patient either flex or extend her back may alleviate this problem. The same technique can be utilized if difficulty is encountered during removal of the catheter.
2. Small incremental doses of local anesthetic titrated to the desired sensory level should be used. The use of both isobaric and hyperbaric agents may be needed to provide an adequate anesthetic, especially in patients with anatomic abnormalities of the spine.
3. Small doses of anesthetics with higher concentrations may provide a better block than larger doses of weaker concentrations.
4. More total drug may be required when using combined isobaric and hypobaric agents than with hyperbaric agents alone.

DOSAGE

Any of the local anesthetic agents used for single-dose subarachnoid anesthesia may be used for CSA. However, an advantage of CSA is the ability to tailor the level and duration of anesthesia. Ultra-short-acting local anesthetics are extremely useful for minimizing hemodynamic changes and subarachnoid opioids may also be added as desired. It must be remembered that morphine is approximately 10 times more potent in the subarachnoid space than in the epidural space; recommended dosages range from 0.1 to 0.5 mg for achieving 12 to 24 hours of analgesia. The respiratory rate must be continuously monitored for 24 hours because of the possibility of delayed respiratory depression associated with subarachnoid morphine administration. The administration of fentanyl in doses of 10 to 25 μg will supplement the local anesthetic effect and provide 2 to 4 hours of analgesia. Because of the greater lipid solubility of fentanyl, there is less incidence of delayed respiratory depression.

PRECAUTIONS

All precautions previously stated for subarachnoid anesthesia earlier in this chapter should be taken with CSA.

Again, care must be taken to avoid kinking or bending of the microcatheter during placement and to avoid accidental removal following successful insertion. There is also the danger that the microcatheter may be inserted directly into a blood vessel; negative aspiration of blood is not a guarantee that the catheter has not been placed or migrated into a vessel. The amount of local anesthetic used for subarachnoid anesthesia is small enough so that accidental intravascular injection is usually without consequence but will be reflected by the lack of a developing anesthetic effect. Following surgery or delivery, it is important to remember to position the patient so that her back is either flexed or extended while the microcatheter is being removed. If the microcatheter seems difficult to remove, excessive force or traction should not be applied, as it may break, resulting in the need for further patient manipulation.

COMPLICATIONS

All complications discussed earlier for subarachnoid anesthesia apply to CSA. Other disadvantages associated with the use of the microcatheter in CSA are mostly technical and include the following:

1. Inability to thread the catheter
2. Inability to inject the anesthetic
3. Catheter breakage
4. Unintentional removal of the catheter
5. Inadequate anesthesia
6. Possible inability to aspirate CSF from the subarachnoid space because of increased resistance in the catheter

7. Microcatheters have been noted to bend, kink, twist, and even knot

The larger 19- to 21-gauge epidural catheters can usually be placed into the subarachnoid space with minimal difficulty. Since these catheters are larger and more rigid than the microcatheters, they thread easier and are not prone to catheter lumen occlusion. The microcatheter, however, is very different. Hurley and Lambert[6] reported a 20 percent failure rate with their early trials during the development of the microcatheter.

Catheter breakage, always a concern with any catheter in the subarachnoid space, may readily occur if the catheter should be withdrawn through the needle. When a catheter is unable to be advanced, both the catheter and needle must be removed together. The breakage of two microcatheters during attempted catheter removal has been reported.[6] The catheter should be protected at all times by carefully securing it properly, minimizing patient movement, especially during operating and delivery room positioning; and careful removal of the catheter with minimal force. Should a catheter break, roentgenography or computed tomography may be helpful in analyzing the location of the remaining fragment. Full explanation of the complications to the patient is prudent. Surgical retrieval is usually not advised unless there are neurologic findings.

Except for post-dural puncture headache, neurologic complications following CSA are rare. The incidence of post-dural puncture headache in parturients has been noted to be as high as 16 to 21 percent when a 19-gauge spinal needle and large catheter are used.[7,8] During CSA using a 25- or 26-gauge spinal needle and a 32-gauge microcatheter, a 4 percent incidence of post-dural puncture headache was reported.[6] Other neurologic sequelae, including adhesive arachnoiditis, transverse myelitis, cauda equina syndrome, and septic meningitis, are rare following subarachnoid anesthesia.

INDICATIONS

The advantages of CSA over single-dose subarachnoid anesthesia and, in some cases, continuous epidural anesthesia for labor and delivery include the following:

1. Dosage requirements of local anesthetics are greatly decreased; 10 to 15 times less local anesthetic is needed for CSA than is needed for epidural anesthesia, thus virtually eliminating the possibility of systemic toxic reactions.
2. Greater control of effects and sensory level achieved is possible.
3. Cardiovascular complications are minimized since careful titration of sensory anesthesia (and sympathetic block) is possible.
4. Respiratory complications are minimized.
5. The duration of anesthesia can be prolonged indefinitely.
6. The definite flow of CSF through the catheter confirms the placement in the subarachnoid space.
7. Subarachnoid opioids may be administered during or at the completion of the procedure to provide postoperative pain relief.

The following indications for CSA with a microcatheter for labor and delivery anesthesia should be considered:

1. Anatomic abnormalities, such as kyphoscoliosis, which might make identification or access to the epidural space very difficult.
2. Previous back surgery, including laminectomy and placement of Harrington rods, which might result in altered spinal anatomy making it very difficult to achieve epidural catheter placement.
3. The morbidly obese parturient, in whom anatomic identification of the epidural space may be difficult and single-dose subarachnoid anesthesia undesirable because of the possibility of an unintentional "high spinal" causing respiratory arrest and complications of airway management. In addition, complications from severe hypotension associated with the sudden onset of a massive sympathetic blockade are often encountered in this patient group when single-dose subarachnoid anesthesia is used.

When a 25- or 26-gauge spinal needle is used in the placement of a microcatheter, the occurrence of post-dural puncture headache has been observed by Hurley and Lambert[6] to be the same as that observed after single-dose spinal anesthesia using a 26-gauge needle. Although results with the microcatheter in the obstetric patient are preliminary, if the incidence of complications proves to be no greater than that for single-dose subarachnoid or epidural anesthesia, then CSA with a microcatheter would prove very useful for analgesia or anesthesia during labor and delivery

CONTRAINDICATIONS

The absolute and relative contraindications are the same as those previously discussed for single-dose subarachnoid anesthesia. Other contraindications to CSA include the possibility of cord or nerve root damage, the possibility of the introduction of infection, and the already-discussed possible higher incidence of post-dural puncture headache in the parturient.

REFERENCES

1. Dean HP: Discussion on the relative value of inhalation and injection methods of inducing anesthesia. Br Med J 2:869, 1907
2. Tuohy EB: Continuous spinal anesthesia: its usefulness and technique involved. Anesthesiology 5:142, 1944
3. Bizzarri DV, Giuffrida JG, Bondoc L, Fierro FE: Continuous spinal anesthesia using a special needle and catheter. Anesth Analg 43:393, 1964
4. Shroff PK, Skerman JH, Blass NH: Continuous spinal blockade: an old technique revisited. South Med J 81:178, 1988
5. Huckaby T, Skerman JH, Hurley RJ, Lamburt DH: Sensory analgesia for vaginal deliveries: a preliminary report of continuous spinal anesthesia with a 32 gauge catheter. Reg Anesth 16:150, 1991
6. Hurley RJ, Lambert DH: Continuous spinal anesthesia with a microcatheter technique: preliminary experience. Anesth Analg 70:97, 1990
7. Giuffrida JG, Bizzarri DV, Masi R, et al: Continuous procaine spinal anesthesia for cesarean section. Anesth Analg 51:117, 1972
8. Peterson DO, Borup JL, Chestnut JS: Continuous spinal anesthesia: case review and discussion. Reg Anesth 8:109, 1983

PUDENDAL NERVE BLOCK AND LOCAL INFILTRATION FOR VAGINAL DELIVERY

ANATOMY AND LANDMARKS

The pudendal nerve originates from S2–S4 (Fig. 7-19). It leaves the pelvis by way of the lower part of the greater sciatic foramen, curves around the spine of the ischium, crosses the sacrospinous ligament close to its attachment to the ischial spine, and then re-enters the pelvis alongside the internal pudendal artery at the lesser sciatic foramen. The pudendal nerve then branches into the inferior hemorrhoidal (rectal) nerve, and perineal nerve, and the dorsal nerve of the clitoris. These nerves are best blocked at the ischial tuberosity. Because it is also easily palpable, the ischial tuberosity constitutes an important anatomic landmark.

The perineal area derives additional innervation from the pudendal branch of the posterior femoral cutaneous nerve, which supplies mostly the posterior labial portion of the perineum.

Although the major innervation to the anterior aspect of the perineum is carried by the perineal nerve and the dorsal nerve of the clitoris, a secondary nerve supply is also provided by the ilioinguinal (L1) and genitofemoral (L1–L2) nerves. Therefore, these must be blocked by supplemental infiltration if thorough anesthesia of the anterior portions of the labia majora and the mons pubis is needed.

PATIENT POSITION

For the pudendal block the patient is placed in the lithotomy position.

MATERIALS

The following are needed:

One pair of sterile gloves
Antibacterial solution for cleansing the skin
One sterile cup for the antibacterial solution
Forceps
Sterile gauze pads
Sterile towels
One 25-gauge, 1.6- to 3.8-cm needle for skin infiltration
Two 22-gauge, 7.5- to 10-cm short-beveled needles for the pudendal block and infiltration of the labia and perineum.
One 10-ml syringe with finger rings. These materials are required for a unilateral pudendal block. In obstetrics, bilateral pudendal blocks are necessary.

If the transvaginal technique is chosen, the special transvaginal needle with the appropriate guide, such as the Kobak needle or Iowa trumpet with a 15.2-cm, 20-gauge needle, is used.

One disposable pudendal block/local infiltration tray usually contains all of the above items.

TECHNIQUE

The pudendal block can be performed by either the perineal or transvaginal route.

Perineal Route

The advantages of the perineal route are that the branches of both the pudendal nerve and the posterior femoral cutaneous nerve can be blocked from the same injection point because they are both close to the ischial tuberosity. With the patient in the lithotomy position, the perineal area is cleansed with an aqueous antibacterial solution and the ischial tuberosity is palpated. An

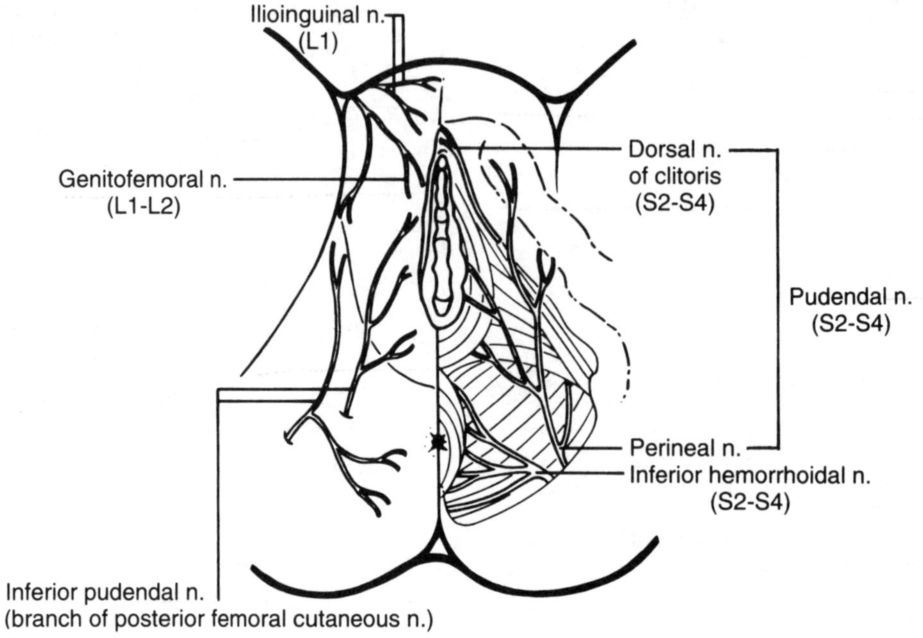

Fig. 7-19. Innervation of the perineum.

intradermal wheal is raised at the site of the ischial tuberosity, and a small amount of a local anesthetic is injected through a 25-gauge needle. The 10-ml syringe is filled with the local anesthetic and is attached to the 7.5- to 10-cm needle. The needle is then inserted through the wheal at a right angle to the skin. The needle is advanced slowly into the tissues, with small amounts of the local anesthetic injected as the needle is advanced. The index finger of the left hand is inserted into the vagina or rectum and the tuberosity of the ischium is palpated.

This index finger now guides the needle toward the ischial tuberosity. This structure is usually encountered at a depth of 2.5 to 4 cm from the skin, depending on the size of the patient. With the needle in place, 5 to 10 ml of the local anesthetic solution is injected at the anterolateral aspect of the ischial spine as well as under the tuberosity to block the inferior pudendal branch of the posterior femoral cutaneous nerve. The syringe then has to be detached from the needle, refilled, and reattached.

The needle then is advanced to the medial aspect of the ischial spine, where another 5 to 10 ml of the local anesthetic solution is injected to block the branches of the pudendal nerve. Since the pudendal artery and vein run parallel to the pudendal nerve in this area, the injection of the local anesthetic should be intermittent, with an aspiration performed between the injection of each 2 to 3 ml of the local anesthetic solution. This will prevent an intravascular injection of a significant amount of local anesthetic drug. If blood is seen upon aspiration, the needle should be repositioned until no more blood is observed on aspiration. The syringe is refilled again and about 5 to 10 ml of the local anesthetic is injected as the needle is advanced about 2.5 cm past the ischial tuberosity into the ischiorectal fossa. This blocks the pudendal nerve in Alcock's canal. The syringe is refilled one last time and the point of the needle is advanced posteriorly to the ischial spine using the index finger in the vagina or rectum as guide. The finger can palpate the sacrospinous ligament and it guides the needle in this direction until the "popping" sensation indicates that the needle has pierced the ligament. The needle is advanced another 0.5 cm and 5 to 10 ml of the local anesthetic solution is injected at this point to block the pudendal nerve before it branches. The needle is then withdrawn. The other side is then blocked. When the contralateral pudendal block is completed, the obstetrician prepares to block the secondary innervation of the perineum.

Using a sterile, 7.5- to 10-cm needle, the area 1.5 cm lateral and parallel to the labium majorum, from the middle of the labium to the mons pubis can then be infiltrated. This blocks the secondary innervation from the iliohypogastric, ilioinguinal, and genitofemoral nerves. This infiltration, too, is usually performed bilaterally. Aspiration must be accomplished between each 2- to 3-ml injection of local anesthetic during local infiltration in the lateral vaginal area or in the perineum. Often, perineal infiltration will be the only method used during vaginal delivery. Frequent aspiration is essential to avoid intravascular injection in the edematous and engorged perineum.

Transvaginal Route

The transvaginal technique utilizes the same anatomic landmarks. A specialized transvaginal needle and guide assembly is needed, such as the Kobak needle or Iowa trumpet with a 20-gauge, 15.2-cm needle.

The patient is in the lithotomy position and the perineum is prepared with an antibacterial solution. The index and middle fingers of one hand are inserted into the vagina until the ischial spine and the sacrospinous ligament can be palpated. With the transvaginal needle withdrawn into the shaft of the guide, the Kobak needle or the Iowa trumpet is inserted into the vagina and its point is positioned on the sacrospinous ligament as it attaches to the ischial spine (Fig. 7-20). The needle is then advanced about 1.6 cm past the surface of the mucosa until it "pops" through the mucous membrane and the sacrospinous ligament. About 5 to 10 ml of the local anesthetic solution is injected into this location, with an aspiration test after the injection of each 2 to 3 ml to ensure that the solution is not being injected into the pudendal artery or vein that lies in close proximity. If a bloody return is observed in the syringe, the needle is moved until no blood is observed on aspiration. In obstetrics, the block is then repeated on the other side.

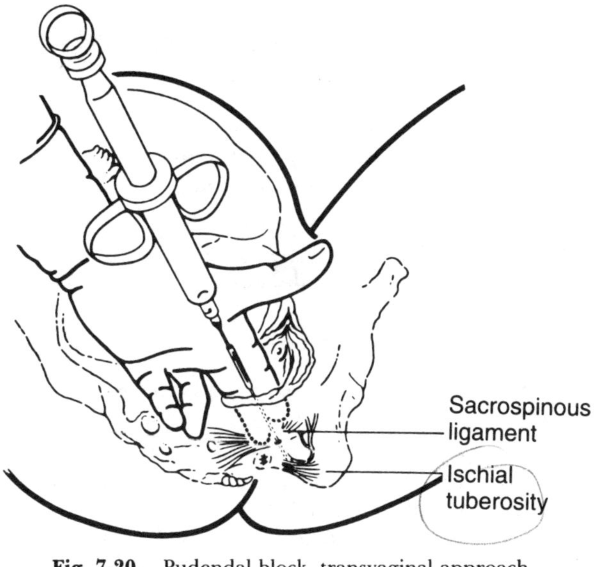

Fig. 7-20. Pudendal block, transvaginal approach.

A supplemental infiltration of the area lateral to the labia majora to provide anesthesia of the anterior perineum may be performed as described previously. See Table 7-9 for dosages.

In practice, the transvaginal technique is most commonly used.

Table 7-9. Local Anesthetics for Pudendal Block[a]

Local Anesthetic[b]	Onset of Action (min)	Duration of Action (min)
Bupivacaine 0.25%–0.5%	5–10	60–180
Chloroprocaine 1–2%	3–5	45–90
Lidocaine 0.5%–1.0%	5–10	60–120
Mepivacaine 0.5%–1.0%	5–10	60–120

[a] Total milligram dosage of the local anesthetic should not exceed manufacturer's recommendations.

[b] Without epinephrine.

PRECAUTIONS

Frequent aspirations must be performed when injecting the local anesthetic solution to ensure that the drug is not injected into the pudendal vessels that lie close to the pudendal nerve.

If the block is done outside the delivery room, cardiopulmonary resuscitation equipment must be immediately available. Delivery rooms must be fully supplied with the same anesthesia and resuscitative equipment found in the operating suite.

COMPLICATIONS

When the needle is in the vicinity of the ischial spine, care must be taken that the rectal mucosa is not pierced. Although the ischial spine can be palpated through the vagina as well as the rectum, the technique of palpating the anatomic landmarks through the rectum is superior because it ensures that the rectal mucosa is not pierced.

INDICATIONS

1. Anesthesia of the perineum for the second stage of an uncomplicated obstetric delivery. It should be noted, however, that the uterine contractions are not painless when this method of anesthesia is used, as they would be if a subarachnoid, epidural, or caudal block were performed.

2. Perineal and rectal surgery, with premedication according to the needs of the patient.
3. Differential diagnosis of perineal pain.
4. Relief of pain and perineal pruritus, as in carcinoma of the vulva.

CONTRAINDICATIONS

A contraindication of this block would be localized infection at the site of needle puncture.

LOCAL INFILTRATION FOR CESAREAN DELIVERY

In 1974, Ranney and Stanage advocated local anesthesia for cesarean delivery because "local field block of the abdominal wall is the least complicated, most direct anesthetic technique which will provide the necessary relief from pain, yet least adversely modify the maternal-fetal physiology."[1] These authors cited two neonatal deaths of term infants in 1951 and 1952 as motivation for learning the technique of local anesthesia for cesarean delivery. Now, 40 years later, the availability of safe regional or general anesthetic techniques in most hospitals renders the need for local anesthesia for abdominal delivery almost obsolete. Consequently, few obstetricians or anesthesiologists in practice today have ever seen or administered local anesthesia for a cesarean delivery. Nonetheless, on rare occasions, knowledge of the procedures for local infiltration for cesarean delivery may prove lifesaving for the mother and fetus.

Indications for use of local anesthesia for cesarean delivery are limited. In some hospitals, personnel trained in general or regional anesthesia may be on call from home. In such a setting, should a parturient present with severe fetal distress, the obstetrician may be required to begin delivery under local anesthesia. Also rare, but conceivable, is the parturient with an inaccessible or compromised airway combined with a failed or contraindicated regional block. While these may be very rare circumstances, the need to supplement a "patchy" or partial intraspinal anesthetic may be the most common indication for local infiltration.

The opinions expressed in this manuscript are those of the author and not necessarily those of the United States Air Force or the Department of Defense.

ANATOMY

Sensory innervation of the lower abdominal wall originates from the anterior division of the T7–T11 intercostal nerves. These nerves run in the neurovascular bundle beneath the inferior margin of each rib and then medially between the aponeuroses of the internal oblique and transverse adominis muscles. As each approaches the semilunar line, or lateral margin of the rectus abdominis muscle, it turns anteriorly to penetrate the posterior aspect of the inferolateral rectus sheath (Fig. 7-21). These major fibers course medially about halfway through the rectus muscle, then again turn anteriorly to penetrate the anterior rectus sheath. These arborize to become the anterior cutaneous branches of the thoracic nerves. Additionally, each of these thoracic nerves gives off a lateral cutaneous branch that supplies the skin from the mid-axillary line to the semilunar line. The T12, iliohypogastric, and ilioinguinal nerves all pass more toward the mons pubis. The iliohypogastric nerve courses between the internal and external oblique muscles to supply the skin from the anterior superior iliac crest, medially to the area just superior to the pubic bone. The ilioinguinal nerve descends within the inguinal canal, exits at the external ring, and branches superficially to supply the skin over the symphysis pubis, mons, and labia majora. In general, the areas near the pubic bone and mons are more densely innervated than the areas supplied by the T7–T11 nerves. Finally, regarding the relative density of nerve endings in the different layers, the skin is the most sensitive, followed by the fascia second, muscle third, and subcutaneous tissue last.

METHODS FOR LOCAL AND LOCAL–REGIONAL BLOCK

Multiple techniques for local or local–regional anesthesia of the lower abdominal wall have been described. Most, however, are modifications of one of four specific techniques: (1) intercostal–paravertebral nerve block; (2) lateral intercostal–thoracoabdominal nerve block; (3) rectus abdominis block; and (4) direct local infiltration.

Intercostal–Paravertebral Block

As previously described, on rare occasion the need for cesarean delivery may arise in a patient for whom both intraspinal and general anesthesia are contraindicated. In such a circumstance, if personnel trained in regional anesthesia are available, and if the fetus is not in extremis mandating emergent delivery, an intercostal–paravertebral block may be performed. This pro-

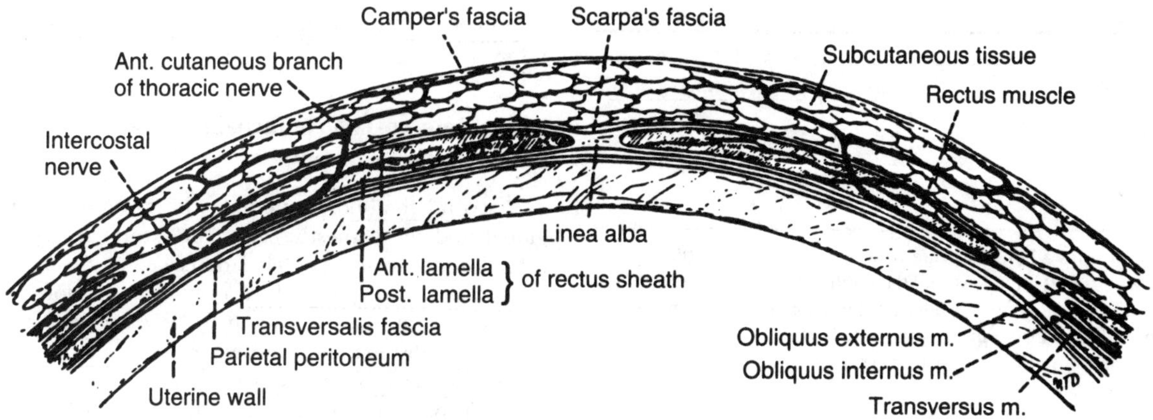

Fig. 7-21. Anatomy. Schematic diagram showing the course of the thoracic nerves as they supply the various layers of the anterior lower abdominal wall. (From Bonica,[2] with permission.)

cedure offers the advantage of more complete anesthesia and relaxation of the abdominal wall, yet requires less total anesthetic solution than other methods. Possible complications include pneumothorax, intravascular injection, and hypotension as a result of peripheral vasodilation from the paravertebral block.[2]

The procedure, as described by Bonica, is performed as follows.[2] The patient is placed on the operating table on her side such that the plane of her back makes a 45-degree angle with the floor, allowing access to all points required for the block (Fig. 7-22). While a number of anesthetic solutions may be used, that favored by Bonica

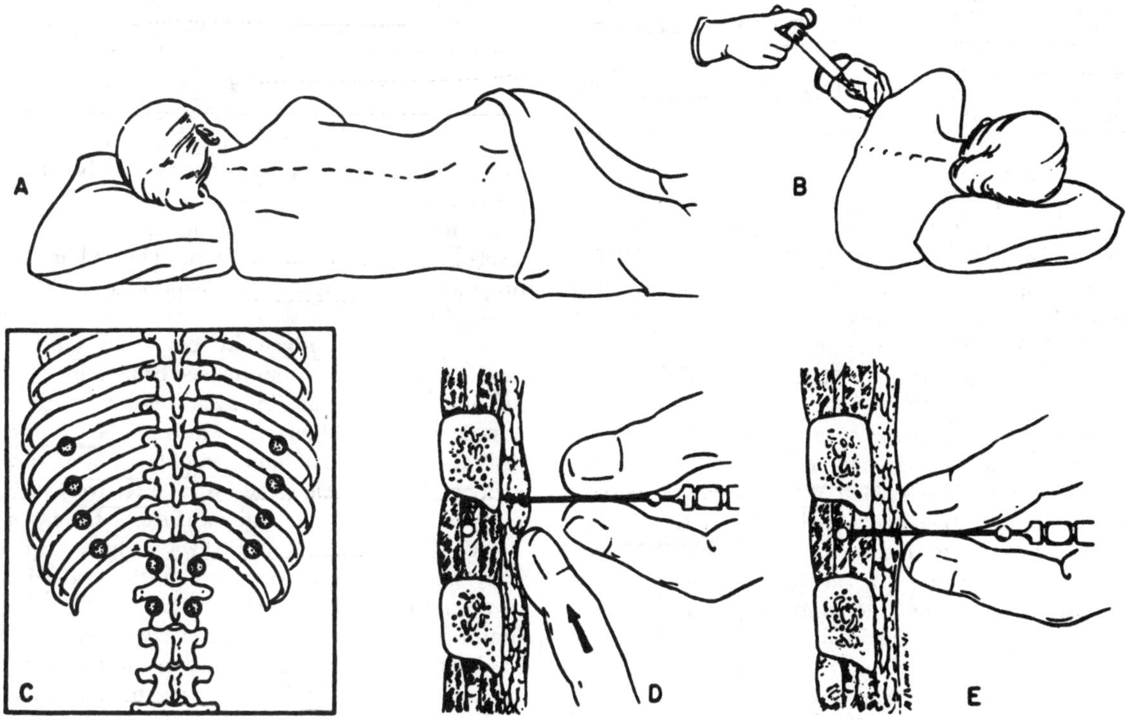

Fig. 7-22. Intercostal paravertebral block. **(A & B)** Positioning of the patient. **(C)** Points for intercostal and paravertebral injections. **(D & E)** Technique for intercostal injection. (From Bonica,[2] with permission.)

Table 7-10. Maximal Recommended Doses of Common Local Anesthetics

Local Anesthetic	Without Epinephrine (mg/kg)	With Epinephrine[a] (mg/kg)
Lidocaine	4.0	7.0
Chloroprocaine	11.0	14.0
Bupivacaine	2.5	3.0
Mepivacaine	5.0	—
Tetracaine	1.5	—

[a] Assumes all epinephrine concentrations are 1:200,000.

(Modified from Chestnut DH, Gibbs CP: Obstetric anesthesia. p. 493. In Gabbe SG, Niebyl JR, Simpson JL (eds): Obstetrics: Normal and Problem Pregnancies. 2nd Ed. Churchill Livingstone, New York, 1991, with permission.)

is a mixture of 1 percent chloroprocaine combined with 0.1 percent tetracaine, which produces 2 to 3 hours of anesthesia. Other suggested local anesthetics are given in Table 7-10. The intercostal blocks are placed at the most prominent part of the posterior aspect of each rib bilaterally at the T8, T9, T10, and T11 segments. A finger is used to protect the intercostal space and push the skin just cephalad. A short needle then is advanced to the inferior margin of the rib, the skin is released, and the needle advanced another 5 mm into the neurovascular bundle, where the anesthetic is deposited. Paravertebral block is then carried out at the T11–T12 and L1 areas to block the iliohypogastric nerve, ilioinguinal nerve, and fibers supplying the uterus, respectively.

To perform the paravertebral block, the patient is placed briefly in the sitting position. The spinous processes of the T11–T12 and the L1 vertebrae are located by counting cephalad from L4. This is easily palpated in a horizontal line between the iliac crests. With a marker, horizontal lines are drawn on the skin through the most cephalad point of each spinous process of the three target vertebrae. A vertical line is then drawn parallel to the spine 3.2 to 3.8 cm on both sides of the spine depending on the size of the patient. The resulting six intersections are the points of entry for the paravertebral block.[3] After a skin wheal is raised at each point, a 3.8-cm, 22-gauge needle is used to infiltrate directly down to the transverse process that should lie below each wheal. Next, a 7.5-cm, 22-gauge needle is advanced in the same tract until it impinges on the transverse process. At this point, a distance of 3 cm is visualized or measured from the surface of the skin and marked on the needle. With care taken to remain in the parasaggital plane, the needle is angled caudad, little by little, until it passes just beneath the transverse process, upon which the needle is advanced until the mark reaches the skin. Ten to 20 ml of the above local anesthetic solution should be injected in each of the six sites.

Lateral Intercostal–Thoracoabdominal Nerve Block

A second method, combining the advantages of regional and local anesthesia, is the lateral intercostal–thoracoabdominal nerve block described by Busby.[4] The advantage of this procedure over that previously described is that this method may be employed by the delivering obstetrician. The expertise needed for paravertebral block is not required.

The procedure, beginning with the arrowhead field block, is described by Busby as follows (Fig. 7-23A). A point midway between the inferior costal margin and the iliac crest is located in the mid-axillary line. A 2-inch, 22-gauge needle is used to penetrate the fascia of the internal and external oblique muscles, depositing 5 to 8 ml of local anesthetic to block the 11th intercostal nerve. The needle is withdrawn to just beneath the skin, angled 45 degrees cephalad, and again advanced through the aponeuroses to access the 10th intercostal nerve. Finally, this same needle is again withdrawn to just beneath the surface of the skin, angled 45 degrees caudad, and advanced, thus depositing the local anesthetic in the vicinity of the 12th intercostal nerve. Because the area over the mons is also innervated by the iliohypogastric and ilioinguinal nerves, these must be blocked as they exit the inguinal ring (Fig. 7-23B). To accomplish this, the skin over the pubic tubercle is pierced, angling the needle 45 degrees down and laterally for 2 to 3 cm, depositing the anesthetic at the level of the external oblique fascia. The abdomen is then draped for a midline incision. A "pigskin" wheal is raised along the line of incision with care taken to place the local anesthetic intradermally, not in the subcutaneous fat. Next, the fascia is anesthetized by piercing the raised line and slowly injecting the local anesthetic as the needle advances through the fascia, which can be felt as a slight resistance. A small amount, roughly 1 ml, of anesthetic is deposited just below the fascia, effectively lifting the peritoneum off of the undersurface of the fascia (Fig. 7-23C). The needle is withdrawn slightly, angled caudally, and again advanced through the fascia, injecting slowly as the needle traverses the fascia. This is repeated until the complete line is infiltrated. After the incision has been carried through the fascia and the peritoneum has been entered, Busby advocates the placement of 10 ml of anesthetic freely into the peritoneal cavity, effectively anesthetizing the serosal surfaces in the pelvis. Although probably not necessary, a small amount of

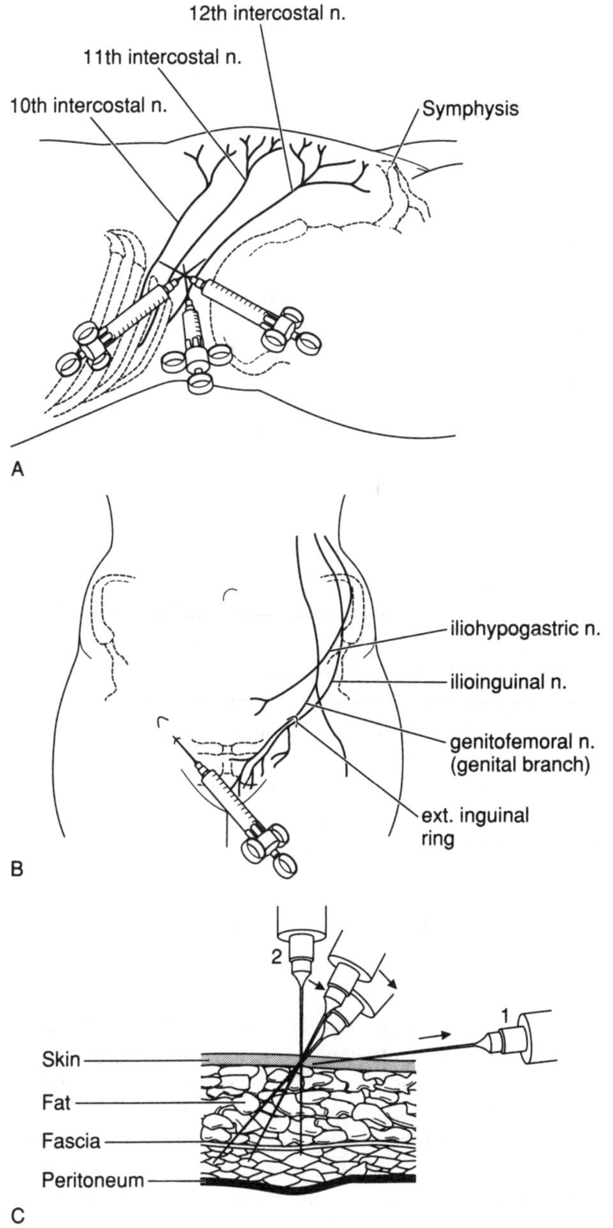

Fig. 7-23. Lateral intercostal thoracoabdominal nerve block. **(A)** Arrowhead field block. **(B)** Injection to block the iliohypogastric and ilioinguinal nerves. **(C)** Technique for midline skin and fascial injection. (From Busby,[4] with permission.)

anesthetic may also be injected just beneath the proposed bladder flap to facilitate dissection of the tissue planes and provide additional visceral anesthesia.

Like the intercostal–paravertebral block, the lateral intercostal–thoracoabdominal procedure may be complicated by pneumothorax or intravascular injection. Additionally, while Busby reported reasonable results in 28 patients, others have not been able to achieve the same success with this procedure. Ranney and Stanage wrote of this method, "... it [lateral intercostal block] seemed that more time and procaine were wasted than the process was worth."[1]

Rectus Abdominis Block

The rectus block takes advantage of the fact that the thoracoabdominal nerves course through the rectus sheath before branching to supply the lower abdominal wall. Ranney and Stanage suggest that by using this technique the amount of local anesthetic required is minimal with 1 percent procaine 60 ml usually providing adequate cesarean anesthesia.[1] (The author suggests the use of 1 percent chloroprocaine or 0.5 percent lidocaine.) They describe the procedure as follows (Fig. 7-24).

The anesthetic is first drawn up in 10-ml syringes fitted with 1.5-inch, 25-gauge needles. After raising a skin wheal 4 cm lateral to the umbilicus, the needle is directed just beneath the skin toward the umbilicus, infiltrating 2 ml as the needle advances. As the needle is withdrawn, the operator stops at three points to angle the tip just deep to the rectus fascia, as shown in Fig. 7-24. Approximately 1 ml of anesthetic is injected at each spot. Before the needle is fully withdrawn, its point is directed toward the pelvis, advanced beneath the skin, and used to create the next skin wheal, as shown in the figure. This process is repeated down to the pubis, the same process being repeated on the contralateral side. Next, a continuous subcutaneous wheal is created in the midline without deep infiltration. Finally, after the skin and subcutaneous tissues are opened, the fascia is directly infiltrated and incised. The visceral peritoneum may be handled as in the previous procedures.

In experienced hands, patient acceptance of this technique is remarkable. Ranney and Stanage reported that of 141 women who had had a cesarean delivery under rectus block anesthesia, 77 underwent a repeat cesarean and only three asked for a general anesthetic.[1] Despite this apparent patient approval, there are disadvantages to the rectus block. First, the procedure is associated with several complications, including toxic reactions from excessive doses or intravascular injection, unintentional injection directly into the uterus, and hematomas from laceration of abdominal wall vessels.[2] Second, while the theory behind injection into the rectus sheath may sound attractive, this anatomic compartment may be very hard to identify in the pregnant woman with a distended abdomen, diastasis recti, or marked obesity.

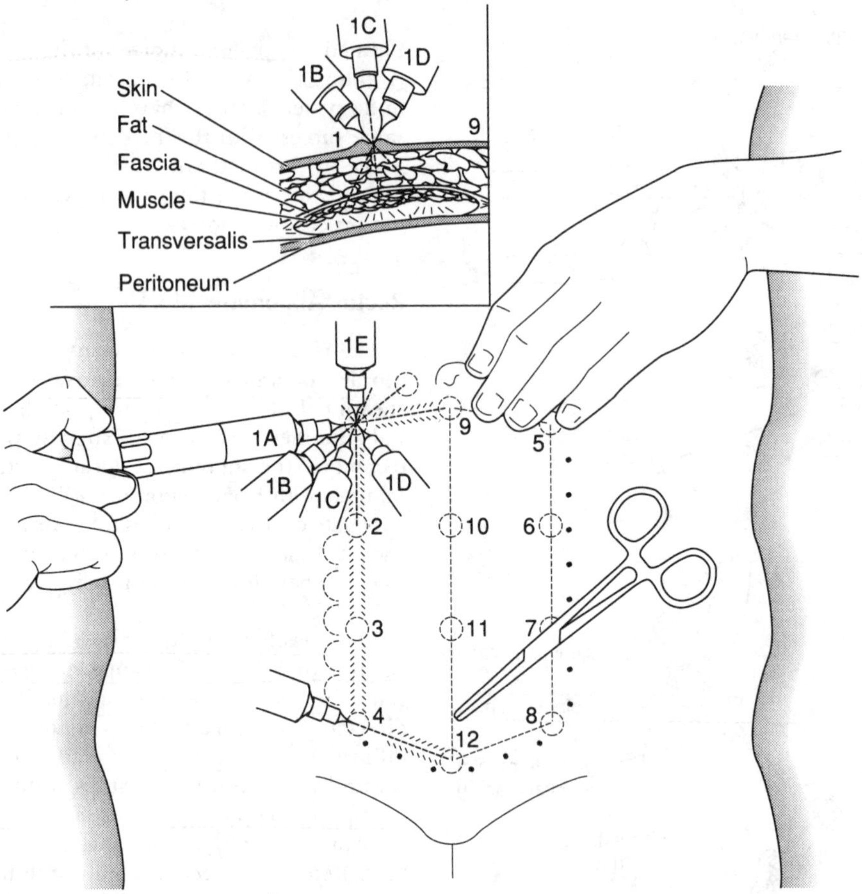

Fig. 7-24. Rectus block. Schematic diagram showing points for injection. (Inset: Detail of rectus compartment infiltration.) (From Ranney and Stanage,[1] with permission.)

In recognition of this, some authors recommend that rectus block anesthesia be performed only by persons with extensive experience with this technique in the nonpregnant patient, effectively excluding most obstetricians.[2]

Direct Local Infiltration

When a laboring patient must be delivered emergently and no one trained in anesthesia is available, the most reliable technique for anesthetizing the lower abdominal wall is simple local infiltration. This method requires no special knowledge of regional anesthesia and is not dependent on operator experience. Because local infiltration does not require repositioning of the patient or redraping of the sterile field, the procedure may be carried out rapidly by the delivering obstetrician.

The most important consideration in local infiltration for abdominal delivery is an awareness of the maximum recommended dose of the specific agent used. The maximum recommended dose of the local anesthetic agents commonly available in labor and delivery suites are reviewed in Table 7-10. Because the limits for toxicity for most agents will be rapidly achieved with the 200 to 300 ml needed for adequate anesthesia, Zuspan suggests that concentration of the available solutions should be halved, noting that this will not compromise the block needed for cesarean delivery.[5]

Local infiltration for cesarean delivery, as modified from Zuspan[5] and Bonica,[2] is begun by raising a 2-cm skin wheal just inferior to the umbilicus using a 5-cm, 25-gauge needle. Directed parallel to the skin, this needle is then used to infiltrate the intracutaneous tissue toward the pubis in a series of four to five injections (Fig. 7-25A). Using one hand for countertraction, care is taken to keep the needle just beneath the skin, not in the subcutaneous fat. Next, using a 10-cm, 22-gauge needle, the subcutaneous tissue is infiltrated with 6 to 8 ml of solution, again using countertraction and direct pressure on the needle point to ensure the tract con-

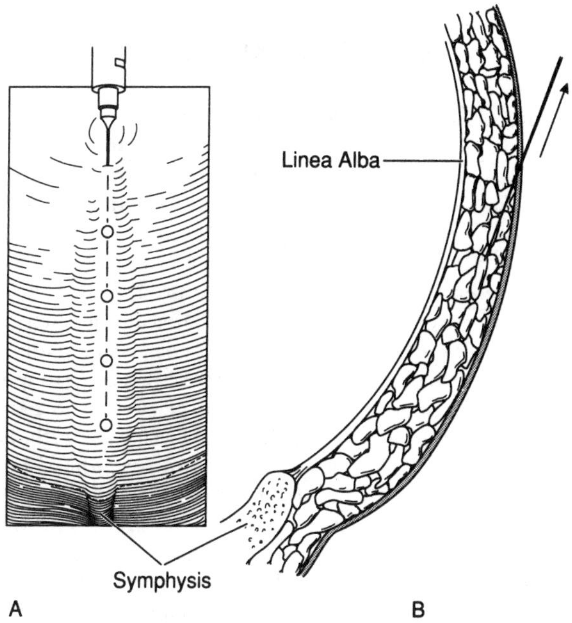

Fig. 7-25. Local infiltration of **(A)** the skin and **(B)** the subcutaneous tissue. (Modified from Bonica,[2] with permission.)

forms to the contour of the abdomen (Fig. 7-25). After 3 to 4 minutes, the skin may be gently incised. Lateral infiltration of the skin and subcutaneous tissue is not required. By gently separating the wound edges the fascia of the anterior medial border of each rectus sheath may be exposed for the next step. Using an 8-cm, 22-gauge needle, the rectus sheath is pierced, directing the needle laterally and down approximately 10 to 15 degrees (Fig. 7-26A). The needle is advanced 3 to 5 cm until its point is thought to be at the lateral posterior margin of the muscle. Two milliliters of solution are then injected and the needle slowly withdrawn while injecting another 1 to 2 ml. By repeating this step at 3-cm intervals toward the symphysis, a continuous layer of anesthetic is placed in the potential space between the muscle and the posterior fascia (Fig. 7-26B). This blocks the thoracoabdominal nerves as they traverse the rectus compartment, and produces anesthesia between the lateral margins of the two rectus muscles. After 3 to 5 minutes the fascia may be incised, exposing the parietal peritoneum. If the peritoneum is still sensitive, this may be anesthetized with direct infiltration or topical application of a local anesthetic. The visceral layers are handled as described for the previous methods.

SURGICAL CONSIDERATIONS

Realizing that with any of these local techniques the patient will be awake, anxious, and aware of her surroundings, the obstetrician has several additional responsibilities. First, he or she must ensure that all persons in the delivery room remain as quiet and calm as possible. The patient must be told to expect some minor discomfort and pressure intermittently throughout the operation. Additionally, she may experience moderate back pain with delivery of the fetus through the uterine incision. Importantly, surgical technique should be gentle. Retraction and stretching of tissues should be absolutely minimized. In modern obstetrics, there is no

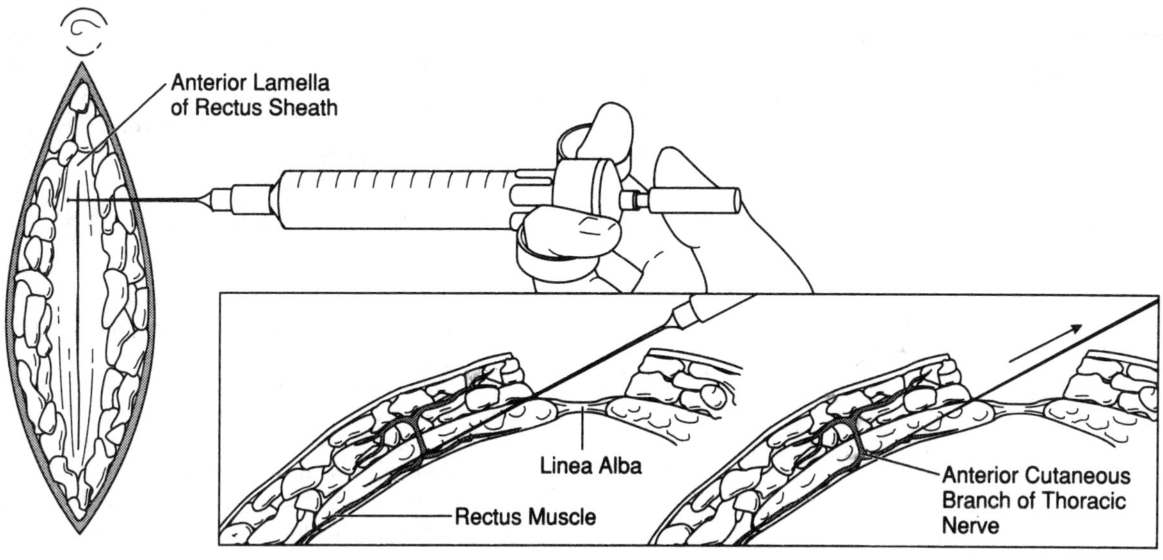

Fig. 7-26. **(A)** Local infiltration block. Injection of rectus muscle. (*Figure continues.*)

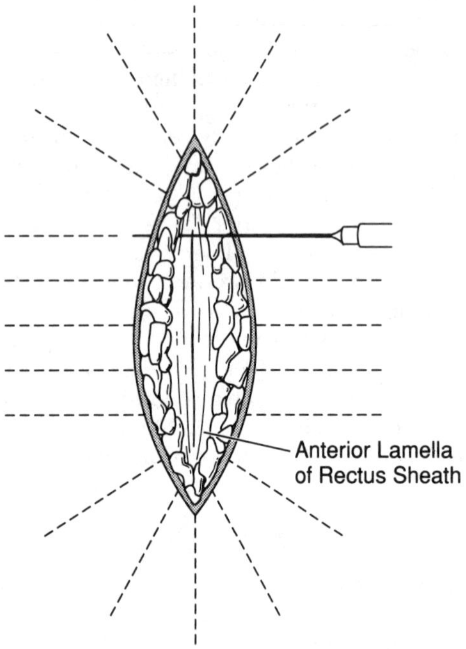

Fig. 7-26. (*Continued*). **(B)** Local infiltration block. Placement of successive rectus compartment injections. (From Bonica,[2] with permission.)

place for a transverse or Pfannenstiel incision when the delivery must be performed under local anesthesia. These incisions take longer, require more dissection, are associated with a greater potential for bleeding, and are not suited for any of the anesthetic techniques described in this section. Finally, although the operation may have already begun, the obstetrician should ensure that someone continues to try and reach trained anesthesia personnel.

REFERENCES

1. Ranney B, Stanage WF: Advantages of local anesthesia for cesarean section. Obstet Gynecol 45:163, 1975
2. Bonica JJ: Principles and Practice of Obstetric Analgesia and Anesthesia. p. 527. FA Davis, Philadelphia
3. Moore DC: Regional Block: A Handbook for Use in the Clinical Practice of Medicine and Surgery. 4th Ed. p. 280. Charles C Thomas, Springfield, IL, 1965
4. Busby T: Local anesthesia for cesarean section. Am J Obstet Gynecol 87:399, 1963
5. Zuspan KJ: Anesthesia and analgesia. p. 147. In Zuspan FP, Quilligan EJ (eds): Douglas-Stromme Operative Obstetrics. 5th Ed. Appleton & Lange, East Norwalk, CT

PARACERVICAL BLOCK

Paracervical block (PCB) involves injection of a local anesthetic, usually via the bilateral transvaginal approach, into the mucosae of the cervicouterine junction. Here lie fibers of the T10–T11 and L1 nerves, thus pain relief for the first stage of labor may be achieved by PCB. However, the uterine blood vessels and the fetal presenting part also lie in close proximity to these nerves. Consequently, maternal complications such as intravascular injection of local anesthetic and hematoma formation have been reported with PCB. Fetal complications such as bradycardia, acidosis, seizures, and perinatal death are hazards of PCB, owing to local anesthetic absorption by the uteroplacental unit and the fetus. Continuous monitoring of fetal heart rate and uterine contractions is mandatory if PCB is utilized. The immediate availability of adequate facilities for vaginal or cesarean delivery is essential if PCB is administered.

Because of the aforementioned maternal and fetal complications, PCB has not been used for obstetric pain relief at the Boston Hospital for Women and the Brigham and Women's Hospital for over 20 years. Therefore, although PCB is an excellent block for gynecologic procedures, it is not described or discussed in any more detail.

RESUSCITATIVE EQUIPMENT

Resuscitative equipment must be immediately available if a regional block is administered outside the delivery room. Of course, the delivery room must have the same type and quality of anesthetic equipment as a surgical operating room.

ADULT RESUSCITATIVE EQUIPMENT

1. Oxygen apparatus, including a source of 100 percent oxygen and a delivery system such as a bag and mask or any one of several commercially available reinflatable bag and mask kits.
2. Suctioning apparatus, essential to help clear the airway of secretions or other material if regurgitation of gastric contents of active vomiting occurs.
3. Airways: oral, nasal, and endotracheal. If the airway becomes compromised, then intubation should be performed with the aid of succinylcholine (1 to 1.5 mg/kg).

4. Laryngoscopes, with a variety of blades and sizes.
5. Electrocardiograph/cardiac defibrillator in combination and portable.
6. Board to be placed on the bed under the patient's chest to allow optimal closed-chest cardiac compression.

DRUGS

1. General: intravenous fluids, vasopressors, diphenhydramine, succinylcholine.
2. For central nervous system toxic reaction from unintentional intravascular injection or rapid systemic absorption: succinylcholine for endotracheal intubation and thiopental or diazepam for central nervous system depression.
3. For cardiopulmonary depression or arrest: vasopressors (epinephrine for myocardial stimulation/ephedrine for hypotension unresponsive to bolus infusion of intravenous fluids), sodium bicarbonate, calcium chloride, atropine, lidocaine, propranolol, isoproterenol, potassium chloride, digoxin, etc. Cardiopulmonary resuscitation must be initiated if a central nervous system toxic reaction or myocardial depression leads to severe cardiopulmonary collapse or arrest.

UNINTENTIONAL INTRAVASCULAR INJECTION

Treatment of a central nervous system reaction secondary to unintentional intravascular injection includes the following steps:

1. Maintain an adequate airway for effective ventilation (endotracheal intubation may be necessary).
2. Administer 100 percent oxygen by mask and bag or by intermittent positive-pressure ventilation if necessary.
3. Use succinylcholine to facilitate endotracheal intubation if necessary.
4. Administer an ultra-short-acting barbiturate (e.g., thiopental) in incremental doses of 50 mg or intravenous diazepam in incremental doses of 2.5 mg to stop the convulsions.
5. Monitor maternal vital signs.
6. Monitor fetal heart rate.
7. Place the parturient in the lateral position and continue to administer oxygen.
8. Treat hypotension with an infusion of crystalloid solution and/or ephedrine in increments of 10 mg intravenously as needed.
9. Expedite delivery if the mother and/or fetus is in jeopardy, otherwise delay delivery to permit maternal disposal of local anesthetic.
10. Continue cardiopulmonary resuscitation as needed.
11. If closed-chest cardiac compression is necessary because of low cardiac output or cardiac arrest, raise the legs and manually displace the uterus to increase venous return.
12. Emergency vaginal or cesarean delivery may be necessary to maximize venous return for effective cardiopulmonary resuscitation.

Oxygenation is the key to the successful management of this problem. It is *mandatory* that resuscitative equipment and appropriate drugs be immediately available when any local anesthetic is administered by whatever route.

UNINTENTIONAL SUBARACHNOID INJECTION

The same technique as for treatment of unintentional intravascular injection is utilized, with the exception that depression of the central nervous system with diazepam or thiopental is not necessary. Thiopental may be used to induce sleep, however, which is then maintained by an inhalational technique.

1. Place the patient in the Trendelenberg position as soon as possible after the injection occurs to attempt to limit the spread, since most epidural anesthetic solutions are hypobaric in the subarachnoid space.
2. If possible, attempt to aspirate at least 10 ml of cerebrospinal fluid and local anesthetic from the subarachnoid space to decrease the amount of local anesthetic in contact with the spinal cord and nerves.

CARDIAC ARREST AND CARDIOPULMONARY RESUSCITATION IN THE OBSTETRIC PATIENT

Cardiac arrest in late pregnancy or during delivery is a rare event. Unfortunately, when it occurs, maternal survival is very low because the etiology of the arrest is not often reversed and the physiologic changes present in late pregnancy often hamper effective cardiopulmonary resuscitative efforts.

Some causes of cardiac arrest in the parturient at term include:

1. Total spinal anesthetic
2. Local anesthetic toxicity from unintentional intravascular injection
3. Trauma
4. Pulmonary embolism
5. Amniotic fluid embolism

PHYSIOLOGIC CHANGES OF PREGNANCY AS THEY RELATE TO CARDIOPULMONARY RESUSCITATION

Term pregnant patients are at a distinct disadvantage during cardiac arrest. They become hypoxic more readily because of a 20 percent decrease in their functional residual capacity and a 20 percent increase in their resting oxygen consumption.[1] The enlarged uterus along with the resultant upward displacement of the abdominal viscera will decrease compliance during controlled ventilation. The most serious problem is the effect of aortocaval compression in the supine position. During closed-chest cardiac compression (CCCC) in adults, the best cardiac output that can be achieved is between one-fourth to one-third of normal. Although many factors contribute to this, poor venous return to the heart is of paramount importance. At term, the vena cava is completely occluded in 90 percent of supine pregnant patients, resulting in a decrease in cardiac stroke volume of as much as 70 percent.

TREATMENT OF MATERNAL CARDIAC ARREST

The resuscitation of a pregnant patient at term is unlikely to be successful unless this vena caval compression can be eliminated. To accomplish this, a wedge must be placed under the right hip to displace the gravid uterus to the left. Rees and Willis[2] have shown that effective CCCC can be accomplished with a patient tilted at a 30 degree angle to the left. Cardiopulmonary resuscitation should begin immediately by securing the airway and following current advanced cardiac life support guidelines. If aggressive cardiopulmonary resuscitation with a properly positioned patient is not successful after 5 minutes, cesarean delivery must be performed as soon as possible.[3,4] This procedure will immediately relieve the vena caval obstruction from the gravid uterus and increase the chance of survival for both the infant and the mother. Cardiopulmonary resuscitation must be continued throughout the procedure until spontaneous and effective cardiac activity occurs. Controlled ventilation may have to be continued for a longer period of time. This aggressive approach to management will increase survival rates for mothers and neonates.

REFERENCES

1. Zakowski MI, Ramanathan S: CPR in pregnancy. Cur Rev Clin Anesth (Review) 10:106, 1990
2. Rees GAD, Willis BA: Resuscitation in late pregnancy. Anesthesia 43:347, 1988
3. Oates S, Williams GL, Rees GAD: Cardiopulmonary resuscitation in late pregnancy. Br Med J 297:404, 1988
4. Marx G: Cardiopulmonary resuscitation of late pregnant women. Anesthesiology 56:156, 1982

THE BRIGHAM AND WOMEN'S HOSPITAL EXPERIENCE

Table 7-11. Obstetric Anesthesia Statistics

	Vaginal Deliveries					Cesarean Deliveries		Total
Year	Epidural	Subarachnoid	Inhalational	Other[a]	Total	No.	%	Deliveries
1962–63[b]	246	3,789	1,034[c]	396	5,465	501	8	5,966
1968–69	1,198	4,563	256	645	6,662	594	8	7,256
1969–70	2,007	4,128	322	799	7,256	687	9	7,943
1970–71	2,299	3,145	293	817	6,554	743	10	7,297
1971–72	2,070	2,171	107[d]	810	5,158	700	12	5,858
1972–73	2,414	1,606	44	1,011	5,075	907	15	5,982
1973–74	2,319	1,462	40	1,071	4,892	1,159	19	6,051
1974–75	2,345	1,122	56	1,317	4,840	1,195	20	6,035
1975–76	2,492	923	32	1,467	4,914	1,255	20	6,169
1976–77	2,451	709	32	1,701	4,893	1,359	22	6,242
1977–78	2,571	570	30	2,196	5,367	1,455	21	6,822
1978–79	2,223	391	23	2,005	4,642	1,383	23	6,025
1979–80	2,303	346	18	2,099	4,766	1,512	24	6,278
1980–81	2,236	277	12	2,914	5,439	1,509	22	6,948
1981–82	2,319	237	12	3,074	5,642	1,784	24	7,426
1982–83	2,432	200	4	3,614	6,250	1,841	23	8,091
1983–84	2,755	149	7	3,633	6,544	2,103	24	8,647
1984–85	3,025	143	2	3,747	6,917	2,324	25	9,241
1985–86	3,518	134	3	3,526	7,181	2,547	26	9,728
1986–87	3,818	111	3	3,324	7,256	2,622	26	9,878
1987–88	3,927	83	6	3,459	7,475	2,643	26	10,118
1988–89	4,208	46	3	3,364	7,621	2,409	24	10,030
1989–90	4,413	43	6	3,460	7,922	2,422	23	10,344

[a] Includes local infiltration and pudendal block.
[b] Inadequate statistics available for 1963 to 1968.
[c] Mask or endotracheal intubation.
[d] Endotrachial intubation only.

Table 7-12. Statistics for Anesthesia for Cesarean Delivery

	Epidural		Subarachnoid		General		Total	
Year	No.	%	No.	%	No.	%	No.	% of all deliveries
1974–75[a]	118	10	524	44	552	46	1,195	20
1975–76[b]	171	14	529	42	566	44	1,266	20
1976–77	288	21	483	36	588	43	1,359	22
1977–78[a]	286	20	609	42	559	38	1,455	21
1978–79	358	26	502	36	523	38	1,383	23
1979–80	429	28	477	32	606	40	1,512	24
1980–81	477	32	568	38	453	30	1,509	22
1981–82[a]	586	33	758	42	439	25	1,784	24
1982–83	735	40	656	36	450	24	1,841	23
1983–84	844	40	760	36	499	24	2,103	24
1984–85	1,239	53	651	28	434	19	2,324	25
1985–86	1,300	51	792	31	455	18	2,547	26
1986–87	1,336	51	914	35	372	14	2,622	26
1987–88	1,399	53	944	36	300	11	2,643	26
1988–89	1,272	53	927	38	210	9	2,409	24
1989–90	1,307	54	921	38	194	8	2,422	23

[a] One hypnosis.
[b] Approximate.

Table 7-13. Obstetric Anesthesia Statistics for the Period October 1989 to September 1990

Primary Anesthetic	No.	%
Vaginal delivery		
Subarachnoid[a]	43	0.5
Epidural	4,413	55.7
General	6	0.08
Local	2,445	30.9
No anesthesia	1,015	12.8
Unrecorded	0	0.0
TOTAL	7,922	100.0
Cesarean delivery		
Subarachnoid[a]	921	38.0
Epidural	1,307	54.0
General	194	8.0
TOTAL	2,422	100.0

[a] 27 g. Quincke needle.

Table 7-14. Adequacy of Anesthesia According to Type of Delivery and Type of Anesthesia for the Period October 1989 to September 1990

Type of Anesthesia	No.	%
Vaginal Delivery		
Epidural		
Adequate anesthesia	4,050	91.8
Suppl./local	350	7.7
Suppl./subarach.	13	0.3
Suppl./general	0	0.0
TOTAL	4,413	100.0
Subarachnoid		
Adequate anesthesia	43	100.0
Supplement with local	0	0.0
Supplement with general	0	0.0
TOTAL	43	100.0
Cesarean delivery		
Epidural		
Adequate anesthesia	1,189	91.0
Supplement with subarachnoid	49	3.7
Supplement with general	69	5.3
TOTAL	1,307	100.0
Subarachnoid		
Adequate anesthesia	906	98.4
Supplement with general	15	1.6
TOTAL	921	100.0

Table 7-15. Post-Dural Puncture Headache and Treatment with Blood Patch

Type of Anesthesia	No. Patients (%)	Type of Anesthesia	No. Patients (%)
Subarachnoid	1,027[a]	Epidural	5,720
Headaches	34 (3.3)	Dural punctures	140
Blood patches	13 (1.3)[b]	Headaches	96 (1.7)[c]
		Blood patches	66 (1.2)[d]

[a] Includes 1 case of subarachnoid anesthesia as a failed continuous spinal anesthesia and 62 cases in which subarachnoid anesthesia was used as supplementation.
[b] 38.2% of headaches were treated with a blood patch.
[c] 68.6% of dural punctures resulted in headache.
[d] 68.8% of headaches were treated with a blood patch.

Table 7-16. Dural Puncture, Headache and Epidural Blood Patch Incidence in Epidural Anesthesia

Year	No. Epidural Anesthesias	No. Dural Punctures (%)	No. Headaches (%)	No. Epidural Blood Patches (%)
1984–85	4,264	81 (1.9)	52 (64.2)	33 (63)
1985–86	4,818	75 (1.6)	53 (70.7)	32 (60.4)
1986–87	5,154	70 (1.4)	50 (71.4)	30 (60)
1987–88	5,326	75 (1.4)	53 (70.7)	41 (77.4)
1988–89	5,480	97 (1.8)	65 (67)	45 (73.8)
1989–90	5,720	140 (2.4)	96 (68.6)	66 (68.8)

Table 7-17. Post-Dural Puncture Headache and Epidural Blood Patch Incidence in Subarachnoid Anesthesia

Year	No. Subarachnoid Anesthesia	No. Headaches (%)	No. Patches (%)
1984–85[a]	857	59 (6.9)	14 (23.7)
1985–86[a]	997	79 (7.9)	15 (18.9)
1986–87[a]	1,079	72 (6.7)	19 (26.4)
1987–88[a]	1,027	60 (5.6)	18 (30.0)
1988–89[a]	1,031	48 (4.7)	17 (35.4)
1989–90[b]	752	20 (2.7)	6 (30)
1990–1991[c,d]	709	9 (1.3)	1 (11.1)

[a] 26g Quincke point B–D spinal needles.
[b] 27g Quincke point B–D spinal needles.
[c] 25g Whitacre pencil point B–D spinal needles.
[d] October 1990 through June 1991.

Table 7-18. Incidence of Post-Dural Puncture Headache According to Medication Used and Needle Size for the period October 1989 to September 1990

	No. Patients	No. Headaches	%
Medication			
Bupivacaine	43	2	4.7[a]
Tetracaine/procaine	0	0	0.0
Lidocaine	18	3	16.7[a]
Bupivacaine/fentanyl	875	26	2.9[a]
Lidocaine/fentanyl	14	1	7.1[a]
Medication unrecorded	34	2	5.9
Tetracaine/fentanyl	0	0	0.0
No medication given	1	0	0.0
Bupivacaine/lidocaine	1	0	0.0[a]
Bupivacaine/alfentanil	22	0	0.0
Bupivacaine/sufentanil	18	0	0.0
Bupivacaine/lidocaine/fentanyl	1	0	0.0[a]
Needle size			
17-gauge needle			
Bupivacaine/lidocaine	1	0	0.0
Bupivacaine/lidocaine/fentanyl	1	0	0.0
22-gauge needle			
Lidocaine/fentanyl	1	0	0.0
26-gauge needle			
Bupivacaine	1	0	0.0
Lidocaine	2	0	0.0
Bupivacaine/fentanyl	1	0	0.0

[a] Continuous spinal anesthesia.

POST-DURAL PUNCTURE HEADACHE

The first use of subarachnoid anesthesia is often attributed to Corning because of his experiments with intraspinal injections of cocaine in 1885. In 1891, Quincke reported on the diagnostic and therapeutic use of lumbar dural puncture to drain cerebrospinal fluid (CSF) from patients with hydrocephalus. The first diagnosis of post-dural puncture headache (PDPH) was made by August Bier in 1898, when he observed four of six patients on whom he had performed subarachnoid anesthesia develop headaches.[1] As with many early investigators of regional anesthesia, he experimented on himself. His assistant, Dr. Hildebrandt, attempted to administer a subarachnoid anesthetic to Bier using a "fine hollow needle." Unfortunately, the syringe did not fit properly and much CSF, along with the cocaine, was lost, resulting in an ineffective anesthetic. Bier then successfully performed a subarachnoid anesthetic on Hildebrandt.

"After these experiments on our own bodies we both went to dinner without any physical complaints. We drank wine and smoked several cigars. I went to bed at 11 o'clock and slept well throughout the night. I awoke, feeling refreshed and well the next morning, and went for a walk for an hour. Toward 3 P.M., my face turned pale; the pulse was rather faint but remained regular, and was about 70 beats per minute. Furthermore, I had the sensation of a very strong pressure in my head and felt dizzy when I arose quickly from my chair. All these symptoms disappeared as soon as I lay down horizontally but they returned when I arose in the late afternoon. Therefore, I had to go to bed, and I stayed in bed for nine days, since all the described symptoms returned whenever I tried to arise."

"Dr. Hildebrandt felt very well when he went to bed at 11 P.M., however, he could not fall asleep because he was affected by restlessness. At midnight, violent headaches occurred, which increased gradually to an unbearable degree. At 1 A.M. vomiting began, which recurred once during the night. Dr. Hildebrandt felt very poor the next morning, but with great physical effort he was able to do his work, which consisted mainly in operating and dressing of wounds. He had to go to bed in the afternoon, but he arose again the next morning and did his work although he still did not feel well for three or four days. He again had headaches."

Even though this experiment was performed in 1898, Bier's observations and conclusions are still valid today. He noted the headache was postural and that it was related to loss of CSF, and not to the local anesthetic itself (not in the above quote, however).

CLINICAL FEATURES

The PDPH is classically described as beginning when the patient sits or stands upright, and it is relieved upon reclining or assuming the supine position. It is aggravated by coughing and sudden movements. The headache is usually a dull aching pressure or heaviness, which characteristically begins in the occipital region and often spreads over the top of the head to the frontal region behind the eyes. Reflex spasm of the cervical muscles may occur and the pain also may radiate down the neck. It can be mild to incapacitating and the patient usually describes it as unlike any previous headache.

The onset of PDPH can occur immediately or up to several days after dural puncture. Vandam and Dripps reported the average time to be within the first 48 hours of the postoperative period.[2] This may correlate with the time the patient begins to ambulate. The duration of the headache can be from hours to months (if left untreated). However, Vandam and Dripps found that most headaches resolved after 4 days.[2]

The associated symptoms include nausea and vomiting, depression, visual changes, and auditory disturbances. Vandam and Dripps reported a triad that consisted of a PDPH in association with ocular and auditory dysfunction and called it "the syndrome of decreased intracranial pressure."[2] They noted a 0.4 percent incidence of visual difficulties, including diplopia, blurred vision, and photophobia. They also observed six cases of transient lateral rectus muscle paralysis. These symptoms may be secondary to cranial nerve (abducens VI) stretching associated with decreased CSF volume.[3] They also described 0.4 percent incidence of auditory difficulties, including decreased acuity, tinnitus, and a sensation of "ear popping." These symptoms might also be secondary to decreased CSF pressure, as there are anatomic communications between endolymph canals and CSF.[4]

Headache in the setting of a recent dural puncture may not necessarily be a PDPH. There are other serious causes for headache that should be ruled out (Tables 7-19 and 7-20).

Table 7-19. Differential Diagnosis of Headache

Meningitis
Cerebral hemorrhage (subdural, subarachnoid)
Cerebral infarction (cortical vein thrombosis)
Hypertensive crises
Migraine
Metabolic (electrolyte imbalance, hypoglycemia)
Psychogenic (postpartum)
Hormonal imbalance

Table 7-20. Evaluation of Headache Not Caused by Dural Puncture

History
Characteristics
Prior history of headaches
Family history of headaches
History of depression
Associated symptoms
Physical examination
Vital signs: temperature, blood pressure, heart respiratory rate
General appearance
Neck signs
Neurologic exam
Mental status
Sensory, motor and reflexes
Gait/positional alterations of headache symptoms
Laboratory work-up
Complete blood count, electrolytes, glucose, electrocardiogram
Computed tomography scan, diagnostic dural puncture, electromyelogram (neurologic consult)

PATHOPHYSIOLOGY

The etiology of PDPH is complex and multifactorial. One of the major components is loss of CSF through the dural puncture site with resultant reduction in CSF pressure. Normal lumbar CSF pressure is 5 to 15 cmH_2O in the horizontal position. It increases to over 40 cmH_2O in the erect position, whereas the pressure in the epidural space remains close to atmospheric in either position. Therefore, in the erect position a pressure gradient of 40 to 50 cmH_2O exists, favoring leakage of CSF from the subarachnoid space into the epidural space.[5] Multiple studies have supported the correlation between PDPH and reduction in CSF volume (and pressure).[6–8] Kunkle et al. found they were consistently able to induce the symptoms of PDPH in normal human subjects in the erect position by free drainage of 20 ml of CSF.[9] The headache could then be decreased in intensity by tipping the patient to the horizontal position, and completely relieved by artificially raising the CSF pressure to normal with a subarachnoid injection of saline solution. Other investigators have found the headache symptoms could be relieved by raising the epidural space pressure with saline[10] or blood.[11]

The acute reduction of CSF volume reduces the CSF's cushioning effect on the brain. Theoretically, this can cause downward traction on pain-sensitive structures (intracranial sinuses, vessels, nerves, and cerebral tentorium). Above the tentorium, the pain is referred via the trigeminal nerve to the frontal region of the head. Below the tentorium, the pain is referred via the vagus and glossopharyngeal nerve to the occiput. Pain in the upper neck and shoulder regions is referred via the upper three cervical nerves.[12]

Another component of PDPH may be cerebral vasodilatation. The intracranial pressure is determined by the volume of three compartments within the fixed intracranial space: cerebral blood volume (5 to 8 percent), brain tissue (85 percent), and CSF (7 to 10 percent). A loss of CSF volume leads to a reflex vasodilatation of the cerebral vessels to increase cerebral blood volume. A reduction in the volume of one of the intracranial components is balanced by an increase in the volume of another. This vasodilatation may stimulate perivascular stretch receptors similar to one of the mechanisms of migraine headache.

Certain patient populations seem to be at increased risk for PDPH. These include younger patients, female patients, and pregnant or postpartum patients.[2,5,13,14] The incidence of PDPH is remarkably lower in the elderly (age greater than 60 years). Although the reasons are not clearly understood, older patients do have a less dynamic CSF circulation and lower CSF pressures. A lower initial CSF pressure at the time of dural puncture may result in a reduced gradient for leakage. In addition the cerebrospinal vessels of the elderly may be less reactive to volume changes. Finally, the constitution of connective tissue (and possibly, the dura) changes with age and this may aid in rapid closure of the dural leak.

The incidence of PDPH in the obstetric patient is about twice the incidence observed in the nonobstetric population. At our institution, there has been about a 6 percent incidence of PDPH after subarachnoid anesthesia in our obstetric population over a 5-year period (see Table 7-17 in the previous section). The higher incidence of PDPH in the obstetric patient is also multifactorial.[14] The peripartum patient is predisposed to intravascular volume depletion from diuresis, vomiting, diaphoresis, blood loss with delivery, and oral fluid restriction. This may contribute to slower CSF regeneration. During labor, the CSF pressure is transiently increased with bearing down, and this may favor a leak gradient across a dural puncture site. The increase in abdominal pressure during pregnancy results in distended epidural vessels and concomitant reduction of the epidural volume. With resolution of the aortocaval compression after delivery, epidural venous engorgement subsides, resulting in a reduction of epidural space pressure. This may also favor a leakage gradient. The higher incidence of PDPH in young women persists even when obstetric patients are excluded from consideration.

PREVENTION

The use of small-gauge needles for dural puncture and needle insertion with the bevel parallel to the dural fibers are techniques reported to reduce the incidence of PDPH. Other technical factors that may reduce the incidence of PDPH include bevel design, angle of needle approach, patient positioning, anesthetic agents used, and possibly, the use of a catheter for continuous infusion.

Needle Diameter

Many studies have correlated spinal needle diameter and the incidence of PDPH (Table 7-21). In 1968, Phillips et al. reviewed 10,440 subarachnoid anesthetics.

Table 7-21. Relationship of Needle Size to Incidence of Headache

Study	Needle Size	Headache Incidence (%)
Green (1950)[15]	20 g	33.3
	26 g	0.4
Vandam and Dripps (1956)[2]	16 g	18.0
	20 g	14.0
	24 g	6.0
Tarrow (1963)[16]	16 g	18.0
	19 g	10.0
	25 g	0.2
White (1962)[17]	22 g	9.5
	25 g	5.1
Phillips et al. (1968)[13]	25/26 g	3.5

This study was comparable in magnitude, data gathering, and protocol to the Vandam and Dripps study of 1956. However, Phillips et al. obtained a significantly lower overall incidence of PDPH (3.5 percent versus 11 percent). They attributed this difference to needle size as 82 percent of the spinal needles they used were 25- and 26-gauge, whereas 82 percent of the needles used by Vandam and Dripps were 20- and 22-gauge. Their finding was noteworthy considering the susceptibility of the patient population studied (99 percent were female, with a mean age of 25).[13]

Other studies have demonstrated an extremely small incidence of PDPH when 29- to 32-gauge needles are used.[18–20] These ultrafine needles require an introducer system because they are so flexible and fragile, and may have a higher failure rate.

Bevel Direction

In 1926, Green postulated that dural puncture with the needle bevel parallel to the dural fibers would result in a smaller defect, and that this would decrease the amount of CSF leak.[21] Dural punctures with the bevel perpendicular to the fibers are likely to cause greater anatomic damage, thus hindering rapid closure of the leak. In 1946, Franksson and Gordh confirmed this hypothesis by examining dura from patients who underwent dural puncture just prior to death. They found, using light microscopy, approximately twice the number of severed fibers when the dura was punctured at right angles.[22]

Mihic, in 1985, provided additional clinical evidence by reporting a significantly higher number of PDPH when the dura was punctured perpendicularly. In fact, he stopped piercing the dura with the bevel perpendicular after 62 patients because of the extremely high incidence of PDPH (16.1 percent versus 0.24 percent).[23] Norris et al. recommend identifying the epidural space with the needle bevel oriented parallel to the dural fibers, as they found a lower incidence of PDPH if unintentional dural puncture occurred.[24]

Bevel Design

The configuration of the needle point may affect the incidence of PDPH. A needle with a cutting bevel edge may cause more damage to the dura than a conical-point needle (Whitacre). This needle may separate instead of lacerate the dural fibers, resulting in less CSF leak.[23,24] These needles have been seldom used because of the difficulty with needle positioning associated with a dull point.[25] However, our initial experience with a disposable 25-gauge Whitacre needle is extremely encouraging.

Needle Angle

The angle at which the dura is pierced might influence the size and nature of the dural hole. In 1977, Hatfalvi reported a series of over 600 subarachnoid blocks using a 20-gauge needle in which he had no PDPH and attributed this finding to the paramedian approach.[27] Using an in vitro model with samples of human dura, Ready et al. found a 30 degree angle of approach to the dural resulted in significantly lower CSF leak rates than with a similar needle used at 60 or 90 degrees.[28] Since the holes made in the contiguous layers of the dura by a paramedian approach do not overlap, a seal might be formed (Fig. 7-27).

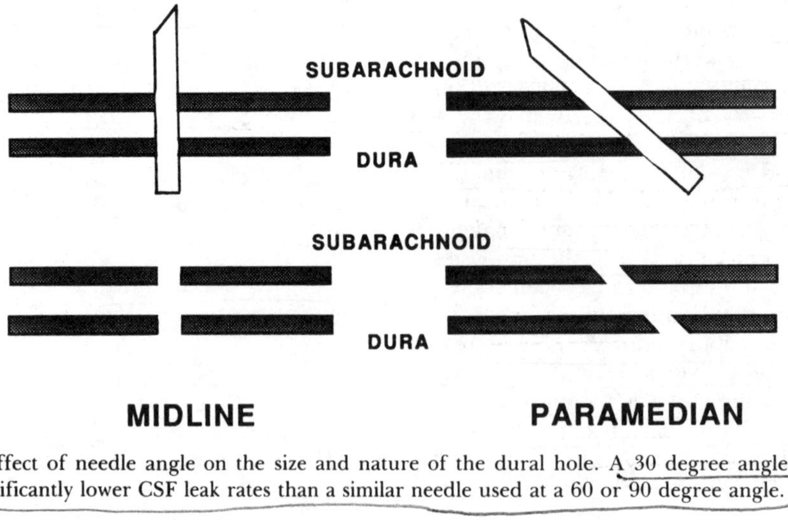

Fig. 7-27. Effect of needle angle on the size and nature of the dural hole. A 30 degree angle of approach results in significantly lower CSF leak rates than a similar needle used at a 60 or 90 degree angle.

Patient Position

Patients are generally placed in a flexed position to facilitate the insertion of a spinal needle through the midline. This position may place tension on the dura, resulting in an extended tear at the dural puncture site. Ash, in 1955, and Rosser and Schneider, in 1956, suggested that there may be an advantage to an "unflexed back position."[29,30] Ash observed a 6 percent incidence of PDPH when using the prone position to perform subarachnoid blocks. Rosser found only a 0.54 percent incidence by keeping the back in a "comfortably neutral" position (i.e., the patient was in the lateral position with the back neither flexed or extended). These reported incidences of PDPH are lower than expected considering both investigators used 20- to 22-gauge spinal needles and 40 percent of Rosser's patients were pregnant. The fact that these investigators often used the paramedian approach when the midline approach was unsuccessful (in the unflexed back position) may account for their low reported incidence of PDPH.

Agent Used

In their 1956 review, Vandam and Dripps concluded that the particular local anesthetic agent used for subarachnoid block had no relationship to the incidence of PDPH[2]; this concept is still accepted. However, in a recent abstract, Naulty et al. suggested that certain local anesthetic agents may correlate with a higher incidence of PDPH (lidocaine > bupivacaine > tetracaine-procaine mixture).[31] They also implicated the use of dextrose in the anesthetic solution as possibly increasing the incidence of PDPH. Other investigators have noted the addition of epinephrine[32] or fentanyl[33] may lower the incidence of PDPH.

Continuous Subarachnoid Anesthesia

Until recently, continuous subarachnoid anesthesia (CSA) has not been a popular technique because of the concern that dural puncture with a large-bore needle would result in an unacceptably high incidence of PDPH. However, with the exception of the Guiffrida et al. study in 1972, recent work has indicated that the incidence of PDPH after CSA might be surprisingly low[34–39] (Table 7-22).

It can be argued that a CSA catheter may stent open the dural puncture, resulting in greater CSF leak. Conversely, the catheter may actually occlude the dural hole while in place, thus minimizing CSF leakage into the epidural space. Finally, the catheter may precipitate an inflammatory reaction, which may hasten the closure of the dural defect when it is removed.

Table 7-22. Incidence of Headache following Dural Puncture According to Needle Size

Study	Needle Size	Headache Incidence (%)
1972—Giuffrida et al. (cesarean delivery patients)[34]	21 g	16
1972—Kallos and Smith[35]	18 g	0
1983—Peterson et al.[36]	18 g	0
1987—Denny et al.[37]	18 g	<1
1988—Giuffrida et al. (Vascular surgery patients)[38]	21 g	<2
1989—Hurley and Lambert[39]	26 g	4

The data on CSA are difficult to interpret because the patient populations vary and the group of patients selected for CSA may already have been at low risk for PDPH because of their age. Giuffrida et al. found a relatively high incidence of PDPH. Their patient population were pregnant women undergoing cesarean delivery.

Microcatheters (32-gauge) are presently being developed and tested for use with 26- and 28-gauge spinal needles, which may further diminish the incidence of PDPH,[39] although it is too early to tell.

MANAGEMENT OF AN UNINTENTIONAL DURAL PUNCTURE ("WET TAP") AND POST-DURAL PUNCTURE HEADACHE

Unintentional Dural Puncture

The incidence of unintentional dural puncture ("wet tap") associated with epidural placement is 1 to 2 percent at the Brigham and Women's Hospital, and the associated incidence of PDPH in the obstetric population is about 70 percent[12,40,41] (see Table 7-16 in the previous section). When an unintentional dural puncture occurs, the needle should be withdrawn and replaced at a more cephalad interspace with the catheter directed cephalad or at a more caudad interspace with the catheter directed caudad. Obtaining a block at a different level may reduce the incidence of PDPH. This is probably because the volume of local anesthetic in the epidural space reduces the pressure gradient between the subarachnoid space and the epidural space, minimizing CSF leak and optimizing early dural closure. In this situation, it is important to use a minimal amount of air if the loss-of-resistance technique is being used. Air injected into the epidural space may transverse across the dural puncture, resulting in an immediate, severe headache from an unintentional pneumoencephalocele. When inserting the catheter at the different interspace, it is wise to direct it away from the interspace where the unintentional dural puncture occurred. Careful observation is required as injection of local anesthetics into the epidural space may result in some local anesthetic transversing the dural hole, resulting in subarachnoid instead of epidural anesthesia.[42,43]

Post-Dural Puncture Headache

Conservative Therapy. Conservative treatment is used first because PDPH is usually self-limiting and often only mild to moderate in intensity. The first rule of conservative therapy for PDPH is bed rest in the supine position. Having the patient lie flat after dural puncture will not prevent PDPH and is no longer recommended.[44–46] In fact, longer recumbency predisposes the patient to an increased incidence of nausea,[46] delayed diagnosis of PDPH, and possible thromboembolism. The role for recumbency is *after* the diagnosis of PDPH is made, as most patients get excellent relief by lying supine. Other conservative therapy includes oral or intravenous hydration to allow increased CSF production and analgesics (acetominophen, ibuprofen, or other nonsteroidal anti-inflammatory drugs (NSAIDs) to relieve symptoms. The authors and the editor have had excellent success with NSAIDs instead of aspirin-like compounds. The editor does not use Fiorinal because many patients complain of a "barbiturate hangover." Abdominal binders and varying the patient's position to increase venous return are not well tolerated and have not proven effective.[46,47]

Caffeine. Some investigators have reported that intravenous caffeine therapy (caffeine benzoate 500 mg) at multiple intervals reduces the duration and extent of PDPH.[48,49] Camann et al. used a single oral dose of caffeine (300 mg) and found improvement in PDPH, although this effect was transient in 30 percent of their patients.[50] The basis of using caffeine in the treatment of PDPH comes from the observation that a loss in CSF volume leads to a reflex vasodilatation in the cerebral vessels. It is postulated that the pain of PDPH is due to this reactive hyperemia and subsequent stretch of vascular receptors in the cerebral vessels, similar to the etiology of migraine headache. Therefore, caffeine may work by constricting such vessels.

Saline Infusion. Studies have shown that bolus injection or continuous infusion of saline into the epidural space via epidural catheter may be effective in reducing the pain of PDPH, especially when the dural puncture is secondary to a misadventure with a 17-gauge epidural needle.[51,52] Such infusions probably work by increasing volume and, therefore, pressure in the epidural space, thereby reducing the transdural gradient and the extent of the CSF leak. Unfortunately, the rise in epidural pressure with saline is transient and the PDPH often recurs.[10] Whether given by bolus injection or continuous infusion for treatment or prophylaxis the results with epidural saline are not as good as the epidural blood patch with autologous blood.[51,53–55]

Epidural Blood Patch. Use of an autologous epidural blood patch (EBP) as a treatment for PDPH was first described by Gormley in 1960 and has been widely practiced since.[14,56,57] The success rate of the EBP is excellent (above 90 percent). The blood should be

Table 7-23. Protocol for Epidural Blood Patch

1. Review chart, obtain written informed consent
2. Check baseline vital signs
3. Insert IV line; acute hydration with warm crystalloid (about 1 L)
4. IV sedation/narcotics prn (fentanyl, 50–100 μg, midazolam 1 mg, metoclopramide 10 mg)
5. Oxygen by mask prn (5–6 L/min)
6. Position patient slowly, preferably in lateral position to avoid worsening headache
7. Identify epidural space, preferably with loss of resistance to fluid technique. Hanging-drop technique is less preferable because the "vacuum" in the epidural space may be lessened after a dural puncture. If using loss of resistance to air technique, use minimal amount (see text).
   a) Use same space as dural puncture
   b) If more than one dural puncture, use lowest interspace
   c) Preferable to use midline approach
8. Using sterile technique, withdraw 20 ml blood from arm opposite the IV line. It is easier to draw from the dependent arm.
9. Maintaining sterile technique, inject blood into the epidural space about 1 ml/3–4 seconds. Usual dose is 10–20 ml. If pain or pressure (back, leg, buttock) is noted before 15 ml, stop and let pressure recede. Continue only if there is no exacerbation of discomfort.
10. Turn patient supine; place blankets under knees to flatten lumbar lordosis
11. Let patient rest 30 minutes and continue IV fluids (remainder of first liter)
12. After 30 minutes, raise head of bed in stages while continually assessing patient for PDPH symptoms.
13. After patient is sitting upright, post EBP orders:
    a) Avoid straining (from vomiting, stool, etc.) and heavy lifting for 5 days
    b) Limited activity (encourage bed rest) first 24 hours
    c) Compazine 5 mg PO/IM
    d) Encourage oral intake
    e) Tell patient to contact anesthesia department if headache symptoms recur

injected in close approximation to the puncture site, if possible. There is greater cephalad spread of blood in the epidural space, therefore, in the presence of more than one dural puncture, the lowest puncture site should be chosen[58] (Table 7-23). Valsalva maneuvers after a recent EBP have been reported to "blow out" the patch with resultant redevelopment of PDPH. The rate of success for repeated EBP are even better (95 percent), possibly because the first EBP creates a matrix to which the second can adhere. After several unsuccessful EBPs, other etiologies for headache must be pursued (e.g., cortical vein thrombosis).[59,60]

The EBP is probably effective initially because it increases pressure in the epidural space, thus reducing the pressure gradient between the subarachnoid space and epidural space. The increase in epidural pressure is transmitted across the dura to the subarachnoid space, causing an increase in the subarachnoid pressure.[11] This mechanism is probably responsible for the immediate relief of symptoms. The epidural blood occludes the dural hole via clot formation and serves as a matrix for connective tissue repair (Fig. 7-28). Epidural blood appears to be more effective than saline because its increased viscosity and hypertonicity reduces the rate of resorption into the general circulation and the clot must be resolved over time. Investigators have proposed dextran 40 to be more effective than normal saline for treatment of PDPH if one accepts the increased viscosity and hypertonicity concepts.[61]

The use of a prophylactic EBP via the epidural catheter or spinal needle has been described.[62] However, studies have shown that the incidence of PDPH does not change significantly with a prophylactic or early (sooner than 24 hours) EBP.[63,64] More recent studies have challenged these earlier findings,[65,66] but no large-scale study has demonstrated the efficacy of a prophylactic EBP. Since it is impossible to predict which patient will develop a PDPH, only a portion of patients with dural puncture (including unintentional epidural needle puncture) develop PDPH. Many of these patients can be treated conservatively. Therefore, the use of a prophylactic EBP is not currently performed routinely.

No permanent sequelae from a therapeutic EBP have been reported, however, transient back stiffness and paresthesias are relatively common. Other rare complications include meningismus, abdominal cramps, tinnitus, vertigo, fever, epidural hematoma, and subcutaneous hematoma at the injection site. Contraindications to an EBP include septicemia or local infection in the area of injection, blood dyscrasias or anticoagulation, and the presence of active central axis neurologic disease. There is no contraindication to performing epidural or subarachnoid anesthesia in patients with a previous EBP.[67,68] The success of subsequent epidural or subarachnoid anesthesia does not appear to be altered,[68] although there are a few anecdotal reports to the contrary. Since the EBP should be resolved in a matter of days, one is

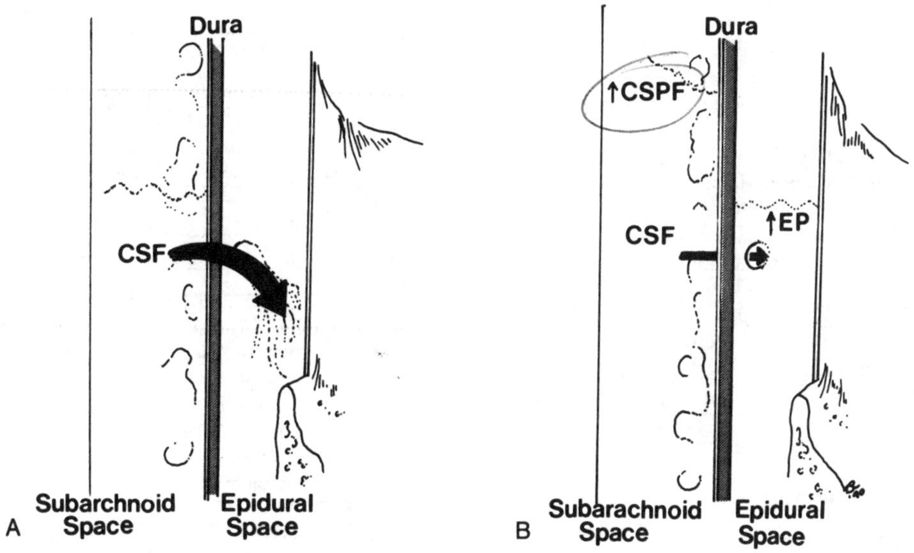

Fig. 7-28. **(A, B)** The epidural blood patch works by increasing pressure in the epidural space, thus reducing the pressure gradient between the subarachnoid space and the epidural space and causing an increase in subarachnoid pressure.

hard pressed for an explanation of subsequent epidural or subarachnoid failure.

REFERENCES

1. Bier A: Versuche Ober/cocaineisirung des ruckenmarkes. Deut Z Chir 51:361, 1899
2. Vandam LD, Dripps RD: Long term follow-up of patients who received 10,098 spinal anesthetics. JAMA 161:586, 1956
3. Wolff E: A bend in the sixth cranial nerve and its possible significance. Br J Opthalmol 12:22, 1928
4. Hughsen W: A note on the relationship of cerebrospinal and intralabrinthine pressures. Am J Physiol 101:396, 1932
5. Tourtellotte WW, Haerer AF, Heller GL, Somers JE: Post-lumbar Puncture Headaches. p. 87. Charles C Thomas, Springfield, IL, 1964
6. Glesne OG: Lumbar puncture headaches. Anesthesiology 11:702, 1950
7. Jacobaeus HC, Frumerie K: About the leakage of spinal fluid after lumbar puncture and its treatment. Acta Med Scand 58:102, 1925
8. Alpers B: Lumbar puncture headache. Arch Neurol 14:806, 1925
9. Kunkle EC, Ray BA, Wolfe HG: Experimental studies on headache. Arch Neurol 49:323, 1943
10. Usubiaga JE, Brea LM, Goyena R: Effect of saline injections on epidural and subarachnoid space pressures and relation to postspinal anesthesia headache. Anesth Analg 46:293, 1967
11. Coombs DW, Hooper D: Subarachnoid pressure with epidural blood "patch." Reg Anesth 4:3, 1979
12. Brownridge P: The management of headache following accidental dural puncture in obstetric patients. Anaesth Intens Care 11:4, 1983
13. Phillips OC, Ebner H, Nelson AT,, Black MH: Neurologic complications following spinal anesthesia with lidocaine: prospective review of 10,440 cases. Anesthesiology 30:284, 1969
14. Ostheimer GW: Headache in the post-partum period. p. 27. In Marx GF (ed): Clinical Management of Mother and Newborn. Springer-Verlag, New York, 1979
15. Green BA: A 26 gauge lumbar puncture needle: its value in the prophylaxis of headache following spinal anesthesia for vaginal delivery. Anesthesiology 11:464, 1950
16. Tarrow AB: Post spinal headache. Anaesthetists 1963
17. White CW, Weiss JB, Niver EC, Heerdegen DK: Anesthesia and post partum headache. Obstet Gynecol 20:734, 1962
18. White Flaatten H, Rodt SA, Vannes J, et al: Postdural puncture headache using 26- or 29-gauge needles in young patients. Reg Anesth 11:5, 1988
19. Frumin MJ: Spinal anesthesia using a 32 gauge needle. Anesthesiology 30:599, 1969
20. Ditman M, Renkel F: Spinal anesthesia with extremely fine needles. Anesthesiology 70:1035, 1989
21. Green HM: Lumbar puncture and the prevention of post puncture headache. JAMA 86:391, 1926
22. Franksson C, Gordh T: Headache after spinal anesthesia and a technique for lessening its frequency. Acta Chir Scand 94:443, 1946
23. Mihic D: Postspinal headache and relationship of needle bevel to longitudinal dural fibers. Reg Anesth 10:76, 1985
24. Norris MC, Leighton BL, DeSimone CA: Needle bevel direction and headache after inadvertent dural puncture. Anesthesiology 70:729, 1989
25. Kreuscher HP, Sandmann G: Prevention of postspinal headache by using Whitacre's pencil-point needle. Reg Anesth 11:5, 1988
26. Abouleish E, Yamaoka H, Hingson R: Evaluation of a tapered spinal needle. Anesth Analg 53:258, 1974
27. Hatfalvi BI: The dynamics of post-spinal headache. Headache J 17:64, 1977
28. Ready LB, Cuplin S, Haschke RH, Nessly M: Spinal needle determinants of rate of transdural fluid leak. Anesth Analg 69:457, 1989
29. Ash WH: Lateral approach for spinal anesthesia. Anesthesiology 16:455, 1955
30. Rosser BH, Schneider M: The unflexed back and a low incidence of severe spinal headache. Anesthesiology 17:288, 1956
31. Naulty JS, Hertwig L, Datta S, et al: Influence of local anesthetic solution on post-dural puncture headache. Anesthesiology 63:A454, 1985
32. Gielen MJM, Meulman H, VanBeern H, Bridenbaugh PO: Does the addition of epinephrine to hyperbaric bupivacaine .5% in spinal anesthesia decrease the incidence of tourniquet induced pain? Abstract F3, ESRA, Malmo, Sweden, 1986
33. Johnson MD, Hertwig L, Vehring PH, Datta S: Intrathecal fentanyl may reduce the incidence of spinal headache. Anesthesiology 71:A911, 1989
34. Giuffrida JG, Bizzarri DV, Masi R, Bondoc R: Continuous procaine spinal anesthesia for cesarean section. Anesth Analg 51:117, 1972
35. Kallos T, Smith TC: Continuous spinal anesthesia with hypobaric tetracaine for hip surgery in lateral decubitus. Anesth Analg 51:766, 1972
36. Peterson DO, Borup JL, Chestnut JS: Continuous spinal anesthesia case review and discussion. Reg Anesth 8:109, 1983
37. Denny N, Masters R, Pearson D, Reed J, et al: Postdural puncture headache after continuous spinal anesthesia. Anesth Analg 66:791, 1987
38. Giuffrida JG, Bizzarri DB, Dalsania J: Continuous spinal anesthesia—experience with 535 patients. Abstract II, 9th World Congress of Anesthesiology, Washington, D.C., 1988
39. Hurley RJ, Lambert DH: Continuous spinal anesthesia with a microcatheter technique: preliminary experience. Anesth Analg 70:97, 1990
40. Craft CB, Epstein S, Coakley CS: Prophylaxis of dural puncture headache with epidural saline. Anesth Analg 52:228, 1973
41. Ostheimer GW: Prophylactic epidural blood patch. Reg Anesth 4:17, 1979
42. Hodgkinson R: Total spinal block after epidural injection into an interspace adjacent to an inadvertent dural perforation. Anesthesiology 55:593, 1981

43. Leach A, Smith GB: Subarachnoid spread of epidural local anaesthetic following dural puncture. Anaesthesia 43:671, 1988
44. Jones RJ: The role of recumbency in the prevention and treatment of post spinal headache. Anesth Analg 53:788, 1974
45. Carbaat PAT, Crevel HV: Lumbar puncture headache: controlled study on the preventative effect of 24 hours bed rest. Lancet 2:1133, 1981
46. Vilming ST, Schrader H, Monstad F: Post-lumbar-puncture headache: the significance of body posture. Cephalalgia 8:75, 1988
47. Hander CE, Smith FR, Perkin GD, Clifford RF: Posture and lumbar puncture headache: a controlled trial in 50 patients. J R Soc Med 75:404, 1982
48. Sechzer PH, Abel L: Post-spinal anesthesia headache treatment with caffeine. I. Evaluation with demand method. Curr Ther Res 24:307, 1978
49. Jarvis AP, Greenwalt JW, Fagraeus L: Intravenous caffeine for post dural puncture headache. Anesth Analg 65:316, 1986
50. Camann WR, Murray RS, Mushlin PS, Lambert DH: Effect of oral caffeine on post dural puncture headache. A double-blind placebo-controlled trial. Anesth Analg 70:181, 1990
51. Crawford JS: The prevention of headache consequent upon dural puncture. Br J Anaesth 44:598, 1972
52. Gibson BE, Wedel DJ, Faust RJ, Peterson RC: Continuous epidural saline infusion for the treatment of low CSF pressure headache. Anesthesiology 68:789, 1988
53. Rice GG, Dabbs CH: The use of epidural and subarachnoid injections of saline solution in the treatment of severe postspinal headache. Anesthesiology 11:17, 1950
54. Craft JB, Epstein BS, Coakley CS: Prophylaxis of dural puncture headache with epidural saline. Anesth Analg 52:228, 1973
55. Bart AJ, Wheeler AS: Comparison of epidural saline placement and epidural blood placement in the treatment of post lumbar puncture headache. Anesthesiology 48:221, 1978
56. DiGiovanni AJ, Galbert MW, Wahle WM: Epidural injection of autologous blood for postlumbar puncture headache. Anesth Analg 51:226, 1972
57. Gormley JB: Treatment of post-spinal headache. Anesthesiology 21:565, 1960
58. Szeinfeld M, Ihmeidan IH, Moser MM, et al: Epidural blood patch: Evaluation of the volume and spread of blood injected into the epidural space. Anesthesiology 64:820, 1986
59. Zandstra GC, Veigas OJ: Post partum headache following regional analgesia: a symptom of cerebral venous thrombosis. Can J Anaesth 36:705, 1989
60. Younker D, Jones MM, Adenwala J, et al: Maternal cortical vein thrombosis and the obstetric anesthesiologist. Anesth Analg 65:100, 1986
61. Barrios-Alarcan J, Aldrete JA, Paragoas-Tapia D: Relief of post lumbar puncture headache with epidural dextran 40: a preliminary report. Reg Anesth 14:78, 1989
62. Ozdil T, Powell WF: Post lumbar puncture headache: an effective method of prevention. Anesth Analg 44:542, 1965
63. Loeser EA, Hill GE, Bennett GM, Sedeberg JH: Time vs success rate for epidural blood patch. Anesthesiology 49:147, 1978
64. Palahniuk RJ, Cumming M: Prophylactic blood patch does not prevent post-lumbar puncture headache. Can Anaesth Soc J 26:132, 1979
65. Anderson EF: Immediate blood patching after inadvertent dural puncture. Anesthesiol Rev 122:49, 1985
66. Coldunna-Ramano P, Shapiro BE: Unintentional dural puncture and prophylactic epidural blood patch in obstetrics. Anesth Analg 69:522, 1989
67. Abouleish E, Wadhwa RK, Vega S, et al: Regional anesthesia following epidural blood patch. Anesth Analg 54:634, 1975
68. Naulty JS, Herold R: Successful epidural anesthesia following epidural blood patch. Anesth Analg 57:272, 1978

POSTOPERATIVE ANALGESIA AFTER CESAREAN DELIVERY

The therapeutic choices for treatment of pain following cesarean delivery include PCA (patient-controlled analgesia), and epidural, subarachnoid, and traditional intramuscular opioids. The obstetric patient's needs are different from those of the general surgical patient. After cesarean delivery, women desire to remain alert in order to bond with their neonates. Therefore, the optimal analgesic modality should provide maximum pain relief with minimal sedation in order to promote maternal-neonatal bonding.

PATIENT-CONTROLLED ANALGESIA

Intermittent IM dosing of opioids does not reliably produce satisfactory postoperative analgesia.[1] Variable absorption from intramuscular injection sites results in fluctuating, unpredictable plasma concentrations.[1] This uneven absorption accounts for the wide variations in peak plasma concentration (Cmax) and the time to reach the peak plasma concentration (Tmax) following intramuscular injections.[2] Pain relief occurs when the plasma opioid concentration reaches a minimum effective analgesic concentration (MEAC). MEAC is relatively consistent for a given patient but varies two- to fivefold among patients.[2] When narcotics are given via timed, scheduled intramuscular dosing, plasma concentrations are in excess of MEAC only 35 percent of the time during any 4-hour dosing interval.[2]

The response to PCA has been enthusiastic from both patients and obstetricians. Because PCA delivers opioids intravenously, the wide swings in plasma concentration seen with intramuscular dosing are avoided. On-demand self-administration of small amounts of opioid can accommodate highly variable analgesic requirements. PCA allows patients to "titrate" their specific analgesic needs. The immediate accessibility of analgesia also decreases the anxiety associated with the normal delay in receiving conventional IM medication. Patients use PCA to maintain plasma opioid concentrations within range of their respective MEAC.[3] The therapeutic window is narrow, and very small fluctuations in opioid concentration (0.5 μg/ml of meperidine) can mean the difference between discomfort and adequate analgesia.[1]

It is presently hypothesized that an individual patient's MEAC is determined by his or her preoperative endogenous opioid content in the cerebrospinal fluid (CSF).[4] Patients with low quantities of endogenous opioids in the CSF use PCA to administer liberal amounts of exogenous opioid in order to maintain higher plasma opioid concentrations. Conversely, patients with high preoperative endogenous opioid content in the CSF use PCA more sparingly to maintain lower plasma opioid concentrations. A recent report suggests that this may not apply in obstetric patients, however.[5]

At present, the most commonly used modes of administration of PCA are demand dosing (a fixed dose is self-administered) and constant-rate infusion plus demand dosing (a background infusion is supplemented by patient demand). Infusion demand modes (where demands are granted as an infusion) and variable-rate infusion plus demand dosing modes (where a microprocessor monitors demand and controls the infusion rate accordingly) are presently under study.[6]

INTRASPINAL OPIOIDS

Alternatively, intraspinal (epidural or subarachnoid) opioids may be used to provide potent analgesia after cesarean delivery. The sites of action of both epidural and subarachnoid opioids are the opioid receptors in the dorsal horn of the spinal cord.[7] Both the onset and duration of analgesia correlate with CSF opioid concentration, not plasma concentration.[8] Since epidural opioids must passively diffuse across the dura into the CSF, higher lipid solubility is associated with faster onset. Clearance from the CSF determines the duration of action. Highly lipid-soluble opioids (fentanyl, sufentanil, meperidine, methadone, butorphanol) are quickly absorbed into adjacent tissues, particularly the vasculature. Hence, a more segmental block of relatively short duration is obtained with increasing lipophilicity, as the opioid does not diffuse widely throughout the epidural and subarachnoid space.[9]

The low lipid solubility of morphine, by contrast, accounts for its slower onset but extremely long duration of action (12 to 24 hours). Morphine spreads widely in the epidural and subarachnoid spaces, causing a nonsegmental block. The quality of analgesia is similar with both lipophilic and hydrophilic opioids, though the onset and duration differ greatly.[9]

Concomitant with the use of morphine is the possibility for delayed respiratory depression. Late respiratory depression is due to rostral spread, which affects medullary respiratory centers. Though this feared complication is rare and usually gradual in onset, patients should be closely monitored for 24 hours following injection. The lipid-soluble opioids are not associated with delayed respiratory depression because their cephalad spread is limited.[9]

COMPARISON OF TECHNIQUES FOR ANALGESIA AFTER CESAREAN DELIVERY

Epidural morphine provides superior analgesia as compared to either PCA or intramuscular morphine following cesarean delivery.[10] (A similar trial using lipophilic opioids has not been performed.) The duration of analgesia with epidural morphine is variable, however. Approximately 40 percent of patients require systemic narcotics within 12 hours and 50 percent by 24 hours after administration of a single bolus dose of epidural morphine.[11] Addition of parenteral narcotics for breakthrough pain may increase the chance of respiratory depression when using intraspinal opioids.

Overall, patients are more satisfied with PCA-administered morphine. Although epidural morphine provides more profound analgesia, it is associated with frequent bothersome side effects (pruritus, nausea, and vomiting). The incidence of pruritus requiring treatment may be as high as 45 percent, compared to 5 percent for patients receiving either PCA or intramuscular morphine after cesarean delivery.[10]

A significant percentage of patients may also experience pruritus with epidural administration of lipophilic opioids. This pruritus, however, is usually transient and mild and does not require treatment. The incidence of nausea is similar among PCA, epidural, and intramuscular routes.

ANALGESIC PRACTICE AT THE BRIGHAM AND WOMEN'S HOSPITAL

For alleviation of post-cesarean delivery pain at our institution, both techniques are sequentially used in combination. Because of the rare but real risk of respiratory depression, use of agents via intraspinal administration has been restricted to the lipid-soluble opioids. If cesarean delivery is performed with subarachnoid anesthesia, the opioid is given during administration of the block. If a patient elects epidural anesthesia, a single dose of lipid-soluble opioid is administered immediately after birth. Occasionally, a second dose may be given in the postanesthesia care unit.

The addition of opioids to local anesthetics for subarachnoid anesthesia improves both intraoperative and immediate postoperative analgesia. Subarachnoid administration of as little as 6.25 μg of fentanyl with hyperbaric bupivacaine results in 3 to 4 hours of postoperative analgesia.[12] This is similar to the duration of analgesia obtained from epidural fentanyl but with much lower dose of opioid. For subarachnoid block, fentanyl 10 μg is customarily added to hyperbaric bupivacaine. In contrast, subarachnoid morphine provides approximately 24 hours of postoperative analgesia[13] This prolonged pain relief must be weighed against the risk of delayed respiratory depression.

The minimum reliably effective dose of epidural fentanyl is 50 μg, which results in 3 to 7 hours of analgesia.[14] Dilution of fentanyl in at least 10 ml of preservative-free normal saline or local anesthetic has been shown to shorten the onset time and increase the duration of analgesia as compared to administration of lesser volumes.[15] The minimum effective dose of epidural sufentanil has not been determined, although 25 to 50 μg provides 3.5 to 5.6 hours of analgesia.[16] Increasing doses of fentanyl or sufentanil will not prolong duration, but may reduce total narcotic requirement for up to 24 hours after cesarean delivery.[14]

After admission to the postanesthesia care unit, a PCA infuser is connected to the patient. The patient may begin to self-administer opioids when pain is first perceived. Patients typically use PCA for 24 to 48 hours after surgery.

REFERENCES

1. Austin KL, Stapleton JV, Mather LE: Relationship between blood meperidine concentrations and analgesic response: a preliminary report. Anesthesiology 53:460, 1980
2. Austin KL, Stapleton JV, Mather LE: Multiple intramuscular injections: a major source of variability in analgesic response to meperidine. Pain 8:47, 1980
3. Tamsen A, Hartvig P, Fagerlund C, Dahlström B: Patient-controlled analgesic therapy. Part II. Individual analgesic demand and analgesic plasma concentrations of pethidine in postoperative pain. Clin Pharmacokinet 7:164, 1982
4. Tamsen A, Sakurda T, Wahlström A, et al: Postoperative demand for analgesics in relation to individual levels of endorphins and substance P in cerebrospinal fluid. Pain 13:171, 1982
5. Eisenach JC, Dobson CE II, Inturissi CE, Hood DD: Do spinal enkephalins mediate analgesia in pregnancy? (abstract) Anesth Analg 68:S78, 1989
6. Mather LE, Owen H: The pharamcology of patient-administered opioids. p. 27. In Ferrante FM, Ostheimer GW, Covino BG (eds): Patient-Controlled Analgesia. Blackwell Scientific Publications, Boston, 1990
7. Game CJ, Lodge D: The pharmacology of the inhibition of dorsal horn neurones by impulses in myelinated cutaneous afferents in cats. Exp Brain Res 23:75, 1975
8. Nordberg G, Hedner T, Mellstrand T, Dahlström B: Pharmacokinetic aspects of epidural morphine analgesia. Anesthesiology 58:545, 1983
9. Cousins MJ, Mather LE: Intrathecal and epidural administration of opioids. Anesthesiology 61:276, 1984
10. Harrison DM, Sinatra R, Morgese L, Chung JH: Epidural narcotics and patient-controlled analgesia for post-cesarean section pain relief. Anesthesiology 68:454, 1988
11. Eisenach JC, Grice SC, Dewan DM: Patient-controlled analgesia following cesarean section: a comparison with epidural and intramuscular narcotics. Anesthesiology 68:444, 1988
12. Hunt CO, Naulty JS, Bader AM, et al: Perioperative analgesia with subarachnoid fentanyl-bupivacaine for cesarean delivery. Anesthesiology 71:535, 1989
13. Rosen MA, Hughes SC, Shnider SM, et al: Epidural morphine for the relief of postoperative pain after cesarean delivery. Anesth Analg 62:666, 1983
14. Naulty JS, Datta S, Ostheimer GW, et al: Epidural fentanyl for post cesarean delivery pain management. Anesthesiology 63:694, 1985
15. Birnbach DJ, Johnson MD, Arcario T, et al: Effect of diluent volume on analgesia produced by epidural fentanyl. Anesth Analg 68:808, 1989
16. Rosen MA, Dailey PA, Hughes SC, et al: Epidural sufentanil for postoperative analgesia after cesarean section. Anesthesiology 68:448, 1988

NURSING CARE OF THE PARTURIENT RECEIVING EPIDURAL ANESTHESIA

NURSING CARE PLAN

Communication between the anesthesiologist and the nursing service is vital to ensure quality patient care. Institutions that provide epidural block as a form of obstetric anesthetic should provide detailed in-service education for the nursing staff. These programs should review the physiologic changes of pregnancy, pharmacology and basic pharmacokinetics of local anesthetic agents, physiology of sympathetic blockade, complications of regional anesthetic, treatment of complications, and both maternal and neonatal resuscitation. This would provide the information needed to create a functional nursing care plan for the obstetric patient receiving epidural anesthesia.

ASSESSMENT

Nursing care of the obstetric patient receiving epidural anesthetic begins with a thorough patient assessment that should provide the following information:

1. Does the obstetric history include any medical problems or allergies?
2. Did the patient attend prepared childbirth classes?
3. Has the patient planned on receiving analgesia or anesthesia?
4. Is the patient aware of the types of analgesia and anesthesia available for labor and vaginal or cesarean delivery in this institution?
5. Does the patient have a previous history of anesthetic complications?
6. Has the patient ever had back problems or neurologic symptoms?
7. When did the patient last eat or drink?
8. Will a significant other be in attendance during labor and at delivery?

EXPLAINING THE PLANNED PROCEDURE

If the parturient chooses major regional anesthesia, an explanation of the procedure provides her with information that may alleviate fear and promote compliance for initiation of the block.

Explanation of the technique and procedure to the patient in active labor should be informative but concise when the patient's attentiveness is not interrupted by painful contractions.[1]

PREPARATION

Antacid

Maternal aspiration is a major complication of obstetric anesthetic. Previous studies indicate that a patient with 25 ml of gastric volume with a pH $\leq$ 2.5 is at risk for acid aspiration.[3] Clear antacids are given by mouth to decrease gastric acidity by raising the pH of gastric juice. Sodium citrate (0.3 mol/L) or its equivalent has replaced particulate antacids because of the possible hazards of aspirating the particulate matter.[3,4] Oral antacids given to the pregnant patient when she is sitting or lying in the semi-Fowler's position will begin to neutralize the gastric contents of the stomach. The gravid uterus divides the stomach into two separate compartments, the fundal sac and the antral sac. Holdsworth demonstrated that turning the patient through 360 degrees allows antacid passage to the antral sac and adequate mixing.[5] It is standard procedure to administer 30 ml of a clear antacid prior to the initiation of the epidural block. The patient is placed in the right lateral position for the administration of the epidural block to assist in distributing the antacid to the lower sac of the stomach, after which the patient is turned supine with a wedge under the right hip to provide left uterine displacement. (Neutralization of gastric fluid [raising pH above 3.0] has been documented by the editor within 6 minutes of administering 30 ml of a clear antacid.)

Intravenous Infusion

Placement of an intravenous catheter in the distal forearm allows movement of the hand and wrist without interfering with the continuous intravenous infusion. A 16- or 18-gauge catheter is preferred. An intravenous infusion set containing a hand pressure chamber facilitates rapid infusion of crystalloid for acute intravascular volume expansion to prevent or treat hypotension due to sympathetic blockade, peripheral vasodilation, or hemorrhage. Lactated Ringer's solution or normal saline 1,000 ml is infused rapidly prior to initiation of the epidural block in labor. Before an epidural or subarachnoid block is initiated for cesarean delivery, at least 1,500 ml is given. Glucose solutions are not used because of the placental transfer of glucose which causes fetal hyperglycemia and hyperinsulinemia that results in neonatal hypoglycemia.[6]

Table 7-24 provides a checklist for nursing care of patients receiving epidural anesthetic.

ADMINISTRATION OF THE EPIDURAL BLOCK

A bath sheet or large square cotton bed pad is placed under the patient. This will help in moving her and prevent dislocation of the epidural catheter after insertion. Vital signs and fetal heart rate (FHR) are checked prior to positioning the patient in the lateral position. A fetal scalp electrode is placed to provide continuous FHR monitoring throughout the procedure if the cervix is sufficiently dilated. The patient should bring her back to the edge of the bed closest to the anesthesiologist. (The editor prefers the parturient to be in the right lateral position.) The patient is assisted in assuming the fetal position by having her knees bent and brought as close to her abdomen as possible. The patient should be

Table 7-24. Nursing Checklist for Epidural Anesthesia

Available and functioning oxygen equipment, including bag, mask, and tubing to connect to an oxygen outlet
Available and functioning suction equipment
Adequate lighting
Hospital bed or stretcher in "locked" neutral position with the ability to be placed in the Trendelenberg position
Epidural cart, including Epidural trays Local anesthetic agents Antiseptic solution Gloves Tape Intravenous solutions and infusion sets Resuscitation equipment, including laryngoscopes and endotracheal tubes Drugs
Clear plastic tape to aid in viewing the epidural catheter and less skin irritation
"Crash cart" for emergencies
Expiration dates for the epidural tray and all medications should be checked

instructed to envisage the letter "C" and to place her chin down to her chest and push the midsection of her back out toward the anesthesiologist.

The patient is coached with the appropriate breathing technique during contractions. The "coach" should be within her view and provide gentle support under her knees and behind her neck to help maintain position. Sensations should be explained as they occur: the cold antiseptic backwash, burning or stinging as the local anesthetic skin wheal is raised, pressure during the insertion of the epidural needle and the possibility of a twinge or "electric shock" when the catheter is passed into the epidural space. The anesthesiologist should be assisted in taping the epidural catheter securely to the patient's back.

The patient is told to move to the center of the bed and to dig her heels into the bed; she is then lifted over onto her back. If it is explained that brushing against the bed will dislodge the epidural catheter, the patient will understand the need to lift up and over. The bed is adjusted to a semi-Fowler's position and a blanket roll is placed under the right hip to initiate left lateral displacement of the uterus, which decrease aortocaval compression.

MONITORING

Maternal blood pressure and pulse rate and the FHR are monitored immediately. Blood pressure measurements are repeated every minute for 5 minutes, then every 3 to 5 minutes, five times. If the blood pressure remains stable at 30 minutes after the injection, routine vital sign checking may be resumed (checked and recorded at least every 15 minutes). Symptoms of hypotension or local anesthetic toxicity usually occur within the first few minutes after administration, therefore vital signs should be monitored and noted frequently.

If the patient experiences any symptoms of local anesthetic toxicity ("ringing" in the ears, circumoral numbness, a metallic taste, dizziness, nausea, or sudden anxiety or confusion), it should be reported to the anesthesiologist immediately. Hypotension after the block or suspected local anesthetic toxicity is treated by increasing the degree of left lateral tilt, administration of oxygen (6 to 8 L/min) via mask, increasing the intravenous fluid infusion rate, placing the bed in the Trendelenberg position and elevating the patient's legs to promote venous return. Vital signs should then be rechecked. The anesthesiologist and the obstetrician should be notified of the patient's change in status. The anesthesiologist is responsible for the medical treatment of hypotension and should be immediately available.

Fetal heart sounds should be auscultated at least every 5 minutes if continuous external or internal monitoring is not used. It is the policy of the Brigham and Women's Hospital that any parturient receiving an epidural block must have continuous electronic or ultrasonic FHR monitoring. The contractions should be monitored by hand if tocodynamometry is not available. The uterus should be palpated for frequency, strength, and duration of contractions to assess progress in labor.

Labor is often induced or augmented with intravenous oxytocin. The oxytocin infusion should be discontinued during the placement of the epidural block and resumed infusion when an adequate sensory block is achieved.

MAINTENANCE OF ANESTHESIA

The degree of motor block varies and the patient may be unable to move her legs with an epidural block. Use of pillows or blankets will help to avoid compression pressure points and cushion and support joints. When moving or turning a patient, bend her knees and protect her legs and feet from injury. A pillow placed against her back will provide support when the patient is lying on her side.

The patient should be encouraged to rest when she is comfortable and relaxed. Questions about the epidural anesthetic, impending delivery, or postpartum procedures should be anticipated and answered, and emotional support provided as necessary. Status of the bladder must be assessed frequently, as the sensory block associated with epidural anesthetic decreases the sensation of distension and the urge to void. The patient should be encouraged to void; if she is unable to void, straight catheterization may be required. Perineal hygiene should be maintained

The duration of action of the local anesthetic agent used must be known. The anesthesiologist should be notified for reinforcement as needed; as it is easier to maintain an effective level than to restart the epidural block. The anesthesiologist should be called upon to reevaluate the block when necessary and prior to vaginal or cesarean delivery. If a continuous epidural infusion of local anesthetic with or without opioid is administered, the concentration of the drugs and the rate of infusion should be recorded. (The editor believes that the labor nurse can ascertain the level of sensory and motor block at regular intervals, although this concept is difficult for nursing administrations to accept.)

TRANSFERRAL TO THE DELIVERY ROOM

If the delivery takes place in a delivery or operating room the patient is moved from bed or stretcher to the delivery table. A roller can be employed or a team can lift the patient on the bed sheet. The patient should be instructed to lift her head and to keep her arms folded across her chest during transfer. Intravenous tubing, indwelling Foley catheter, and the epidural catheter must be protected when moving the patient. Proper body alignment should be maintained. Proper lifting technique will prevent injury to the nursing staff and others involved in patient transfer. We advocate the labor-delivery-recovery (LDR) concept at our institution.

POSTPARTUM CARE

In the postpartum period, the site of the epidural catheter should be examined for bleeding, oozing, or possible infection. An unintentional dural puncture may result in a postpartum headache. If this occurs, the anesthesiologist should be notified, appropriate analgesics given as ordered, intravenous or oral fluids increased, and the patient encouraged to lie flat in bed. The anesthesiologist will determine what therapy (e.g., epidural blood patch) will be employed.

REFERENCES

1. Nicolls ET, Corke BC, Ostheimer GW: Epidural anesthetic for the woman in labor. Am J Nursing 81:1826, 1981
2. Roberts RB, Shirley MA: Reducing the risk of aspiration during cesarean section. Anesth Analg 53:859, 1974
3. Gibbs CP, Schwartz DJ, Wynne JW, et al: Antacid pulmonary aspiration in the dog. Anesthesiology 51:380, 1979
4. Gibbs CP, Spohr L, Schmidt D: In vitro and in vivo evaluation of sodium citrate as an antacid. Anesthesiology 55:A311, 1981
5. Holdsworth JS, Johnson K, Mascall G, et al: Mixing antacids with stomach contents. Anaesthesia 35:641, 1980
6. Kenepp NB, Shelley WC, Gabbe SG, et al: Fetal and neonatal hazards of maternal hydration with 5% dextrose before caesarean section. Lancet 1:1150, 1982

8

The High-Risk Parturient

OBSTETRIC HEMORRHAGE

Hemorrhage is a major cause of maternal mortality in the obstetric patient. Significant bleeding occurs in 3 percent of all pregnancies, and can be massive.[1] The causes of peripartum hemorrhage include:

1. Placenta previa
2. Abruptio placentae
3. Placenta accreta/increta/percreta
4. Uterine rupture
5. Uterine inversion
6. Uterine atony
7. Retained placenta
8. Coagulopathy
   (a) Disseminated intravascular coagulation (DIC) (related to intrauterine fetal demise), chorioamnionitis, amniotic fluid embolism, abruption, or preeclampsia
   (b) HELLP syndrome (hemolysis, elevated liver enzymes, and low platelet [count])
   (c) pre-existing factor deficiencies and hematologic abnormalities
9. Cervical and vaginal lacerations
10. Cervical and uterine abnormalities (polyps, tumors, varicosities)
11. Trauma
12. Advanced ectopic pregnancy

Placenta previa and abruptio placentae account for one-half to two-thirds of all cases of antepartum hemorrhage.

If hemorrhage is severe and uncontrollable, the patient will require a cesarean hysterectomy. The role of the anesthesiologist is to recognize the patient at increased risk for peripartum hemorrhage, make the appropriate anesthetic choice, and be prepared to manage hemorrhage when it occurs.

When a patient presents with obstetric hemorrhage the initial anesthetic approach is essentially the same regardless of etiology. A brief history should be obtained, including the patient's gestational age; etiology of bleeding (if known); drug allergies; medical, surgical, obstetric, and anesthetic history; and family history of problems with anesthesia. A brief physical examination should be performed, with special attention to the airway (i.e., can this patient be intubated if a rapid-sequence induction of general anesthesia becomes necessary—cf. the section on management of the obstetric patient with a difficult airway in Chapter 6), the vital signs (i.e., does the patient have orthostatic hypotension, if this can be evaluated, the amount of blood loss, which is not always externally apparent, and the ease of intravenous access. Depending on the amount of bleeding, at least one large intravenous catheter should be placed and a blood sample sent for type and crossmatch, hematocrit, and DIC/coagulopathy hematologic profile. Finally, the anesthesiologist must communicate with the obstetrician and be aware of his or her plans for delivery. If the patient is unstable with massive hemorrhage, the anesthetic management consists, first and foremost, of intravascular volume resuscitation, which is essentially the same regardless of the etiology of the hemorrhage.

PLACENTA PREVIA

Pathophysiology

Placenta previa occurs when the placenta implants in the lower uterine segment, and partially or completely overlies the cervical os. It is classified as *total*, *partial*, or *marginal* depending on the location of the placenta relative to the os (Fig. 8-1).

In 1985, Clark et al. reported an overall incidence of placenta previa of 0.3 percent.[2] Incomplete separation of the placenta previa accounts for one-third of all third-trimester bleeding. The classic presentation is painless vaginal bleeding; however, placenta previa can also present as a problem during labor. Associated factors include increased maternal age (it is three times more common in women over 35) and increased parity. The most important risk factor is a prior cesarean delivery or uterine scar. Clark et al. found the incidence of placenta previa to increase from 0.26 percent in patients with no prior cesarean deliveries to 10 percent in patients with four or more prior cesarean deliveries.[2]

In this age of increased prenatal screening, placenta previa is often diagnosed on routine prenatal ultrasound with 95 percent accuracy.[3] Although maternal mortality has decreased to less than 1 percent fetal mortality can be as high as 20 percent.[1]

Anesthetic Management

If a patient presents at term with vaginal bleeding and a suspected placenta previa but is stable and there is no sign of fetal distress, an ultrasound examination should be performed. In the unlikely event that ultrasound is not available, a double set-up examination should be performed in the delivery room with the anesthesia care team ready in case an emergency cesarean delivery becomes necessary.

Preoperative preparation includes the following:

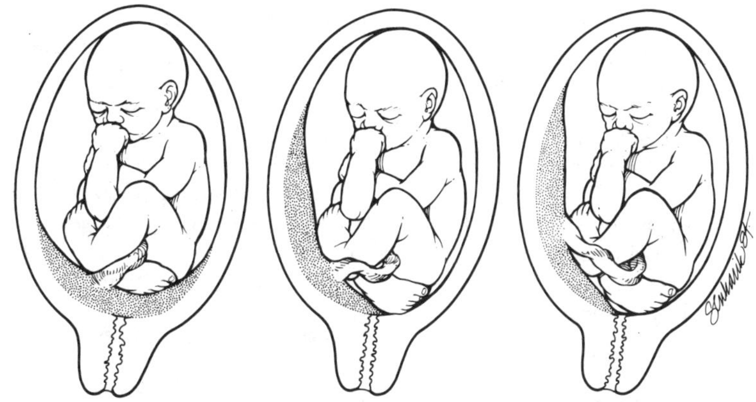

Fig. 8-1. Three variations of placenta previa. (From Benedetti,[21] with permission.)

1. Two large (14- or 16-gauge) intravenous catheters
2. Two to four units of packed red cells in the operating room
3. A blood pump, blood warmer, and warming blanket immediately available
4. Administration of an oral nonparticulate antacid to the patient before the start of the procedure
5. Oxygen
6. Left uterine displacement
7. An assistant prepared to apply cricoid pressure if administration of general anesthesia for an emergency cesarean delivery becomes necessary

Once the diagnosis of placenta previa is made, if the vaginal bleeding stops, the patient is stable, and there is no fetal distress, the patient should be placed at bedrest and undergo an elective cesarean delivery when the fetus is at term or more mature. At that time, regional anesthesia is appropriate as long as the mother is not bleeding and the anesthesiologist is aware of the potential for increased blood loss. If it is a documented placenta previa and a primary cesarean delivery, it is our policy to proceed with either subarachnoid or epidural anesthesia after placing two large intravenous catheters and ensuring that the patient's blood has been typed and crossmatched for at least two units of packed red cells. If the patient has a known placenta previa and history of prior cesarean deliveries, and is therefore at increased risk for placenta accreta and cesarean hysterectomy, we proceed with continuous epidural anesthesia or general anesthesia only after placing two large intravenous catheters and having two to four units of packed red cells available in the delivery or operating room (cf. Gravid Hysterectomy, below).

If, in the rare event that a double set-up examination is necessary and bleeding develops, the patient becomes unstable, or there is fetal distress, it will be necessary to proceed with administration of general anesthesia for an emergency cesarean delivery while initiating vigorous intravascular volume resuscitation. General anesthesia should be preceded by acute oxygenation (denitrogenation) using a rapid-sequence induction utilizing cricoid pressure. The patient should have left uterine displacement and have been given a clear, nonparticulate antacid prior to induction. Intravenous metoclopromide 10 mg should be considered, especially for patients who have eaten recently. General anesthesia is induced with sodium thiopental 3 to 4 mg/kg or ketamine 0.5 to 1.0 mg/kg and succinylcholine 1 to 1.5 mg/kg as long as the patient is not hypotensive or severely hypovolemic. If the patient is hypotensive ketamine 0.5 to 1.0 mg/kg can be used instead of thiopental. However, if the patient is severely hypovolemic secondary to prolonged bleeding, ketamine should be avoided, because its myocardial depressant effects will lead to further hypotension in a patient who already has a maximally stimulated sympathetic nervous system. After induction, the patient is given 100 percent oxygen. Nitrous oxide and halogenated agents are added only if the patient can tolerate them. One must be aware that halogenated agents can decrease blood pressure and uterine tone, which will lead to further bleeding postpartum. After the baby is delivered, the anesthetic is converted to a nitrous oxide-oxygen mixture with supplemental narcotic according to the tolerance of the patient. If there is profuse bleeding, the patient can go into hemorrhagic shock. Resuscitation may be difficult because bleeding will continue until after the placenta is removed. Central venous catheterization is frequently necessary to help manage fluid administration. It is important to maintain left uterine displacement, until after the baby is delivered, even if the mother requires cardiopulmonary resuscitation. Often the neonate will require resuscitation, which should be performed by another qualified individual, as the primary responsibility of the anesthesiologist is to the mother.

Patients with placenta previa have an increased incidence of postpartum hemorrhage due to the fact that the lower uterine segment has less vasoconstrictor capability and can continue to bleed as the result of uterine atony.[4,5]

PLACENTA ACCRETA (PERCRETA AND INCRETA)

Pathophysiology

Placenta accreta, percreta, and increta are conditions of abnormal placentation that are frequently associated with placenta previa. With placenta accreta, the placental villi attach directly to the myometrium without decidua basalis, but do not invade the myometrium. With placenta increta, the placenta invades the myometrium; whereas with placenta percreta, the placenta penetrates through the myometrium and into the serosa and other surrounding structures, including bladder, bowel, and large vessels. It may be total, partial, or focal depending on how much placenta is involved. The overall incidence varies widely, but has been reported to be as high as 1 in 2,562 pregnancies.[6] The etiology is unknown, but a number of factors that adversely affect the endometrium may contribute to the development of an accreta, including placenta previa, prior cesarean delivery, prior manipulation of uterus (dilation and currettage, myomectomy, etc.), congenital malformations of uterus, uterine tumors, multiparity, and perhaps smoking and being the daughter of a mother who was given diethylstilbestrol. Of these, the best-documented and most important is the association with placenta previa and prior cesarean delivery. Clark et al. reported a 5 percent risk of accreta in patients with placenta previa in an unscarred uterus, which increased to 24 percent in patients with placenta previa and one prior cesarean delivery and to 67 percent in patients with placenta previa and four or more prior cesarean deliveries.[2] The overall incidence of accreta has been rising, which is most likely due to the increasing numbers of cesarean deliveries being performed.[7]

The clinical presentation of accreta is by hemorrhage, usually diagnosed at the time of delivery of the placenta. The placenta can be difficult to remove, and this can be accompanied by massive blood loss (i.e., 1,000 ml or more). The clinical severity of the accreta is also associated with the presence of uterine scars. There is an increased incidence of percreta and increta in patients with uterine scars, and there is an increased need for cesarean hysterectomy.[2]

Conservative management of accreta includes oversewing the implantation site, uterine artery ligation, currettage, manual removal, local excision and repair, administration of prostaglandins and oxytoxics, and hypogastric artery ligation.[2] However, in the majority of cases, a cesarean hysterectomy is required.

Anesthetic Management

If placenta accreta is diagnosed during delivery secondary to hemorrhage, two large intravenous catheters should be immediately placed and blood pump tubing connected to the infusing solution. Oxygen should be administered. Blood should be drawn for type and crossmatch. Blood should be sent to the operating room as soon as possible. Vigorous intravascular volume resuscitation should be initiated, with appropriate monitoring if needed. Assistance should be requested. If the patient has no anesthetic, a clear antacid and intravenous metoclopramide 10 mg should be given, especially if the patient has eaten recently. If this has not already been done, a brief history should be obtained, either from the patient or the physicians involved, and examination of the patient's airway must be accomplished. If a continuous regional anesthetic is already functioning, it may be continued as long as one can maintain hemodynamic stability and intravascular volume replacement while the patient is awake. If the patient has not already received anesthesia or is unstable, one must proceed with an emergency general anesthetic utilizing a rapid-sequence induction, as previously described.

If a patient presents with a known placenta previa and a history of prior cesarean deliveries, one must have a high index of suspicion for an accreta and recognize the increased risk for a cesarean hysterectomy. In most instances, the patient will have had a prenatal ultrasound examination that identified the accreta. In this situation, it is our practice to proceed with continuous epidural anesthesia, as long as the patient desires regional anesthesia and there is no suspicion of increta or percreta, after placing two large intravenous catheters and having two to four units of packed red cells in the operating room, and blood warmers and a warming blanket immediately available (see Gravid Hysterectomy, below).

ABRUPTIO PLACENTAE

Pathophysiology

Abruptio placentae (abruption) is the premature separation of an abnormally implanted placenta after the 20th week of gestation. The reported incidence varies from 0.5 to 2.5 percent and represents one-third of all antepartum hemorrhages.[1] It is classified as mild to severe depending on the degree of separation. Maternal mortality is reported to be less than 3 percent with very high perinatal mortality, approaching 60 percent in some studies.[1,5] Abruption is thought to occur secondary to underlying disease of the decidua and uterine blood vessels. Associated factors include hypertensive disorders of pregnancy, chronic hypertension, multiparity, uterine abnormalities, previous abruption (0.1 percent recurrence rate), and preterm rupture of membranes. More than one-half of cases occur before 36 weeks.[1] Abruption classically presents as abdominal pain. The degree of separation determines the severity of symptoms, which include uterine irritability and vaginal bleeding. However, the amount of vaginal bleeding often underrepresents the amount of blood loss because there may be hemorrhage behind the placenta, into the myometrium or broad ligaments, or behind the fetus (concealed abruption). Diagnosis is made clinically and/or by ultrasound.

Complications include hypotension and hemorrhagic shock; coagulopathy secondary to DIC (20 to 40 percent of severe abruptions); acute renal failure (1 to 4 percent); concurrent pregnancy-induced hypertension (50 percent of severe abruptions); postpartum hemorrhage; and ischemic organic necrosis.[5,8] DIC, which occurs secondary to release of tissue thromboplastin from necrotic tissues, involves activation of circulatory plasminogen, which leads to fibrinolysis and consumption of platelets, clotting factors, and fibrinogen.[9] The diagnosis of DIC is made by the presence of hypofibrinogenemia, thrombocytopenia, increased prothrombin time (PT) and partial thromboplastin time (PTT), decreased factors V and VIII, and fibrin split products.

Anesthetic Management

The anesthesiologist presented with a patient having an abruption should first ascertain the severity of the abruption, as anesthetic management depends on the stability of the patient. If the patient is stable and there is no fetal distress, evaluation should proceed as with any patient with obstetric hemorrhage, with emphasis on ruling out hypovolemia and assessing the magnitude of blood loss (remembering the possibility of concealed abruption), and ruling out coagulopathy and DIC. All patients should have left uterine displacement and be given oxygen and an oral nonparticulate antacid. One large intravenous catheter should be inserted and blood for type and crossmatch should be requested, along with a complete hematologic and coagulation profile. The anesthesiologist should be prepared for the possibility of aggressive intravascular volume replacement. If the patient is stable and not hypovolemic, and there is no fetal distress or coagulopathy, then it is appropriate to provide continuous epidural anesthesia for labor and vaginal or cesarean delivery. Contraindications to regional anesthesia include a platelet count of less than 100,000, abnormal bleeding time, increased fibrin split products, fibrinogen less than 200 and abnormal PT and PTT.[10]

If the abruption is severe and the patient is unstable and hypovolemic, or if there is fetal distress or DIC, then one must proceed with a general anesthetic for an emergent cesarean delivery utilizing a rapid-sequence induction. The management is essentially the same as that for an emergency general anesthetic for placenta previa. It is important to remember that ketamine can increase uterine tone, and therefore could theoretically worsen an abruption and cause or increase fetal distress.[5]

If DIC is present, the anesthesiologist must have available large quantities of blood products, including whole blood (if possible), packed red cells, fresh frozen plasma, platelets, and cryoprecipitate, and must watch for hemorrhage from other sites. DIC usually will be corrected with removal of the cause (i.e., the placenta and fetus). Postpartum hemorrhage can occur secondary to uterine atony and DIC. Fibrin split products can inhibit the action of oxytoxin and cause uterine relaxation, contributing to uterine atony.[5]

UTERINE RUPTURE

For further discussion, see Vagina Birth after Cesarean Delivery, later in this chapter.

Pathophysiology

Uterine rupture can occur ante-, intra-, or postpartum. The incidence is 0.08 to 0.1 percent.[5] Maternal mortality varies from 5 to 60 percent if rupture is secondary to prolonged labor. Overall fetal mortality is 50 percent.[11] A complete rupture into the abdomen presents as sudden intense abdominal pain and hypotension. An incomplete rupture can present as mild abdominal or shoulder pain (caused by subdiaphragmatic irritation from blood), vaginal bleeding, or peritonitis. Rupture is also marked by fetal distress, frequently demonstrated by a sudden prolonged bradycardia or the disappearance of fetal heart tones.

Associated maternal factors include:

1. Uterine scar (a low transverse scar is associated with a 0.5 percent incidence, a vertical scar, 2.1 percent)[1]
2. Previous difficult delivery
3. Rapid, spontaneous, tumultuous labor
4. Prolonged labor with excessive oxytoxin stimulation

5. Weak uterine muscles secondary to multiple gestations, multiparity, or polyhydraminios
6. Trauma secondary to forceps or intrauterine manipulation or external version
7. Cephalopelvic disproportion

Obstetric management consists of emergent laparotomy and delivery, with either uterine repair or hysterectomy, depending on the degree of rupture.

Anesthetic Management

The anesthetic management involves an emergent administration of general anesthesia, as described previously, unless the patient already has an epidural catheter in place. It is appropriate to continue to utilize the epidural anesthetic as long as the anesthesiologist is able to maintain hemodynamic stability and intravascular volume replacement, and the patient is awake and reasonably comfortable. One must keep in mind that sympathetic blockade is going to aggravate hypotension secondary to blood loss. If the patient becomes unstable, it may become necessary to convert to a general anesthetic. (See Gravid Hysterectomy, below.)

PUERPERAL UTERINE INVERSION

Pathophysiology

Puerperal uterine inversion is a rare cause of peripartum hemorrhage, but when it occurs, it can be associated with massive hemorrhage and high maternal morbidity and mortality. Inversion is classified as first, second, or third degree, depending in the amount of inversion.[12] It can occur acutely after delivery before the cervical ring has contracted, subacutely, or chronically (more than 4 weeks postpartum).[13] The reported incidence varies widely. A recent review by Shah-Hosseini reported an incidence of 1 per 6,407 pregnancies.[12] The incidence is higher in nulliparous patients.[12–14] Although many factors have been proposed as predisposing to inversion, most, including improper traction on the umbilical cord,[12] are insufficiently documented. Those factors found to be most consistently associated with inversion are fundal implantation of the placenta (55 percent),[12] antepartum use of magnesium sulfate,[15] and uterine atony. It is thought that some patients may have a congenital weakness or anomaly of the uterus that predisposes them to inversion.[14]

The patient with uterine inversion presents with hemorrhage, shock, and pain. The degree of blood loss is frequently underestimated.[14]

Treatment consists of restoring intravascular volume and reducing the inversion. The key to successful replacement of the uterus includes speed of recognition and institution of therapy, preservation of antiseptic technique which may offer a role for prophylactic antibiotics and anesthesia sufficient to allow the required manipulation.[14] One must have a high index of suspicion for inversion even though this is a rare event. Several recent series have reported a maternal mortality of zero which is attributed to early recognition and treatment.[13–15]

If inversion is diagnosed before cervical ring contraction, the uterus can often be replaced manually. If this is not possible, a paracervical or intra-abdominal surgical approach and uterine relaxation are necessary.[14]

The degree of blood loss is related to the time the uterus remains inverted. Average estimated blood loss is 1,775 ml (reported range 200 to 3,000 ml).[14] If the placenta is still adherent after inversion, the uterus should be replaced before removing the placenta to decrease blood loss.[12–14] Primiparous patients have greater blood loss.

Oxytocics should not be given before the inverted uterus is replaced, because the resulting cervical contraction will prevent manual replacement. Once the uterus is replaced, uterine atony can be a major problem and there is a risk of reinversion. Vigorous uterine massage, administration of high doses of oxytocics, and uterine packing are often required.

Complications include reinversion, sepsis, urinary retention, anemia, and pituitary necrosis.[14]

Anesthetic Management

The need for vigorous resuscitation must be anticipated. Large intravenous catheters should be placed; blood typed, crossmatched, and prepared for infusion; and fluids and blood warmed prior to administration. Oxygen should be administered. Blood loss is often underestimated and can be very rapid.

Regional or local anesthesia may be adequate for manual replacement of an acute inversion diagnosed early before the cervix contracts.

Subacute or chronic inversion after cervical and uterine contraction has occurred requires uterine relaxation for uterine replacement.[12,14] This can be accomplished with general anesthesia using a volatile agent. If it is a subacute inversion, the patient must still be considered to have a full stomach, therefore a rapid-sequence induction with placement of endotracheal tube is indicated after administration of an oral antacid. The patient must have acute intravascular volume resuscitation first in order to tolerate the high dose of volatile agent needed to obtain uterine relaxation. A major problem arises when uterine inversion is not recognized as the cause of postpartum hemorrhage and the hemorrhage is treated with massage and oxytocics. The patient continues to hemorrhage and a contracted, but inverted, uterus and cervix are produced, rendering manual replacement impossible. The patient, who is still bleeding, will be unable to tolerate the use of high doses of volatile agents because of hypotension.

POSTPARTUM UTERINE ATONY

Pathophysiology

Postpartum uterine atony is the major cause of postpartum hemorrhage. It occurs in 2 to 5 percent of all vaginal deliveries.[4,16] Maternal mortality is less than 1 percent.[4] Associated factors include increased parity, multiple births, large infants, polyhydramnios, excessive oxytocic use, retained placenta, uterine inversion, precipitous labor, chorioamnionitis, prolonged labor, and a prior history of postpartum hemorrhage secondary to uterine atony.[17] The presenting symptom is painless vaginal bleeding or a rising fundus if the os is occluded by clots.

Anesthetic Management

Anesthetic management consists of administering oxygen; giving a nonparticulate oral antacid; inserting a large intravenous catheter; type and crossmatch of blood (if not already done); and aggressive volume resuscitation with crystalloid, colloid, and blood, if necessary, and monitoring urine output and central venous pressure. If bleeding is severe, the uterus is vigorously massaged and occasionally packed. Intravenous oxytocin 20 U/1,000 ml is administered. If atony is severe, an intravenous bolus of oxytocin 1 to 2 U may be given, keeping in mind that rapidly administered oxytocin can cause vasodilation and hypotension. If atony does not improve quickly after starting oxytocin the patient may be given methergine 0.2 mg. Methergine can only be given intramuscularly, as it can cause severe hypertension and resultant intracranial hemorrhage if given intravenously. Prostaglandin $F_{2}\alpha$ given directly into the uterus is another alternative. This can produce maternal nausea and vomiting. If the above measures are not successful, emergency laparotomy with either ligation of the internal iliac arteries or a gravid hysterectomy is indicated. (For anesthetic management, see Gravid Hysterectomy; below.) *Warning*: blood loss can be massive.

RETAINED PLACENTA

Pathophysiology

Retained placenta occurs in 1 percent of all vaginal deliveries.[11] Management requires manual exploration of the uterus, which usually requires at least some analgesia, if not anesthesia.

Anesthetic Management

If regional (i.e., epidural) anesthesia is in place, it may be continued during removal of the placenta, maintaining a T10 level. The anesthesiologist must recognize that if the bleeding becomes severe, the sympathetic block from the epidural anesthesia will exacerbate hypotension.[11] If an epidural anesthetic is not in place or functioning, the anesthetic options include subarachnoid block, general anesthesia, or monitored anesthesia care with intravenous sedation, depending on the patient. A general anesthetic must include a rapid-sequence induction with endotracheal intubation, as the patient is still at increased risk for aspiration. All patients should receive an oral nonparticulate antacid. Regardless of the anesthetic choice, ketamine should be avoided, as it can increase uterine tone, making manual exploration difficult.[11] Before initiating any anesthetic, the hematocrit and occasionally coagulation studies should be checked, if possible. In practice, this is not always easy to accomplish, therefore, the clinical judgment of the anesthesiologist is essential. The patient should have a functioning intravenous catheter in place. Using crystalloid solution or, on occasion, packed red cells may be necessary for volume replacement.

CERVICAL OR VAGINAL LACERATIONS AND TEARS

The patient with a cervical or vaginal laceration presents with postpartum bleeding although her uterus is firm. Lacerations are most common after a precipitous vaginal delivery, instrumental (i.e., forceps) delivery, or delivery of large infant. Anesthetic management is essentially the same as for retained placenta.

GRAVID HYSTERECTOMY

Pathophysiology

Gravid or cesarean hysterectomy or a hysterectomy performed within 24 hours postpartum is the definitive therapy for postpartum hemorrhage refractory to other more conservative measures. Gravid hysterectomy can be performed for either elective or emergent indications, although in recent years there has been a decrease in the number of elective cesarean hysterectomies. The overall incidence of cesarean hysterectomy is 0.11 percent according to the most recent prospective study by Chestnut et al.[18] The indications for elective gravid hysterectomy include[19]:

1. Carcinoma in situ
2. Cervical cancer
3. Dysmenorrheal menorrhagia

4. Uterine tumors or myomata
5. Chronic pelvic inflammatory disease
6. Breast cancer with therapeutic oophorectomy
7. Sterilization procedure in a patient with prior cesarean deliveries (uncommon today)

Indications for an emergent gravid hysterectomy include:[19]

1. Placenta previa
2. Placenta accreta
3. Uterine rupture
4. Uterine atony
5. Chorioamnionitis (less common)
6. DIC
7. Broad ligament hematoma complicating cesarean delivery
8. Fibroids precluding uterine closure
9. Extension of uterine incision secondary to macrosomia

Placenta previa and accreta are the two most common reasons for a cesarean hysterectomy, followed by uterine rupture and atony.[19]

With the increase in the number of cesarean deliveries being performed and the association between placenta previa/accreta and prior cesarean deliveries demonstrated by Clark et al. (see the discussion of placenta accreta, above) there are an increased number of patients at risk for emergent cesarean hysterectomy.[2,7] The risk of placenta previa increases from 0.2 percent in patients with an unscarred uterus to 10 percent in patients with four or more prior cesarean deliveries.[2] The risk of an accreta is 5 percent in a patient with an unscarred uterus and previa, and increases to 70 percent in patients with four or more prior cesarean deliveries and previa.[2] In a study by Clark et al., 82 percent of patients with previa/accreta and a prior uterine incision underwent a gravid hysterectomy, in comparison to 58 percent of patients with a previa/accreta and an unscarred uterus.[2]

Clark et al. identified a number of risk factors for cesarean hysterectomy[7]:

1. History of prior cesarean delivery with placenta previa/accreta
2. Uterine atony preceded by
   (a) Amnionitis
   (b) Cesarean delivery for arrest of labor
   (c) Oxytocic augmentation of labor
   (d) Magnesium sulfate
   (e) Increased fetal weight

However, in this study, only 74 percent of patients with a hemorrhagic complication requiring cesarean hysterectomy could be identified prior to delivery. In other words, 26 percent of all patients requiring emergent cesarean hysterectomy will be a surprise.[7]

There is an increased morbidity and mortality associated with cesarean hysterectomy (both elective and emergent) because of the increased duration of the procedure and the increased blood loss and fluid and transfusion requirements. Clark et al. reported that emergent gravid hysterectomy required a mean duration of 2 to 4 hours and the mean estimated blood loss was 2,000 to 5,000 ml (in comparison to 1,500 ml for an elective cesarean delivery).[7] Ninety-six percent of patients required a transfusion.[7] Chestnut et al., in a recent large prospective study, however, found a maternal mortality of zero.[19]

Anesthetic Management

In the past it was thought that regional anesthesia was contraindicated in patients at risk for emergent cesarean hysterectomy or in those patients undergoing an elective cesarean hysterectomy. This was because of the increased duration of surgery, increased complications of the surgery, and the frequent need for regional anesthetics to be converted to general anesthesia because of increased interoperative nausea, vomiting, and pain secondary to intraperitoneal manipulation.[19] However, recent studies by Chestnut et al.[19] and Arcario et al.[20] have shown that there is a role for regional anesthesia in managing these patients. The study of Arcario et al. even suggested that epidural anesthesia may decrease the amount of blood loss and fluid replacement needed in these cases.[20] However, this observation has not been borne out in other studies.

At our institution, elective cesarean hysterectomy is not a contraindication to continuous epidural anesthesia as long as there is (1) aggressive maintenance of a T4 level, (2) use of prophylaxis against nausea and vomiting such as metoclopramide and droperidol as needed, (3) judicious intravenous sedation to combat restlessness associated with a long procedure; and (4) adequate preparation to manage large blood losses. In the prospective study by Chestnut et al., no patient receiving regional anesthesia had to receive a supplemental general anesthetic intraoperatively.[19] We also believe epidural anesthesia is appropriate management for the normovolemic patient undergoing elective repeat cesarean delivery for placenta previa despite the fact that these patients are at high risk for placenta accreta and emergent gravid hysterectomy. The anesthesiologist must be prepared for major hemorrhage and the need for intravascular volume replacement with blood, colloid, and crystalloid solutions. A preoperative ultrasound may help identify those patients with an accreta (epidural anesthesia must be carefully considered in any patient with a suspected placenta percreta or increta).

We routinely place two large intravenous catheters in these patients and have two to four units of crossmatched blood (usually packed red cells) available before induction of anesthesia. An oral nonparticulate antacid is given with or without intravenous metoclopramide preoperatively. It is most important to keep these patients warm by using warming blankets and fluid warmers. The mother is given 100 percent oxygen throughout the procedure if a regional anesthetic is administered. When a patient presents with massive, uncontrollable peripartum hemorrhage requiring a cesarean hysterectomy, general anesthesia is usually necessary. Management is essentially the same as has already been outlined throughout this section. If the patient has not been in labor or has received a continuous epidural anesthetic, a brief history should be obtained. Left uterine displacement should be used and a large intravenous catheter inserted. Oxygen and an oral nonparticulate antacid should be administered and a rapid-sequence induction of general anesthesia performed. Ketamine should be considered for induction. If the patient is profoundly hypotensive, it may be necessary to proceed with a minimal induction agent coupled with succinylcholine to facilitate intubation.

Massive blood loss and the need for aggressive intravascular volume resuscitation must be anticipated. The need for keeping the patient as warm as possible must be appreciated.

REFERENCES

1. Chantigian RC: Antepartum hemorrhage. p. 236. In Datta S, Ostheimer GW (eds): Common Problems in Obstetric Anesthesia. Year Book Medical Publishers, Chicago, 1987
2. Clark S, et al: Placenta previa/accreta and prior cesarean section. Obstet Gynecol 66:89, 1985
3. Pritchard JA: Obstetric hemorrhage. p. 389. In Pritchard JA, McDonald PC (eds): Williams Obstetrics. 17th Ed. Appleton & Lange, East Norwalk, CT, 1984
4. Plumer M: Bleeding problems. p. 309. In James F, et al (eds): Obstetric Anesthesia: The Complicated Patient. 2nd Ed. FA Davis, Philadelphia, 1988
5. Gatt SP: Anesthetic management of the obstetric patient with antepartum or intrapartum hemorrhage. In Clinics in Anesthesiology. Vol. 4, No. 2, April 1986
6. Read J, et al: Placenta accreta: changing clinical aspects and outcome. Obstet Gynecol 56:31, 1980
7. Clark SL, Yeh SY, Phelan JP, et al: Emergency hysterectomy for obstetric hemorrhage. Obstet Gynecol 64:376, 1984
8. Hibbard BM, Jeffcoate TN: Abruptio placentae. Obstet Gynecol 27:155, 1966
9. Pritchard JA: Haematological problems associated with delivery, placental abruption, retained dead fetus, and amniotic fluid embolism. Clin Haematol 2:563, 1973
10. Datta S: The high-risk parturient. p. 244. In Ostheimer GW (ed): Manual of Obstetric Anesthesia. Churchill Livingstone, New York, 1984
11. Biehl DR: Antepartum and postpartum hemorrhage. In Shnider SM, Levinson G (eds): Anesthesia for Obstetrics. Williams & Wilkins, Baltimore, 1987
12. Shah-Hosseini R: Puerperal uterine inversion. Obstet Gynecol 73:567, 1989
13. Watson P, et al: Management of acute and subacute puerperal inversion of the uterus. Obstet Gynecol 55:12, 1980
14. Kitchin J, et al: Puerperal inversion of the uterus. Am J Obstet Gynecol 123:51, 1975
15. Platt L, et al: Acute puerperal inversion of the uterus. Am J Obstet Gynecol 141:187, 1981
16. Newton M: Postpartum hemorrhage. Am J Obstet Gynecol 54:51, 1967
17. Pritchard JA, et al: Abnormalities of the third stage of labor. p. 707. In Pritchard JA, McDonald PC (eds): Williams Obstetrics. 17th Ed. Appleton & Lange, East Norwalk, CT, 1985
18. Chestnut DH, Eden RD, Gall SA, Parker RT: Peripartum hysterectomy: a review of cesarean and postpartum hysterectomy. Obstet Gynecol 65:365, 1985
19. Chestnut DH, et al: Anesthetic management for obstetric hysterectomy—a multi-institutional study. Anesthesiology 70(14):607, 1989
20. Arcario T, Greene M, Ostheimer GW, et al: Risks of placenta previa/accreta in patients with previous cesarean deliveries (abstract). Anesthesiology 69:A659, 1988
21. Benedetti TJ: Obstetric hemorrhage. p. 485. In Gabbe SJ, Neibyl JR, Simpson JL (eds): Obstetrics: Normal and Problem Pregnancies. Churchill Livingstone, New York, 1986

VAGINAL BIRTH AFTER CESAREAN DELIVERY

In October 1988, the American College of Obstetricians and Gynecologists (ACOG) decided that vaginal birth after a previous cesarean delivery, or the trial of labor (TOL), was an acceptable alternative to elective repeat cesarean delivery.[1] The guidelines established by ACOG have not adequately addressed the risks of epidural anesthesia for the relief of labor pain during a TOL; however, reports in the obstetric literature have suggested that it is safe. The purpose of this section is

The text and tables of this section are reproduced with modification from Regional Anesthesia. 15:304, 1990, with permission.

to review the literature on trial of labor and examine the role of epidural anesthesia.

CESAREAN DELIVERY

Between 1970 and 1984, the cesarean delivery rate increased from 5.5 percent to 18 percent in the United States.[2] In 1985, cesarean delivery was the most frequently performed major operation in America, exceeding the combined total of all tonsillectomies, appendectomies, and mastectomies.[3] The most common reason for performing a cesarean delivery in this country is a history of a prior cesarean delivery. The origin of the elective repeat cesarean delivery came from the belief that the risk of uterine rupture in a laboring "scarred" uterus outweighed the maternal and neonatal risks of an elective repeat cesarean delivery.[4] It was determined that the type of uterine incision played a significant role in the severity of uterine rupture during labor after cesarean delivery.[5,6] A uterine incision on the upper segment of the uterus (classical incision) is more likely to rupture without warning. The classical incision is 10 times more likely to rupture than the low transverse uterine incision, resulting in excessive hemorrhaging and extrusion of the fetus into the abdomen.[5,6] Ruptured incisions of the lower uterine segment form a dehiscence or window that is relatively avascular; these incisions rarely result in abdominal extrusion of the fetus and rarely interfere with the birthing process.[5,6]

TRIAL OF LABOR

In 1981, the National Institutes of Health decided that vaginal birth after cesarean delivery in patients with a lower-segment uterine scar should be considered the reasonable alternative to elective repeat cesarean delivery.[7] Since that time, numerous retrospective and prospective studies have been performed examining the last 30 years of obstetrics in the United States. The results of such studies have shown that a TOL can be safely tolerated by patients with low transverse uterine incisions, by patients with more than one prior low transverse cesarean delivery, and by those with oxytocic induction or augmentation of labor.[8–12] The overall success rate for a TOL is 60 to 80 percent and increases to 90 percent when the indication for the previous cesarean delivery was a breech presentation. When the indication for the previous cesarean delivery was fetopelvic disproportion or failure to progress, the success rate is 55 to 65 percent.[8–13] The rationale for attempting a TOL is the decreased maternal and fetal morbidity and mortality from vaginal delivery when compared with the elective repeat cesarean delivery.[1,8,9,14] The increase in maternal morbidity associated with cesarean delivery is due to a 0.31 percent incidence of bladder laceration, a 0.09 percent incidence of ureteral injury, a 30 to 50 percent increase in blood loss, increased chance of wound infection, increased hospital stay (from 2.5 to 4.5 days), increased risk of postoperative thrombophlebitis (from 0.25 to 0.1 percent with vaginal delivery to 2 to 10 percent with cesarean delivery), and longer postoperative recovery period compared to a successful TOL.[1,5,8,9,14]

In this era of cost containment, economic factors need to be considered. In a 1984 study performed by Flamm et al.,[13] the total cost for a vaginal delivery after cesarean delivery was $2,087, compared to $5,101 for elective repeat cesarean delivery.

Cesarean delivery may not be a benign event for the fetus or neonate. Poorly timed elective cesarean delivery can result in iatrogenic prematurity, which causes fetal morbidity or death. Elective cesarean delivery has been associated with persistent fetal circulation in term infants, which can be a fatal condition.[15–16] However, with the use of amniocentesis and biochemical evaluation of amniotic fluid to determine fetal lung maturity, the occurrence of iatrogenic prematurity should be a rare event.

There are two types of uterine separation associated with a TOL: incomplete rupture and complete rupture. Incomplete rupture is a relatively benign event and is not associated with increased maternal or fetal morbidity or mortality. It is usually an incidental finding, detected by vaginal palpation of the uterine scar after a vaginal delivery or noted during direct visualization at cesarean delivery. The incidence of incomplete rupture with a TOL is 0.5 to 3.0 percent.[8,19–22] Complete uterine rupture is associated with significant maternal morbidity and fetal morbidity or mortality.[34] The incidence of complete rupture is 0.3 to 0.5 percent with a TOL, compared to 1 per 800 to 1 per 3,000 (0.125 to 0.3 percent) for spontaneous rupture of unscarred uteri.[8,9,35–38] In our review of 10,967 patients, presented in 14 studies from 1980 to 1989, there were no maternal deaths related to the TOL. There were a total of nine fetal deaths secondary to scar rupture during the TOL. This gives a perinatal mortality rate (PMR) of less than 1 per 1,000 births. In a study by Meehan et al.,[23] the PMR in 1,498 patients with one or more cesarean delivery scars delivered between 1972 and 1982 was analyzed. Repeat elective cesarean delivery was performed in 654 of the patients, and the PMR was 4.5 per 1,000 births. TOL was attempted in 844 patients, and the PMR dropped from 40 per 1,000 births to 20 per 1,000 births by the end of the study. In view of the improvement in the PMR and the added risk to the mother with elective cesarean delivery, obstetricians advocate a policy of TOL with informed consent in selected cases.[23]

Analysis of the Meehan et al. study looking at PMR secondary to complete uterine rupture reveals a PMR of only 4.7 per 1,000 births. Combination of the present study with the Meehan et al. study yields a PMR resulting from complete uterine rupture of 1 per 1,000 to 4.7 per 1,000 births, which is equal to the PMR for elective cesarean delivery. Thus, complete uterine rupture is not a significant contributor to the PMR resulting from a TOL.

THE USE OF EPIDURAL ANESTHESIA

The American College of Obstetricians and Gynecologists[1] have adopted the following guidelines for trial of labor. "A woman with a low transverse uterine incision in the absence of a contraindication (classical incision) should be encouraged to attempt a trial of labor. There are insufficient data to assess the safety or danger of labor for women with a previous low vertical incision. Likewise, the effects of labor on patients with more than one fetus, a breech presentation, or an estimated fetal weight greater than 4,000 g have not been substantiated. Continuous electronic fetal monitoring and 24-hour blood banking capabilities could be available. Anesthesia coverage and an obstetrician capable of evaluating labor and performing an emergency cesarean delivery should be in house."

Although the "classic" signs and symptoms of rupture are abdominal pain between contractions or a severe tearing sensation followed by cessation of uterine contractions, the majority of ruptures usually present with signs of fetal distress diagnosed by continuous fetal heart rate (FHR) monitoring.[34] FHR patterns heralding complete rupture are severe variable decelerations or a prolonged deceleration. Associated with the FHR changes can be loss of pressure tracing on the internal uterine pressure monitor.[8–11,24] In Tables 8-1 and 8-2, data are presented from 14 TOL studies between 1980 and 1989. There were 10,967 patients who attempted a vaginal birth after a cesarean delivery. A total of 41 complete uterine ruptures occurred, giving a rupture incidence of 0.37 percent. Of the 10,967 patients undergoing a TOL, 1,623 of them had epidural catheters placed for relief of labor pain (Table 8-1). The presentation of 37 of the 41 ruptures is shown in Table 8-2. The Meehan et al.[25] study failed to mention the presenting signs and symptoms of their four ruptures and none of them had epidural anesthesia.

The incidence of uterine rupture in patients with epidural anesthesia (14 of 1,623) was 0.86 percent. The incidence of uterine rupture in patients without epidural anesthesia (23 of 9,344) was 0.25 percent. The incidence of rupture in the epidural group is three times greater than the incidence in the nonepidural group. However, because of the small sample size of uterine ruptures, the increased incidence of ruptures in the epidural group is not clinically significant. Three of the 14 ruptures presented with "classic" abdominal pain alone, 7 with fetal distress alone, and 2 with both fetal distress and abdominal pain; 1 was an incidental finding at cesarean delivery, and 1 presented with postpartum bleeding.

Table 8-1. Trial of Labor Data from 14 Studies

Study	Year	No. Patients	With Epidural	Without Epidural	Complete Rupture	Rupture Incidence (%)
Carlsson[29]	1980	119	77	42	2	1.7
Demianczuk[19]	1982	92	41	51	2	2.2
Meier[21]	1982	207	19	188	0	0
Martin[32]	1983	717	98	619	3	0.42
Uppington[31]	1983	222	71	151	4	1.8
Rudick[28]	1984	115	115	0	1	0.87
Flamm[13]	1984	230	73	157	0	0
Horenstein[27]	1985	732	0	732	2	0.27
Stovall[10]	1987	272	153	119	1	0.37
Molloy[33]	1987	1,781	85	1,696	8	0.45
Phelan[9]	1987	1,796	178	1,618	5	0.28
Flamm[8]	1988	1,776	181	1,595	3	0.17
Meehan[25]	1989	1,498	187	1,311	4	0.27
Meehan[23]	1989	1,350	345	1,005	6	0.44
TOTAL		10,967	1,623	9,344	41	
Overall rupture incidence						0.37

Table 8-2. Presenting Signs of Uterine Rupture[a]

Presenting Signs of Rupture	Number of Patients Who Ruptured	With Epidural (n = 1,623)	Without Epidural (n = 9,344)
Abdominal pain	4	3	1
Fetal distress	21	7	14
Incidental finding at cesarean delivery	3	1	2
Fetal distress and abdominal pain	5	2	3
Postpartum bleeding	4	1	3
Total	37	14	23
Rupture incidence		0.86%	0.25%

[a] Data from Table 8-1. The four ruptures from Meehan[25] are not included because their presentation is not mentioned in the study.

It is interesting that 5 of 14 (35 percent) complete ruptures in the epidural group presented with abdominal pain, compared to 4 of 23 (17 percent) in the nonepidural group (Table 8-2). Two of the five ruptures in the epidural group presented with abdominal pain associated with monitored fetal distress. All of the studies alluded to the fact that satisfactory epidural anesthesia was obtained. However, none gave specific levels of epidural sensory or motor block at the time of uterine rupture. Overall, abdominal pain alone or in association with monitored fetal distress was present in only 9 of the 41 (22 percent) of all uterine ruptures (Table 8-2). Fetal distress alone was the presenting sign of rupture 50 percent of the time in the epidural group and 61 percent of the time in the nonepidural group. Overall, uterine rupture presented with signs or symptoms other than abdominal pain 76 percent of the time, with fetal distress presenting by itself 52 percent of the time (Table 8-2). Thus, the single most reliable sign of uterine rupture is fetal distress rather than abdominal pain. Of note, however, is the fact that if abdominal pain is going to occur with complete uterine rupture, there will be the development of "breakthrough pain" despite the presence of epidural anesthesia. Crawford[26] referred to this phenomenon as the "epidural sieve."

The presentation of uterine rupture as it relates to the presence or absence of epidural anesthesia, oxytocin, and prostaglandin administration is shown in Table 8-3. Twenty-three of the 41 (56 percent) ruptures occurred in patients without epidural anesthesia, compared to only 18 of 41 (44 percent) ruptures in patients with epidural anesthesia. This suggests that there is no increased incidence of uterine rupture in patients with epidural anesthesia. Nineteen of the 41 (46 percent) ruptures occurred in patients who did not receive any agent for induction or augmentation of labor (oxytocin or prostaglandin). Twenty-two of 41 (54 percent) patients developing ruptures received either intravenous oxytocin or vaginal prostaglandin, which does not represent a significant clinical difference from the nonoxytocin group.

Horenstein and Phelan[27] studied the risks and benefits of oxytocin usage in 732 patients who underwent a TOL. In their study, 40 percent of the patients received oxytocin for either induction or augmentation of labor and 60 percent did not receive oxytocin. The incidence of incomplete rupture in the oxytocin and nonoxytocin groups was 3 percent and 2 percent, which is not clinically significant. There were only two complete ruptures, one with oxytocin and one without oxytocin. Flamm et al.[8] performed a similar study and found no increased incidence of incomplete rupture with oxytocin usage in a TOL. There were three complete ruptures in their study, one with oxytocin and two without oxytocin.

The present review of the literature confirms the obstetric clinical impression that complete uterine rupture is not significantly increased with oxytocin use for induction/augmentation of labor. Nine of the 41 (22 percent) ruptures occurred in patients who received epidural anesthesia and induction/augmentation of labor, compared to 10 of 41 (24 percent) ruptures in patients who received no epidural anesthesia and no induction/augmentation of labor. There appears to be no increased risk of complete uterine rupture with the combination of epidural anesthesia and oxytocin.

Studies have shown that epidural anesthesia does not have a negative effect on the success rate of vaginal delivery with trial of labor. Phelan et al.[9] studied 1,796 women undergoing a TOL. Epidural anesthesia was administered to 178 patients, all of whom also received oxytocin for augmentation of labor. When the cesarean delivery rate for the combination of epidural anesthesia and oxytocin was compared to that for patients who received oxytocin alone, there was no significant difference (approximately a 31 percent incidence of cesarean delivery for both groups). Flamm et al.[8] had similar results. Among 1,776 patients who underwent a TOL, 181 patients received epidural anesthesia for relief of labor pain. One hundred thirty-four (74 percent) delivered vaginally. The success rate in this group did not differ from those who did not have epidural anesthesia (1,180 of 1,595, or 74 percent).

Table 8-3. Rupture Presentation Related to Epidural Anesthesia, Oxytocin, and Prostaglandin Use

Presentation	Epidural	Epi + Oxy	Oxy	PG	Nothing	Epi + PG
Abdominal pain alone	0	3	0	1	0	1
Abdominal pain and fetal distress	1	1	2	0	1	0
Fetal distress alone	7	3	5	0	5	0
Incidental finding at cesarean delivery	1	0	2	0	0	0
Postpartum bleeding	0	1	0	0	3	0
Presentation not given[a]	0	0	3	0	1	0
TOTAL	9	8	12	1	10	1

Epi, epidural; oxy, oxytocin; PG, prostaglandin.
[a] Meehan.[25]

CLINICAL RECOMMENDATIONS

We recommend that sensory analgesia with intraspinal opioids or sensory anesthesia with local anesthetics with or without opioids rather than complete anesthesia be the goal for relief of labor pain. The lowest possible local anesthetic concentration and dose—with or without opioids—should be considered. We prefer continuous epidural anesthesia using bupivacaine 0.0625 to 0.125 percent with fentanyl 1 to 2 μg/ml. This mixture is administered at a rate of 8 to 12 ml/h after the establishment of the anesthetic using a variety of drugs. It is our conclusion from the literature and our practice that epidural anesthesia is safe during a TOL provided appropriate fetal and uterine contraction monitoring are used.

REFERENCES

1. Committee on Obstetrics: Maternal and Fetal Medicine: Guidelines for Vaginal Delivery after a Previous Cesarean Birth. American College of Obstetricians and Gynecologists Newsletter No. 64, 1988
2. Notzon FC, Placek PJ, Taffel SM: Comparison of national cesarean-section rates. N Engl J Med 316:386, 1987
3. Nation Center for Health Statistics Monthly Vital Statistics Report: Advance Report of Final Natality Statistics. Vol. 34, p. 6. U.S. Government Printing Office, Washington, DC, 1985
4. Cragin EB: Conservatism in obstetrics. NY State J Med 104:1, 1916
5. Hibbard L: Cesarean section and other surgical procedures. p. 517. In Gabbe SG, Neibyl JR, Simpson JL (eds): Obstetrics: Normal and Problem Pregnancies. Churchill Livingstone, New York, 1986
6. Pritchard JA, MacDonald PC: Williams Obstetrics. 16th Ed. p. 861. Appleton & Lange, East Norwalk, CT, 1980
7. National Institutes of Health: Cesarean Childbirth. NIH Publication No. 82-2067. Bethesda, MD, 1981
8. Flamm BL, Lim OW, Jones C, et al: Vaginal birth after cesarean: results of a multicenter study. Am J Obstet Gynecol 158:1079, 1988
9. Phelan JP, Clark ST, Diaz F, Paul RH: Vaginal birth after cesarean. Am J Obstet Gynecol 157:1510, 1987
10. Stovall TG, Shaver DC, Solomon SK, Anderson GD: Trial of labor in previous cesarean section patients, excluding classical cesarean sections. Obstet Gynecol 70:713, 1987
11. Pruett KM, Kirshon B, Cotton DB, Poindexter AN: Is vaginal birth after two or more cesarean sections safe? Obstet Gynecol 72:163, 1988
12. Induction of Labor. Technical Bulletin No. 49. American College of Obstetricians and Gynecologists, Washington, D.C., 1978
13. Flamm BL, Dunnett C, Fischermann E, Quilligan EJ: Vaginal delivery following cesarean section: use of oxytocin augmentation and epidural anesthesia with internal tocodynamic and internal fetal monitoring. Am J Obstet Gynecol 148:759, 1984
14. Eisenkop SM, Richman R, Platt LD, Paul RH: Urinary tract injury during cesarean section. Obstet Gynecol 64:376, 1982
15. Chervenk FA, Herslinger R, Freedman R, Lamastra P: Current perspectives on iatrogenic neonatal respiratory distress syndrome. J Reprod Med 31:53, 1986
16. Heritage CK, Cunningham MD: Association of elective repeat cesarean delivery and persistent pulmonary hypertension of the newborn. Am J Obstet Gynecol 152:627, 1985
17. Hjalmarson O, Krantz B, Jacobson B, et al: The importance of neonatal asphyxia and cesarean sections as risk factors for neonatal respiratory disorders in an unselected population. Acta Paediatr Scand 71:403, 1982
18. Evard JR, Gold EM: Cesarean section: risk/benefit. Perinatal Care 2:4, 1978
19. Demianczuk NN, Hunter DJ, Taylor DW: Trial of labor after previous cesarean section: prognostic indicators of outcome. Am J Obstet Gynecol 142:640, 1982
20. Gibbs CE: Planned vaginal delivery following cesarean section. Clin Obstet Gynecol 23:507, 1980
21. Merrill BS, Gibbs CE: Planned vaginal delivery following cesarean section. Obstet Gynecol 52:50, 1978
22. Case BD, Corcoran R, Jeffcoate N, Randle GH: Cesarean and its place in modern obstetric practice. J Obstet Gynaecol Br Commonw 78:203, 1981
23. Meehan FP, Magani IM: True rupture of the cesarean scar (a 15-year review. 1972–1987). Eur J Obstet Gynecol Reprod Biol 30:129, 1989

24. Uppington J: Epidural analgesia and previous cesarean section. Anaesthesia 38:336, 1983
25. Meehan FP, Burke G, Casey C, Sheil JG: Delivery following cesarean section and perinatal mortality. Am J Perinatol 6(1):90, 1989
26. Crawford JS: The epidural sieve and MBC (minimal blocking concentration): a hypothesis. Anaesthesia 31:1277, 1976
27. Horenstein JM, Phelan JP: Previous cesarean section: the risks and benefits of oxytocin usage in a trial of labor. Am J Obstet Gynecol 151:564, 1985
28. Rudick V, Niv D, Hetman-Perl M, et al: Epidural analgesia for planned vaginal delivery following previous cesarean section. Obstet Gynecol 64:621, 1984
29. Carlsson C, Nybell-Lindahl G, Ingemarsson I: Extradural block in patients who have previously undergone cesarean section. Br J Anaesth 52:827, 1980
30. Eckstein KL, Oberlander SG, Marx GF: Uterine rupture during epidural blockade. Can J Anaesth 20:566, 1973
31. Martin JN, Harris BA, Huddleston JF, et al: Vaginal delivery following previous cesarean birth. Am J Obstet Gynecol 146:255, 1983
32. Meier PR, Porreco RP: Trial of labor following cesarean sections: a two-year experience. Am J Obstet Gynecol 144:671, 1982
33. Molloy BG, Sheil O, Duigan NM: Delivery after cesarean section: review of 2,176 consecutive cases. Br Med J 294:1645, 1987
34. Eden RD, Parker RT, Gall SA: Rupture of the pregnant uterus: a 53-year review. Obstet Gynecol 68:671, 1986
35. Brudell M, Chakmavarti S: Uterine rupture in labor. Br Med J 1:122, 1975
36. Smith AM: Uterine rupture in labor. Br Med J 1:446, 1975
37. Schrinsky DC, Benson RC: Rupture of the pregnant uterus: a review. Obstet Gynecol Surv 33:217, 1978
38. Caggiano AP, Breen JL: Uterine rupture. Int Surg 50:368, 1968

PREMATURITY

Prematurity is defined as birth occurring between 20 and 37 completed weeks of gestation. The incidence ranges between 7 and 8 percent in the United States.[1] Prematurity accounts from more than 80 percent of all perinatal deaths either directly or indirectly.[2] A distinction is now made between the fetus or neonate that is "preterm" (born before the 38th week of gestation) and that which is "small for gestational age" (birthweight below the 10th percentile for gestational age).[3] Outcome is closely tied to both gestational maturity and birthweight (Fig. 8-2).[4] Preterm infants who survive may require prolonged intubation and extremely expensive and long-term neonatal intensive care for treatment of such problems as respiratory distress syndrome, bronchopulmonary dysplasia, intracranial hemorrhage, and necrotizing enterocolitis. After discharge, they remain at risk for morbidity from recurrent respiratory infections, cardiovascular disease, delayed growth, and poor neurodevelopmental outcome. Attempts to delay delivery through pharmacologic tocolysis entail additional risks to mother and fetus that must be balanced against the potential benefits. The obstetric, anesthetic, social, economic, and ethical challenges posed by the problem of prematurity remain formidable. This section focuses on the obstetric and anesthetic issues.

OBSTETRIC CONSIDERATIONS

Etiology

The precise mechanisms responsible for the timing and initiation of labor are complex and poorly understood. A recent study suggested that an early "up regulation" of myometrial responsiveness to oxytocin may play a role in preterm onset of labor.[5] Other factors implicated include oxytocin receptor concentrations and use of prostaglandins, progesterone, estrogen, and catecholamines. A variety of clinical factors have been associated with preterm labor (Table 8-4), including fetal, uterine, cervical, and placental abnormalities, uterine overdistension, infection, and maternal trauma or disease. Currently the ability to predict preterm labor is limited, but when one or more of the factors listed in Table 8-4 is present, increased antenatal surveillance is appropriate.

Associated Problems

Breech presentation is much more common in preterm labor (25 percent compared to 3 percent at term).[6] The incidence of maternal hemorrhage is also higher during preterm birth because of associated placenta previa, abruption, or uterine atony from residual tocolytic effect. Prolapsed cord and fetal distress are also more common in the preterm fetus, which is less tolerant of asphyxia or maternal hypotension. In addition, infection is more common because of the association between premature rupture of membranes and preterm labor.[7] Signs of infection may be obscured by concurrent administration of glucocorticoids to enhance fetal lung maturity.

Obstetric Management of Preterm Labor

The first challenge in obstetric management is early recognition of preterm labor. Early signs of labor may be subtle and the distinction between false and true labor can be difficult. The estimated 20 to 40 percent

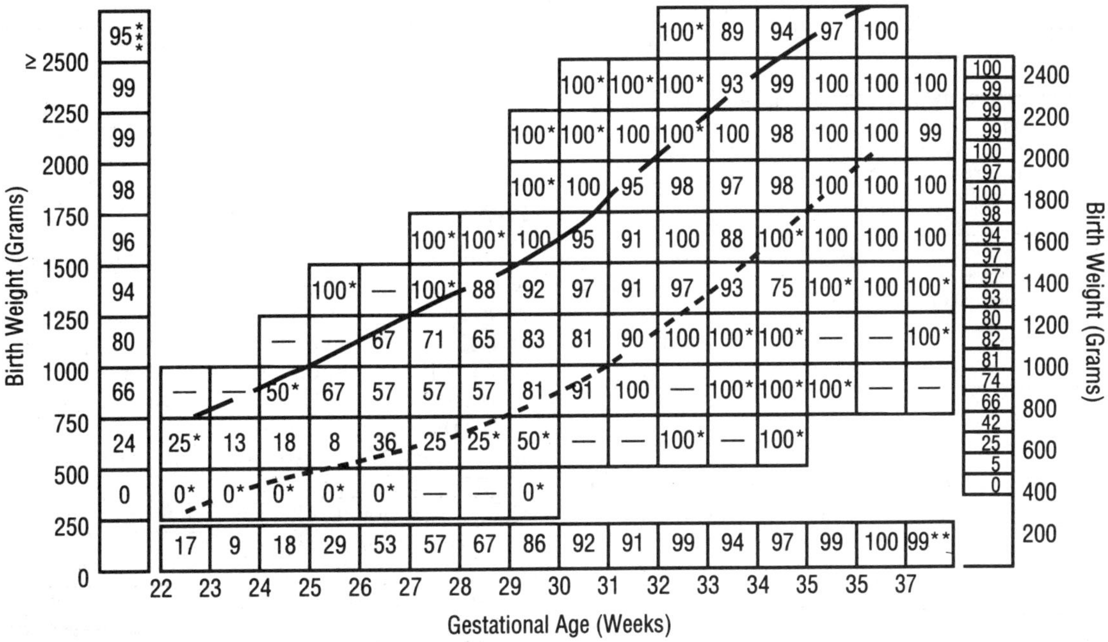

Fig. 8-2. The survival rate by birthweight and gestational age at the University of Alabama from 1979 to 1981. The dotted line represents the 10th percentile of birthweight for gestational age, and the solid line represents the 90th percentile. *, less than 5 values; **, greater than 37 weeks but less than 2,500 g; ***, more than 2,500 g but less than 37 weeks. (From Goldenberg et al.,[4] with permission.)

overdiagnosis rate subjects many women to the risk of tocolytic therapy unnecessarily. However, if one delays making the diagnosis by 3 to 5 hours, cervical dilation may progress to the point where tocolytics are ineffective.

Initial obstetric management usually calls for bedrest and intravenous fluid administration (crystalloid 500 ml) to suppress pituitary oxytocin production, although these maneuvers are rarely effective.[8] A history and physical examination of the mother should be performed to screen for maternal complications or conditions that might contraindicate tocolysis. A baseline cardiovascular examination, electrocardiogram (ECG), and early anesthetic consultation are commended because of the important side effects and interactions of tocolytic agents (see Ch. 5). Assessment of the fetus usually begins with fetal heart rate monitoring.

Table 8-4. Factors Associated with Preterm Labor

Prior history of preterm delivery or abortion
Preterm rupture of membranes
Incompetent cervix
Uterine anatomic abnormalities
Overdistended uterus (multiple gestation, polyhydramnios, etc.)
Placental abnormalities (previa, abruption)
Fetal malformations
Fetal demise
Maternal systemic disease (uncontrolled diabetes, hyperthyroidism, cardiovascular disease, etc.)
Retained intrauterine device
Trauma or surgery
Low socioeconomic status
Coitus
Tobacco use
Cocaine use

Tocolysis

Armed with the abovementioned evaluations of both mother and fetus, the obstetrician must decide whether the interests of the mother and fetus are best served by delivery or tocolysis. Absolute and relative contraindications to pharmacologic tocolysis are listed in Table 8-5. When prolongation of pregnancy or the side effects of tocolytic agents are sufficiently threatening to the health of the mother, or when a hostile intrauterine environment threatens the fetus, preterm labor should be allowed to progress to delivery. In the absence of contraindications, pharmacologic tocolysis may be em-

Table 8-5. Contraindications to Inhibition of Preterm Labor

Absolute Contraindications
Significant maternal hemorrhage
Acute fetal distress (that is not due to tetanic contractions)
Chorioamnionitis
Eclampsia/severe pregnancy-induced hypertension
Fetal anomaly incompatible with life
Intrauterine death
Relative Contraindications
Mild pregnancy-induced hypertension
Maternal cardiovascular disease
Fetal growth retardation
Diabetes
Uncontrolled hyperthyroidism
Severe renal disease

ployed on a long-term basis or for a short term to allow administration of glucocorticoids (see below) or for transfer to a high-risk obstetric facility.

Enhancement of Fetal Lung Maturity

A major cause of morbidity and mortality in premature infants is respiratory distress syndrome. Prior to 34 weeks gestation, insufficient alveolar surfactant production by fetal type II pneumocytes leads to impaired oxygenation, increased pulmonary vascular resistance, hyaline membrane disease, and right-to-left shunting of blood. Maternal administration of glucocorticoids (betamethasone or dexamethasone) may decrease the incidence of respiratory distress syndrome in the premature infant according to Liggins and Howie.[9] Clinical studies may be found that both support[10] and refute[11] their efficacy. The mechanism by which glucocorticoids accelerate surfactant production is unknown. The beneficial effects of glucocorticoids are transient and are diminished if birth occurs more than 7 days after administration.[12] Delivery must be delayed at least 24 hours to allow administration of glucocorticoids. The efficacy of glucocorticoid therapy in patients with premature rupture of membranes has been questioned.[13] Interestingly, premature rupture of membranes itself may accelerate fetal lung maturation,[14] although this is a matter of controversy.

The difficult decision as to whether or not to employ glucocorticoids must involve consideration of the risks. Pregnancy-induced hypertension and the hyperglycemia of diabetes may be exacerbated by steroids. In addition, there is an increased risk of infection or of masking an infection in patients receiving steroids. The metabolic side effects associated with β-adrenergic tocolytics (hyperglycemia and hypokalemia) are often exaggerated by concurrent administration of steroids. Pulmonary edema has been reported during combined therapy of steroids together with terbutaline, ritodrine, or magnesium, but it is not clear that glucocorticoids increase the risk above that which already exists with those tocolytic agents. Concerns about impaired fetal development based on studies in animals[15] have not proved significant in humans.[16]

Premature Rupture of Membranes

Controversy surrounds the management of patients with premature rupture of membranes (PROM). Eighty to 90 percent of such women will go into preterm labor within 7 days. There is some sentiment that delay of delivery in this population would expose patients to an increased risk of chorioamnionitis. One recent study found that infants born to women with chorioamnionitis had a fourfold increase in the incidence of respiratory distress, neonatal sepsis, and intraventricular hemorrhage.[17] Antibiotic therapy prior to overt chorioamnionitis has been shown to reduce these complications.[18] Another study found no increase in neonatal sepsis or intraventricular hemorrhage following prophylactic tocolysis in women with PROM.[19] However, they also found that tocolytic therapy in women with PROM was not more effective than expectant management. Moreover, as previously mentioned, the efficacy of glucocorticoid therapy in this population has been questioned.

OBSTETRIC CONSIDERATIONS FOR DELIVERY

If tocolysis fails, or if preterm delivery is elected, the chief obstetric considerations after maternal safety are the avoidance of fetal asphyxia and trauma. The preterm fetus is less tolerant of asphyxia and the premature skull is less calcified and offers less protection against intracerebral hemorrhage from the trauma of birth. Although malpresentations are more common in preterm deliveries, fetopelvic disproportion is seldom a problem except with a transverse lie. However, the resistance of the cervix or vagina may cause trauma to the neonate and a liberal episiotomy is often recommended. For this same reason, cesarean delivery is often preferred and an ample uterine incision helps minimize fetal trauma. Cesarean delivery is often elected for breech presentation of an infant older than 32 weeks gestation because of concern for the risk of entrapment of the aftercoming head. Following rupture of membranes, cord entrapment and compression is more common during premature deliveries. Personnel skilled in neonatal resuscitation should be present at delivery.

ANESTHETIC CONSIDERATIONS

The anesthesiologist may be asked to administer anesthesia to parturients prior to term under the following conditions: (1) for labor and vaginal delivery if tocolysis fails or is contraindicated, (2) for elective cesarean delivery if indicated for maternal or fetal well-being, and (3) for emergent cesarean delivery for fetal distress. Maintenance of maternal safety, avoidance of fetal asphyxia, and provision of maternal comfort remain the preeminent goals of the obstetric anesthesiologist. In addition, for vaginal delivery of the preterm fetus, it is extremely important to inhibit the reflex urge to bear down in order to avoid a precipitous and traumatic delivery. Uncontrolled precipitous delivery markedly increases the risk of intracerebral hemorrhage in the preterm neonate. As mentioned above, the preterm fetus is less tolerant of asphyxia. Fetal or neonatal asphyxia markedly increases the risk of respiratory distress syndrome, intracerebral hemorrhage, and necrotizing enterocolitis in the preterm neonate. The anesthesiologist must be aware of the increased risk of maternal hemorrhage due to the higher incidence of placenta previa, abruption, or the residual effects of tocolytic agents. Because the preterm fetus has a decreased tolerance of asphyxia and an increased incidence of placenta previa, abruption, prolapsed cord, and infection, a trial of preterm labor may very suddenly, and not uncommonly, result in fetal distress and the need for emergent cesarean delivery. The side effects of recently administered tocolytic agents may importantly impact on anesthetic management (see discussions of individual tocolytic agents, below).

Most textbooks state that preterm fetuses are more susceptible to the depressant effects of analgesic/anesthetic drugs for the following reasons: (1) premature fetuses, with their less developed lungs, kidneys, and liver have a slower rate of drug metabolism and excretion; (2) premature infants have decreased protein binding capacity; (3) the premature fetal blood–brain barrier is more permeable; and (4) the premature fetus is more likely to be acidotic and, therefore, more vulnerable to the phenomenon of "ion trapping" of local anesthetic drugs. Recent studies in preterm sheep fetuses question the significance of these effects with regard to lidocaine in the absence of fetal acidosis.[20] Further work remains to be done to clarify this issue in humans. In the meantime, the prudent anesthesiologist should limit dosages of local anesthetics and narcotics to the minimum necessary to achieve the desired effects.

ANESTHETIC MANAGEMENT

Vaginal Delivery

Lumbar epidural anesthesia is generally the anesthetic of choice for preterm labor and vaginal delivery. It provides all the advantages previously mentioned for full-term delivery, including reduction of maternal pain, anxiety, catecholamine levels, and hyperventilation as well as preservation of maternal awareness and maintenance of intact airway reflexes to protect against aspiration of gastric contents. It also obviates the need for systemic narcotics or other anesthetic agents to which the preterm fetus may be more susceptible. Perhaps most importantly, the relaxation of the pelvic floor and diminution of the reflex expulsive efforts facilitates the smooth, controlled, and atraumatic delivery of the fragile preterm fetus. An epidural level between T8 and T10 allows the mother to push and stop pushing at the request of the obstetrician. It also provides anesthesia for a wide episiotomy and, if necessary, forceps or vacuum extraction. In addition, it can be rapidly extended to provide anesthesia for cesarean delivery if indicated. In comparison to general anesthesia, there are few interactions between epidural anesthesia and tocolytic agents.

The basic principles for the safe administration of an epidural block, including acute intravascular volume expansion, nonparticulate antacid administration, left uterine displacement, continuous fetal heart rate monitoring, and frequent blood pressure monitoring with prompt treatment of hypotension, all apply to the parturient in preterm labor as well as to the full-term parturient. The details of technique and choice of agent(s) are discussed elsewhere. Only a few caveats should be added when applied to preterm labor. First, the aforementioned poor tolerance of the preterm fetus for asphyxia places an even higher priority on avoidance and prompt treatment of hypotension. Second, in contrast to term labor, diminution of the reflex urge to bear down is desirable in the final minutes of the second stage of preterm labor, and preservation of maximal motor strength is relatively less important. Therefore we recommend a more dense local anesthetic block (e.g., 0.5 percent bupivacaine or 1.5 to 2.0 percent lidocaine). When delivery is imminent, a low subarachnoid anesthetic to T10 with hyperbaric 5 percent lidocaine (30 to 50 mg), hyperbaric 0.75 percent bupivacaine (5 to 8 mg), or hyperbaric 0.5 percent tetracaine (4 to 6 mg) is an acceptable alternative. The final caveat is that the anesthesiologist must be fully cognizant of any coexisting side effects of tocolytic agents (see below).

Cesarean Delivery

Regional Anesthesia. Cesarean delivery may be indicated for the preterm fetus either emergently because of fetal distress or electively because of malpresentation or in an effort to protect the extremely premature infant from birth trauma. Whenever time permits, either subarachnoid or epidural anesthesia is preferable to general anesthesia for reasons previously elucidated. Techniques, dosages, and choice of agents are not different from those described for the term parturient. If the preterm fetus is breech, however, performing the block with the parturient in the sitting position may predispose to prolapse of the umbilical cord. Maternal hypotension is more likely to occur when establishing a T4 level of anesthesia for cesarean delivery than when establishing a T10 level for vaginal delivery. Prior to establishing the block, patients should be acutely administered crystalloid 1.5 L (1,500 ml) to prevent hypotension. More judicious hydration is called for in the parturient who is received β-adrenergic tocolytics because they are at risk for pulmonary edema (see below). Hypotension may be more common following the rapid sympathectomy of subarachnoid anesthesia compared to the slow, controlled rise of an epidural block. When time constraints preclude an epidural block, however, subarachnoid anesthesia may be administered safely if meticulous attention is paid to adequate intravascular volume expansion and prompt treatment of early signs of decreasing blood pressure. Depression of the premature neonate due to fetal exposure to anesthetic agents is theoretically possible following an epidural anesthetic, but far less likely following a subarachnoid anesthetic because of the lower dosages required. When fetal distress is suspected in a patient in preterm labor with a functioning epidural catheter in place, chloroprocaine is the agent of choice for rapidly raising the level to T4 to allow emergent cesarean delivery. The short maternal half-life of this ester (21 seconds) together with the low tendency to be ion trapped and accumulate in the fetal circulation make it extremely safe for both the mother and the premature fetus. Given the controversy over prior reports of neurotoxicity associated with the low pH and preservative in earlier preparations of chloroprocaine,[21] it should not be used for subarachnoid anesthesia or in any epidural anesthetic in which there is suspicion of a dural tear or subarachnoid migration of the catheter.

General Anesthesia. General anesthesia may occasionally be indicated for abdominal delivery of the preterm fetus in cases of severe fetal distress where for technical or time reasons, intraspinal anesthesia cannot be accomplished, or when regional anesthesia is either contraindicated or refused. The maternal potential hazards of failed intubation, aspiration, hypertension, and awareness under anesthesia all apply to the preterm parturient subjected to general anesthesia as well as to the term parturient. In addition, the preterm fetus may be at greater risk of neonatal depression due to exposure to anesthetic agents than the term fetus. Term infants delivered abdominally under general anesthesia are more likely to be depressed at birth, have low 1-minute Apgar scores, and require active resuscitation than those whose mothers receive regional anesthesia.[22] The preterm fetus would be expected to be more vulnerable to depression from maternally administered general anesthetics. Preterm fetal lambs have a lower MAC (minimal alveolar concentration) to halothane than older lambs.[23] Any anesthetic-related depression of premature neonates may be minimized by a well-conducted general anesthetic (as described in Ch. 6), minimal induction to delivery time, and neonatal oxygenation and ventilation to speed the elimination of residual inhaled anesthetics.

Anesthetic management may be greatly complicated by the side effects of recently administered tocolytic agents. A full understanding of the spectrum of agents currently in use as well as their mechanism and side effects is essential.

TOCOLYTIC AGENTS

A list of the various classes of tocolytic agents and their maternal and fetal side effects is provided in Table 8-6. Currently, the most widely used agents are the β-adrenergic agents, magnesium sulfate, and, to a lesser extent, the prostaglandin synthetase inhibitors and calcium channel blockers. Ethanol has been abandoned because of its excessive side effects. Similarly, phosphodiesterase inhibitors such as theophylline are rarely used because of the narrow margin between therapeutic and toxic dosages, and the availability of safer agents. The common mechanism by which these agents cause relaxation of uterine smooth muscle involves a reduction of intracellular calcium either by direct action or via an increase in cyclic AMP (Fig. 8-3).

β-Adrenergic Tocolytic Agents

Terbutaline and ritodrine are currently the most commonly used tocolytics in the United States. Although they have some preferential β_2 action, significant β_1 activity remains and accounts for most of the undesirable side effects (see Table 8-6). Table 8-7 lists some relative contraindications to β-adrenergic therapy.

Tachycardia is the most common side effect of these agents, with heart rates occasionally exceeding 120 beats/min (bpm). If the anesthetic can be delayed by 30 minutes after the last dose of β-adrenergic agonist, the tachycardia may subside substantially. If general anesthesia is required, care should be taken to avoid agents that exacerbate tachycardia (e.g., ketamine) or predispose to arrhythmias (halothane). Extreme tachycardia should be brought under control with short-acting β-blockers (esmolol, labetalol) prior to a rapid-sequence induction. Lead II should be monitored on the ECG for arrhythmias. Patients with heart disease should be mon-

Table 8-6. Side Effects of Drugs Used to Stop Labor

Drug	Maternal Effects	Fetal and Neonatal Effects
β-Adrenergic agents	Hypotension Tachycardia Chest pain/tightness Pulmonary edema Congestive heart failure Arrhythmias (atrial and ventricular) Anxiety, nervousness Nausea and vomiting Headache Hyperglycemia Metabolic (lactic) acidosis Hypokalemia	Tachycardia Fetal hyperglycemia/rebound neonatal hypoglycemia Increased free fatty acids Fetal asphyxia with large doses due to maternal hypotension or increased uterine vascular resistance resulting in decreased uterine blood flow
Magnesium sulfate	Pulmonary edema Chest pain/tightness Nausea and vomiting Flushing Drowsiness Blurred vision Increased sensitivity to muscle relaxants	Hypotonia Drowsiness Decreased gastric motility Hypocalcemia
Ethanol	Central nervous system depression with hypotension, disorientation and agitation Increased gastric secretion and acidity Nausea and vomiting Headache Hypoglycemia Metabolic acidosis	Fetal and neonatal depression Neonatal respiratory depression Hypotonia Metabolic acidosis Hypoglycemia Temperature instability Gastric irritation and vomiting Fetal alcohol syndrome (withdrawal)
Prostaglandin synthetase inhibitors	Gastrointestinal irritation Inhibition of platelet function Reduced factor XII Depressed immune system	Premature closure of the ductus arteriosus Pulmonary hypertension
Calcium channel-blocking agents	Hypotension Reduced cardiac contractility Reduced cardiac conduction Inhibition of platelet aggregation	? Decreased uterine blood flow
Diazoxide	Tachycardia Hypotension Hyperglycemia	Decreased uterine blood flow Hyperglycemia Tachycardia
Phosphodiesterase inhibitors	Tachycardia Arrhythmias Narrow therapeutic index Hypotension Tremulousness, nausea and vomiting Hyperglycemia Hypokalemia	Tachycardia Hyperglycemia Rebound hypoglycemia

itored for signs of myocardial ischemia. One should remember that the tachycardia makes it more difficult to judge anesthesia depth or adequacy of intravascular volume expansion.

Pulmonary edema is seen in about 5 percent of patients receiving β-adrenergic tocolysis, usually occurring 24 to 48 hours after therapy is initiated. The cause of such pulmonary edema remains a matter of controversy. Risk factors include pre-existing cardiac disease, multiple-gestation pregnancy, anemia, overyhydration, prolonged tocolytic therapy with β-adrenergic agonists, hypokalemia, sepsis, and, possibly, combined therapy with magnesium. Concurrent use of glucocorticoids is no longer thought to increase the risk of pulmonary edema.[6] There is speculation in the literature about both cardiogenic and noncardiogenic etiologies. Attempts to document left ventricular failure echocardiographically or with pulmonary artery catheterization

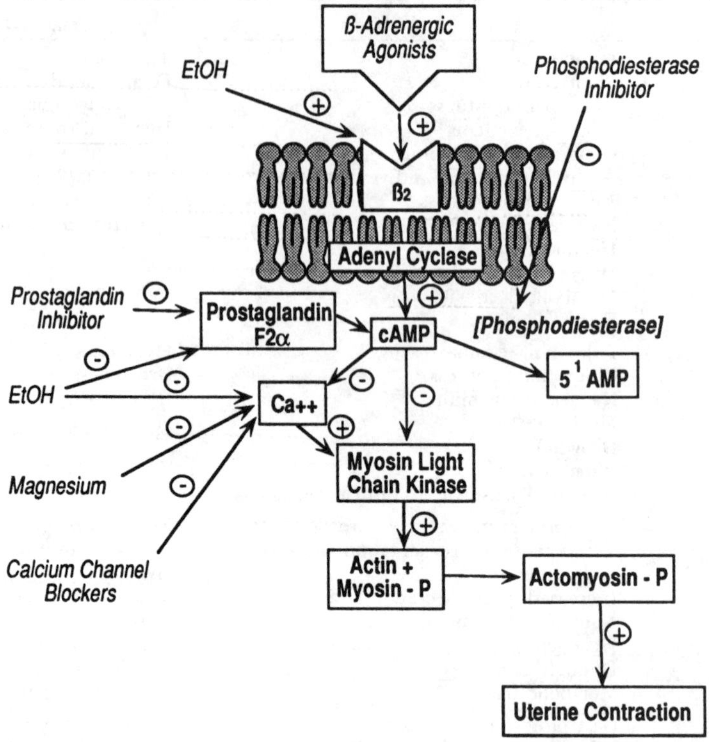

Fig. 8-3. Mechanisms of tocolysis. (Modified from Dailey,[31] with permission.)

have failed.[24,25] Currently the balance of evidence favors a noncardiogenic mechanism for β-adrenergic agonist-associated pulmonary edema in the patient without preexisting cardiac disease. The relative contributions of fluid overload, decreasing plasma oncotic pressure, and increasing pulmonary capillary permeability remain in question and probably vary from patient to patient. During concurrent sepsis, increased pulmonary capillary permeability is likely to be a prominent contributing factor, and it has been speculated that many cases of pulmonary edema may have been precipitated by occult chorioamnionitis while receiving β-adrenergic therapy.[25] Hypoxic pulmonary vasoconstriction appears to be impaired by β-adrenergic tocolytics,[26] and this may account for the observation that hypoxia is exaggerated out of proportion to the radiographic demonstration of pulmonary edema in these patients.

Table 8-7. Relative Contraindications to β-Adrenergic Therapy

Hyperthyroidism
Unstable diabetes mellitus
Asthma
Uncontrolled hypertension
Severe pregnancy-induced hypertension
History of migraine headaches
Significant cardiac disease (AS, MS, IHSS)

Because of the risk of pulmonary edema, intravascular fluids should be limited, if possible, to 2 to 2.5 L/24 h. If pulmonary edema occurs, treatment should include discontinuation of the β-adrenergic agent, fluid restriction, sitting position, supplemental oxygen by mask, and judicious diuresis guided by central venous and, if possible, pulmonary artery information.

In the setting of mild pulmonary edema, epidural anesthesia for labor and vaginal delivery should be preceded by cautious acute intravascular volume expansion with dextrose-free crystalloid 250 to 500 ml. The vasodilation induced by the epidural block should be a major concern and, if delivery is necessary, the anesthetic level must be cautiously raised to T4. Subarachnoid anesthesia is relatively contraindicated in this situation because the attendant rapid sympathectomy may be poorly tolerated because of the patient's tenuous intravascular volume status, tachycardia, and diminished cardiovascular reserve. Emergent anesthesia for cesarean delivery for the patient in florid pulmonary edema requires a rapid-sequence induction for general anesthesia, positive-pressure ventilation and, possibly, positive end-expiratory pressure (PEEP).

Hypotension due to the peripheral vasodilatory side effects of β-adrenergic tocolytics may occur during regional or general anesthesia. The premature fetus is less tolerant of asphyxia than the term fetus and hypotension must be corrected quickly. Rapid infusion of crystalloid is relatively contraindicated as it may precipitate pulmonary edema. If the patient is significantly tachycardic (heart rate > 120 bpm), ephedrine or other sympathomimetics with primarily β-agonist activity may have a reduced efficacy and exacerbate the tachycardia. Agents with primarily α-agonist activity had been traditionally avoided in parturients because of fears that they would cause a reduction in uterine blood flow based on animal studies.[27] Recent human studies in term parturients in whom hypotension during regional anesthesia for cesarean delivery was treated with either phenylephrine or ephedrine failed to reveal any significant adverse neonatal outcomes (including acid–base status, Apgar scores, and early neonatal neurobehavioral examinations) attributable to the use of the α-agonist, phenylephrine.[28,29] Proof that phenylephrine may be applied safely to the parturient in preterm labor to correct hypotension awaits further studies.

Metabolic side effects of β-adrenergic agonists include increased glycogenolysis and lipolysis, hyperglycemia, increased insulin release, and hypokalemia as potassium shifts into the intracellular compartment. Since total-body potassium stores are preserved, this hypokalemia generally does not require treatment. Hyperventilation and alkalosis may worsen the hypokalemia and are to be avoided, whereas hypoventilation and acidosis may increase the possibility of arrhythmias. The hyperglycemia resulting from β-adrenergic tocolytic therapy may require treatment with insulin in diabetic patients. Concurrent administration of glucocorticoids to accelerate fetal lung maturation will further exacerbate the hyperglycemia. Neonatal rebound hypoglycemia may be profound.

Myocardial ischemia, infarction, and death have been reported in association with β-adrenergic tocolytics.[30] In the absence of pre-existing heart disease, however, the incidence of myocardial ischemia would appear to be low. Each patient should be carefully screened for cardiac disease with a thorough history, physical examination, and baseline ECG prior to initiating therapy with β-adrenergic tocolytics.

Magnesium Sulfate

Magnesium is thought to attenuate uterine smooth muscle contraction by competing with calcium at the cell membrane level and preventing an increase in free intracellular calcium.[31] Its efficacy as a tocolytic agent has been favorably compared to ritodrine.[32] However, magnesium and β-adrenergic agonists have many side effects in common.

The principal cardiovascular side effect is decreased blood pressure due to relaxation of peripheral vascular smooth muscle. Unlike β-adrenergic agonists, magnesium does not possess direct positive chronotropic properties, although reflex tachycardia may occur. At toxic levels (greater than 10 mg/dl) depression of myocardial contractility and conduction may occur, with heart block at serum magnesium levels greater than 12 mg/dl.[33] In the absence of toxicity, magnesium is generally thought to have milder cardiovascular consequences than β-adrenergic agonists. Interestingly, Chestnut et al. demonstrated in pregnant ewes subjected to hemorrhage that therapeutic magnesium levels blunted the compensatory hemodynamic response to hypovolemia more severely than did ritodrine.[34] Pulmonary edema is less frequently seen in patients receiving magnesium therapy than in patients receiving β-adrenergic tocolytics (approximately 1 percent compared to 5 percent). Combination therapy of magnesium together with β-adrenergic agents increases the likelihood of pulmonary edema.[35]

The anesthetic implications with regard to hypotension and pulmonary edema are similar to those previously mentioned for patients receiving β-adrenergic agents. In the absence of florid pulmonary edema, hemorrhage, or a coagulopathy, regional anesthesia is usually preferable to general anesthesia for labor and vaginal or cesarean delivery for the reasons outlined above. Acute hydration should be performed with caution and an awareness of the potential for pulmonary edema. Hypotension should be promptly treated with ephedrine. Unlike patients receiving β-adrenergic agonist, tachycardia is seldom significant and α-agonists are rarely required to treat hypotension.

Magnesium also causes striated muscle weakness by a combination of three mechanisms: (1) decreased release of acetylcholine from the neuromuscular junction, (2) decreased sensitivity of end plates to acetylcholine, and (3) decreased excitability of the muscle membrane.[36] This results in a heightened sensitivity to both depolarizing and nondepolarizing muscle relaxants. Administration of calcium does not reliably prevent this effect. Both degree and duration of muscle relaxation may be increased, and attempts to reverse a nondepolarizing muscle relaxant, even with large doses of an anticholinesterase, may be incomplete. Therefore, a nerve stimulator is recommended to guide use of muscle relaxants and to judge adequacy of reversal prior to extubation. The fasciculations following succinylcholine may be attenuated by the effects of magnesium. It should be emphasized that, because the degree of interaction between succinylcholine and magnesium is unpredictable, and because the concerns about aspiration far outweigh the consequences of prolonged intubation, the full intubating dose of succinylcholine should be used when performing a rapid-sequence induction of general anesthesia for the patient receiving magnesium therapy. Interactions between magnesium and muscle relaxants are further discussed in Chapter 5.

Other side effects associated with magnesium include nausea, vomiting, flushing, drowsiness, and blurred vision. Respiratory depression may occur with toxic levels. In the presence of renal insufficiency, toxicity from magnesium is more likely to occur. Finally, the anesthesiologist should be alert to the possibility of postpartum uterine atony and hemorrhage in the patient who receives magnesium therapy.

Calcium Channel Blockers

Calcium channel blockers are being administered with increasing frequency for inhibition of preterm labor. Nifedipine, the most extensively studied in this class, has been found to be as effective as ritodrine but with fewer maternal and fetal side effects.[37,38] In a recent study, Ferguson et al.[36] found that in doses sufficient to achieve tocolysis, nifedipine caused minimal cardiovascular alterations. Peripheral vasodilation led to a mild (4 percent) decrease in mean blood pressure compared to ritodrine (14 percent). The increase in heart rate associated with nifedipine was mild (less than 10 percent) and attributed to the baroreflex, whereas ritodrine caused a marked tachycardia (40 percent above baseline) through both reflex and direct β_1 stimulation. The mild negative inotropic effects of calcium channel blockers are usually offset by the reflex increase in heart rate. Caution should be exercised in the use of potent inhaled agents as they may cause enhanced myocardial depression and vasodilation as well as blunting of the compensatory baroreceptor reflex, resulting in significant hypotension.

Metabolic effects of nifedipine are similarly mild compared to ritodrine. Although some hemodilution occurs because of vasodilation, potassium levels remain unaltered. Serum glucose levels are minimally elevated compared to patients receiving ritodrine, possibly making nifedipine a preferred tocolytic agent for diabetic patients.

One case report described a patient who developed weakness and difficulty swallowing while receiving concomitant magnesium and nifedipine tocolytic therapy.[39] It was speculated that since both agents interfere with the intracellular flux of calcium ions into skeletal muscle, their effects may be additive. However, no other reports of such an interaction have appeared and animal studies on this subject have yielded conflicting results.[40]

The use of calcium channel blockers, like all tocolytics, may result in postpartum uterine atony and hemorrhage. Atony due to residual calcium channel blockers, however, may be unresponsive to oxytocin or prostaglandin $F_2\alpha$.

Use of calcium channel blockers for tocolysis had been limited by concerns that uterine blood flow might be impaired by the vasodilation and reduction in mean arterial blood pressure. Such an effect was seen in the awake pregnant ewe receiving sufficient verapamil to cause significant hypotension.[41] However, more recent studies in humans using Doppler measurements of umbilical artery blood flow demonstrated no significant effect of nifedipine on uteroplacental circulation.[38,42] It is probable that as long as mean arterial pressure is preserved, uteroplacental blood flow is not compromised by calcium channel blockers.

In the absence of an overdose of calcium channel blockers with significant hypotension, both regional and general anesthesia may be applied safely. Care should be taken to avoid hypotension from the synergistic cardiac depression that may occur when inhaled anesthetics combine with calcium channel blockers. Finally, attention must be given to monitor for postpartum uterine atony and hemorrhage due to residual tocolytic effect.

Prostaglandin Synthetase Inhibitors

Prostaglandins soften the cervix and stimulate the uterus to contract during labor and preterm labor.[43] Prostaglandin synthetase inhibitors (PSIs) have been proven effective for inhibition of preterm labor in multiple clinical trials.[44] Maternal side effects are minimal in comparison to other tocolytic agents. They include occasional gastrointestinal irritation (nausea, gastritis, peptic ulcer disease), impaired platelet function, and mildly impaired renal function. PSIs should be avoided in patients with bleeding disorders, renal disease, or peptic ulcers. Fever is suppressed by these agents, so low-grade infections such as early chorioamnionitis may go unnoticed. Prolonged use of indomethacin may cause oligohydramnios, and, in fact, has been used to treat idiopathic polyhydramnios. Widespread use of PSIs is currently limited by concerns over the potential fetal side effects.

Because prostaglandins are involved in maintaining the patency of the ductus arteriosus prior to birth, it is feared that inhibition of these prostaglandins by agents like indomethacin might lead to premature closure of the ductus arteriosus and might consequently lead to persistent fetal circulation after birth. Animal models suggest that the risk is greater if indomethacin exposure takes place late in gestation,[45,46] possibly because transplacental passage of indomethacin is greater near term in the rat.[47] On this basis, most recommend that a short course of indomethacin for tocolysis prior to 34 weeks gestation is safe for the fetus. Multiple clinical studies support this position.[44,48] Recently, however, Moise et al. demonstrated that in humans, unlike rats, transplacental transfer of indomethacin takes place easily regardless of gestation age[49] and that echocardiographic evidence of in utero transient premature ductal closure was common following low-dose, short-course indomethacin therapy as early as 26.5 weeks of gestation.[50] Therefore, if a parturient received a prolonged course of PSIs prior to birth, it would be prudent to have personnel available who could evaluate and treat signs of persistent fetal circulation.

Of more direct concern to anesthesiologists is the effects of PSIs on platelets. Thromboxane A_2, a potent stimulator of platelet aggregation, is derived from arachidonic acid. Cyclo-oxygenase, the initial enzyme in this cascade, is inhibited permanently by aspirin and reversibly by indomethacin. Platelet function may be impaired if aspirin was administered within 10 days or indomethacin within 24 hours. Patients are therefore at risk for postpartum bleeding, especially if platelet dysfunction coexists with uterine atony. Great controversy surrounds the question of whether PSI therapy contraindicates regional anesthesia. The risk of an epidural hematoma is presumed increased in patients with an abnormal bleeding time. It is recommended that a bleeding time be obtained prior to institution of a regional block. Recognizing the extreme rarity of epidural hematomas, I (and the editor) regard PSI usage to be a relative rather than an absolute contraindication to regional anesthesia. Whenever intraspinal anesthesia is employed in a patient who is receiving aspirin or indomethacin, the risks versus benefits justification should be clearly stated in the chart and made clear to the patient. Frequent neurologic evaluations after resolution of the block should be performed to detect as early as possible any signs of an epidural hematoma. If seen, early surgical decompression will be necessary to prevent permanent neurologic damage.

Parenthetically, a recent case report described two women with pregnancy-induced hypertension treated with β-blockers who became profoundly hypertensive after receiving indomethacin for inhibition of preterm labor.[51] Therefore, PSI should be avoided in patients receiving β-blockers for hypertension.

REFERENCES

1. Gonik B, Creasy RK: Preterm labor: its diagnosis and management. Am J Obstet Gynecol 154:3, 1986
2. Rush RW, Davey DA, Segall ML: The effects of preterm delivery on perinatal mortality. Br J Obstet Gynecol 85:806, 1978
3. Cunningham FG, MacDonald PC, Gant NF: Preterm and post term pregnancy and inappropriate fetal growth. p. 741. In Pritchard JA, MacDonald PC (eds): Williams Obstetrics. 18th Ed. Appleton & Lange, East Norwalk, CT, 1989
4. Goldenberg RL, Nelson KG, Hale CD, et al: Survival of infants with low birth weight and early gestational age, 1979–1981. Am J Obstet Gynecol 149:508, 1984
5. Garfield RE, Beier S: Increased myometrial responsiveness to oxytocin during term and preterm labor. Am J Obstet Gynecol 161:454, 1989
6. Gutsche BB, Samuels P: Anesthetic considerations in premature birth. Int Anesthesiol Clin 28:33, 1990
7. Hack M, Fanaroff AA: Outcomes of extremely low birthweight infants between 1982 and 1988. N Engl J Med 321:1642, 1989
8. Percon RA, Strassner HT, Kirz DS, Towers CV: Controlled trial of hydration and bedrest versus bedrest alone in the evaluation of preterm uterine contractions. Am J Obstet Gynecol 161:775, 1989
9. Liggins GC, Howie RN: A controlled study of antepartum glucocorticoid treatment of the respiratory distress syndrome in premature infants. Pediatrics 50:515, 1972
10. Howie RN, Liggins GC: Clinical trial of antepartum betamethasone therapy for prevention of respiratory distress in preterm infants. Proceedings of Fifth Study Group, Royal College of Obstetricians and Gynecologists, October: 281, 1977
11. Quirk, JG, Raker RK, Petri RH, Williams AM: The role of glucocorticoids, unstressful labor, and atraumatic delivery in the prevention of respiratory distress syndrome. Am J Obstet Gynecol 1134:768, 1979
12. Liggins GC, Howie RN: The prevention of RDS by maternal steroid therapy. p. 415. In Gluck L (ed): Modern Perinatal Medicine. Year Book, Chicago, 1974
13. Garite TJ, Freeman RK, Linzey EM, et al: Prospective randomized study of corticosteroids in the management of premature rupture of the membranes and the premature gestation. Am J Obstet Gynecol 141:508, 1981
14. Yoon JJ, Harper RG: Observations on the relationship between duration of rupture of the membranes and the development of idiopathic respiratory distress syndrome. Pediatrics 52:161, 1973
15. Mosier HD, Dearden LC, Tanner SM, et al: Dispropor-

tionate organ growth in the fetus after betamethasone administration, abstracted. Pediatr Res 13:486, 1979
16. Liggins GC: Report on children exposed to steroids in utero. Contemp Obstet Gynecol 19:205, 1982
17. Morales WJ: The effects of chorioamnionitis on the developmental outcome of preterm infants at one year. Obstet Gynecol 70:183, 1987
18. Amon E, Lewis SV, Sibai BM, et al: Ampicillin prophylaxis in preterm premature rupture of the membranes: a prospective randomized study. Am J Obstet Gynecol 159:539, 1988
19. Garite TJ, Kirk A, Keegan KA, et al: A randomized trial of ritodrine tocolysis versus expectant management in patients with premature rupture of membranes at 25–30 weeks of gestation. Am J Obstet Gynecol 157:388, 1987
20. Pedersen H, Santos AC, Morishima HO, et al: Does gestational age affect the pharmacokinetics and pharmacodynamics of lidocaine in mother and fetus? Anesthesiology 68:367, 1988
21. Gissen AJ, Datta S, Lambert D: The chloroprocaine controversy. II. Is chloroprocaine neurotoxic? Reg Anesth 9:135, 1984
22. Ong BY, Cohen MM, Pahalniuk RJ: Anesthesia for cesarean section: effects on neonates. Anesth Analg 68:270, 1989
23. Gregory FA, Wagde JG, Biehl DR, et al: Fetal anesthetic requirements (MAC) for halothane. Anesth Analg 62:9, 1983
24. Philipsen T, Eriksen PS, Lynggard F: Pulmonary edema following ritodrine-saline infusion in premature labor. Obstet Gynecol 58:304, 1981
25. Benedetti TJ: Life threatening complications of betamimetic therapy for preterm labor inhibition. Clin Perinatol 13:843, 1986
26. Conover WB, Benumot JL, Key TC: Ritodrine inhibition of hypoxic pulmonary vasoconstriction. Am J Obstet Gynecol 159:1467, 1988
27. Ralston DH, Shnider SM, DeLorimier AA: Effects of equipotent ephedrine, mephentermine and methoxamine on uterine blood flow in the pregnant ewe. Anesthesiology 40:354, 1974
28. Ramanathan S, Grant GJ: Vasopressor therapy for hypotension due to epidural anesthesia for cesarean section. Acta Anesthesiol Scand 32:559, 1988
29. Moran DH, Perillo M, LaPorta RF, et al: Phenylephrine in the prevention of hypotension following spinal anesthesia for cesarean delivery. J Clin Anesthesia 3:301, 1990
30. Benedetti TJ: Maternal complications of parenteral β-sympathomimetic therapy for premature labor. Am J Obstet Gynecol 145:1, 1983
31. Dailey PA: Anesthesia for preterm labor. p. 243. In Shnider SM, Levinson G (eds): Anesthesia for Obstetrics. 2nd Ed. Williams & Wilkins, Baltimore, 1987
32. Hollander DI, Nagey DA, Pupkin MJ: Magnesium sulfate and ritodrine hydrochloride: a randomized comparison. Am J Obstet Gynecol 156:631, 1987
33. Stoelting RK: Pharmacology and Physiology in Anesthetic Practice. JB Lippincott, Philadelphia, 1987
34. Chestnut DH, Thompson CS, McLaughlin GL, Weiner CP: Does the intravenous infusion of ritodrine or magnesium sulfate alter the hemodynamic response to hemorrhage in gravid ewes? Am J Obstet Gynecol 159:1467, 1988
35. Ogburn P, Hansen C, Williams P, et al: Magnesium sulfate and betamimetic dual agent tocolysis in preterm labor after single agent failure. J Reprod Med 30:583, 1985
36. Foldes FF: Factors which alter the effects of muscle relaxants. Anesthesiology 20:464, 1959
37. Ferguson JE, Dyson DC, Schutz T, Stevenson DK: A comparison of tocolysis with nifedipine or ritodrine: analysis of efficacy and maternal, fetal and neonatal outcomes. Am J Obstet Gynecol 163:105, 1990
38. Meyer WR, Randall HW, Graves WL: Nifedipine vs ritodrine for suppression of preterm labor. J Reprod Med 35:649, 1990
39. Snyder SW, Cardwell MS: Neuromuscular blockade with magnesium sulfate and nifedipine. Am J Obstet Gynecol 161:35, 1989
40. Bikhazi GB, Leung I, Flores C, et al: Potentiation of neuromuscular blocking agents by calcium channel blockers in rats. Anesth Analg 67:1, 1988
41. Murad HN, Tabsh KMA, Shilyanski G, et al: Effects of verapamil on uterine blood flow and maternal cardiovascular function in the awake pregnant ewe. Anesth Analg 64:7, 1985
42. Mari G, Kirshan B, Moise KJ, et al: Doppler assessment of the fetal and uteroplacental circulation during nifedipine therapy for preterm labor. Am J Obstet Gynecol 161:1514, 1989
43. Grieves S, Liggins GC: Phospholipase A activity in human and ovine uterine tissue. Prostaglandins 12:229, 1976
44. Niebyl JR, Witter FR: Neonatal outcome after indomethacin treatment for preterm labor. Am J Obstet Gynecol 155:747, 1986
45. Rudolph AM, Heyman MA: Hemodynamic changes induced by blockers of prostaglandin synthesis in the fetal lamb in utero. Adv Prostaglandin Thromboxane Leukotriene Res 4:231, 1978
46. Sharpe GL, Larsson KS, Thalme B: Studies on closure of the ductus arteriosus. XII. In utero effect of indomethacin and sodium salicylate in rats and rabbits. Prostaglandins 9:585, 1975
47. Klein KL, Scott WJ, Clark KE, Wilson JG: Indomethacin-placental transfer, cytotoxicity and teratology in the rat. Am J Obstet Gynecol 141:448, 1981
48. Dudley DK, Hardie MJ: Fetal and neonatal effects of indomethacin used as a tocolytic agent. Am J Obstet Gynecol 151:181, 1985
49. Moise KJ, Ou C, Kirshon B, et al: Placental transfer of indomethacin in the human pregnancy. Am J Obstet Gynecol 162:549, 1990
50. Moise KJ, Huhta JC, Sharif DS, et al: Indomethacin in the treatment of premature labor: Effects on the fetal ductus arteriosus. New Engl J Med 319:327, 1988
51. Schoenfeld A, Freedman S, Hod M, Ovadia Y: Antagonism of antihypertensive drug therapy in pregnancy by indomethacin. Am J Obstet Gynecol 161:1204, 1989

BREECH DELIVERY

Obstetric management of the patient with breech presentation remains controversial. Some centers favor vaginal breech delivery under certain conditions, whereas in other institutions abdominal delivery is routinely performed for all breech infants. The anesthesiologist must be prepared to administer anesthesia for a trial of labor, vaginal delivery, or cesarean delivery (either elective or emergent).

OBSTETRIC CONSIDERATIONS

Breech presentation occurs in approximately 3.5 percent of pregnancies. The causes of breech presentation are unknown. Certain abnormalities predispose to this presentation, notably prematurity, multiparity, uterine anomalies, and multiple gestation. Three types of breech presentation are described (Fig. 8-4):

1. Frank breech: Lower extremities flexed at the hips and extended at the knees.
2. Complete breech: Lower extremities are flexed at both the hips and knees.
3. Incomplete breech: One or both extremities are extended and one or both feet are present in the vagina.

About 60 percent of breeches are frank, 30 percent incomplete, and 10 percent complete. The type of breech presentation has implications for delivery. The incidence of successful vaginal delivery is highest for a frank breech. Prolapsed umbilical cord occurs most commonly with incomplete presentation.[1,2]

Analysis of data from studies in the 1950s and 1960s has encouraged a growing trend toward abdominal delivery for all breeches. For breech versus vertex vaginal deliveries, these studies reported a fourfold increase in perinatal mortality and a 12-fold increase in trauma to the baby during delivery.[3] Cord prolapse and asphyxia were also more common.[4] Premature infants, with their relatively large head: body size ratio, have an increased incidence of head entrapment.[4] Compression of the aftercoming head may cause intracranial hemorrhage, and is a principal cause of perinatal mortality. At the present time in the United States, approximately 80 percent of breech-presenting term infants are delivered abdominally.[5]

Recent studies have reported that vaginal delivery was successful in 72 percent of *selected* term patients without any increase in fetal or maternal morbidity and mortality.[5] Patients selected for a trial of labor had both an

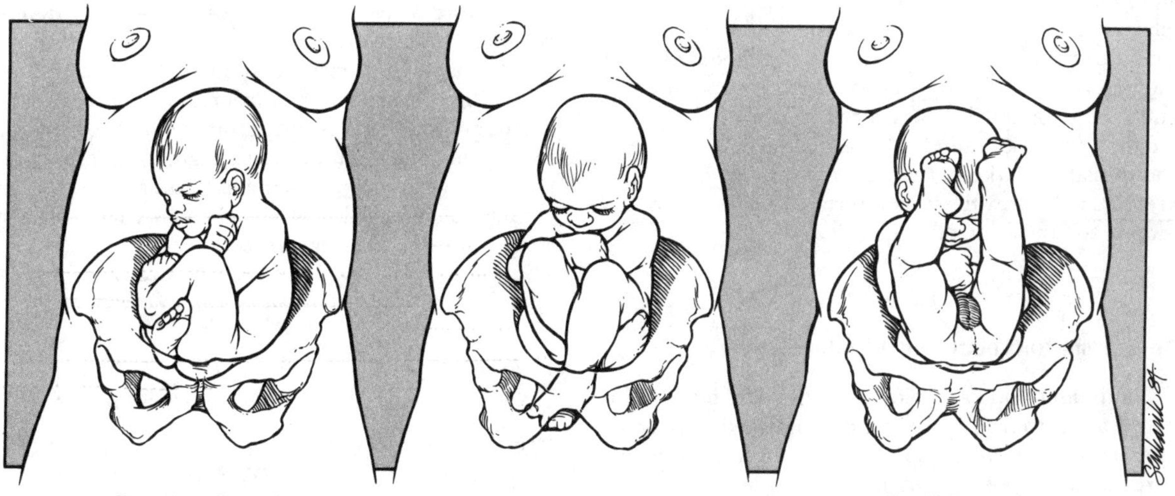

Complete Breech | Incomplete Breech | Frank Breech

Fig. 8-4. Three possible breech presentations. The complete breech demonstrates flexion of the hips and flexion of the knees. The incomplete breech demonstrates intermediate reflexion of one hip and knee. The frank breech demonstrates flexion of the hips and extension of both knees. (From Seeds JW: Malpresentations. p. 539. In Gagge SG, Niebyl JR, Simpson JL (eds): Obstetrics: Normal and Problem Pregnancies. 2nd Ed. Churchill Livingstone, New York, 1986, with permission.)

adequate pelvic outlet documented by radiologic pelvimetry and an estimated fetal weight of between 1,500 and 4,500 g. Viable fetuses weighing less than 1,500 g are generally delivered abdominally.[6]

ANESTHETIC CONSIDERATIONS

Three potential problems are of concern to the anesthesiologist for a breech delivery: (1) prematurity, (2) difficult or traumatic delivery, and (3) coexisting maternal/fetal illness or anomalies. The anesthesiologist should evaluate the patient, review the history and physical examination, and discuss with the obstetrician the probable obstetric and possible anesthetic needs for each parturient. Patient care can be optimized if this can be done as soon as possible after admission to the labor and delivery suite.

A trial of labor for breech presentation may necessitate emergency cesarean delivery. For example, umbilical cord prolapse may occur in 2 percent of frank breeches at term.[1] Therefore, an anesthesiologist must be immediately available. Overall, 70 to 84 percent of trials of labor result in successful vaginal delivery.[7]

Continuous lumbar epidural anesthesia has advantages and disadvantages in the patient laboring with a breech presentation. Epidural anesthesia usually does not prolong the first stage of labor if initiated in the active phase of labor. Although the second stage of labor may be prolonged with epidural anesthesia, full breech extraction is not more frequent and perinatal morbidity is not increased.[8] Epidural anesthesia, by relaxation of the pelvic floor, lessens pressure on the fetal head and may decrease the likelihood of fetal trauma. In addition, surgical anesthesia can rapidly and safely be obtained in the event of fetal distress, thus avoiding the risks attendant to the induction of general anesthesia. For these reasons, epidural anesthesia is preferred. It provides a comfortable patient who can cooperate for a controlled delivery.

ANESTHETIC MANAGEMENT

Anesthesia for Labor and Vaginal Delivery

Continuous lumbar epidural anesthesia may be induced after appropriate antacid prophylaxis and acute intravenous hydration. The addition of a lipid-soluble narcotic to a dilute solution of local anesthetic may relieve the profound "rectal pressure" frequently noted by patients with a breech-presenting fetus. Narcotics should be used with caution in the gravida with a premature infant, who is more sensitive to respiratory depression. More-concentrated solutions of bupivacaine may also be used to alleviate the rectal pressure, but motor block of the perineal muscles will be exaggerated. Some advocate delay in the "block" of sacral segments to minimize motor block and maintain the effectiveness of the maternal "pushing" effort.

General anesthesia after a rapid-sequence induction and tracheal intubation is indicated should uterine relaxation be required for full breech extraction. After tracheal intubation, uterine relaxation is obtained with a volatile anesthetic agent (up to 2 MAC [minimal alveolar concentration] as needed). There is no difference in uterine relaxation properties of halothane, enflurane, or isoflurane. After delivery, volatile agents should be discontinued to allow efficient oxytocin-induced uterine contractions. Anesthesia is maintained with intravenous narcotics and a mixture of nitrous oxide and oxygen until extraction of the placenta and surgical repair are complete. A succinylcholine infusion (0.1 percent) may be used for muscle relaxation.

Should Dührssen's incisions of the cervix be necessary, severe maternal hemorrhage may occur. Bleeding into the pelvis is common. Blood exiting from the vagina is *not* the only blood loss occurring.

Anesthesia for Cesarean Delivery

Regional or general anesthesia may be indicated by maternal preference and/or fetomaternal well-being. The anesthesiologist must be prepared to induce general anesthesia using a volatile agent to relax the uterus if necessary. The patient should breathe 100 percent oxygen before delivery to avoid possible delay in denitrogenation if uterine relaxation is requested.

External version may be attempted in patients with known breech presentation prior to the onset of labor. Although anesthesia is not recommended for this procedure, immediate availability of an anesthesiologist is necessary when external version is attempted. External version has risks of fetomaternal hemorrhage, placental abruption, or umbilical cord compression.

REFERENCES

1. Pritchard JA, MacDonald PC, Gant NF (eds): Williams Obstetrics. 17th Ed. Appleton & Lange, East Norwalk, CT, 1985
2. Rovinsky JR, Miller JA, Kaplan S: Management of breech presentation at term. Am J Obstet Gynecol 115:497, 1973
3. Morgan HS, Kane SH: An analysis of 16,327 breech births. JAMA 187:262, 1964
4. Potter MG Jr, Heaton CE, Douglas GW: Intrinsic fetal risk in breech delivery. Obstet Gynecol 15:158, 1960
5. Flanagan TA, Mulchahey KM, Korenbrot CC, et al: Management of term breech presentation. Am J Obstet Gynecol 156:1492, 1987

6. Confino E, Ismajovich B, Sherzer A, et al: Vaginal versus cesarean section oriented approaches in the management of breech delivery. Int J Gynaecol Obstet 23:1, 1985
7. Bingham P, Lilford RJ: Management of the selected term breech presentation: assessment of the risks of selected vaginal delivery versus cesarean section for all cases. Obstet Gynecol 69·965, 1987
8. Confino E, Ismajovich B, Rudick V, et al: Extradural analgesia in the management of singleton breech delivery. Br J Anaesth 57:892, 1985

MULTIPLE GESTATION

Multiple gestation is associated with increased maternal, fetal, and neonatal morbidity. Twins occur in about 1 percent of all pregnancies, triplets in 0.01 percent. Multiple gestation is becoming more common as a result of in vitro fertilization and other assisted reproductive technology.

OBSTETRIC CONSIDERATIONS

Maternal morbidity and mortality are increased with multiple gestation because of higher incidence of maternal complications such as:

1. Preeclampsia/eclampsia
2. Placental abruption
3. Preterm rupture of membranes
4. Preterm labor
5. Uterine atony
6. Obstetric trauma
7. Operative delivery (forceps and abdominal)
8. Antepartum and/or postpartum hemorrhage

The rate of primary abdominal delivery may be as high as 50 percent for multiple gestations.[1] Perinatal mortality in twin pregnancies is four to six times greater than in singleton pregnancies.[2] Multiple gestation accounts for 10 percent of all perinatal mortality. This is primary due to the high incidence of preterm delivery and prematurity (40 percent of multiple gestations deliver before the 37th week of gestation).[3] Other fetal and neonatal complications occurring more frequently in multiple gestations include:

1. Congenital anomalies
2. Polyhydramnios
3. Umbilical cord entanglement
4. Umbilical cord prolapse
5. Intrauterine growth retardation
6. Twin–twin transfusion
7. Malpresentation

Monozygous twins have an increased likelihood of cord complications and twin–twin transfusion.[4] Vascular communications present in most monochorionic placentas are responsible for the majority of twin–twin transfusions.[5] Intrauterine and neonatal mortality in multiple gestations with twin–twin transfusion is as high as 80 percent.[6] Antepartum death of one twin occurs in 0.5 to 6.8 percent of twin pregnancies.[7] Morbidity in the surviving twin is common,[8] but has not been demonstrated in triplets.[9] Disseminated intravascular coagulation may develop in the gravida[10,11] or the surviving fetus.[8] Early diagnosis with aggressive antepartum, intrapartum, and postpartum management is the key to decreasing the magnitude of these problems.

Recent work contradicts the previously reported greater incidence of acidosis[12,13] or higher mortality[14] in the second twin (twin B). The acid–base status between twins[15,16] and among triplets[17] is similar. Spellacy et al. reported twins A and B had identical perinatal mortality when they were similar in weight.[2] The use and choice of anesthetic agents or the presence or absence of a nuchal cord may explain the conflicting results.[15] The time interval between vaginal delivery of twin A and twin B does not influence neonatal outcome.[18]

Mode of delivery is an obstetric decision based primarily on gestational age and presentation. Both twins will be in the vertex position only 30 to 50 percent of the time. Some 30 to 40 percent of twin pregnancies will be in the vertex/breech (twin A/twin B) position. In 10 to 20 percent of twins there will be various combinations of breech and transverse lie. Vaginal delivery is more likely if twin A is in the vertex position. Indications for abdominal delivery include:

1. Breech presentation of twin A
2. Prematurity
3. Possibility of interlocking chins
4. Discordance
5. Twin–twin transfusion
6. Congenital anomalies
7. Intrauterine death of one twin
8. Evidence of decreased uteroplacental reserve

Although most obstetricians will deliver twins vaginally, few obstetricians will deliver three or more infants vaginally.

ANESTHETIC CONSIDERATIONS

Multiple gestation exaggerates the physiologic changes of pregnancy. The increased size of the uterus and its contents, especially near term, further decreases total lung capacity, functional residual capacity (FRC), expiratory reserve volume, and residual volume. Decreased FRC allows hypoxemia to develop more rapidly in the parturient, particularly in the supine position.

Cardiovascular changes tend to occur earlier and to a slightly greater extent in multiple gestation. Cardiac output is increased. There is an increased tendency to relative or actual anemia compared with singleton pregnancies.[2] Increased myocardial contractility has been suggested by echocardiography, therefore, cardiac reserve will be limited.[19] The greater combined fetal weight and larger amount of amniotic fluid of the multiple gestation predispose to aortocaval compression and supine hypotension.

Increased gastrin production increases gastric volume and acidity. The larger uterine size may add to lower esophageal sphincter dysfunction, making aspiration pneumonitis a greater hazard. Renal, hepatic, and central nervous system changes are similar to those found in a singleton pregnancy.

The larger size of the uterus may predispose to uterine atony. Increased blood loss after delivery will occur with greater frequency, therefore, adequate intravenous access is essential. Blood for transfusion should be "typed and held" for ready availability.

Preterm labor is common. Therefore, many patients requesting labor analgesia or presenting for abdominal delivery will have received tocolytic agent within the previous 12 hours. This drug therapy may lead to tachycardia, pulmonary edema, or potentiation of neuromuscular blocking agents.

Neither regional or general anesthesia is clearly superior for abdominal delivery. Improved uterine relaxation with general anesthesia may be beneficial for intrauterine manipulation for delivery of premature fetuses and/or abnormal presentations. However, a well-conducted intraspinal anesthetic, with appropriate measures to prevent and immediately treat hypotension, results in good neonatal outcome at delivery.

There are clear benefits from the use of epidural anesthesia, even though labor may be prolonged in multiple gestation[15,16,20] or the frequency of forceps delivery increased.[15,20] The biochemical status of both twins delivered under epidural anesthesia is superior to that of neonates delivered without epidural anesthesia, especially if the maternal bearing-down reflex is obtunded.[15] Perineal relaxation and maternal cooperation decrease fetal and maternal trauma. Abdominal delivery of the second twin is necessary in 4 to 8 percent of gravidas in which the first twin was delivered vaginally.[1,15] If abdominal delivery becomes necessary, surgical anesthesia can be rapidly obtained for a patient with epidural catheter in place to provide anesthesia for labor.

ANESTHETIC MANAGEMENT

Labor

Optimal pain relief is obtained with continuous lumbar epidural anesthesia. Maternal systemic blood pressure and fetal heart rate monitoring are necessary prior to induction of anesthesia. Meticulous attention to hydration (500 to 1,000 ml immediately prior to induction), uterine displacement, and intravenous ephedrine, as necessary, will support uteroplacental perfusion. Bupivacaine 0.125 to 0.5 percent with or without opioid may be used to obtain anesthesia. When less-concentrated local anesthetic solutions are chosen for labor, a "top-up" with a higher concentration is advisable prior to delivery because of the frequent need for operative delivery. (*Operative delivery* is defined as instrument-assisted vaginal delivery or abdominal [cesarean] delivery.)

Vaginal Delivery

The anesthetic management of the delivery of twin A is similar to the vaginal delivery of a singleton except for the increased likelihood of emergency operative delivery. Therefore, oxygen should be administered to the parturient to maximize fetal well-being and to prevent delay should denitrogenation be needed prior to induction of general anesthesia.

The anesthesiologist must be alert and prepared. The time between delivery of twin A and twin B is most likely to present changing obstetric and, therefore, anesthetic situations. An operative delivery may be necessary for the second twin, therefore epidural anesthesia should be maintained after the delivery of twin A. Although the upper dermatomal level of epidural anesthesia may produce adequate anesthesia for and facilitate internal manipulation of the second twin (i.e., version and full breech extraction), it does not produce uterine relaxation. External cephalic version of the second twin may also be facilitated under epidural anesthesia because of the relaxation of the abdominal musculature.[21] However, induction of general anesthesia may have to be considered for internal podalic version followed by a total breech extraction. Following a rapid-sequence induction and endotracheal intubation, a potent halogenated inhaled agent is used to effect maximal uterine relaxation. As soon as delivery is completed the agent should be discontinued.

Abdominal Delivery

Elective abdominal delivery may be performed using regional or general anesthesia. Epidural anesthesia may be preferable to subarachnoid anesthesia because of the slower onset of sympathetic blockade in the gravida particularly susceptible to aortocaval compression. Simultaneous popliteal and brachial blood pressure measurement will allow detection of occult supine hypotension (decreased uterine perfusion due to aortic compression in the presence of normal maternal brachial blood pressure). Particular attention should be paid to administration of oxygen and aspiration prophylaxis in light of the decreased FRC and increased production of gastrin. Intraspinal or general anesthesia induction is otherwise similar to the gravida with a singleton gestation.

REFERENCES

1. Redick LF: Anesthesia for twin delivery. Clin Perinatol 15:107, 1988
2. Spellacy WN, Handler A, Ferre CD: A case-control study of 1253 twin pregnancies from a 1982–1987 perinatal data base. Obstet Gynecol 75:168, 1990
3. Dewan D: Anesthesia for preterm delivery, breech presentation, and multiple gestation. Clin Obstet Gynecol 30:566, 1987
4. D'Alton ME, Newton ER, Cetrulo CL: Intrauterine fetal demise in multiple gestation. Acta Genet Med Gemellol 33:43, 1984
5. Benirschke K: Twin placenta in perinatal mortality. NY State J Med 61:1499, 1961
6. Gonsoulin W, Moise KJ Jr, Kirshon B, et al: Outcome of twin–twin transfusion diagnosed before 28 weeks of gestation. Obstet Gynecol 75:214, 1990
7. Enborm JA: Twin pregnancy with intrauterine death of one twin. Am J Obstet Gynecol 152:424, 1985
8. Syzmonowicz W, Preston H, Yu VYH: The surviving monozygotic twin. Arch Dis Child 61:454, 1986
9. Gonen R, Heyman E, Asztalos E, Milligan JE: The outcome of triplet gestations complicated by fetal death. Obstet Gynecol 75:175, 1990
10. Skelly H, Marivate M, Norman R, et al: Consumptive coagulopathy following fetal death in a triplet pregnancy. Am J Obstet Gynecol 142:595, 1982
11. Romero R, Duffy TP, Berkowitz RL, et al: Prolongation of a preterm pregnancy complicated by death of a single twin in utero and disseminated intravascular coagulation. N Engl J Med 310:772, 1984
12. Young BK, Suidan J, Antoine C, et al: Differences in twins: the importance of birth order. Am J Obstet Gynecol 151:915, 1985
13. James FM III, Crawford JS, Davies P, Naiem H: Lumbar epidural analgesia for labor and delivery of twins. Am J Obstet Gynecol 127:176, 1977
14. Little WA, Friedman EA: Anesthesia for the twin delivery. Anesthesiology 19:515, 1958
15. Crawford JS: A prospective study of 200 consecutive twin deliveries. Anaesthesia 42:33, 1987
16. Gullestad S, Sagen N: Epidural block in twin labour and delivery. Acta Anaesth Scand 21:504, 1977
17. Antoine C, Kirshenbaum NW, Young BK: Biochemical differences related to birth order in triplets. J Reprod Med 31:330, 1986
18. Rayburn WF, Lavin JP Jr, Miodovnik M, Varner MW: Multiple gestation: time interval between delivery of the first and second twins. Obstet Gynecol 63:502, 1984
19. Veille JC, Morton MJ, Burry KJ: Maternal cardiovascular adaptations to twin pregnancy. Obstet Gynecol 153:261, 1985
20. Ogbonna B, Daw E: Epidural analgesia and the length of labour for vaginal twin delivery. J Obstet Gynaecol 6:166, 1986
21. Chervenak FA, Johnson RE, Berkowitz RL, Hobbins JC: Intrapartum external version of the second twin. Obstet Gynecol 62:160, 1983

PREGNANCY-INDUCED HYPERTENSION

Pregnancy-induced hypertension (PIH) occurs in 5 to 7 percent of all pregnancies. PIH is implicated in 20 percent of maternal deaths and in 6 to 10 percent of perinatal deaths. Although primarily a disease of the young primigravida, women with a history of PIH are at risk for its development in subsequent pregnancies.[1–3]

DEFINITION

PIH is defined as hypertension occurring after the 20th week of gestation and resolving by the 6th week postpartum, although it may occur earlier when associated with trophoblastic disease. It is divided into three broad categories based on clinical findings.

1. Gestational hypertension: Hypertension alone. Blood pressure of at least 140/90 or an increase of 30 mmHg systolic or 15 mmHg diastolic above nonpregnant levels noted on two occasions at least 6 hours apart.
2. Preeclampsia: Hypertension with proteinuria (greater than 300 mg/L in 24 hours) and/or generalized edema. Preeclampsia is classified as mild, moderate, or severe. Severe preeclampsia is defined by the presence of one or more of the following:
   a) Systolic blood pressure of at least 160 or diastolic blood pressure of at least 110
   b) Proteinuria of at least 5 g/L in 24 hours
   c) Oliguria: urine output of less than 400 ml in 24 hours
   d) Cerebral or visual disturbances, including headache

e) Pulmonary edema or cyanosis
f) Epigastric pain
g) Presence of the HELLP syndrome (hemolysis, elevated liver enzymes, low platelets)[4,5]

3. Eclampsia: Presence of convulsions or coma, not related to any underlying neurologic disorder.

CLINICAL FINDINGS

The etiology of PIH is not well understood. The pathophysiologic changes appear to result from an imbalance in thromboxane and prostacyclin production, resulting in generalized vasoconstriction, sodium and water retention, vascular endothelial damage, and disruption of the normal coagulation process.[6] All organ systems may be affected.[1–3]

Effects on Blood Volume/Hemodynamic Status

1. Increased total body water.
2. Decreased intravascular volume (up to 30 to 40 percent in severe PIH).[7]
3. Arteriolar vasoconstriction.
4. Decreased central venous pressure (CVP) proportional to the severity of hypertension.
5. Increased vascular permeability, causing a shift of intravascular fluid and protein to extravascular spaces that results in hypovolemia, hypoproteinemia, and generalized edema.
6. Decreased red cell mass, which may be masked by the decreased intravascular volume.
7. Increased sensitivity to vasoactive drugs.

Renal Effects

1. Decreased effective renal blood flow.
2. Decreased glomerular filtration rate.
3. Decreased urea clearance (30 to 50 percent).[8]
4. Glomerular endothelial swelling, compromising capillary lumina.
5. Fibrin deposition along basement membrane.
6. Increased urinary protein loss.
7. Increased serum uric acid proportional to the severity of PIH.[8]
   a) Normal pregnant value: 3 to 3.5 mg/dl
   b) Mild PIH: 4.0 mg/dl
   c) Severe PIH: 7.5 mg/dl
8. Decreased urine output.
9. Rarely, acute renal failure, usually secondary to hemorrhagic hypotension.

Cardiac Effects

1. Increased left ventricular (LV) work secondary to increased systemic vascular resistance.
2. Increased cardiac output (CO), usually due to increased heart rate and increased stroke volume (SV). However, the additional increase in CO seen in the early postpartum period in normal patients does not occur in severe preeclampsia, probably because of the decreased blood volume and increased blood loss.
3. Decreases in CVP of −1 to −4 cmH_2O have been reported in severely preeclamptic patients. CVP may not correlate with pulmonary capillary wedge pressure (PCWP) and pulmonary edema may occur in the presence of a normal CVP.
4. PCWP is variable but is usually normal. High PCWP may indicate LV dysfunction.[9]

Respiratory Effects

1. Marked facial and laryngeal edema may occur and may cause difficulty in intubation.
2. Pulmonary function may be normal in mild preeclampsia.
3. Increased A-a gradient and physiologic shunt have been described in severely preeclamptic patients and may be due to decreased pulmonary blood flow.
4. Pulmonary edema may occur in severe PIH secondary to LV failure or capillary leak from marked hypoalbuminemia (or both).
5. The risk of aspiration during seizures is increased in eclampsia.

Central Nervous System Effects

1. Hyperreflexia.
2. Generalized central nervous system (CNS) edema.
3. CNS hyperirritability.
4. Increased incidence of tonic-clonic seizures (eclampsia); up to 25 percent occur postpartum.
5. Increased sensitivity to CNS depressants.
6. Normal cerebral blood flow.
7. Intracranial hemorrhage is the leading cause of maternal death from PIH.

Effects on Coagulation

1. Decreased platelet count (HELLP syndrome)[4,5]
2. Decreased platelet function in 10 to 25 percent of preeclamptic patients.
3. Increased bleeding time (even in the presence of a normal platelet count).

4. Variable values for clotting time, fibrinogen, and fibrin split products.
5. Disseminated intravascular coagulation is rare unless placental abruption is present. There is an increased incidence of placental abruption in patients with PIH.

Hepatic Effects

1. Increased liver enzymes (HELLP syndrome).
2. Increased bilirubin.
3. Periportal hemorrhage, ischemic lesions, and generalized edema of the liver.
4. Epigastric or right upper quadrant pain, probably due to hepatic swelling.
5. Subcapsular hematoma is rare but often fatal.

Effects on the Uteroplacental Unit

1. Uteroplacental insufficiency exists secondary to increased vascular resistance, decreased plasma volume, increased blood viscosity, and intimal changes decreasing the lumina in placental arteries. Placental perfusion decreases by 50 to 70 percent in PIH.
2. Premature placental aging leads to placental infarcts, uterine hypertonicity, and increased sensitivity to oxytocic drugs.
3. Incidence of placental abruption is 15 times greater than normal.

Perinatal Effects[1–3]

1. Increased incidence of prematurity.
2. Intrauterine growth retardation (less than 25th percentile).
3. Hypoglycemia (less than 30 mg/dl).
4. Fetal asphyxia.
5. Respiratory distress syndrome (usually mild).
6. Hyperbilirubinemia (greater than 15 mg/dl).

OBSTETRIC MANAGEMENT

The obstetric management is guided by the maternal condition and the relative risk to the fetus of premature delivery. The definitive therapy for preeclampsia is delivery of the infant and placenta, and pregnancy should only be allowed to continue if the fetus is tolerating the intrauterine environment and maternal outcome is not threatened. Conditions that mandate delivery are persistent, severe hypertension (for more than 48 hours), the presence of the HELLP syndrome, decreased renal function, and eclampsia.

Mild PIH may be treated with bed rest; sedation; antihypertensive therapy; and monitoring of urine output, weight, and reflexes.

Therapy for more severe PIH prior to delivery should include control of hypertension, reduction of CNS irritability, improvement of renal function, and optimization of fetal status.

Antihypertensives

Many agents have been used for long-term therapy, but for acute treatment of severe maternal hypertension (diastolic blood pressure of more than 110 mmHg) in the labor suite the most commonly used drugs include:

1. Intravenous hydralazine 5 to 10 mg every 20 to 30 minutes.
2. Intravenous labetalol 5 to 10 mg every 5 to 10 minutes.
3. Nifedipine 5 to 10 mg sublingually every 5 to 10 minutes.[10,11]

The goal of therapy is to reduce the diastolic blood pressure to 90 to 105 mmHg.

Anticonvulsants

Magnesium sulfate is currently the mainstay in the United States for reduction of CNS irritability and prevention of seizures. It is administered by continuous intravenous infusion after a loading dose. As it is cleared by the kidneys, monitoring of plasma levels and of renal function is imperative. The therapeutic plasma level is 4 to 8 mEq/L. Plasma levels that exceed this may result in loss of deep tendon reflexes (10 mEq/L), myocardial depression (10 to 15 mEq/L), skeletal muscle relaxation (12 mEq/L) respiratory paralysis (12 to 15 mEq/L), and cardiac arrest (25 to 30 mEq/L). Treatment of severe magnesium toxicity consists of airway management, endotracheal intubation, and administration of calcium.

Magnesium is a mild vasodilator and a reduction in maternal blood pressure may be seen, although this effect is transient and often offset by a reflex tachycardia. It is not an adequate antihypertensive agent. It has a tocolytic effect, which may improve uterine blood flow. Magnesium also may cause maternal sedation, neonatal hypotonia, and respiratory depression.

More recently, diphenylhydantoin has been used for prophylaxis against seizures in preeclamptic patients. Side effects include rash, nausea, and blurred vision.[12]

When seizures occur, intravenous sodium thiopental 75 to 100 mg or intravenous diazepam 5 to 10 mg may be given. Management of the airway is critical and care must be taken to prevent or to rapidly diagnose maternal regurgitation and aspiration.

ANESTHETIC CONSIDERATIONS AND MANAGEMENT

Assessment of Hemodynamic Status

In addition to treatment of hypertension and CNS hyperirritability, hemodynamic status should be optimized. Initially, noninvasive blood pressure monitoring and a Foley catheter for urine output measurement may be adequate. If severe hypertension exists, invasive blood pressure monitoring may be required. Hypovolemia, as evidenced by oliguria, anemia, (hematocrit greater than 37 percent), colloid oncotic pressure (of less than 15 mmHg, or metabolic acidosis, should be treated with careful intravascular volume expansion usually with crystalloid. Initially, intravenous fluids may be administered in 500-ml boluses while monitoring oxygen saturation.

However, if urine output remains low after 2,000 ml of crystalloid or if oxygen saturation (SaO_2) decreases, placement of a CVP catheter is indicated. If initial CVP is greater than 6 cmH_2O or if SaO_2 is less than 90 percent (on room air), pulmonary artery catheterization is probably indicated.

ANESTHESIA FOR LABOR AND VAGINAL DELIVERY

Lumbar Epidural Anesthesia

Lumbar epidural anesthesia (LEA) is the technique of choice for pain relief during labor and delivery. The safety of LEA has been well established.[13–16] Properly administered, it provides good pain relief, thereby reducing plasma catecholamine levels, and aids in the control of maternal hypertension while maintaining uterine and renal perfusion.[13–16] Considerations prior to initiating LEA include:

1. Intravascular volume status. Because most preeclamptic patients are hypovolemic, intravenous hydration is mandatory.[17] Although opinions and methods of care vary, the fluid boluses usually range from 500 to 1,000 ml of a crystalloid solution. As outlined above, if the patient is oliguric or has signs of hypoxemia, CVP and perhaps PCWP monitoring may be necessary for determining intravascular volume status. CVP should be in the 4- to 6-cm H_2O range.
2. Treatment of hypotension. If hypotension occurs, it should be treated with rapid intravenous administration of a crystalloid solution and maintenance of left uterine displacement. Ephedrine and mephentermine have been used safely but doses should be reduced as these patients are more sensitive to the effects of vasopressors. α-Agonists should probably be avoided because they may result in further reductions in the already compromised placental perfusion.
3. Use of epinephrine-containing local anesthetics. Most studies have demonstrated no adverse effect of epinephrine when properly administered in the epidural space.[18] However, intravenous administration of even small doses of epinephrine may result in severe compromise of the uterine blood flow and placental perfusion.[19] For this reason, many anesthesiologists avoid its use in the preeclamptic patient.
4. Contraindications to LEA include infection at the site of insertion, patient refusal, and coagulopathy. Opinions vary with regard to the severity of coagulopathy, but a general rule of thumb is that LEA may be initiated when:
   a) The platelet count is greater than 100,000 and the prothrombin time (PT) and partial thromboplastin time (PTT) are normal.
   b) The platelet count is less than 100,000 and the bleeding time (BT), PT, and PTT are normal.

   If PT, PTT, and BT are prolonged, LEA is generally not performed.

   Coagulation studies should be obtained every 8 hours in the severe preeclamptic parturient.

Subarachnoid Anesthesia

If LEA was not used for labor and an anesthetic is required for vaginal delivery, low subarachnoid anesthesia or saddle block may be performed following all the precautions listed for LEA.

General Anesthesia

Refer to Chapter 6 for the protocol for administering general anesthesia.

ANESTHESIA FOR CESAREAN DELIVERY

Lumbar Epidural Anesthesia

LEA is again the technique of choice unless the previously mentioned contraindications exist. Bupivacaine allows a slower onset of sympathetic block and more time for compensation of hemodynamic changes,

Subarachnoid Anesthesia

Subarachnoid anesthesia may be used but results in a more rapid onset of sympathetic block and derangements in maternal hemodynamics that may be more difficult to control. However, although controversial, some studies suggest that preeclamptic patients may be less sensitive to sympathetic blockade because of the presence of circulating vasopressors such as angiotensin.[20]

General Anesthesia

General anesthesia may be required if regional anesthesia is contraindicated or fetal distress is present. In addition to the usual considerations for general anesthesia for cesarean delivery in the pregnant patient, several conditions specific to preeclampsia exist. Edema of the face, pharynx, and larynx may be present, making laryngoscopy and endotracheal intubation difficult. The marked hypertensive response to laryngoscopy and intubation results in increases of up to 30 percent in mean arterial pressure (MAP) (potentially exceeding the limits of cerebral autoregulation) and in large increases in pulmonary artery pressure and PCWP.[21] Numerous agents have been used to prevent or at least attenuate the cardiovascular response, but an in-depth discussion of each is beyond the scope of this section. Briefly, the β-blocker, labetalol, is efficacious in blunting the response to intubation. It has been shown to preserve uterine blood flow.[22,23] Trimethaphan, the ganglionic blocker, reduces blood pressure but in large doses may prolong the neuromuscular block of succinylcholine. It has a slower onset than other agents but has the advantage of not requiring intra-arterial blood pressure monitoring. Sodium nitroprusside is an excellent agent in this setting because of its rapid onset, short duration, and primarily arterial vasodilating properties.[24] There is a potential for fetal cyanide toxicity over long-term use, so its use should be limited to 5 to 10 minutes at induction of anesthesia.[25] Nitroglycerin has also been shown to be effective and safe.[26] However, in patients who have received a large bolus of fluid, its hypotensive effect may be blunted.[27] The use of infusions of either sodium nitroprusside or nitroglycerin require an arterial catheter for continuous blood pressure monitoring.

In summary, for induction of general anesthesia:

1. Evaluate adequacy of airway: consider awake laryngoscopy for induction of general anesthesia and/or awake fiberoptic intubation if marked facial edema exists. Have several endotracheal tubes available, from 5.0 mm to 7.0 mm. Administer a clear antacid prior to induction (within 30 minutes).
2. Maintain left uterine displacement.
3. Acutely oxygenate and denitrogenate the patient.
4. Induce anesthesia with thiopental 3 to 4 mg/kg, cricoid pressure, and succinylcholine 1.5 to 2.0 mg/kg (100-mg dose commonly used).
5. Prevent and control the hypertensive response. The following agents may be used prior to induction to decrease MAP 20 to 25 percent:
   a) Labetalol
   b) Trimethaphan infusion
   c) Sodium nitroprusside infusion
   d) Nitroglycerin infusion
6. Maintain anesthesia prior to delivery with 33 to 50 percent nitrous oxide in oxygen and add 0.5 to 1.0 percent isoflurane. After delivery, nitrous oxide can be increased to 70 percent if appropriate SaO_2 is maintained and intravenous opioids and anxiolytics can be administered.

REFERENCES

1. Gutsche BB, Cheek TG: Anesthetic considerations in preeclampsia–eclampsia. p. 225. In Shnider SM, Levinson G (eds): Anesthesia for Obstetrics. Williams & Wilkins, Baltimore, 1987
2. James FM III: Pregnancy-induced hypertension. p. 411. In James FM III, Wheeler AS, Dwan DM (eds): Obstetric Anesthesia: The Complicated Patient. FA Davis, Philadelphia, 1988
3. Wright JP: Anesthetic considerations in pre-eclampsia-eclampsia (review article). Anesth Analg 62:590, 1983
4. Weinstein L: Preeclampsia/eclampsia with hemolysis, elevated liver enzymes and thrombocytopenia. Obstet Gynecol 66:657, 1985
5. Weinstein L: Syndrome of hemolysis, elevated liver enzymes and low platelet count: a severe consequence of hypertension in pregnancy. Am J Obstet Gynecol 142:159, 1982
6. Walsh SW: Preeclampsia: an imbalance in placental prostacyclin and thromboxane production. Am J Obstet Gynecol 152:335, 1985
7. Soffranoff EC, Kaufman BM, Connaughton JF: Intravascular volume determinants and fetal outcome in hypertensive disease of pregnancy. Am J Obstet Gynecol 127:4, 1977
8. Hayashi T: Uric acid and endogenous creatinine clearance studies in normal pregnancy and toxemia of pregnancy. Am J Obstet Gynecol 71:859, 1956
9. Benedetti TJ, Cotton DB, Read JC, Miller FC: Hemodynamic observations in severe preeclampsia with a flow directed pulmonary artery catheter. Am J Obstet Gynecol 136:465, 1980
10. Norris MC, Rose JE, Dewan DM: Nifedipine or verapamil counteracts hypertension in gravid ewes. Anesthesiology 65:254, 1986
11. Walters BNJ, Redman CWG: Treatment of severe preg-

nancy-associated hypertension with the calcium antagonist nifedipine. Br J Obstet Gynaecol 91:330, 1984
12. Repke JT, Friedman SA, Lim KH, et al: Magnesium sulfate versus phenytoin in preeclampsia: preliminary results from a randomized clinical trial. Society of Perinatal Obstetricians, Abstract 112, Feb. 1989, New Orleans
13. Moore TR, et al: Evaluation of the use of continuous lumbar epidural anesthesia for hypertensive pregnant women in labor. Am J Obstet Gynecol 152:404, 1985
14. Jouppila P, Jouppila R, Hollmen A, Koivula A: Lumbar epidural analgesia to improve intervillous blood flow during labor in severe preeclampsia. Obstet Gynecol 59:158, 1982
15. Jouppila R, Jouppila P, Hollmen A, Koivula A: Epidural analgesia and placental blood flow during labour in pregnancies complicated by hypertension. Br J Obstet Gynaecol 86:869, 1979
16. James FM III, Davies P: Maternal and fetal effects of lumbar epidural analgesia for labor and delivery in patients with gestational hypertension. Am J Obstet Gynecol 126(2):195, 1976
17. Clark SL, et al: Severe preeclampsia with persistent oliguria: management of hemodynamic subsets. Am J Obstet Gynecol 154:490, 1986
18. Albright G, et al: Epinephrine does not alter human intervillous blood flow during epidural anesthesia. Anesthesiology 54:131, 1981
19. Hood DD, Dewan DM, James FM: Maternal and fetal effects of epinephrine in gravid ewes. Anesthesiology 64:610, 1986
20. Goldkrand JW, Fuentes AM: The relation of angiotensin-converting enzyme to the pregnancy-induced hypertension-preeclampsia syndrome: Am J Obstet Gynecol 154:792, 1986
21. Hodgkinson R, Husain FJ, Hayashi RH: Systemic and pulmonary pressure during cesarean section in parturients with gestational hypertension. Can Anaesth Soc J 27:389, 1980
22. Ramanathan J, et al: The use of labetalol for attenuation of the hypertensive response to endotracheal intubation in preeclampsia. Am J Obstet Gynecol 159(3):650, 1988
23. Michael CA: The evaluation of labetalol in the treatment of hypertension complicating pregnancy. Br J Pharmacol 13:128S, 1982
24. Elis SC, Wheeler AS, James FM III: Fetal and maternal effects of sodium nitroprusside used to counteract hypertension in gravid ewes. Am J Obstet Gynecol 143:776, 1982
25. Naulty J, Cefalo RC, Lewis PE: Fetal toxicity of nitroprusside in the pregnant ewe. Am J Obstet Gynecol 139(6):708, 1981
26. Cotton DB, et al: Role of intravenous nitroglycerin in the treatment of severe pregnancy-induced hypertension complicated by pulmonary edema. Am J Obstet Gynecol 154:91, 1986
27. Hood DD, Dewan DM, James FM III, et al: The use of nitroglycerin in preventing the hypertensive response to tracheal intubation in severe preeclamptics. Anesthesiology 63:329, 1985

AMNIOTIC FLUID EMBOLISM

Amniotic fluid embolism is a rare, unpredictable, and unpreventable obstetric catastrophe. It is initiated by entry of amniotic fluid into the maternal circulation and is characterized by the sudden onset of severe dyspnea, tachypnea, and cyanosis during labor, delivery, or the early puerperium.

Amniotic fluid embolism was first reported by Meyer[1] in 1926. It was reported again in an experiment on laboratory animals by Warden in 1927.[2]

The importance of this condition and these early studies was not established until 1941, when Steiner and Lushbaugh[3] noted the clinical and pathologic findings of eight women who died suddenly during or just after labor. They performed experimental studies on laboratory animals that produced the same severe disturbances of cardiopulmonary function following the entry of amniotic fluid into maternal circulation. Their study was documented with pathologic findings of pulmonary embolism caused by amniotic fluid particulate matter. Schneider et al.[4] in 1968 showed that lethal qualities of human amniotic fluid infused intravenously into dogs were enhanced greatly by the addition of meconium. This description by Steiner and Lushbaugh of a patient with amniotic fluid embolism is classic in its detailed brevity:

> "Profound shock coming on suddenly and unexpectedly in a woman who is usually in severe labor or has just finished such a labor, especially if she is an elderly multipara with an excessively large, perhaps dead, fetus and with meconium amniotic fluid, should lead to a suspicion of the possibility. If, also, the shock is introduced by a chill which is followed by dyspnea, cyanosis, vomiting, restlessness and the like and is accompanied by a pronounced fall in blood pressure and a rapid, weak pulse, the picture is more complete. If pulmonary edema now develops quickly in the known absence of previously existing heart disease the diagnosis is reasonably certain."

Their description is complete except for the development of disseminated intravascular coagulation (DIC) in patients surviving the initial pulmonary insult.

INCIDENCE

The incidence of amniotic fluid embolism has been reported to be between 1 per 8,000 and 1 per 80,000 pregnancies; a more realistic figure is likely between these two extremes.[3,5,6] The mortality rate is very high. Although it is a rare occurrence, it still remains a leading cause of maternal and fetal death. Morgan[7] in 1979 reviewed 272 cases documented in the British medical literature and reported a mortality rate of 86 percent. From the same study, 25 percent of the deaths occurred within the first hour of the onset of symptoms, indicating that, even with optimum critical care management, a high mortality rate persists. Not all sudden deaths in late pregnancy are due to amniotic fluid embolism. We must be careful not to let this diagnosis become the wastebasket for cases of unexplained death in labor, especially without confirmation by autopsy.

ETIOLOGY

Predisposing factors for amniotic fluid embolism include advanced maternal age, multiple pregnancies, fetal macrosomia, short duration of labor, and intense contractions often augmented with an uterine muscle stimulant such as oxytocin.[8] Others suggest that fetal demise, meconium staining of amniotic fluid, amniotomy, pregnancy-induced hypertension (PIH), cesarean delivery, abruptio placentae, placenta previa, ruptured uterus, amniocentesis, insertion of an intrauterine pressure catheter, and pregnancy at term with an intrauterine device present are also causative factors. Recent reviews have documented a significant association of amniotic fluid embolism with advanced maternal age.[7] Documentation of amniotic fluid embolism has also been reported following intrauterine injection of hypertonic saline to induce abortion. Recently a case was reported after use of vaginal prostaglandin E_2.[9]

Amniotic fluid embolus syndrome has been reported in association with a myriad of conditions. These conditions include first- and second-trimester abortion with saline, prostaglandins, and urea, and hysterotomy. It has occurred during labor, at delivery, just after delivery, and in one case even 32 hours postpartum. Most reported cases of amniotic fluid embolism occur during labor; a pattern of vigorous labor or hypertonic uterine contractions or labor further stimulated by use of oxytocin often has been implicated in the pathogenesis. Evidence for this association (use of an oxytoxic) is primarily anecdotal and must be regarded with skepticism. In a review of this subject, Morgan[7] concluded: "In view of the very wide use of accelerated labor and the rarity of amniotic fluid embolism, it must be concluded that there is no direct association between the two." Placental abruption is present in up to 50 percent of cases and may contribute to the pattern of uterine hypertonus associated with amniotic fluid embolism. In 40 percent of cases, fetal death is reported prior to the acute clinical presentation.

In an analysis of data collected in another study,[10] the range of age was from 18 to 43 years, with 22 patients being 30 years old or older; 12 patients were over 35 years of age. The parity of patients ranged from one to eight, with the majority of patients greater than three; however, there were four cases documented in primaparous women. The duration of gestational age of the pregnancies in the patients who subsequently died ranged from 38 to 44 weeks. This excludes those patients who died from amniotic fluid embolism secondary to saline or other fluids injected intra-amniotically to induce abortion.

The characteristics of the labor pattern varied. However, it is of interest to note that four patients developed amniotic emboli without evidence of labor. The majority of patients were in various stages of either spontaneous or augmented labor (in 22 percent labor had been induced and in 11 percent labor had been augmented with an oxytoxic agent). The augmentation or induction of labor was instituted for the usual reasons: ruptured membranes without consistent uterine contractions, postmaturity, PIH, and elective induction. In 10 percent, labor was augmented because of poor progress. Of patients who labored spontaneously, 44 percent had tumultuous and unusually short labors averaging less than 1 hour in duration. No comparably short labors or precipitous deliveries were identified in the patients who received oxytocin stimulation, nor were tetanic contractions reported.

The membranes were documented to be intact in three patients at the time the embolism or onset of symptoms occurred. In most cases studied, the membranes had ruptured either spontaneously or by amniotomy prior to the onset of symptoms. There is documentation, however, indicating that simultaneous rupture of membranes with onset of symptoms of amniotic fluid embolus and meconium fluid was present in approximately 75 percent of these patients.[3]

Concerning fetal factors, no clear pattern of fetal presentation, position, or engagement could be ascertained; most cases documented indicate a vertex presentation. There was generally a lack of documentation associating station of the presenting part with onset of symptoms. It could be assumed, since the onset of symptoms occurred just prior to or during delivery, that the fetal presenting part was engaged.

The size of the infant varied from 5 to 11 pounds, but unfortunately, the data particular to the exact weight of all infants were not available. There is a high incidence of demise and intrapartum death of infants and, unfortunately, of those few infants born alive, a very high percentage expire during the neonatal period. In one study of 21 infants on whom information was available, there were nine diagnoses of demise with five occurring as intrapartum deaths. Ten live births were recorded in this particular study; however, only two infants were documented to have survived. There is a disportionately large number of stillbirths, and some researchers feel that presence of fetal demise reduces the strength of the membranes as well as greatly increases the quantity of particulate matter in the amniotic fluid.[3]

In order for amniotic fluid embolism to occur, the fluid must enter into the maternal circulation. Currently, three recognized conditions must exist for this to result: amniotomy, laceration of endocervical or uterine vessels, and a pressure gradient sufficient to force the fluid into the maternal circulation.

A tear or rent in the membranes such as occurs with amniotomy has been associated with proven embolism.[11] Various sites of entry of amniotic fluid into maternal circulation have been suggested. Laceration of endocervical veins can occur during the normal process of cervical dilation and effacement, although more severe lacerations may occur with a very rapid and tumultuous labor or vigorous cervical manipulation associated with vaginal examination. Uterine vessels can be damaged through surgical procedures such as cesarean delivery or amniocentesis. Trauma is also responsible for causing damage of the uterine vessels. According to Landing,[12] an abnormal opening of the uterine vessels, either decidual or myometrial, which occurs with uterine rupture, placenta accreta, cesarean delivery, or retained placenta, may provide a portal of entry for amniotic fluid. Abruptio placentae, whether marginal or complete, as well as any degree of placenta previa, could also provide a route of entry. If amniotic fluid finds an open maternal venous sinus, it could be pumped by a vigorous contraction through the disrupted amniotic membrane with resultant embolization.

Intra-amniotic injections of fluid (i.e., hypertonic saline, saline, or urea) cause a rise in intrauterine pressure that may be greater than that associated with normal labor. Frost[13] in 1967 reported a patient with a hydatidiform mole who died from trophoblastic embolization of the lungs following injection of intra-amniotic hypertonic saline. A review of deaths following legal abortions in the United States from 1972 to 1978 revealed 15 (12 percent) were due to amniotic fluid embolus; all of these followed intra-amniotic injections, and none followed uterine curettage.[14] Clinically, the symptoms exhibited in these patients were the same as in those with embolism occurring at term. This study also revealed gestational age to be a significant factor. No deaths occurred below 12 weeks of gestation, however, the mortality was 7.2 per 100,000 at 21 weeks or more, representing a risk factor 24 times greater after 21 weeks gestation.[14]

Because of the rarity of the condition combined with the fact that diagnosis is often made during the postmortem examination, it is difficult to determine a definite cause and effect with this catastrophic obstetric event.

PATHOPHYSIOLOGY

The two life-threatening consequences of amniotic fluid embolism, cardiopulmonary collapse and DIC, may occur in sequence or together. The physiology of amniotic fluid embolism results in acute pulmonary hypertension with a sudden reduction of blood flow to the left heart, decreased left ventricular output, and subsequent peripheral vascular collapse. The sudden development of elevated pulmonary artery pressure could precipitate acute cor pulmonale or right ventricular failure. The derangement of the ventilation:perfusion ratio of the lungs produces hypoxemia and acidemia, which in the pattern of a vicious circle further enhances pulmonary artery vasospasm. If severe pulmonary vascular obstruction and cor pulmonale are not immediately fatal, hemorrhage may soon become evident.

The etiology of DIC is controversial. Evidence suggests the potent thromboplastin action of amniotic fluid causes disseminated deposition of fibrin clots and activation of the lysis system. These hemodynamic processes defibrinate the blood,[15] resulting in afibrinogenemia, coagulopathy, and subsequent hemorrhage.[16] The powerful thromboplastin effects of trophoblast are well established; systemic release of trophoblastic material may play an even greater role in the coagulopathy of amniotic fluid embolism than has been appreciated.

Kitzmiller and Lucas have shown that amniotic fluid collected during labor (as compared to fluid collected prior to labor) has greater toxicity when infused into rabbits.[16] The particular substance mediating this reaction is still unknown. Prostaglandins and leukotrienes produce many of the hemodynamic and hematologic effects present in patients with amniotic fluid embolism and have been implicated by some researchers.[17] These metabolites of arachidonic acid are present in increased quantities during labor.[18]

The toxicity of intravenously infused amniotic fluid appears to vary remarkably depending on the particulate matter it contains. This is especially true of meconium-stained fluid. The particulate materials found in amniotic fluid and especially in meconium-stained fluid, according to some investigators, may account for the cause of sudden death associated with this syndrome.[19]

Some researchers postulate that an acute anaphylactoid reaction may play a part in the development of the cardiovascular collapse.[20] For a true anaphylactic reaction to occur, sensitization is required, but evidence for prior sensitization of the parturient to amniotic fluid is lacking. Stefanini and Turpini,[21] in their experiment, noted that an intravenous injection of 15 ml of homologous amniotic fluid in dogs produced no effect, but 1 month later, further administration of a 15-ml aliquot of the same fluid, which had been kept frozen, resulted in hypotension, hypofibrinogenemia, and thrombocytopenia. Therefore, it was suggested the animal had become sensitized to amniotic fluid; this might occur in humans as well. It is possible that penetration of amniotic fluid into the systemic circulation during the antepartum period causes a state of sensitization in humans, and subsequent entry into the circulation during labor and delivery could induce an acute anaphylactic reaction. However, the absence or rarity of pruritus, urticaria, laryngospasm, or wheezing in case reports does not indicate a mast cell-mediated mechanism.

In a recent review on amniotic fluid embolism, Clark[22] concluded the following: some "normal" amniotic fluid may innocuously enter the maternal circulation of many pregnant women. However, amniotic fluid embolism may develop after maternal infusion of "abnormal" amniotic fluid; that is, fluid containing an abnormal substance, possibly one of the arachidonic acid metabolites.

The most significant pathologic findings at autopsy are limited to the lungs. Grossly, the lungs show evidence of pulmonary edema (70 percent in one study),[23] alveolar hemorrhage, and pulmonary embolization of amniotic fluid materials. The presence of embolic particles is essential for diagnosis, but these may be missed on histologic search because of their small size.[19] Amniotic emboli are composed of amorphous debris, fetal epithelial squamous cells (squames), fetal hairs, vernix caseosa, and mucin (from meconium). The emboli tend to lodge in small arteries, arterioles, and capillaries of the lungs.[15] Since uterine trauma is a significant factor in the pathogenesis, signs of uterine laceration or uterine rupture may be evident.[24] Acute right ventricular dilation is usually present. Amniotic fluid elements are sometimes found in the right side of the heart as well as within uterine vessels. Careful evaluation of the other organs may also identify the magnitude of embolization when particulate matter is identified in the maternal brain, kidneys, liver, spleen, and even the hypothalamus.

CLINICAL AND LABORATORY DIAGNOSIS

In a small percentage of patients the onset of symptoms occurred before labor was clinically evident. The majority of patients developed symptoms during the latter part of the first stage of labor and a lesser number became acute during birth. There have been two cases documented that were associated with delivery of the placenta and one case occurred at 32 hours postdelivery. In one series, 45 percent of cases were associated with placental abruption of varying degrees. Many investigators believe this to be one of the primary catalysts in the development of amniotic fluid embolism.

In a review of obstetric patients who developed amniotic embolism,[7] the most common complications that were already present or that developed during delivery are listed in order of frequency of occurrence: severe amnionitis, moderate to severe PIH, cephalopelvic disproportion, and traumatic midforceps delivery.

Prodromal symptoms in amniotic fluid embolism are sudden chills, shivering, sweating, anxiety, and coughing, followed by signs of respiratory distress, shock, cardiovascular collapse, and convulsions. All patients were conscious during the onset of symptomatology. Respiratory difficulty, manifested as cyanosis, tachypnea, and bronchospasm, frequently progresses to fulminant pulmonary edema. Hypoxemia explains the cyanosis and likely accounts for the restlessness, convulsions, and unconsciousness. Reflex tachypnea results from the initial decreased arterial oxygen saturation. Cardiovascular collapse, as heralded by hypotension, tachycardia, and arrhythmia, may end in cardiac arrest. Convulsions may be an early manifestation of central nervous system involvement secondary to cerebral ischemia and may eventually progress to coma and death. If the patient survives this initial episode, bleeding may occur secondary to DIC and uterine atony. In all cases studied, bleeding was never documented as one of the first symptoms.

A definitive diagnosis is usually made at postmortem examination by demonstration of amniotic fluid material in the maternal circulation and the small arteries, arterioles, and capillaries of the pulmonary vessels. In the living patient, diagnosis may be made by identification of lanugo or fetal hair and fetal squames in an aspirate of blood from the right heart.[25] Fetal squames have been recovered in the maternal sputum in some cases.[26] Additional diagnostic tools for confirmation of amniotic fluid embolism suspected by the classic clinical picture include:

1. Chest x-ray, which may show enlargement of the right atrium and ventricle, a prominent proximal pulmonary artery (in massive pulmonary embolism), and pulmonary edema
2. Lung scan, which may demonstrate some areas of reduced perfusion
3. Central venous catheterization, which reveals an

initial rise due to acute pulmonary hypertension and eventually a profound decrease due to severe hemorrhage

4. Measurement of blood coagulation factors

Normally, in pregnancy, blood coagulation factors are increased. However, with amniotic fluid embolism and DIC, the blood fails to clot.

In the differential diagnosis of amniotic fluid embolism, the following entities are to be considered[27]:

1. Pulmonary thromboembolism most often develops postdelivery, is usually caused by a thrombus originating from the lower extremities or pelvic veins, and is usually associated with chest pain.[28]
2. Air embolism may occur following a ruptured uterus, blood transfusion under pressure, or manipulation or placenta previa during labor or cesarean delivery. It is associated with chest pain, but an important differentiating factor from amniotic fluid embolism is the auscultation of a typical water-wheel murmur over the pericardium.[29]
3. Aspiration of gastric contents into the lungs causes cyanosis, tachypnea, coughing, tachycardia, hypotension, and pulmonary edema. However, acid aspiration usually occurs in an unconscious patient with loss of the cough reflex,[28] or during induction or emergence from general anesthesia.
4. Eclamptic convulsions and coma in a pregnant patient may resemble amniotic fluid embolus syndrome, but the presence of hypertension, proteinuria, and edema[29] in the eclamptic patient differentiates these two conditions.
5. Convulsions from a toxic reaction to local anesthetics may be confused with this syndrome, but the close temporal relationship between the onset of symptoms and administration of the drug[29] is the differentiating factor. Also, hypertension is usually present in the early clinical picture of drug toxicity.
6. Acute left heart failure is most commonly seen in pregnant patients with rheumatic heart disease, but the history of rheumatic fever with electrocardiographic changes and other clinical symptoms (i.e., cardiac murmur) helps in the diagnosis.
7. A cerebrovascular accident may be considered in the differential diagnosis, but it is distinguished from amniotic fluid embolism by the absence of cyanosis, hypotension, and pulmonary edema. Also, examination of cerebrospinal fluid should aid in the diagnosis.
8. Hemorrhagic shock in an obstetric patient may be associated with abruptio placentae, placenta previa, or ruptured uterus. Postdelivery hemorrhage may develop from uterine atony, unrepaired cervical laceration, retained products, or uterine inversion. A careful history and physical examination, absence of central cyanosis, and low central venous pressure (if hemodynamic monitoring is used) should guide one to the correct diagnosis and therapy.

OBSTETRIC AND ANESTHETIC MANAGEMENT

To prevent amniotic fluid embolism, trauma to the uterus must be avoided during maneuvers such as insertion of an intrauterine pressure catheter or amniotomy. Unintentional incision of the placenta during cesarean delivery should be avoided if at all possible.[7] Because one of the most frequent predisposing factors is considered to be tumultuous labor, excessively strong and frequent uterine contractions should be controlled by administration of intravenous β-adrenergic drugs[7] or magnesium sulfate with the patient laboring on her left side. Oxytocics, which might precipitate tetanic uterine contractions, should be used appropriately and judiciously.

In most cases, no therapy has been proven effective. Whenever unexplained cyanosis and shock develops during labor, a diagnosis of amniotic fluid embolism should be considered.[30] Assuming a diagnosis could be made prior to death, supportive measures should be focused at cardiopulmonary resuscitation, blood volume replacement, and treatment of coagulopathy.

Resuscitation should begin with endotracheal intubation and mechanical ventilation using inspired oxygen concentrations of 100 percent delivered by positive pressure and positive end-expiratory pressure (PEEP). With the use of PEEP, functional residual capacity should increase and if oxygenation improves, as evidenced by pulse oximetry or arterial blood gas data, a lower PEEP setting may be tried. Careful observation is essential while the patient is receiving high PEEP, as a decrease in cardiac output due to increased intrathoracic pressure may develop and subsequently decrease tissue perfusion. It is hoped that improved oxygenation will reduce pulmonary capillary fragility and thereby decrease the severity of pulmonary edema. To date, there has been no documentation of the use of hyperbaric oxygen, but some feel it would be worth a try in treating the severe tissue hypoxia provided there was time. Careful hemodynamic monitoring is essential. Placement of two large intravenous lines to deliver large volumes of fluid and an intra-arterial catheter to monitor blood pressure, arterial blood gases, and other pertinent chemistries, as well as a central venous or Swan-Ganz catheter to monitor cardiac status, pulmonary pressures, and state of hydration, are of enormous value.

The causes of pulmonary edema have been variably ascribed to vigorous fluid resuscitation, increased pulmonary capillary permeability, and cardiac decompensation due to hypoxia and tachycardia. The severity of pulmonary edema certainly plays an important role in the initial gas exchange abnormality and duration of the aberration. Hemodynamic monitoring is very helpful in preventing fluid overload and directing fluid therapy.

At present there is no clear regimen of drug therapy to reverse the symptoms and complications of amniotic fluid embolism. Drug therapy and other treatment have been supportive and aimed at improving the ventilation/perfusion ratio, maintenance of adequate blood pressure, and treatment of DIC.

The drug used to treat pulmonary complications such as bronchospasm and vasoconstriction of pulmonary arterioles is terbutaline, especially if the patient is undelivered with a viable fetus. Isoproterenol also relieves pulmonary vasoconstriction and improves cardiac function, although it can cause peripheral vasodilation, which will exacerbate the hypotension. Dopamine may be preferable to isoproterenol because it improves cardiac function and increases peripheral and renal perfusion unless given in too large a dose, which would result in decreased renal perfusion. Administration of aminophylline for its bronchodilation and cardiac stimulation effects is controversial, mainly because of the tachycardia it produces. Hydrocortisone in doses up to 2 g/24 hr reduces pulmonary vasospasm and pulmonary edema and potentiates the cardiac response to catecholamines. In the event of heart failure, treatment with intravenous inotropes such as dobutamine is recommended, or digitalization with intravenous digoxin may be instituted.[31] Diuretics can be used if pulmonary capillary wedge pressure is elevated. Indomethacin has been effective in treating severe pulmonary hypertension in laboratory animals and should be considered for use. In a condition with such a high mortality, there would be nothing to lose.

Hypotension should be treated first by left uterine displacement if the patient is undelivered. This can be accomplished easily by insertion of a wedge under the right hip. The vasopressor of choice is ephedrine because it does not decrease uterine perfusion. However, if the fetus has expired or perhaps is already delivered, isoproterenol or dobutamine can be used. The fluid of choice should be lactated Ringer's solution, because its pH is most near that of blood; the rate of infusion will depend on the hemodynamic monitoring. If acidosis is present, as evidenced by arterial blood gas values, sodium bicarbonate should be administered.

Treatment of the bleeding diathesis requires blood replacement using fresh whole blood (when available), as the clotting factors so badly needed are intact. Otherwise, packed red cells and fresh frozen plasma are usually more available and will retain some clotting factors, but the longer they are stored, the more the clotting factors deteriorate. Cryoprecipitate and platelet infusions are also required to help combat the coagulopathy. Heparin therapy is controversial; some patients have been documented to survive with its use, but there is documentation of survival without using heparin.

Uterine bleeding in a patient already delivered should be controlled by massage and use of intravenous oxytocin. If uterine bleeding is unresponsive to these methods, one should consider exploration for retained placenta or membranes or a search for cervical or uterine lacerations. Methylergonovine is also a strong uterine stimulant and can be given intramuscularly or very slowly via intravenous push if considered to be necessary in this life-threatening circumstance. The use of prostaglandins (Hemabat, Upjohn and Co.) to control hemorrhage is controversial and may cause bronchospasm and/or pulmonary hypertension. The use of E-aminocaproic acid and aprotinin is not well documented in the treatment of amniotic fluid embolus, but these agents might be used when rapid reversal of the lytic state is needed before delivery. Aprotinin (Trasylol) should be the drug of choice if the fetus is still viable because it does not cross the placenta as does E-aminocaproic acid, which is teratogenic as well.

When amniotic fluid embolism occurs, the accompanying respiratory distress, cardiovascular collapse, and hemorrhagic tendency are contraindications to any regional techniques, and if severe shock develops, a general anesthetic must be administered with extreme caution. Because immediate delivery is indicated, emergency cesarean delivery is usually required. The choice of anesthetic agents will depend on the patient's condition, and aggressive cardiopulmonary resuscitation may be all that the anesthesiologist can provide.

REFERENCES

1. Meyer JR: Embolis pulmonar-caseosa. Braz Med 2:301, 1926
2. Warden MR: Amniotic fluid as possible factor in etiology of eclampsia. Am J Obstet Gynecol 14:292, 1927
3. Steiner PE, Lushbaugh CC: Maternal pulmonary embolism by fluid as a cause of obstetric shock and expected deaths in obstetrics. JAMA 117:1245, 1941
4. Schneider CC, Henry MM, Chaplick MJ: Meconium embolism in vivo. Am J Obstet Gynecol 101:909, 1968
5. Liban E, Raz S: A clinicopathologic study of fourteen cases of amniotic fluid embolism. Am J Clin Pathol 51:477, 1969

6. Abouleish E: Amniotic fluid embolism: report of a fatal case. Curr Res Anesth Analg 53:549, 1974
7. Morgan M: Amniotic fluid embolism. Anaesthesia 34:20, 1979
8. Courtney LD: Amniotic fluid embolism. Obstet Gynecol Surv 29:169, 1974
9. Less A, Goldberger SB, Bernheim J, et al: Vaginal prostaglandin E_2 and fatal amniotic fluid embolus. JAMA 263:3259, 1990
10. Anderson DG: Amniotic fluid embolism: a re-evaluation. Am J Obstet Gynecol 98:336, 1967
11. Schenken JR, Slaughter GP, DeMay GH: Maternal pulmonary embolism of amniotic fluid. Am J Clin Pathol 20:147, 1950
12. Landing BJ: The pathogenesis of amniotic fluid embolism. II. Uterine factors. N Engl J Med 243:590, 1950
13. Frost ACG: Death following intrauterine injection of hypertonic saline solution with hydatiform mole. Am J Obstet Gynecol 101:342, 1967
14. Guidotti RJ, Grimes DA, Cates W: Fatal amniotic fluid embolism during legally induced abortion in the United States: 1972–1978. Am J Obstet Gynecol 141:257, 1981
15. Russell W, Nicholson J: Amniotic fluid embolism. A review of the syndrome with a report of 4 cases. Obstet Gynecol 26:476, 1965
16. Kitzmiller JL, Lucas WE: Studies on a model of amniotic fluid embolism. Obstet Gynecol 39:626, 1972
17. Azegami M, Mori N: Amniotic fluid embolism and leukotrienes. Am J Obstet Gynecol 115:1119, 1986
18. Karim SN, Devlin J: Prostaglandin content of amniotic fluid during pregnancy and labor. J Obstet Gynaecol Br Commonw 74:230, 1979
19. Holland AJC: Amniotic fluid embolism. Anaesthesia 23:273, 1968
20. Dutta D, Bhargava KC, Chakravarti RN, et al: Therapeutic studies in experimental amniotic fluid embolism in rabbits. Am J Obstet Gynecol 106:1201, 1974
21. Stefanini M, Turpini RA: Fibrinogenopenic accident of pregnancy and delivery: Syndrome with multiple etiological mechanism. Ann NY Acad Sci 75:601, 1959
22. Clark SL: New concepts of amniotic fluid embolism: a review. Obstet Gynecol Surv 45:360, 1990
23. Peterson EP, Taylor HB: Amniotic fluid embolism: An analysis of 40 cases. Obstet Gynecol 35:787, 1970
24. Josey WE: Hypofibrinogenemia complicating uterine rupture: relationship to amniotic fluid embolism. Am J Obstet Gynecol 94:29, 1966
25. Lumley J, Owen R, Morgan M: Amniotic fluid embolism. A report of 3 cases. Anaesthesia 34:33, 1979
26. Schaerf RHM, DeCampo T, Avetta J: Hemodynamic alterations and rapid diagnosis in a case of amniotic fluid embolus. Anesthesiology 46:155, 1977
27. Ziadlourad F, Conklin KA: Amniotic fluid embolism. Semin Anesth 6:171, 1987
28. Abouleish E: Amniotic fluid embolism and disseminated intravascular coagulopathy. p. 160. Abouleish E (ed): Pain Control in Obstetrics. JB Lippincott, Philadelphia, 1977
29. Shnider SM, Moya F: Amniotic fluid embolism. Anesthesiology 22:108, 1961
30. Phillips OC, Weigel JE, McCarthy JJ: Amniotic fluid embolus. Fundamental considerations and a report of cases. Obstet Gynecol 24:431, 1964
31. Mulder JI: Amniotic fluid embolism. An overview and case report. Am J Obstet Gynecol 152:430, 1985

THROMBOEMBOLIC DISEASE

Thromboembolism during pregnancy continues to be a major cause of maternal morbidity.[1,2] The disease has been documented since the early 19th century when dark red patches in the lung or clots in branches of the pulmonary artery were described in Virchow's classic studies.[3] Thromboembolic phenomena usually occur during late pregnancy or during the immediate postpartum period. Both the disease and its treatment produce important physiologic changes that affect anesthetic management.

INCIDENCE

Within the last decade, many epidemiological studies indicate that the disease is 5.5 times more common in women during pregnancy or in the postpartum period than in nonpregnant women, with thrombosis occurring 3 to 6 times more frequently postpartum than antepartum. Interestingly, in women taking oral contraceptives, the occurrence of thromboembolism is increased by a factor of 3.[4] During pregnancy, thromboembolism has been reported to occur in as many as 0.05 to 1.8 percent of deliveries.[5,6] Other recent reports indicate an incidence of deep venous thrombosis of 0.7 per 1,000 pregnancies.[7,8] When a thromboembolic event occurs, it is estimated that there is a 12 percent risk of repeated thrombosis during the same pregnancy and a 5 to 10 percent risk of thromboembolism with subsequent pregnancies. It occurs three times more frequently with cesarean delivery compared to vaginal delivery.

Since the lung is the primary target organ for thromboembolism, it is not surprising that life-threatening conditions frequently result. In the report on Confidential Enquiries into Maternal Deaths in England and Wales, pulmonary embolism was responsible for the deaths of 12 women per year before or immediately after delivery, or 9.4 deaths per million pregnancies; it was second only to abortion as the leading cause of maternal death.[2]

ETIOLOGY

Three major etiologic factors have been described: vessel wall trauma, venous stasis, and alterations of the coagulation mechanism.[3] During pregnancy, all these factors exist. Vessel wall injury does not seem to be necessary to initiate thrombosis because it can occur without a clear history of vessel trauma. However, vessel trauma is frequently sustained by the parturient in the veins of her lower extremities. Thrombophlebitis has been described in each trimester, but is more common in patients who are confined to bed for complications of pregnancy, such as threatened abortion, premature rupture of the membranes, and pregnancy-induced hypertension.

Venous stasis is certainly a risk factor during pregnancy. Venous distensibility increases during the first trimester of pregnancy and, as pregnancy progresses, aortocaval compression by the gravid uterus results in increased venous stasis, which is a major factor predisposing to deep venous thrombosis. This mechanical obstruction is known to result in increased femoral venous pressures beginning in the early part of the second trimester and continuing until term and has been diagnosed by Doppler ultrasound.[9] It is present in the supine and standing positions in the third trimester and partly present in the lateral position as well. The greatest stasis is within the soleus muscles and the valve sinuses in the left iliofemoral segment, with the left lower extremity being involved more frequently than the right; this is probably secondary to compression of the left common iliac vein where it is crossed by the common iliac artery.[8] Other physiologic changes associated with pregnancy that have been implicated in venous stasis include hormonal changes, anemia, pregnancy-induced hypertension, and the hypercoagulable state of pregnancy.

Other risk factors include increased maternal age and parity, obesity, cesarean delivery, prolonged bed rest during pregnancy, estrogen therapy for lactation suppression, blood type other than O, and antithrombin III (AT III) deficiency. Pregnancy causes a number of significant alterations in the coagulation mechanism. All trace protein coagulation factors except XI and XIII are increased during pregnancy. Fibrinolytic activity is decreased in pregnancy and the concentration of soluble fibrin–fibrinogen complexes is increased; increased factor VIII activity contributes to the stabilization of these complexes. The function of platelets in the formation of the thrombus is undetermined because neither the platelet count nor platelet adhesiveness is increased during pregnancy. Venous thrombi contain relatively few platelets so platelets are not believed to be the instigators of the thrombotic process. The decreased number of circulating platelets after delivery is probably related to normal thrombus formation at the placental site.

In patients with hereditary AT III deficiency, AT III activity falls during pregnancy. AT III is the major inhibitor of thrombin, Factor Xa, and other proteases, and inhibits coagulation in vivo.[10,11] AT III deficiency occurs in two forms depending on the level of AT III antigen. The incidence of an autosomal dominant AT III deficiency is between 1 in 2,000 and 1 in 5,000.[12,13] Thromboembolism in AT III deficiency tends to occur during the antepartum period.[14] In classic AT III deficiency, the level of AT III antigen is below 50 percent; whereas in variant AT III deficiency, there is a normal AT III antigen level with abnormalities in the molecule that interfere with function. Women with hereditary AT III deficiency are at risk of developing thromboembolism during pregnancy or when taking oral contraceptives.

PATHOPHYSIOLOGY

Pulmonary thromboembolism produces complex alterations in both pulmonary mechanics and circulatory function. The resulting pathology depends on the quantity and size of the embolus, the site of obstruction, and the presence of any pre-existing cardiopulmonary disease. A single small embolus may have no effect, whereas a large thrombus may break and shower the lungs with multiple emboli producing life-threatening bilateral pulmonary dysfunction. Very small emboli may pass through to the periphery of the lung; if they do not obstruct a branch of the pulmonary artery, rapid lysis occurs, and there are no hemodynamic disturbances nor clinical symptoms. Larger or multiple emboli will occlude the pulmonary artery, resulting in obstruction of the pulmonary circulation (from a large embolus) usually progressing to rapid deterioration and death. With a unilateral pulmonary thromboembolus, the right lower lobe is most frequently the area affected. Recurrent pulmonary emboli often result in pulmonary hypertension.

Pulmonary embolism affects the functioning of both the cardiac and respiratory systems. In the cardiac system, the main abnormalities are a loss of left ventricle preload and an increase in right ventricle afterload, producing an elevation of the right atrial pressure and lowered cardiac output.[15] When left ventricular output is significantly reduced, coronary artery blood flow is decreased. This reduction in coronary artery blood flow is poorly tolerated in patients with limited cardiac reserve. Increased right ventricular pressures can eventually produce right ventricular failure, depending on the pre-existing cardiovascular status. Right coronary blood flow does not seem to decrease during embolization; rather, it seems to increase secondary to local autoregulation. With massive pulmonary embolism or any type of cardiovascular collapse, hypotension and refractory shock may occur. Pulmonary embolism in patients with cardiac disease is often regarded as synonymous with pulmonary infarction; however, this is not always the case, as the ratio of infarct to emboli is about 1:10.

Emboli within the respiratory system produce an increase in dead space ventilation, mismatched ventilation/perfusion, bronchioalveolar constriction of terminal airways, and loss of surfactant, which results in hypoxemia and alveolar atelectasis. The development of regional pulmonary edema further contributes to the hypoxemia. Bronchioalveolar constriction occurs and has been attributed to released humoral factors, including serotonin and/or histamine, and decreased $PaCO_2$. The hypoxemia is not fully corrected by oxygen administration, indicating an intrapulmonary shunt. The resulting hypoxemia and reduction in uterine perfusion will cause fetal distress and emergency cesarean delivery may be required to save the fetus.

CLINICAL AND LABORATORY DIAGNOSIS OF VENOUS THROMBOSIS

Many symptoms mimicking those of deep venous thrombosis, particularly peripheral edema and evidence of stasis, can occur in normal pregnancy. When thrombosis is clinically suspected, a definitive diagnosis is needed. This need often outweighs the side effects and possible complications of venography because it ensures affected patients will receive appropriate therapy, whereas patients with negative studies can avoid the significant hazards of anticoagulation as well as the long-term stigma related to a diagnosis of deep venous thrombosis.

Ascending venography is the most accurate test for deep venous thrombosis. Radiographic contrast dye is injected into a distal dorsal vein of the foot. The leg must be relaxed and non-weight bearing with the patient on approximately a 40 degree incline. This produces a gradual filling of the leg veins and prevents layering of the dye. Visualization of a well-defined filling defect is more than one radiographic view is required for a diagnosis of a venous thrombus. False-positive studies can occur as a result of poor technique, poor choice of injection site, or leg muscle contraction. False-positive results can also occur as the result of pathology such as external compression by a popliteal cyst, hematoma, local cellulitis and edema, or muscle rupture. Ascending venography is suboptimal for examining the deep femoral and pelvic veins because large nonobstructive thrombi may be undetected.

Venography is not without risk, as there are some well-known systemic side effects of radiologic contrast dye. Patients may experience muscle pain, leg swelling, tenderness, and erythema.[16] These side effects can be reduced by lowering the concentration of the contrast medium[17] and using a heparinized saline flush after injection will help prevent the uncommon occurrence of clot formation following venography.

Noninvasive tests without risks or complications include Doppler ultrasound, impedance plethysmography, and thermography. They are, however, much less sensitive for thrombi below the knee. Changes in Doppler tone ("shifts") occur when normal venous blood flow varies with respiration and maneuvers such as the Valsalva maneuver, release of pressure over a distal vein, or squeezing of the muscles. A decrease in amplitude of these shifts can indicate partial venous obstruction, whereas complete occlusion gives no Doppler shift. Doppler ultrasound has a sensitivity of 90 percent and is most useful in the detection of popliteal, femoral, or iliac thromboses.[17] Thrombi that completely occlude proximal veins and those not large enough to obstruct blood flow can escape detection. Because of collateral venous channels, at least 50 percent of small calf thrombi are missed with Doppler ultrasound.[17] Also, results can vary with technique, experience, and patient positioning.

Impedance plethysmography uses changes in electrical resistance to measure changes in blood volume within the limb being tested. With inflation of a thigh cuff, blood is retained in the leg. In the absence of venous obstruction, sudden deflation results in immediate outflow of blood and a concomitant sudden increase in electrical resistance. A much slower change is associated with impaired outflow, which indirectly implies venous thrombosis. A sensitivity of 95 percent and specificity of 98 percent can be achieved with proximal vein thrombi.[17] As in Doppler ultrasound, detection of calf vein thrombi with impedance plethysmography is unreliable. In pregnancy, compression of the inferior vena cava by the gravid uterus can yield false-positive results,[18] and confirmation by venography may be necessary.

Thermography detects deep venous thrombosis by an increase in skin temperature. When blood flow is diverted to superficial collateral vessels or inflammation is present, infrared radiation emission is increased. Other invasive techniques include fibrinogen scanning with Iodine-125 (^{125}I) and radionuclide venography using technetium-99m (^{99m}Tc) particles. Fibrinogen scanning is contraindicated during pregnancy because unbound ^{125}I crosses the placental barrier and enters the fetal circulation. Once in the fetus, it can collect in the fetal thyroid and produce thyroid damage. It is also contraindicated in lactating women because radioactivity has been detected in breast milk and, with a half-life of 60.2 days,[19] temporary interruption of lactation is impractical. In nonlactating postpartum patients, ^{125}I-labeled fibrinogen can be used to identify deep venous thrombosis. It has a longer half-life and gives a smaller radiation dose than did the previously used ^{131}I. Sequential scintillation scanning is performed from 4 hours to 7 days later but usually at 24, 48, and 72 hours. With each scan, radioactivity is compared to background precordial values in search of "a hot spot."

Radionuclide venography using ^{99m}Tc particles is of low risk to the fetus but requires a rapid-sequence gamma camera, which may not be available in many institutions. This technique is more than 90 percent accurate for deep venous thrombosis above the knee.[19]

CLINICAL SYMPTOMS

Frequently the first indication of deep venous thrombosis is embolization to the lung. Clinical manifestations of pulmonary embolism are nonspecific and the diagnosis is frequently missed, even in patients with segmental or larger vessel occlusion. The presenting signs and symptoms include shortness of breath, chest pain (dull substernal tightness), apprehension, altered sensorium, cough, hemoptysis, sweating, syncope, and tachycardia.

A sudden gasping attempt of the patient to breathe during ventilation may be the first indication of an intraoperative pulmonary embolus. If patients are grouped by severity, small emboli are associated with a higher incidence of syncope, whereas sudden massive emboli are associated with a higher incidence of pleural pain. The most common physical findings include tachypnea (at a rate of 30 to 40 shallow breaths per minute), decreased breath sounds, rales, tachycardia, and pyrexia. Other findings that are highly significant include pain, tenderness, swelling and warmth of the affected limb, and Homan's sign (pain in the calf or popliteal region when the knee is flexed and the ankle is dorsiflexed). A chest x-ray may reveal diminished vascular markings, diaphragmatic elevation, and pleural effusion. Electrocardiographic changes consistent with right ventricular failure as well as tachycardia or arrhythmias are also common. However, both chest x-ray and electrocardiogram are frequently normal even in the presence of a pulmonary embolus[20] and their chief value is to rule out other causes of chest pain, such as pneumothorax, rib fracture, tumor, infection, or primary cardiac disease.

DIAGNOSIS OF PULMONARY EMBOLISM

More accurate for the diagnosis of pulmonary embolus is a combined ventilation/perfusion lung scan. The ventilation/perfusion scan can be performed safely during pregnancy, although technetium should be used rather than iodine and uterine shielding is necessary. A mismatch between ventilation and perfusion defects is sufficiently diagnostic of pulmonary vascular occlusion to begin therapy. If the ventilation defects match those seen on the perfusion scan, pulmonary angiography may not be necessary for an absolute diagnosis. Pulmonary angiography is usually avoided because the danger of radiation exposure to the fetus.[20] Serious morbidity can occur in 2 to 4 percent of patients undergoing arteriography.

OBSTETRIC AND MEDICAL MANAGEMENT

Treatment of pulmonary embolism is designed to support cardiopulmonary function and to prevent extension or recurrence of the pulmonary embolism by institution of systemic anticoagulant therapy.[21] Surgical intervention may be indicated in a very few selected cases. Oxygen therapy is essential; intubation may be necessary. The PaO_2 should be maintained at 70 mmHg or above to prevent fetal hypoxia. Morphine may be necessary to relieve pain and anxiety. Fluid status must be monitored closely and pulmonary edema, cardiac failure, or shock must be treated with the necessary drugs as indicated.

Anticoagulation

The cornerstone of therapy is anticoagulation.[22] After one thromboembolic event there is a 12 percent risk of repeat thrombosis during the same pregnancy and a 5 to 10 percent risk of recurrent thromboembolism with subsequent pregnancies.[4,23] The initial anticoagulation should always be induced with intravenous heparin because its effect is immediate. Heparin is a large (20,000-dalton) mucopolysaccharide molecule that acts by combining with AT III (heparin cofactor) to inhibit the formation of thrombin. The lack of thrombin prevents the conversion of fibrinogen to fibrin. Heparin increases the level of activated factor X inhibitor, which again interferes with the production of thrombin from prothrombin and inhibits the activation of factor IX (Christmas factor). Although heparin prevents the formation of further thrombi, it does not act to lyse clots already present. Heparin has a relatively short half-life of 1.5 hours, and, for this reason, continuous intravenous administration is the preferred method for heparin therapy.

A suggested protocol by Bolan[4] is as follows:

1. Draw a baseline complete blood count (CBC), prothrombin time (PT), partial thromboplastin time (PTT), and platelet count.
2. Give a loading dose of 5,000 U of heparin by intravenous bolus.
3. (a) Prepare heparin solution with a concentration of 100 U/ml by adding 50,000 U of heparin to 500 ml of normal saline.
   (b) Start therapy at a rate of approximately 1,000 U/h. Alternatively, the formula of 5 to 20 U/kg/h can be used to calculate the initial dose.
   (c) Adjust infusion rate to achieve a PTT two to three times the control. Check the PTT after any change in infusion rate and once or twice daily after the dosage is stabilized.
   (d) Control the flow of heparin solution with the use of an electronic infusion pump.
4. Check the CBC and urinalysis every other day to monitor for occult hemorrhage.

Heparin is not absorbed from the gastrointestinal tract and intramuscular injection is not advisable because of the risk of hematoma formation at the injection site. In fact, intramuscular injection of any drug should be avoided in a patient undergoing heparin therapy.

The greatest risk with heparin therapy is hemorrhage, which has been noted to occur in between 4 and 33 percent of patients. In addition, heparin can result in allergic reactions, alopecia, osteoporosis, and thrombocytopenia. The etiology of the thrombocytopenia is unknown, but may be related to platelet consumption, as reported by Eldeman et al.[25] Opinions differ regarding the duration of anticoagulant therapy advisable following an acute episode of thromboembolic disease. De Swiet[23] advocates continuing full anticoagulation until 6 weeks after delivery for all patients who had either deep venous thrombosis or pulmonary embolus during pregnancy. Laros and Alger[26] would also continue anticoagulation for the patient with pulmonary embolus into the postpartum period.

Considerable controversy also exists as to which therapeutic agent or regimen is preferable for long-term therapy. The standard method in a nonpregnant patient is to initiate anticoagulation with heparin and then convert gradually to oral anticoagulants. The oral agent most commonly used is sodium warfarin, which acts as a competitive inhibitor of vitamin K in the liver. Warfarin is a small (1,000-dalton) molecule that crosses the placenta readily. In fact, the oral anticoagulants appear to affect the fetus more profoundly than they do the mother because of the fetal immature liver enzyme systems. A number of adverse effects from the use of warfarin agents during the first trimester have significant teratogenic potential. Continued warfarin therapy in the late third trimester can cause fetal bleeding either before or after delivery. Other effects secondary to fetal hemorrhage have reportedly resulted from exposure to warfarin during the second and third trimesters. Bonnar[27] reports an overall fetal mortality between 15 and 30 percent in women taking oral anticoagulants during pregnancy. Because of these adverse effects, most investigators no longer recommend the use of warfarin at any time during pregnancy. Warfarin embryopathy results when the drug is administered during the first trimesters in 15 to 25 percent of cases. The most consistent anomalies are varying degrees of nasal hypoplasia and epiphyseal stapling. Exposure in the second trimester results in a 3 percent or more incidence of severe central nervous system anomalies.[28]

If premature labor develops in a patient taking oral anticoagulants, transfusion of fresh frozen plasma is recommended as the fastest way to replace clotting factors for the mother. Since this therapy will not reverse the fetus's anticoagulated state, cesarean delivery is advised because it is less likely to result in intracranial hemorrhage for the fetus.

If the patient is on heparin therapy at the time of labor and delivery, the situation is much easier to manage. First, the fetus is not affected by the heparin, so fetal hemorrhage is not a risk factor. Second, the half-life of heparin is short; if delivery is anticipated to be more than 4 to 6 hours after the last heparin injection, there is no need to reverse the anticoagulant activity. The usual recommendation is simply to stop the heparin as soon as the patient goes into labor or to omit the heparin dose on the morning of induction or elective cesarean delivery. If an emergency or cesarean delivery is needed while the heparin is still active, protamine, a heparin antagonist, may be given. Protamine forms a stable salt with heparin, with the result that both drugs lose their intrinsic anticoagulant activity. Each milligram of protamine neutralizes 100 U of heparin. The calculated dose of protamine, up to 50 mg, should be slowly administered intravenously over a 3-minute period. Protamine can also be used if the patient develops hemorrhagic complications from heparin therapy, but it must be used with caution as protamine excess may cause anticoagulation. Needless to say, strict attention to circulatory homeostasis during surgery or delivery is essential if anticoagulation is to be resumed in the postpartum period.

Because of its failure to cross the placenta, as well as its easy reversibility, a number of investigators advocate maintaining the patient on heparin therapy throughout the pregnancy. Laros and Alger use 150 to 250 U/kg every 12 hours administered subcutaneously.[26]

Thrombolytic agents recently used for the resolution of a thrombus are currently contraindicated and should be avoided during pregnancy.[28] However, the use of tissue-type plasminogen activator (tPA) may produce thrombolysis with less risk of hemorrhage. tPA is active only when bound to fibrin. Unlike streptokinase and urokinase, which activate plasminogen in the serum and result in the systemic lytic state, tPA is clot specific and activates plasminogen in the thrombus, resulting in thrombolysis without producing a systemic lytic state.[29]

SURGICAL MANAGEMENT

The role of surgery in the treatment of thromboembolic disease during pregnancy is also limited. Procedures that have been used include femoral vein or vena caval interruption and thrombectomy or embolectomy. Femoral vein interruption has been used since 1934 and recently the use of an internal saphenous graft to bypass a thromboembolic region has been reported. Interruption of the vena cava is used to prevent recurrent emboli rising in the lower extremities from reaching the lungs. A number of different procedures have been used for this purpose, including ligation, clipping, plication, and placement of a variety of filters or intraluminal grids,[30] but vena caval–interruption is associated with a postoperative mortality between 1 and 10 percent with a significant risk of long-term morbidity secondary to venous obstruction.

Pulmonary embolectomy is a dangerous procedure but may be life-saving in some patients. The location and extent of the embolus must be confirmed with angiography prior to surgery, and in fact, it has been stated this is the only indication for angiography during pregnancy.[31] Embolectomy should be reserved for the parturient with such massive emboli that she is expected to die before medical therapy would have any effect. Criteria for intervention according to one investigator include a systolic blood pressure of less than 90 mmHg, urine output of less than 20 ml/h and PaO_2 of less than 60 mmHg after 1 hour of nonoperative management. The mortality from embolectomy is high (about 80 percent) and minimal successful use during pregnancy has been described.[31]

ANESTHETIC MANAGEMENT

Anesthetic management depends on when the patient develops her thromboembolism since it may occur any time during the perinatal period: during labor, vaginal or cesarean delivery, or the postpartum period. When thromboembolism has been diagnosed during labor, the primary problem is providing anesthesia for an anticoagulated patient. When it occurs during delivery, the goal is to provide resuscitation, including ventilation and oxygenation (frequently necessitating endotracheal intubation), inotropic support, rapid delivery if indicated, and anticoagulation. The goal of anticoagulation is to prolong the PTT 1.5 to 2.5 times the control. Many fear that this significantly increases the risk of bleeding from regional anesthetic techniques and consider intraspinal anesthetics to be contraindicated in anticoagulated patients. Epidural, subdural, and subarachnoid bleeding resulting in spinal cord compression and neurologic dysfunction has been reported with regional anesthesia in anticoagulated patients.[32] Owens et al.[32] reported 33 cases of spinal hematoma following lumbar puncture or subarachnoid anesthesia. Six of the cases were in association with the administration of a regional anesthetic and 27 of the cases involved lumbar puncture for diagnostic or therapeutic purposes. Forty percent (13 patients) had received anticoagulant therapy (heparin 6, coumadin 1, both 6).

However, regional techniques have been administered to anticoagulated patients without complications. Odoom and Sih[33] reported the results of over 1,000 lumbar epidural blocks in 950 patients undergoing vascular surgery. All patients received oral anticoagulants preoperatively and the majority also received intravenous heparin intraoperatively. Ten percent of patients experienced postoperative backache; however, no side effects were observed that indicated epidural hemorrhage or hematoma and no patient developed neurologic complications. Their conclusion was that epidural anesthesia can be safely used in circumstances similar to their study.

When thromboembolism occurs during labor and delivery in a patient in whom epidural anesthesia has already been initiated, can the epidural be safely continued? Rao and El-Etr[34] reported their results on 3,164 epidural and 847 subarachnoid continuous catheter anesthetics in which all patients received intravenous heparin 1 hour after the institution of the regional anesthetic. The activated coagulation time (ACT) was maintained at twice the baseline. They reported no incidence of peridural hematoma. Matthews and Abrams[35] also reported similar findings on patients receiving subarachnoid morphine prior to heparinization for cardiac surgery.

As with any anesthetic, the risks must be balanced by the benefits to the patient. Although neurologic symptoms associated with regional anesthetics may be rare, the effect of a subarachnoid or epidural hematoma can be catastrophic. There is always the possibility of vascular trauma secondary to needle placement. Phillips and colleagues[36] reported a 3 percent incidence of trauma (bloody tap) with intraspinal procedures, and noted a 6 percent incidence when multiple attempts were required. The incidence of epidural vein cannulation has been noted to be between 1 and 10 percent during epidural procedures.[37] Even in patients receiving low-dose (i.e., "minidose") heparin there are no case reports or prospective studies that provide assurance that intraspinal techniques are safe.[38]

There are some advantages to regional anesthetics in patients at high risk for thromboembolism. The high incidence of thromboembolism following surgery has been related to blood flow stasis during anesthesia and may therefore be modified by anesthetic technique. Several studies have compared the risk of thromboembolism following general anesthesia with that following intraspinal anesthesia in patients undergoing procedures with a high risk of postoperative deep venous thrombosis. In a randomized study by Modig et al.,[39] 67 percent of patients developed proximal deep venous thrombosis and 33 percent of patients developed pulmonary embolism when total hip replacement was performed with general anesthesia. When epidural anesthesia (continued for 24 hours postoperatively) was used, these incidences were reduced to 13 and 10 percent, respectively. Similarly, McKenzie et al.[40] reported a reduction in the incidence of deep venous thrombosis from 76 to 40 percent by the use of subarachnoid anesthesia in patients undergoing repair of femoral neck fractures. A similar effect with epidural anesthesia has been reported in patients undergoing open prostatectomy.[41] The benefit of regional anesthesia for thoracic or general surgical procedures has not been conclusively demonstrated.[42] It is also not known if intraspinal anesthesia has a protective effect that is additive to other methods such as heparin or dextran prophylaxis.

Several mechanisms have been proposed by which intraspinal anesthesia may decrease the incidence of deep venous thrombosis. The major effect is probably reversal of blood flow stasis in the lower limbs due to a reduction in vascular resistance as a result of sympathetic block; there may also be a decrease in blood viscosity due to hemodilution. In contrast to intraspinal anesthesia, general anesthesia definitely reduces lower limb blood flow. The second mechanism for the protective effect of intraspinal anesthesia is prevention of the hypercoagulable state that may follow general anesthesia.

Writer[38] makes the following recommendations for regional techniques in "minidose" anticoagulated parturients:

1. Restrict regional techniques to mothers receiving heparin no more frequently than every 12 hours.
2. Prior to the initiation of the block, the bleeding profile (ACT or PTT) must be normal.
3. Utilize the left lateral position during initiation of anesthetic to reduce aortocaval compression and distention of the epidural veins.
4. Use a midline approach, as lateral techniques will more likely lacerate epidural vessels.
5. Abandon the procedure and proceed to an alternate anesthetic if a traumatic lumbar puncture occurs.

Further recommendations include allowing the epidural block to wear off at intervals to allow for neurologic assessment. Should anticoagulation be instituted following epidural placement, the catheter should be left in place until all systemic anticoagulation is reversed or normalized. After catheter removal, frequent neurologic examinations are necessary to detect early changes indicating hematoma formation. Hematoma diagnosis depends on physical examination, electromyelographic, computed tomographic, and magnetic resonance imaging studies. Should an epidural hematoma occur, recovery is unlikely without surgical intervention.[43]

Considerations for general anesthesia include careful manipulation of the oral mucosa and gentle endotracheal intubation, avoidance of any type of nasal tube placement, avoidance of catheterization of large vessels in the neck unless absolutely necessary, and close observation of intraoperative and postoperative bleeding.

REFERENCES

1. Kaunitz AM, Hughes JM, Grimes DA, et al: Cause of maternal mortality in the United States. Obstet Gynecol 65:605, 1985
2. Turnbull AC: Report on Confidential Enquiries into Maternal Deaths in England and Wales 1979–81. Her Majesty's Statistics Office, p. 30. London, 1986
3. Sabiston DC: Pathophysiology, diagnosis and management of pulmonary embolism. Am J Surg 138:384, 1979
4. Bolan JC: Thromboembolic complications of pregnancy. Clin Obstet Gynecol 26:913, 1983
5. Villasanta U: Thromboembolic disease in pregnancy. Am J Obstet Gynecol 93:142, 1965
6. Aaro LA, Juergens JL: Thrombophlebitis associated with pregnancy. Am J Obstet Gynecol 109:1128, 1971
7. Kierkegaard A: Incidence and diagnosis of deep vein thrombosis associated with pregnancy. Acta Obstet Gynecol Scand 62:239, 1983
8. Bergqvist A, Bergqvist D, Hallbrook T: Deep vein thrombosis during pregnancy: a prospective study. Acta Obstet Gynecol Scand 62:443, 1983
9. Ikard RW, Veland K, Folse R: Lower limb venous dynamics in pregnant women. Surg Gynecol Obstet 132:483, 1979

10. Brandt JT: Current concepts of coagulation. Clin Obstet Gynecol 28:3, 1985
11. Caldwell Dc, Williamson RA, Goldsmith JC: Hereditary coagulopathies in pregnancy. Clin Obstet Gynecol 28:53, 1985
12. Rosenberg RD: Actions and interactions of antithrombin and heparin. N Engl J Med 292:146, 1975
13. Thaler E, Lechner K: Antithrombin III deficiency and thromboembolism. Clin Haematol 10:369, 1981
14. Samson D, Stirling Y, Woolf L, et al: Management of planned pregnancy in a patient with congenital antithrombin III deficiency. Br J Haematol 52:173, 1984
15. Staub MC: Pathophysiology of microembolism lung injury. Anesthesiol Ann Rev Lect p. 302, 1983
16. Bettman MA, Paulin S: Leg phlebography: the incidence, nature and modifications of undesirable side effects. Radiology 122:101, 1977
17. Markisz JA: Radiologic and nuclear medicine diagnosis. p. 41. In Goldhaber SZ (ed): Pulmonary Embolism and Deep Venous Thrombosis. WB Saunders, Philadelphia, 1985
18. Perry PJ, Herron GR, King JC: Heparin half-life in normal and impaired renal function. Clin Pharmacol Res 16:514, 1974
19. Kakkar V: The diagnosis of deep vein thrombosis using the ^{125}I fibrinogen test. Arch Surg 104:152, 1972
20. Moser KM: Diagnosis and management of pulmonary embolism. Hosp Pract 15:57, 1980
21. Morris GK, Mitchell JR: Clinical management of venous thromboembolism. Br Med Bull 34:169, 1978
22. Kalimada P, Rashad MN, Murthy BN, et al: Pulmonary embolism: hemodynamics, diagnosis, prophylaxis and management. Anesthesiol Rev 12:29, 1985
23. de Swiet M: Thromboembolism. Clin Haematol 14:643, 1985
24. Salzman JG, Deykin K, Shapiro RM, et al: Management of heparin therapy—a controlled prospective trial. N Engl J Med 292:1046, 1975
25. Eldeman WL, Barrett RL, Gladney JD, et al: Heparin-induced white clot syndrome. J LA State Med Soc 141:21, 1989
26. Laros RK, Alger LS: Thromboembolism and pregnancy. Clin Obstet Gynecol 22:871, 1979
27. Bonnar J: Venous thromboembolism and pregnancy. Clin Obstet Gynaecol 8:456, 1981
28. LoSasso AM: Pulmonary embolism. p. 165. In Stoelting RK, Dierdorf SF (eds): Anesthesia and Co-existing Disease. Churchill Livingstone, New York, 1983
29. Bounameaux H, Vermylen J, Collen D: Thrombolytic treatment with recombinant tissue-type plasminogen activator in a patient with massive pulmonary embolism. Ann Intern Med 103:64, 1985
30. Barnes AB, Kanarek DJ, Greenfield AJ, et al: Vena cava filter placement during pregnancy. Am J Obstet Gynecol 140:707, 1981
31. Alfrey DD, Benumof JL: Pulmonary diseases. p. 227. In Katz J, Benumof J, Kadis LB (eds): Anesthesia and Uncommon Diseases. WB Saunders, Philadelphia, 1981
32. Owens EL, Kasten GW, Hessel EA: Spinal subarachnoid hematoma after lumbar puncture and heparinization: a case report, review of the literature, and discussion of anesthetic implications. Anesth Analg 65:1201, 1986
33. Odoom JA, Sih IL: Epidural analgesia and anticoagulation therapy: experience with one thousand cases of continuous epidurals. Anaesthesia 38:254, 1983
34. Rao TL, El-Etr AA: Anticoagulation following placement of epidural and subarachnoid catheters: an evaluation of neurologic sequelae. Anesthesiology 55:618, 1981
35. Matthews ET, Abrams LD: Intrathecal morphine in open heart surgery. Lancet 2:543, 1980
36. Phillips OC, Ebner H, Nelson AT, et al: Neurologic complications following spinal anesthesia with lidocaine. Anesthesiology 30:284, 1969
37. Bromage PR: Epidural Anesthesia. WB Saunders, Philadelphia, 1978
38. Writer WDR: Hematologic disease. p. 267. In James FM, Wheeler AS, Dewan DM (eds): Obstetric Anesthesia: The Complicated Patient. FA Davis, Philadelphia, 1988
39. Modig J, Burg T, Karlstrom G, et al: Thromboembolism after total hip replacement: role of epidural and general anesthesia. Anesth Analg 62:174, 1983
40. McKenzie PJ, Wishart HY, Gray I, et al: Effects of anaesthetic technique on deep vein thrombosis: a comparison of subarachnoid and general anaesthesia. Br J Anaesth 57:853, 1985
41. Hendalin H, Mattila MAK, Poikolainen E: The effect of lumbar epidural analgesia on the development of deep vein thrombosis of the legs after open prostatectomy. Acta Chir Scand 147:425, 1981
42. Mellbring G, Dahlgren S, Reiz S, et al: Thromboembolic complications after major abdominal surgery: effect of thoracic epidural analgesia. Acta Chir Scand 149:263, 1983
43. Janis KM: Epidural hematoma following postoperative epidural analgesia: a case report. Anesth Analg 51:689, 1972

VENOUS AIR EMBOLISM

Venous air embolism (VAE) is a recognized complication in many surgical procedures. Classically, VAE has been associated with neurosurgical procedures performed with the patient in the sitting position.[1] However, VAE has also been reported as a complication of abdominal, orthopaedic, plastic, urologic, thoracic, and head and neck surgery. Many of these procedures were performed with the patient in the prone, supine, or lateral position.[1,2]

Numerous case reports of VAE during cesarean delivery have appeared in the medical literature as early as the 19th century. Deaths from VAE during cesarean delivery have been reported as recently as the 1980s.[2] Nonetheless, it was not until 1987 that the occurrence of VAE during cesarean delivery was systematically studied.[3] Subsequently, several studies have documented the occurrence of VAE during cesarean delivery[4–6] as well as during the placement of epidural catheters.[7] VAE may account for signs (e.g., arterial oxygen desaturation, arrhythmias, and hypotension) and symptoms (e.g., dyspnea and chest pain) commonly found in patients during cesarean delivery.[3–6] VAE may even be as common during cesarean delivery as it is during neurosurgical procedures in the sitting position.[1,3,4,6]

INCIDENCE

Precordial Doppler monitoring can detect as little as 0.1 ml of intracardiac air.[1] There is 100 percent correlation between echocardiographic and Doppler evidence of VAE during cesarean delivery, thus demonstrating the specificity of precordial Doppler monitoring.[4] The incidence of Doppler evident VAE during cesarean delivery is 11 to 66 percent.[3–6] The majority of these patients received continuous lumbar epidural anesthesia. In patients receiving general anesthesia for cesarean delivery, the incidence of VAE is 28 to 71 percent.[4,6] VAE may occur throughout the procedure but seems to occur most commonly during hysterotomy or repair of hysterotomy.[3,4,6]

PATHOPHYSIOLOGY

Open venous sinuses and a negative pressure gradient between the surgical wound and heart facilitates entrainment of air into the central venous circulation.[1,2] Gradients as small as -5 cmH_2O have been shown to allow significant amounts of air to enter the venous circulation.[1,8] Routine positioning of patients for cesarean delivery with 10 to 15 degrees of left lateral tilt creates a -10- to -15-cm H_2O pressure gradient between the uterus and the heart.[5] Hysterotomy exposes the uterine sinuses, which may be particularly susceptible to the entrainment of air.[6] Exteriorization of the uterus and traction applied during repair of hysterotomy may distend collapsed veins and exaggerate the pressure gradient with the right heart.[3,6] Although use of a 5- to 10-degree reverse Trendelenberg position does not affect the incidence of VAE during cesarean delivery,[4] use of the Trendelenburg position may further exaggerate the negative pressure gradient.[5,6,9] A decreased central venous pressure increases the risk of venous air entrainment.[2] Factors that decrease central venous pressure include absolute hypovolemia from hemorrhage (placenta previa or placental abruption) and a contracted intravascular volume (prolonged labor with NPO status or pregnancy-induced hypertension) and relative hypovolemia from inadequate acute hydration before the initiation of regional anesthesia with resultant sympathetic block and vasodilation.[2,5–7,9]

Morbidity and mortality resulting from VAE depends on the amount of air entrained, the rate of entrainment, and the site to which the air embolism travels. Small volumes of air entrained slowly are tolerated well without clinical signs or symptoms.[1] However, as little as 0.5 ml/kg/min has been shown to cause symptoms.[7] Large volumes of air (3 to 8 ml/kg) injected rapidly are quickly fatal.[1,6] The most likely cause of death with large VAE is an air lock causing obstruction of the pulmonary outflow tract.[1,2] Smaller amounts of air can result in ventilation/perfusion mismatching with hypoxemia, hypercapnia, right heart failure, arrhythmias, and hypotension.[1,2]

Paradoxical air embolism (i.e., air entering the systemic circulation) can cause coronary or cerebral ischemia, infarction, and death, or permanent neurological deficit.[1] Air may enter the systemic circulation via a patent foramen ovale (10 to 25 percent of the population) or other intracardiac shunts.[1]

CLINICAL PRESENTATION

Massive VAE can present as a devastatingly dramatic event heralded by hypotension, arterial hypoxemia, and electromechanical dissociation leading to cardiac arrest.[9] The clinical picture is routinely much less profound, presumably because of the small volume of VAE.

The etiology of chest pain during cesarean delivery is unclear and is, almost certainly, multifactorial. Complaints of chest pain during cesarean delivery are often dismissed by anesthesiologists and obstetricians as being secondary to surgical traction on the peritoneum. However, it has been demonstrated that there is an association of VAE with subsequent complaints of chest pain by otherwise healthy parturients at routine, elective cesarean delivery.[3,6] Twenty to 50 percent of women with Doppler evident VAE during cesarean delivery will complain of chest pain.[3,6] Less than 2 percent of women will complain of chest pain during cesarean delivery without previous Doppler-evident VAE.[3,6] Patient complaints of chest pain during cesarean delivery should not be ignored. The association of chest pain with VAE should alert the clinician to look for other diagnostic signs.[3,10] The attention of the anesthesiologist should be directed toward making the diagnosis of VAE, a potentially treatable entity.

Arterial oxygen desaturation and dyspnea are associated with VAE.[1,3,4,6,9] Arterial oxygen saturations less than 92 percent are reported in up to 25 percent of parturients during cesarean delivery with Doppler evident VAE.[6] Dyspnea is present in 20 to 40 percent of parturients during cesarean delivery with Doppler-evident VAE.[3,6] Dyspnea associated with arterial oxygen desaturation is unusual in parturients during cesarean delivery without evidence of VAE.[4,6] Other, less frequent clinical presentations associated with VAE during cesarean delivery include cardiac arrhythmias (most often ventricular arrhythmias),[4,9] gasping respirations,[2,9] and hypotension.[2,4,9]

RECOMMENDATIONS

It is evident that VAE is relatively common during cesarean delivery. Although significant mortality and morbidity is rare, about 1 percent of maternal deaths are attributed to VAE.[10]

Given the remote possibility of significant morbidity and mortality, it would seem overly cautious to *mandate* precordial Doppler monitoring in all patients undergoing cesarean delivery. Perhaps, thought, certain groups of patients warrant special attention. Those patients especially prone to develop VAE or in whom otherwise insignificant volumes of VAE would likely cause significant mortality or morbidity might benefit from special preoperative preparation and intraoperative monitoring.

Hypovolemic patients are especially at risk for developing VAE.[2,5,9] A contracted blood volume and low central venous pressure, which enhance entrainment of venous air, could potentially be corrected before delivery.[2] Precordial Doppler monitoring should strongly be considered, if time allows for proper placement before delivery. Patients with a preexisting intracardiac shunt (e.g., patent foramen ovale, atrial septal defect, or ventricular septal defect) require special consideration because of their risk for developing paradoxical air embolism possibly resulting in coronary or cerebral ischemia.[1,2] In these patients, routine precordial Doppler monitoring as well as placement of a multiorificed central venous pressure (CVP) catheter in the upper right atrium to facilitate aspiration of air should be strongly considered.[2]

It is wise to avoid the Trendelenburg position during cesarean delivery because of the increased negative pressure gradient that occurs as well as the associated adverse cardiac and respiratory consequences.[2,6] Flexing the operating room table (dropping the level of the wound toward the level of the heart) before surgery begins might decrease the pressure gradient that would favor venous air entrainment.[2]

Treatment of VAE, either Doppler evident or clinically suspected, should include the following:

1. Further entrainment of air should be prevented by having the obstetricians flood the operative field. Placing the patient in the reverse Trendelenburg position will eliminate the gradient between the heart and the surgical wound. Positioning the patient with the chest tilted to the left will decrease the chance of air lock in the right ventricular outflow tract.[2]
2. Administered 100 percent oxygen to the patient.[2] Discontinue nitrous oxide (if it is being administered).
3. If the patient continues with symptoms of VAE or signs of clinical instability appear, a multiorificed CVP catheter should be inserted and aspiration of intracardiac air attempted. This may be life-saving whenever serious cardiovascular compromise is observed.[2,5]
4. If cardiovascular collapse occurs, immediate delivery of the baby should be accomplished as cardiopulmonary resuscitation according to advanced cardiac life support guidelines is being performed[2] (see Chapter 7).
5. Any patient who becomes comatose or fails to awaken from general anesthesia should be evaluated for intracerebral air with a computed tomographic scan. Hyperbaric pressure oxygen therapy is the only definitive means of treating intracerebral air.[2]

REFERENCES

1. Michenfelder JD: Air embolism. p. 268. In FK Orkin, LH Cooperman (eds): Complications in Anesthesiology. JB Lippincott, Philadelphia, 1983
2. Robinson DA, Albin AS: Parturition and venous air embolism. Obstet Anesth Dig 7:38, 1987
3. Malinow AM, Naulty JS, Hunt CO, et al: Precordial ultrasonic monitoring during cesarean delivery. Anesthesiology 66:816, 1987
4. Fong J, Gadalla F, Pierri MK, et al: Incidence of venous air embolism during cesarean section (Abstract). Anesthesiology 69:A655, 1988
5. Karuparthy VK, Downing JW, Husain FJ, et al: Incidence of venous air embolism during cesarean section is unchanged by the use of a 5 to 10 degree head-up tilt. Anesth Analg 69:620, 1989
6. Vartikar JV, Johnson MD, Datta S: Precordial Doppler monitoring and pulse oximetry during cesarean delivery: detection of venous air embolism. Reg Anesth 14:145, 1989
7. Naulty JS, Ostheimer GW, Datta S, et al: Incidence of venous air embolism during epidural catheter insertion. Anesthesiology 57:410, 1982
8. Babinski MF, Gilbert J, Smith SL: Venous air embolism is not restricted to neurosurgery! (Correspondence). Anesthesiology 59:151, 1983
9. Younker D, Rodriguez V, Kavanaugh J: Massive air embolism during cesarean section. Anesthesiology 65:77, 1986
10. Kaunitz AM, Hughes JM, Grimes DA, et al: Causes of

maternal mortality in the United States. Obstet Gynecol 65:605, 1985

CARDIAC DISEASE

VALVULAR DISEASE

Maternal mortality due to cardiac disease in parturients continues to decline with earlier diagnosis, improved monitoring, and better interventional modalities. There are an increasing number of women of childbearing age with cardiac disorders. The prevalence of heart disease during pregnancy ranges from 0.4 to 4.1 percent. Patients with severe valvular disease[1,2] require a team approach involving anesthesiology, obstetrics, nursing, and cardiology personnel. If possible patients with surgically correctable lesions should undergo repair prior to pregnancy, thereby improving maternal and fetal prognosis. It is absolutely essential for the anesthesiologist to have a thorough understanding of the altered cardiovascular dynamics as well as the disease process prior to the institution of any anesthetic technique.

PREANESTHETIC ASSESSMENT AND PREPARATION

A thorough review of old records, a detailed history, and a thorough physical examination should be performed by the anesthesiologist if time permits. This may elucidate evidence of early cardiac decompensation. Pain and anxiety increase serum catecholamine levels, leading to tachycardia and a reduction in uteroplacental blood flow. A quaternary anticholinergic, glycopyrrolate, which does not cross the placenta to any great extent, should be considered if an antisialogogue is necessary.

Elective surgical procedures should be delayed until after delivery. This annuls possible (and still unknown) dangers of teratogenesis and premature labor. If surgery is necessary but not urgent it is wise to wait until the second or third trimester, thus avoiding the critical period of organogenesis. Finally, delivery of the parturient should be planned at a time of day when the maximal number of consultants are available if at all possible.

MATERNAL MONITORING

All parturients with heart disease(s) warrant continuous monitoring[3] during labor and delivery, and in the postpartum period. If patients are New York Heart Association Class I or II they may not require invasive monitoring. Class III and IV patients will benefit by management at a high-risk obstetric center, where invasive monitoring is employed. An arterial catheter not only provides for continuous monitoring of blood pressure but facilitates the taking of serial arterial blood gas samples if necessary during labor and delivery. Central venous pressure (CVP) monitoring may help guide fluid management. One must remember that CVP measurements reflect right-sided pressures (of the heart) and may not accurately reveal left-sided pressures. Flow-directed pulmonary artery catheters may permit better assessment of left-ventricular (LV) filling pressure by monitoring pulmonary capillary wedge pressure and allow estimates of cardiac output to be made by thermodilution techniques. These invasive modalities may guide the clinician's interventions specifically directed at preload, afterload, and/or myocardial contractility. A review of the cardiovascular changes that accompany pregnancy can be found in Chapter 1.

The risk of thromboembolism is increased in cardiac patients and one should consider the use of elastic stockings or a mechanical compression device.

ANESTHETIC MANAGEMENT

Because of the significant risk of aspiration we choose to employ a regional technique with minimal sedation if not contraindicated for labor and vaginal or cesarean delivery. All parturients in our institution receive a nonparticulate antacid (some variant of 0.3 mol/L sodium citrate) 30 ml by mouth within 30 minutes prior to induction regardless of the technique, be it regional or general anesthesia. If a general anesthetic is planned we recommend an adequate period of denitrogenation with 100 percent oxygen for a minimum of 3 minutes. A rapid-sequence technique for induction is used. Intubation is accomplished with a cuffed endotracheal tube while cricoid pressure is applied and *not* released until confirmation of the correct placement of the endotracheal tube is established. Then, and only then, do we give permission for the surgeon to begin the procedure. Pulse oximetry and capnography are essential in addition to the routine monitoring devices commonly used.

All patients are positioned with left uterine displacement to optimize uterine blood flow and increase venous return. The fetal heart rate is monitored pre- and intraoperatively. This allows for the evaluation of the drugs or events that may interfere with uterine blood flow. Tocodynamometry should be used to monitor uterine contractions.

If a regional technique is employed, adequate preanesthetic intravascular volume expansion should be accomplished with 1 to 2 L of a physiologic solution (e.g., lactated Ringer's solution not D5W). Uterine blood flow is directly proportional to the maternal systemic pressure. Hypotension is treated aggressively with fluids and intravenous ephedrine or, in some instances, phenylephrine if not contraindicated.

MITRAL VALVE PROLAPSE

Pathophysiology

Mitral valve prolapse[4,5] (MVP), also known as myxomatous degeneration, ballooning mitral valve, Barlow's syndrome, precordial honk, or whoop, among others, is characterized by prolapse of the mitral valve leaflet(s), usually the posterior leaflet into the left atrium during ventricular systole. MVP is a very common finding, estimated to have a prevalence of 5 percent among the general population and up to 20 percent in women. The diagnosis is suggested upon auscultation, which reveals a loud midsystolic snap and possible late systolic murmur heard best at the cardiac apex and confirmed by angiography or echocardiography. The etiology is unknown but it is thought to be autosomal dominant with reduced male expressivity. The classic patient with MVP is thin and tall and may possess other marfanoid features. Although the prevalence is high, few patients are symptomatic and fewer are on chronic medical management unless transient ischemic episodes or premature ventricular contractions prevail. If the MVP is severe, they are treated similarly to patients with mitral regurgitation (see the following section). Sudden death is commonly discussed but is quite rare and probably results from an arrhythmia. Prophylactic antibiotics should be administered for protection from subacute bacterial endocarditis when cesarean delivery is anticipated. For uncomplicated vaginal delivery in an asymptomatic patient, we follow the cardiologist's[6] suggestions.

Anesthetic Management

The anesthetic goals in these patients are to minimize sympathetic stimulation. We will use a regional technique if not contraindicated. If a general anesthetic is necessary, we would choose to avoid the use of ketamine and/or pancuronium so as to minimize sympathetic stimulation. The cardiovascular response to laryngoscopy and intubation can be blunted with the administration of labetalol or esmolol, however, patients with coexistent LV dysfunction may not tolerate these medications. Prompt correction and optimization of intravascular volume is instituted to minimize the occasional cardiac arrhythmia and, if necessary, these patients are treated with intravenous lidocaine or esmolol. If vasopressors are needed and the MVP is severe, one should consider using phenylephrine rather than ephedrine.

RHEUMATIC HEART DISEASE

Despite the discovery and widespread use of penicillin, rheumatic heart[7,8] disease still comprises the bulk of cardiac abnormalities in the childbearing population. The mortality in this group of patients is primarily secondary to heart failure with resultant respiratory failure. Valvular lesions are 75 to 90 percent mitral stenosis, 6 to 12 percent mitral regurgitation, 2 to 5 percent aortic regurgitation, and 1 percent aortic stenosis.

MITRAL STENOSIS

Pathophysiology

The murmur of mitral stenosis[9] (MS) is usually best heard using the bell of the stethoscope over the apex of the heart when the patient is in the supine position. It has a characteristic low pitch and rumbling sound not unlike a drum roll. Frequently the murmur is accompanied by a thrill with palpation of the apex in the left lateral position.

MS is the most common rheumatic valvular lesion in pregnancy and a thorough history and physical examination may reveal signs and symptoms of dyspnea, hemoptysis, orthopnea, or paroxysmal nocturnal dyspnea. Consultation with the cardiologist and anesthesiologist is encouraged in all these patients. If the MS is severe and a gradient in excess of 20 to 25 mmHg exists, decompensation is increasingly likely, especially with the onset of atrial fibrillation. Monitoring to diagnose paroxysmal atrial tachycardia, atrial fibrillation, or an increase in the pulmonary capillary wedge pressure is helpful. Signs of LV dysfunction may be suggestive of concomitant aortic valvular incompetence or mitral insufficiency. Associated complications include pulmonary embolism and pulmonary infarction, which tend to occur between 28 and 32 weeks. One must remember that this time frame is when the blood volume is at its peak. Pulmonary embolic phenomena may also occur during the onset of labor or the immediate postpartum period.

Anesthetic Management

The primary goal in the patient with mitral stenosis is to maintain a slow heart rate. Rates greater than 110 beats/min are not tolerated well. Therefore, we choose to avoid drugs such as atropine, scopolamine, glycopyrrolate, pancuronium, meperidine, ketamine, and nifedipine. If the patient has atrial fibrillation with a rapid ventricular response, we consider either digitalization or cardioversion. β-blockers can also be employed. We choose to start with esmolol because it has a short half-life. If this is tolerated well, one may consider longer-acting β-blockers such as propranolol.

Blood pressure should be carefully monitored. An acute drop in afterload may produce reflex tachycardia with resultant cardiac failure. Caution should also be exercised in the rapid infusion of intravenous fluids, which may precipitate atrial fibrillation or heart failure.

Hypercarbia and hypoxia are not desirable but, in these patients, may be catastrophic, producing an increase in pulmonary vascular resistance and placing undue strain on the right heart. We prefer a functioning continuous epidural technique and will raise the sensory level gradually[10] to minimize the cardiovascular changes, decrease the painful sensation of contractions, and prevent concomitant tachycardia. We do not use epinephrine in the local anesthetic. A single-shot subarachnoid block is not the regional technique of choice because of difficulty in controlling the level and the abrupt changes in the cardiovascular response that are so frequently seen. However, a continuous subarachnoid anesthetic can be considered since the sensory anesthetic level can be raised slowly, if necessary, to provide anesthesia for cesarean[11] delivery.

As stated previously, if a general anesthetic is employed, we avoid the use of a anticholinergic. A rapid-sequence induction utilizes thiopental, a neuromuscular blocker such as vecuronium, and a small dose of narcotic such as fentanyl to supplement the general anesthetic. We again would avoid drugs such as ketamine, pancuronium, and meperidine that are known to produce tachycardia.

Chesley claims that the mortality of parturients with mitral stenosis is equal to that of women who have never conceived. Atrial fibrillation is a common sequelae of MS and does result in an increased mortality in either pregnant or nonpregnant patients.[12]

MITRAL REGURGITATION

Pathophysiology

Mitral regurgitation (MR) is probably the second most common cardiac valvular abnormality present during pregnancy. The ausculatory findings include a soft S_1 and a widely split S_2. The murmur is high pitched and holosystolic, usually best heard at the apex with radiation into the left axilla. The increased blood volume that results from pregnancy is physiologically helpful to the parturient with MR. In chronic mitral regurgitation, in contrast to acute mitral regurgitation, the left atrium dilates and accommodates the regurgitant load. LV dilation and hypertrophy accompanies the dilated left atrium. The LV end-diastolic pressure increases. A reduction in the ejection fraction may result, eventually progressing to left heart failure. The left atrial dilation may result in atrial fibrillation, which may cause more serious consequences such as pulmonary edema with an associated maternal mortality as high as 17 percent. Another serious complication of atrial fibrillation is embolization.

Anesthetic Management

We prefer a functioning continuous epidural or subarachnoid anesthetic for labor and vaginal or cesarean delivery. The sympathetic blockade that accompanies these techniques results in a decrease in the afterload favoring the forward flow of blood. As with all major regional techniques, there is an increase in the venous capacitance and adequate intravascular volume expansion must occur prior to induction. Lateral displacement[13] of the uterus is essential to prevent aortocaval compression. These patients should receive antibiotic prophylaxis against the development of endocarditis. We strongly encourage a close working relationship with a cardiologist so that the addition of hydralazine, a low-sodium diet, and aggressive diuretic therapy may be instituted.

If surgical intervention must occur, timing is critical to avoid perioperative morbidity and mortality. Undue delay may result in irreversible left ventricular failure. In the United States, the treatment of choice for this lesion is valve replacement.

AORTIC STENOSIS

Pathophysiology

Aortic stenosis[14] is symptomless until constriction of the orifice becomes critical, resulting in a decline in stroke volume. Exercise or labor may induce angina, syncope, or dyspnea.

Auscultation reveals an ejection crescendo–decrescendo murmur occurring after S_1 and ending before S_2, usually heard best at the second right interspace with radiation to the carotid arteries. This murmur differs from that of mitral regurgitation, which is holosystolic.

Stroke volume is compromised and there is an increase in LV systolic pressure (LVSP), which results in hypertrophy of the left ventricle. With an increase in LVSP, subendocardial blood flow is compromised, which may result in ischemia. Tachycardia and vasodilation must be avoided. Sufficient time is required for ejection through a narrowed outflow tract. A decrease in the mean aortic pressure along with a concomitant decrease in coronary artery perfusion pressure is perilous.

Anesthetic Management

These patients tolerate the increase in catecholamines during labor much better than patients with MS, as stated above. An acute decrease in systemic vascular resistance (SVR) can result in ischemia and sympathetic blockade and should be avoided. We do not use a subarachnoid block but may choose a continuous epidural block provided adequate acute intravascular hydration has been performed using 1 to 2 L of fluid. A gradual increase in the level of the block is sought. Some would argue that an arterial catheter should be placed to allow continuous blood pressure monitoring. Hypotension should be aggressively treated with fluids and, if necessary, with intravenous phenylephrine rather than ephedrine. Some would suggest that a volatile anesthetic with thiopental, a nitrous oxide-oxygen mixture, and vecuronium for muscle relaxation be employed for cesarean delivery. Regardless of the technique chosen, good intravenous access is necessary. We prefer two 14 to 16 gauge catheters. A five-lead electrocardiograph monitor can be used to detect signs of myocardial ischemia.

AORTIC REGURGITATION

Pathophysiology

Unlike the lesion of aortic stenosis, the derangement in aortic insufficiency produces a high-pitched blowing murmur immediately following S_2, during diastole. Occasionally the murmur is faint but can be accentuated by having the patient lean forward. The backward flow results in diastolic and systolic overloading; therefore, the goals should be to decrease SVR and maintain a more rapid heart rate to decrease the time for regurgitation.

Anesthetic Management

Continuous epidural or subarachnoid anesthesia is recommended and will produce a decrease in SVR by sympathetic blockade. Bradycardia is avoided and treated if necessary. If hypotension develops, ephedrine is the drug of choice because it will tend to increase or maintain heart rate as well increase the vascular tone.

IDIOPATHIC HYPERTROPHIC SUBAORTIC STENOSIS

Pathophysiology

Idiopathic hypertrophic subaortic stenosis (IHSS) is a relatively common autosomal-dominant inherited disorder, and although considered a congenital heart lesion, it will be considered here for completeness. The pathophysiology of this disorder is best thought of as a pressure gradient across the ventricular outflow tract. Therefore, anything that increases the gradient across the aortic valve will further stress the cardiovascular system. An increase in the contractility may further worsen the obstructive effect of the hypertrophied muscle. A decrease in the LV end diastolic volume (LVEDV) or preload or an acute reduction in SVR will worsen the obstructive effect. Tachycardia will also reduce the cardiac output by effectively reducing the ventricular filling time and ejection fraction. Pregnancy and its associated physiologic changes may effect this disorder in conflicting ways. Initially, the expanded intravascular volume may have a beneficial effect by increasing LVEDV but, as gestation advances, the increase in SVR may have a detrimental effect. We recommend the use of β-blocking agents during pregnancy, and most of these patients have been taking them chronically. They act to reduce the contractility, thereby improving the obstruction. The slower heart rate will permit a greater ventricular filling period and ejection fraction.

Anesthetic Management

We avoid the use of sympathomimetic agents, including calcium chloride, epinephrine, ephedrine, and digoxin, because of their propensity to increase the occlusive effect of the lesion. Other agents to avoid would be the diuretics that may adversely affect preload. Direct blood pressure monitoring with the use of an arterial catheter and the use of CVP monitoring is helpful in serious lesions. We encourage intravascular volume expansion with warmed crystalloid solution and continuation of β-blockade. These patients should receive prophylactic antibiotics for subacute bacterial endocarditis. Continuous epidural anesthesia is initiated early in labor and maintained with a mixture of local anesthetic and narcotic. If emergent cesarean delivery is required, a regional anesthetic technique is *not* contraindicated. However, a slowly titrated continuous epidural or subarachnoid anesthetic with aggressive hemodynamic support aided by continuous invasive monitoring may be used. As the chemically induced sympathectomy resolves, it will result in an increase in SVR and autologous transfusion. A rapid induction or a single-dose epidural or subarachnoid anesthetic is discouraged. We also believe that IHSS patients should be monitored in an intensive care unit setting for 24 hours postoperatively. If a continuous epidural or subarachnoid catheter can be continued postoperatively, postoperative opioid analgesia may be employed if available. Patient-controlled analgesia is another option to be considered.

HEART SURGERY DURING PREGNANCY

Surgical management of an acutely decompensated parturient with valvular or congenital heart disease may be the best or the only effective treatment after vigorous medical therapy. Over the years, an increasing number of successful open-heart procedures have been reported during pregnancy, many of which employed cardiopulmonary bypass (CPB). Definitive cardiac surgery is remarkably safe and effective during pregnancy and fetal survival is reasonable, especially considering the 100 percent mortality with either maternal demise or therapeutic abortion to reduce the stress of pregnancy on maternal cardiac decompensation.

The optimal timing of cardiac surgery during pregnancy is in the second trimester, prior the 30th week gestation. At this time, fetal drug exposure is not a problem since organogenesis is complete. This time frame avoids the time of increased cardiovascular demands of the growing fetus. The danger of spontaneous labor unresponsive to tocolysis is also increased as the parturient approaches term.

Anesthetic Management

The goals of anesthesia include avoiding uterine aortocaval compression prior to, during, and after cardiopulmonary bypass, and the prevention of gastric aspiration. A high-dose narcotic induction and anesthetic technique is our choice. It is reasonable to avoid benzodiazepines during the first trimester because of their possible teratogenic effects. Narcotics (fentanyl and morphine), neuromuscular blocking agents (succinylcholine and pancuronium), and volatile agents (enflurane and isoflurane) have an excellent safety record for use during pregnancy. Hypotension should be aggressively treated with intravenous fluids, ephedrine, and/or phenylephrine as governed by the cardiac lesion. The fetus tolerates the nonpulsatile flow of CPB very well. Fetal heart rate monitoring[15] and tocodynamometry should be used intraoperatively and postoperatively. During CPB, the fetal heart rate variability is reduced as well as the baseline heart rate. This is probably secondary to high-dose narcotics, nonpulsatile flow, and hypothermia. If labor begins, tocolysis should be started with magnesium sulfate or β-agonists such as terbutaline or ritodrine as governed by the lesions and maternal cardiovascular status.

The risks associated with heparin anticoagulation and protamine are comparable to those of nonpregnant patients undergoing CPB. Heparin does not cross the placenta, whereas warfarin is contraindicated because it is teratogenic, and does cross the placenta. Protamine does not cross the placenta.

GENERAL OBSTETRIC MANAGEMENT OF THE PREGNANT CARDIAC PATIENT

If a patient has severe cardiac disease in the nonpregnant state, one can assume that her cardiac reserve during pregnancy will be nonexistent. The cardiologist, obstetrician, and the patient should discuss and critically explore the cardiac obstacles and the residual cardiac reserve available so that a wise decision regarding the termination or continuation of pregnancy can be made.

Regardless of the cardiac lesion(s) that a parturient may have, the avoidance of intrauterine asphyxia is one of the primary goals AFTER the well-being of the mother is achieved. Many factors may decrease uterine blood flow. Maternal hypoxia and hypercarbia decrease uterine blood flow, so one should ensure an adequate FiO_2, correct position of the endotracheal tube, and attention to hypoventilation and airway obstruction, as well as avoidance of drugs or maneuvers that may induce laryngospasm or bronchospasm. If a regional anesthetic technique is chosen, particular care must be taken to avoid intravascular injection of a local anesthetic, which will induce convulsions resulting in hypoxia.

Hypotension from hemorrhage, sepsis, excessively deep inhalational anesthesia, or uncontrolled sympathetic blockade from regional anesthesia diminish uteroplacental blood flow. Uterine artery vasoconstriction may be caused by a metabolic and/or respiratory alkalosis, a markedly high endogenous level of circulating catecholamines, or iatrogenically induced vasoconstriction from phenylephrine, dopamine, methoxamine, or ketamine. Uterine hypotonus[16] may be produced by toxic doses of local anesthetic, resulting in a decrease in uterine blood flow.

REFERENCES

1. Sullivan JM, Ramathan KB: Management of medical problems in pregnancy-severe cardiac disease. N Engl J Med 313:304, 1985

2. Rahimtoola SH: Perspective on valvular heart disease: an update. J Am Coll Cardiol 14:1, 1989
3. Duzlin ML: Antepartum fetal heart rate monitoring state of the art. Clin Perinatol 16:627, 1989
4. Devereux R: Diagnosis and prognosis of mitral valve prolapse. N Engl J Med 320:1077, 1989
5. Sokolow M, McIlroy MD: Clinical Cardiology. 4th Ed. p. 386. Lange Med Publications, Los Altos, CA, 1986
6. Kopriva C: The cardiologist as a consultant to the anesthesiologist. 1990 Annual Refresher Review Course Lectures 164:1, 1990
7. Bisno A, Shulman S, Dajani A: The rise and fall (and rise?) of rheumatic fever. JAMA 259:728, 1988
8. Denny F: T. Duckett Jonesvand rheumatic fever in 1986. Circulation 76:963, 1989
9. Clark SL, Phelan JP, Greenspoon J et al: Labor and delivery in the presence of mitral stenosis.
10. Grundy EM, Zamora AM, Winnie AP: Comparison of spread of epidural anesthesia in pregnant and nonpregnant women. Anesth Analg 57:644, 1979
11. Datta S, Alper MH: Anesthesia for cesarean section. Anesthesiology 53:142, 1980
12. Sullivan JM, Ramanathan KB: Management of medical problems in pregnancy—severe cardiac disease. N Engl J Med 313:304, 1985
13. Eckstein KL, Marx GF: Aortocaval compression and uterine displacement. Anesthesiology 40:92, 1974
14. Easterling TR, Chadwick HS, Oho CM, Benefetti TJ: Aortic stenosis in pregnancy, Obstet Gynecol 72:113, 1988
15. Carter MC: Fetal monitoring. J Biomed Eng 10:527, 1988
16. Munson ES, Embro W: Enflurane, isoflurance and halothane and isolated human uterine muscle. Anesthesiology 46:11, 1977

ARRHYTHMIAS

Pregnancy is associated with an increased incidence of benign arrhythmias, such as atrial premature contractions. Fortunately, serious arrhythmias are rare in pregnancy. In general, arrhythmias occurring during pregnancy should be approached similarly to arrhythmias occurring in nonpregnant women. The presence of triggering causes, coexisting cardiac disease, and most importantly, the hemodynamic status of the patient should determine both the nature and urgency of workup and treatment. One special consideration in treating arrhythmias in pregnancy is the effect of therapeutics on fetal well-being. Although all drugs used to treat arrhythmias have potential deleterious effects on the fetus, a wide array of drugs have been used with safety (Table 8-8).

DISTURBANCE OF SINUS RHYTHM

Sinus tachycardia is common during pregnancy. Normal maternal heart rate increases from 10 to 20 percent during pregnancy. The stress of labor and delivery causes further increases in heart rate. In addition, tocolytic therapy with β-adrenergic drugs will increase heart rate. In the absence of hypoxia, hypotension, anemia, or fever, sinus tachycardia requires no specific therapy.

Sinus bradycardia is rare in pregnancy in the absence of organic cardiac disease. Underlying causes such as hypothyroidism, coronary artery disease, cardiomyopathy, and drug effects should be considered and treatment should be directed at these conditions if the patient is symptomatic.

SUPRAVENTRICULAR ARRHYTHMIAS

The incidence of *premature atrial contractions* (PACs) is increased in pregnancy, as is the likelihood of their causing symptoms of palpitations or anxiety.[1] PACs are usually benign and are often related to fatigue, stress, and caffeine or alcohol consumption. Removal of the precipitating factor often alleviates the arrhythmia. In patients with rheumatic heart disease, PACs may precede the development of atrial flutter or fibrillation.

Paroxysmal atrial tachycardia (PAT) is a rapid re-entrant rhythm, beginning and ending with a PAC. Heart rates usually range from 140 to 220 beats/min (bpm) with this rhythm. Pregnant women seem to have increased susceptibility to developing PAT. In particular, women with a prior history of PAT tend to have more frequent and more severe episodes during pregnancy. In nearly all cases, the rhythm is well tolerated, unless there is underlying cardiac disease. In this situation, the development of PAT may be an early indicator of cardiac compromise or impending failure.

Carotid sinus massage may help distinguish this rhythm from sinus tachycardia (no effect or gradual slowing) or atrial flutter with 2:1 block (increased degree of block) and may be therapeutic, abruptly converting the aberrant rhythm to sinus rhythm. Other vagal maneuvers may also be employed. Edrophonium and phenylephrine have been used to slow the heart rate in symptomatic patients, and refractory cases may require digoxin, verapamil, or β-blockades. Patients with PAT and hypotension or other cardiac instability should be treated with synchronized cardioversion.[2]

Paroxysmal atrial tachycardia with block usually occurs in the setting of digoxin toxicity. Digoxin levels should be checked, and hypokalemia should be corrected if it exists.

Atrial flutter is quite uncommon in pregnant women. In this rhythm, the atrial discharge rate, seen as flutter waves, ranges from 220 to 340 bpm, whereas ventricular response rates are often 150 bpm. Carotid sinus massage increases the atrioventricular (AV) block and can make the diagnosis more clear.

Table 8-8. Guide to Antiarrhythmic Drugs in Pregnancy

Drug	Route of Administration	Clinical Application	Therapeutic Concentration	Use in Pregnancy	Comment
Lidocaine	Parenteral	"Choice in ventricular tachyarrhythmias, digitalis toxicity	2–4 μg/ml	Safe	Toxic doses and fetal acidosis may cause CNS and cardiovascular depression in the neonate
Quinidine	Oral	Paroxysmal atrial tachyarrhythmias[a]	2–5 μg/ml	Relatively safe	Excessive doses may lead to premature labor, very occasionally neonatal thrombocytopenia
Procainamide	Oral, parenteral	Termination and prophylaxis in atrial tachyarrhythmias	4–8 μg/ml (+NAPA 8–16 μg/ml)[b]	Relatively safe	High incidence of maternal antinuclear antibodies and lupuslike syndrome with chronic use
Phentoin	Oral, parenteral	Digitalis toxicity, refractory ventricular tachyarrhythmias	10–18 μg/ml	Not recommended for clinical use[c]	High risk of malformations ("fetal hydantoin syndrome"), bleeding disorder
Disopyramide	Oral, parenteral	Atrial and ventricular tachyarrhythmias	3–7 μg/ml	Probably safe[d]	One report documents uterine contractions in association with the drug
Verapamil	Oral, parenteral	Paroxysmal supraventricular tachycardia, rate control in chronic atrial fibrillation	15–30 ng/ml[e]	Probably safe[d]	Rapid IV injection may occasionally cause maternal hypotension and fetal distress
Digoxin	Oral, parenteral	Paroxysmal supraventricular tachycardia, rate control in chronic atrial fibrillation	1–2 μg/ml[e]	Safe	Adjust dosage when quinidine is given concomitantly
Propranolol	Oral, parenteral	Termination and prophylaxis in atrial and ventricular tachyarrhythmias, rate control in chronic fibrillation	75–100 ng/ml[e]	Relatively safe	Chronic administration may be associated with IUGR, premature labor, neonatal hypoglycemia, bradycardia, and respiratory depression

[a] Prior digitalization recommended.
[b] NAPA, N-acetylprocainamide.
[c] Probably safe as acute therapy of digitalis-induced arrhythmias.
[d] These drugs have not been studied extensively enough in pregnant patients to establish absolute safety, but no serious adverse effects have been reported.
[e] Large interindividual variation.
(Modified from Rotmensch HH, Elkayam U, Frishman W: Am J Cardiol 27:445, 1971, with permission.)

Hyperthyroidism, chronic pulmonary disease, and organic heart disease are disorders often associated with this rhythm disturbance in pregnancy. Therapy should be directed toward the underlying condition and emphasis should be placed on slowing the ventricular response. Digoxin, verapamil, quinidine, and procainamide have all been used to treat atrial flutter.

Atrial fibrillation is characterized by the absence of P waves and an irregularly irregular ventricular response. Ventricular response rates range from 140 to 200 bpm in untreated patients to 90 to 100 bpm in patients on chronic therapy.

Atrial fibrillation is rare in pregnancy except in patients with mitral valve disease. Other associated conditions include cardiomyopathy, coronary artery disease, chronic obstructive pulmonary disease, pulmonary embolism, and hyperthyroidism.

In chronic atrial fibrillation, progressive dilation of the left atrium with development of mural thrombi and eventual systemic embolization is a persistent risk. Anticoagulation should be considered in these patients. During pregnancy this usually consists of heparinization to avoid coumarin-associated embryopathy.

Digoxin is the mainstay of chronic therapy for atrial fibrillation. Verapamil may also be used acutely to slow the ventricular rate. As with PAT, synchronized cardioversion should be employed promptly if the patient becomes unstable.

VENTRICULAR ARRHYTHMIAS

The incidence of *premature ventricular contractions* (PVCs) is increased during pregnancy. Isolated, asymptomatic PVCs require no therapy. Symptomatic PVCs in women without intrinsic cardiac disease are best treated by removing possible precipitating factors such as caffeine or alcohol. If PVCs are frequent, echocardiography may be useful to rule out previously undiagnosed mitral valve prolapse or asymmetric septal hypertrophy. In women with underlying cardiac disease, new onset of PVCs may herald the development of cardiac failure.

Serum lidocaine levels in women receiving epidural anesthesia with lidocaine range from 2 to 4 μg/ml. This is comparable to therapeutic serum lidocaine levels achieved with continuous intravenous infusions of lidocaine. Indeed, there is a case report of improvement of ventricular ectopy in a parturient receiving lidocaine epidural anesthesia.[3] Although epidurally administered lidocaine cannot be recommended as primary therapy for PVCs in labor, its reported efficacy in this regard might influence the anesthesiologist's selection of local anesthetic to use in a patient with PVCs.

Ventricular tachycardia (VT) is rare in pregnancy, but does occur more frequently in patients with a history of PVCs. Most pregnant women with VT have underlying cardiac disease such as coronary artery disease, cardiomyopathy, valvular heart disease, asymmetric septal hypertrophy, mitral valve prolapse, or congenital prolonged QT syndrome.

The treatment of VT depends entirely on the condition of the patient. An unstable patient should be treated with direct countershock. "Stable" patients (usually those with slower heart rates) may respond to lidocaine. Bretylium and phenytoin are second-line drugs. Correction of any underlying problems such as hypokalemia, hypomagnesemia, and hypoxia are essential. Drugs such as procainamide and quinidine are used to control chronic or recurrent VT.

Ventricular fibrillation, though rare in pregnancy, is the most common cause of death in pregnant women, as well as the remainder of the population. Therapy consists of immediate application of direct current countershock and institution of advanced cardiac life support.

Both cardioversion and defibrillation have been used successfully in pregnancy, at voltages ranging from 10 to 360 J. Other than transient fetal arrhythmias, which resolve spontaneously, fetal outcomes have been good.[4,5] This is probably because the amount of electrical energy reaching the fetus is relatively small, and the fetal heart has a high fibrillatory threshold.

Considerations for anesthetizing a pregnant woman undergoing cardioversion include all of the usual considerations of anesthetizing a parturient, such as minimizing the risk of aspiration and avoidance of aortocaval compression. In addition, in the later stages of pregnancy, lateral displacement of the mediastinum and heart by the enlarging uterus requires placement of the apical defibrillator paddle slightly more lateral than usual to deliver the electrical current directly over the heart.

It should also be noted that in a cardiac arrest situation in which a parturient does not respond to the initial series of defibrillation and resuscitation, emergent cesarean delivery will improve both the mother's and baby's outcome from cardiopulmonary resuscitation (CPR).[6] Delivery of the infant will make maternal CPR and ventilation more effective, and will also decrease maternal oxygen consumption. The infant can be cared for more effectively once it is delivered, as decreased uterine perfusion during arrest situations leads rapidly to fetal acidosis and distress.

CONDUCTION ABNORMALITIES

Bundle branch blocks (BBB) are rare in pregnancy. Right BBB is found more often than left BBB in women in childbearing age. Cardiac diseases that may produce

BBB include cardiomyopathy, coronary artery disease, and valvular disease. In the absence of underlying cardiac disease, no specific therapy is required.

Women with *Wolff-Parkinson White* (WPW) syndrome may be more likely to experience arrhythmias during pregnancy. WPW is characterized by a short PR interval, and wide QRS complex with a δ-wave. Re-entrant tachycardias via a variant conduction pathway (the bundle of Kent) are the most common, often with ventricular rates exceeding 200 bpm. Therapy includes countershock for unstable rhythms, and procainamide and β-blockers for chronic control. Digoxin may favor conduction through the variant pathway by blocking conduction through the AV node, and may not treat the re-entrant arrhythmia.

First-degree AV block consists of a prolonged PR interval (greater than 0.20 second). No specific therapy is required for this rhythm disturbance, which may be transient, as a result of increased vagal tone (i.e., drugs such as digoxin or β-blockers) or permanent, as a result of AV node disease.

Second-degree AV block has two subsets. Mobitz I heart block is caused by a delay in conduction at the AV node. Progressive lengthening of the PR interval, eventually followed by a dropped ventricular beat, is seen. Mobitz I block rarely causes significant bradycardia. It can be associated with digoxin use, increased vagal tone, inferior myocardial infarction, and myocarditis. Therapy should be directed at the underlying problem if the patient is symptomatic. Otherwise, close monitoring will suffice, as this block rarely progresses to higher-degree blocks.

Mobitz II block is caused by a delay in conduction below the AV node. Ventricular rates can be quite slow, causing symptoms such as fatigue, dyspnea, and syncope. Mobitz II block often progresses to a higher-level block, and permanent pacemaker insertion is often necessary.

Third-degree AV block is characterized by dissociation of atrial and ventricular conduction. Ventricular rates are frequently in the 40 to 50 bpm range. Third-degree AV block is very rare in women of childbearing age. When seen, it is often associated with rheumatic heart disease, inferior myocardial infarction, acute myocarditis, and congenital heart block. Patients with congenital heart block often have associated ventricular septal defects.

Symptoms such as fatigue, syncope, orthopnea, and dyspnea result from low cardiac output associated with the slow heart rate, loss of synchronized atrial contraction for ventricular filling, and the underlying disease state. Permanent pacemaker insertion is the treatment of choice.

ANESTHETIC CONSIDERATIONS

Anesthetic considerations for pregnant women with arrhythmias are essentially the same as those for pregnant patients with underlying organic heart disease that results in arrhythmias. The reader is referred to the sections of this book dealing with those specific considerations.

REFERENCES

1. Meller J, Goldman ME: Rhythm disorders and pregnancy. In Elkayam U, Gleicher N, (eds): Cardiac Problems in Pregnancy: Diagnosis and Management of Maternal and Fetal Disease. Alan R. Liss, New York, 1982
2. Mangano DT: Anesthesia for the pregnant cardiac patient. p. 345. In Shnider SM, Levinson G, (eds): Anesthesia for Obstetrics. Williams & Wilkins, Baltimore, 1987
3. Juneja MM, Ackerman WE, Kaczorowski DM, et al: Continuous epidural lidocaine infusion in the parturient with paroxysmal ventricular tachycardia. Anesthesiology 71:305, 1989
4. Vogel JHK, Pryor R, Blount SG: Direct current defibrillation during pregnancy. JAMA 193:970, 1965
5. Sussman HI, Duque D, Lesser ME: Atrial flutter with 1:1 conduction. Report of a case in a pregnant woman successfully treated with DC countershock. Dis Chest 49:99, 1966
6. Johnson MD, Saltzman DH: Cardiac disease. In Datta S (ed): Anesthetic Obstetric Management of High Risk Pregnancy. CV Mosby–Year Book, St. Louis, 1991

CONGENITAL HEART DISEASE

Obstetric anesthesiologists are increasingly called upon to care for parturients with congenital heart disease. Congenital heart lesions are being diagnosed and successfully corrected at earlier stages, and, therefore, increasing numbers of women who might have succumbed to their heart lesions just years ago are now surviving to childbearing age. Congenital heart disease is seen with increased frequency relative to rheumatic heart disease.

A detailed discussion of each congenital heart lesion is beyond the scope of this section. Instead, the common left-to-right shunts are considered as a group, followed by the right-to-left shunts. Aortic coarctation is discussed separately. For a discussion of valvular lesions the reader is referred to the pertinent sections earlier in this chapter.

LEFT-TO-RIGHT SHUNTS

Left-to-right shunts include atrial septal defects, ventricular septal defects, and patent ductus arteriosus. All of these lesions result in increased pulmonary blood flow, as blood from the left heart passes to the right heart through the defect. This situation exists as long as left-sided pressures are higher than right-sided pressures, which is the usual case early in the course of the disease. Over time, right ventricular hypertrophy and, eventually, pulmonary hypertension develop. If the lesion remains uncorrected, progressive medial hypertrophy and intimal fibrosis of the pulmonary vasculature may result with ensuing right ventricular failure.[1]

Pregnancy creates an additional burden by increasing intravascular blood volume, heart rate, and cardiac output. Parturients with small shunts who are asymptomatic prior to pregnancy may be able to tolerate this additional stress without sequelae. However, patients with large shunts and/or diminished myocardial reserve may develop symptoms of congestive heart failure. In addition, patients with these lesions who become compromised and have pulmonary hypertension may develop bidirectional or right-to-left shunting (known as Eisenmenger's syndrome, see below). In some instances, this may be due to the decreased systemic vascular resistance occurring during pregnancy as a result of an increase in circulating prostacyclins.

Proper care for these patients should include close follow-up by an obstetrician, cardiologist, and anesthesiologist with open discussion of method of delivery, options for analgesia/anesthesia, and contingency plans for maternal or fetal emergencies. Baseline investigations should include a 12-lead electrocardiogram, chest X-ray, echocardiogram, hematocrit, and serum creatinine.

Anesthetic Considerations

Anesthetic considerations vary with the severity of the lesion and the degree of myocardial dysfunction and pulmonary hypertension. In all cases, precautions must be taken with intravenous-access devices and fluids to avoid air bubbles and thrombi, which may paradoxically embolize right to left though the shunt and eventually reach the brain. Prophylaxis against bacterial endocarditis may be necessary. Electrocardiographic monitoring is important to detect arrhythmias in patients who are susceptible (e.g., patients with atrial septal defect). Pulse oximetry is valuable, providing continuous information regarding status of oxygenation, and can alert the caretakers to the onset of right-to-left shunting. Patients with evidence of pulmonary hypertension, congestive heart failure, or shunt reversal may require intra-arterial and pulmonary artery pressure monitoring.

Other considerations include careful attention to repleting blood loss and avoiding systemic hypotension, which may encourage shunt reversal. In addition, conditions that increase pulmonary vascular resistance, such as hypoxemia, hypercarbia, and acidosis, should be avoided or treated promptly. Avoidance of aortocaval compression is a main priority; left uterine displacement is necessary throughout labor and delivery.

For labor and delivery, epidural anesthesia can provide a pain-free labor, thereby decreasing catecholamine levels and possible increases in systemic vascular resistance caused by pain plus minimize hemodynamic changes seen with contractions. Meticulous attention to blood pressure, judicious fluid administration prior to the initiation of the anesthetic, and slow titration of local anesthetic level to prevent precipitous decreases in systemic vascular resistance (which might produce shunt reversal in patients with pulmonary hypertension) are essential. In addition, a technique employing loss of resistance to saline rather than air should probably be used to avoid the chance of injecting air into the epidural vein. An existing epidural anesthetic can easily be dosed for cesarean delivery should the need arise.

If general anesthesia is used, the precautions for a patient with a full stomach and the necessity of securing the airway with an endotracheal tube apply.

Many anesthetic choices have been employed safely for cesarean delivery. Those patients who are asymptomatic can probably tolerate any anesthetic technique. Patients who are more severely compromised require careful attention to avoiding myocardial depression and decreases in systemic vascular resistance. A nitrous oxide–oxygen plus opioid-based technique is often used in this situation, although other choices may be acceptable as well.

RIGHT-TO-LEFT SHUNTS

Right-to-left shunts are also described as cyanotic heart defects and include tetralogy of Fallot, transposition of the great arteries, tricuspid atresia, and Eisenmenger's syndrome. Historically, a few women with these lesions reached childbearing age, but with earlier and improved corrective surgery, more women with these lesions are reaching childbearing age.

Patients whose lesions have been successfully surgically corrected and who have no residual lesions should tolerate pregnancy without increased risk. Their mode of delivery and anesthetic management may include epidural, subarachnoid, or general anesthesia without any particular consideration. Prophylaxis against bacterial endocarditis may be indicated, however.

Uncorrected or palliated patients are at high risk for maternal and fetal problems during pregnancy and require special care throughout their pregnancy. They should be followed closely by their obstetrician and cardiologist. Consultation with an anesthesiologist with expertise in this area should occur early in pregnancy and a plan of care developed for both the expected mode of delivery and any emergencies that might develop.

Pregnancy increases the morbidity of patients with uncorrected right-to-left shunts.[3] The decrease in systemic vascular resistance occurring in pregnancy promotes increased right-to-left shunting and cyanosis, particularly immediately postpartum, when systemic vascular resistance may be at its lowest. The stress and pain associated with labor may increase pulmonary vascular resistance and increase right-to-left shunting as well. Blood loss and ensuing hypotension at the time of delivery may potentiate shunting and contribute to increasing cyanosis and hypoxia. Maintenance of stable intravascular volume and close control of blood pressure are vitally important.

Monitoring consists of electrocardiography, pulse oximetry, and, in nearly all cases, intra-arterial and central venous catheterization. Oxygen should be provided and hypoxemia, hypercarbia, and acidosis avoided because of their deleterious effects on pulmonary vascular resistance.

Anesthetic Considerations

Controversy exists over the best choice for pain relief during labor and anesthesia for cesarean delivery. It is of prime importance to avoid myocardial depression and to maintain normal systemic vascular resistance, venous return, and circulating blood volume regardless of the technique selected.

If regional anesthesia is chosen, epidural anesthesia allows a more gradual onset of the block and sympathectomy, and is preferred over subarachnoid anesthesia.[5] As emphasized previously, decreases in systemic vascular resistance are undesirable, therefore prevention of aortocaval compression by left uterine displacement, judicuous fluid administration, and slow incremental dosing of the epidural anesthetic to provide a slow onset of hemodynamic alterations are essential. Prompt treatment of any decrease in systemic blood pressure is important. Phenylephrine is the drug of choice to raise the blood pressure and systemic vascular resistance. Another advantage to carefully administered epidural anesthesics is the ability to employ epidural opioids, which will improve the quality of the block, and allow the use of lower concentrations or local anesthetic for sensory pain relief during labor.[4] In addition, epidural opioids can be employed for the treatment of postoperative or postpartum pain, avoiding the need for systemic opioids.

If general anesthesia is chosen, particular concern must be given to prevention of aspiration, as the typical rapid-sequence induction may not be well tolerated by these patients. Administration of a nonparticulate antacid, metoclopramide, and histamine (H_2)-receptor antagonist may be useful to decrease the likelihood of pulmonary aspiration syndrome. Use of inhaled agents must be tempered by concern over the myocardial depression and vasodilation they produce. Finally, the hemodynamic responses to laryngoscopy, intubation, and positive-pressure ventilation must be considered.[4]

COARCTATION OF THE AORTA

Coarctation of the aorta is a high-grade narrowing of the aorta, frequently occurring just distal to the left subclavian artery. Other cardiac anomalies and cerebral aneurysms can coexist with this lesion. Hypertension is nearly always present. Recent trends toward early surgical correction have resulted in fewer women with coarctation of the aorta reaching childbearing age prior to surgical correction. Once surgically corrected, pregnancy can be undertaken without increased fetal or maternal morbidity. However, pregnancy in untreated patients is associated with a maternal mortality of 3 to 9 percent, and fetal mortality is even higher, about 20 percent.

Cardiac output is rate limited with this lesion because of the fixed obstruction produced by the coarctation. Although bradycardia is poorly tolerated, severe tachycardia may result in left-ventricular decompensation. The increased intravascular volume and metabolic demands of pregnancy can be compensated for only by an increase in the heart rate. Also, the progressive decline in systemic vascular resistance may not be well tolerated because the compensating tachycardia may result in symptoms of congestive heart failure. Aortic rupture or dissection are also possible because of intimal damage caused by turbulent flow beyond the coarctation. The stresses of labor and delivery do not seem to increase the risk of rupture, although changes in the aortic anatomy have been documented in pregnancy. Most deaths from aortic rupture or dissection occur prior to labor and delivery.

Patients with surgically corrected coarctation of the aorta may undergo labor and delivery and anesthesia without increased risk. Patients with uncorrected, uncomplicated coarctation who are asymptomatic require routine monitoring and careful attention to maintaining systemic vascular resistance and adequate left-ventricular filling (i.e., avoidance of bradycardia, aortocaval compression, and hypovolemia).

Patients who have symptoms of congestive heart failure or aneurysmal dilatation of the aorta should have intra-arterial and pulmonary artery pressure monitoring. The sympathectomy that occurs with epidural and subarachnoid anesthetics must be carefully managed. If regional anesthesia is necessary, an epidural technique, with or without opioids, is preferred over subarachnoid anesthesia. Other alternatives include epidural or subarachnoid opioids (without local anesthetics) with pudendal block for labor and delivery, or general anesthesia for cesarean delivery. Regardless of the technique chosen, careful monitoring of heart rate and blood pressure is essential. Decrease in heart rate or blood pressure should be treated promptly and systemic vascular resistance maintained.

REFERENCES

1. Fink BW: Congenital Heart Disease. Year Book Medical Publishers, Chicago, 1980
2. Cobb T, Gleicher N, Elkayam U: Congenital heart disease and pregnancy. In Elkayam U, Gleicher N (eds): Cardiac Problems in Pregnancy. Diagnosis and Management of Maternal and Fetal Disease. Alan R. Liss, New York, 1982
3. Gleicher N, Medwall J, Hochberger D, et al: Eisenmenger's syndrome and pregnancy. Obstet Gynecol Surv 34:721, 1979
4. Johnson MD, Saltzman DH: Cardiac Disease. In Datta S (ed): Anesthetic and Obstetric Management of High Risk Pregnancy. CV Mosby–Year Book Medical Publishers, St. Louis, 1991
5. Spinnato JA, Kraynack BT, Cooper MW: Eisenmenger's syndrome in pregnancy. Epidural anesthesia for elective cesarean section. N Engl J Med 304:1215, 1981
6. Mangano DT: Anesthesia for the pregnant cardiac patient. p. 345. In Shnider SM, Levinson G (eds): Anesthesia for Obstetrics. Williams & Wilkins, Baltimore, 1987

MYOCARDIAL INFARCTION

Myocardial infarction complicating an otherwise normal pregnancy is a rare event.[1,2] First described in 1922,[3] only 84 additional cases have been reported, yielding an incidence of 1 in 10,000 deliveries.[4–14] The coronary anatomy of over 30 percent of these cases has been delineated, either by angiography or postmortem studies.[15] Although arteriosclerosis was found in 40 percent of the patients, most vessels that were evaluated did not demonstrate severe disease. Thrombus formation and spasm is the primary cause of myocardial infarction in the parturient. Myocardial infarction during pregnancy is associated with a mortality of 30 percent and the incidence will probably increase over the next decade as older parturients undergo labor and delivery. Appropriate anesthetic management can help to reduce the morbidity and mortality of myocardial infarction during pregnancy.

FACTORS AFFECTING THE RISK OF MYOCARDIAL INFARCTION

The risk of myocardial infarction during pregnancy can be attributed to factors unrelated to the pregnancy and the intrinsic physiologic changes characteristic of a normal pregnancy. The former account for the increasing incidence of myocardial infarction now being seen in this population. Increasing maternal age is one of the more notable trends. The older parturient is more likely to have an elevated cholesterol level, high blood pressure, and work-related stress. Therefore, she is a candidate for arteriosclerotic coronary disease. In addition, tobacco consumption among women has increased over the last 30 years. Smoking enhances platelet aggregation, making the parturient hypercoagulable, and predisposed to coronary thrombosis.[16] Finally, use of illicit drugs is much more pervasive in our society and ingestion of cocaine may compromise coronary circulation by acutely provoking coronary spasm.

Numerous physiologic changes occur during a normal pregnancy that drastically alter the balance of myocardial oxygen supply and demand. The resultant myocardial ischemia increases the risk of myocardial infarction. Of all the organ systems, the cardiovascular system undergoes some of the most profound changes. The pregnant state imposes additional hemodynamic demands on the heart: the 30 percent increase in plasma volume, 40 percent increase in cardiac output, and 50 percent increase in metabolic demand all satisfy the increasing metabolic needs of both fetus and mother. The increase in cardiac output peaks at 28 to 32 weeks of gestation and remains elevated at that level until the onset of labor.[17,18] At that point, cardiac output may further increase by 25, 50 and 80 percent during the first, second, and third stages of labor, respectively.[19] A cardiac output two to three times that of the baseline nonpregnant state can be attained in the postpartum period. These changes may occur even more acutely during a cesarean delivery, in which the blood volume of the previously parallel fetal circuit is returned to the maternal circulation almost instantaneously.[20] These tremendous increases in myocardial oxygen demand must be met or myocardial ischemia will result.

Coincident with increased myocardial demand, other physiologic changes simultaneously decrease myocardial oxygen supply and increase the risk of myocardial ischemia. Pulmonary and hematologic changes may lower oxygen content. The enlarging uterus impinges on the diaphragm and lungs, reducing both functional residual capacity and residual volume. This causes inappropriate matching of ventilation and perfusion as well as increased physiologic shunt, which decreases the hemoglobin saturation during periods of stress. A dramatic increase in the plasma volume outstrips increases in the red cell mass, leading to the relative anemia of pregnancy, which further decreases oxygen content. At the cellular level, unloading of oxygen is hampered in the parturient because oxygen is more tightly bound to the hemoglobin molecule. Mild alkalosis secondary to chronic hyperventilation and lower 2,3-DPG levels shifts the oxyhemoglobin dissociation curve "leftward."

Coronary perfusion may also be compromised. A lower diastolic pressure reflects the progressive decrease in peripheral vascular resistance that occurs during the course of the pregnancy. Left coronary artery perfusion may fall as the gradient between systemic diastolic and left ventricular end-diastolic pressure narrows. Coronary artery thrombosis or vasospasm may also reduce myocardial oxygen supply. The parturient is in a hypercoagulable state because of an increase in most of the clotting factors, and this may predispose her to thrombus formation.[21,22] Coronary spasm may also be more problematic. The chorion, which contains 160 times the renin concentration of maternal plasma, may release renin during transient episodes of uterine ischemia, provoking coronary spasm.[23,24] Abnormal vasomotor responses may compromise even minimally diseased coronary arteries, especially during periods of increased demand.[25]

Familiarity with the dynamics of maternal physiology allows one to anticipate when the parturient is at increased risk for myocardial infarction, or extension and subsequent decompensation, and what maneuvers might ameliorate the situation. Specifically, the parturient is most at risk at 32 weeks, right at the time of delivery, and immediately postdelivery. Not only do the majority of myocardial infarctions occur during the third trimester, but death is twice as likely.[4]

IMMEDIATE MEDICAL MANAGEMENT

The immediate management of an acute myocardial infarction can be divided into patient stabilization and invasive cardiac intervention. The principles of treatment mirror those guiding therapy for any patient presenting with an acute myocardial infarction, tempered by cognizance of relevant maternal changes and potential fetal toxicities.

Stabilization necessitates admission to an intensive care unit, where oxygen therapy should be provided, along with continuous electrocardiographic, fetal heart rate, and invasive hemodynamic monitoring. Initial therapy is designed to relieve ongoing ischemia and prevent extension of myocardial injury. There is no evidence that narcotics, nitrates, calcium channel blockers, or β-blockers have any adverse fetal effects, and these agents should be utilized for their sedative, antianginal, and antihypertensive effects as needed.[26–28] It has been reported that fewer neonatal complications have been reported following the use of selective, as compared to nonselective, β_1-blockers.[29–32] Calcium channel blockers may have special utility because of the prominent vasospastic component in the pathogenesis of myocardial infarction in the parturient.

The complications of myocardial infarction should be treated aggressively. After 32 weeks of gestation, the cardiovascular system is already stressed from coping with the increased demands imposed on it. Decompensation is quite likely should the heart become ischemic or markedly dysfunctional. The resultant congestive failure is best treated first with afterload-reducing agents such as hydralazine or labetalol.[33] A report suggests that captopril may be teratogenic and the marginal experience with other angiotensin converting enzyme inhibitors in this population precludes their use.[34] Although nitroglycerin is appropriate for the treatment of pulmonary congestion, sodium nitroprusside is relatively contraindicated because thiocyanate and cyanide may accumulate in the fetus after prolonged use.[35] Digoxin is a safe initial inotrope but clearly more potent agents should be utilized, if needed.

Rapid supraventricular or ventricular arrhythmias may also compromise maternal circulation and, hence, placental perfusion. Digoxin is the drug of choice for the treatment of rapid ventricular response in atrial fibrillation or flutter. A higher volume of distribution secondary to increased serum protein binding may mandate greater doses than usually employed. Lidocaine is the preferred agent for the treatment of ventricular arrhythmias, although procainamide, quinidine, and disopyramide all can be used safely in the parturient. All local anesthetics cross the placenta. Lidocaine has been demonstrated to have no lasting adverse effects on the fetus[28] and the same should be true of the other local anesthetics.

Anticoagulation should be considered after a myocardial infarction, especially since the parturient is hypercoagulable. Low-dose heparin may prevent further thrombosis in inflammed coronary vessels. Severe anterior wall hypokinesis, with or without mural thrombus, may necessitate treatment with systemic anticoagulation. Furthermore, bed rest during an admission to the hospital increases the risk of deep venous thrombosis and secondary pulmonary embolus, which could be catastrophic. Heparin is the preferred agent because it does not cross the placenta and its reversibility reduces the risk of hemorrhage at the time of delivery. The logistics of coumarin therapy are less problematic. The drug is teratogenic,[36] may cause retroplacental and fetal intracranial hemorrhage,[37] and may lead to central nervous system defects.[38]

Occasionally, more drastic cardiac intervention may be necessary. If the mother is viable, emergency cardiac catheterization should be considered in the acute phase to determine the feasibility of percutaneous angioplasty or surgical revascularization if a large segment of myocardium is at risk. The role for clot lysis with either streptokinase or tissue plasminogen activator has not been established. If the fetus is viable, and the mother has not responded to appropriate resuscitative efforts, than consideration should be given to cesarean delivery of the fetus. This decision must be made with alacrity to avoid unnecessary prolongation of fetal hypoxia or asphyxia.

OBSTETRIC CONSIDERATIONS

Key obstetric considerations during this period are ensuring fetal viability timing the delivery, and deciding on the mode of delivery. After 24 weeks of gestation, the fetus is considered viable, and should be adequately monitored with ultrasound at the time of all maternal interventions that potentially could affect it. The goal of optimizing uterine perfusion is achieved by careful attention to left uterine displacement, assuring adequate hydration, and treating the sequelae of myocardial infarction as outlined above. Failure to use appropriate medications to "protect" the fetus at the expense of maternal hemodynamic stability is unjustifiable. Improving oxygen delivery may necessitate oxygen administration, blood transfusion to treat anemia, phenylephrine to raise systemic pressure, and nitroglycerin to reduce left ventricular end-diastolic pressure. In fact, recent studies suggest that fetal acidosis may actually be alleviated when a vasoconstrictive agent such as phenylephrine is used to restore blood pressure to baseline.[39]

The timing of delivery is not as clear-cut as one might suppose. Waiting beyond the acute period avoids early myocardial irritability, which is manifest by ventricular arrhythmias and conduction disturbances, and the patient is more apt to be hemodynamically stable. On the other hand, the cardiovascular stresses of pregnancy will increase and the risk of rupturing myocardial scar tissue will be higher.

Historically, cesarean delivery has carried at higher risk. Normal vaginal delivery avoids surgical stress, is associated with less blood loss and a lower rate of infection, and allows earlier ambulation. On the other hand, a cesarean delivery is predictable, allows more meticulous hemodynamic control, and avoids the prolonged stress of labor. Even a well-controlled labor, with a functioning epidural anesthetic providing an adequate surgical block, is still marked by significant fluctuations in vascular tone and cardiac output that appear to be hormonally mediated. If a vaginal delivery is contemplated, the length of labor, how much stress the patient can tolerate, and consideration of a low forceps delivery should be discussed in advance.

ANESTHETIC CONSIDERATIONS

The key elements of anesthetic management are ensuring that the patient is optimally prepared for delivery and the provision of a safe anesthetic course. Preparations must always begin with a complete anesthetic evaluation. An accurate assessment of cardiovascular reserve is the ideal, although not always obtainable, goal. Maximizing the oxygen supply and demand balance should be well under way, with provision of oxygen, maintenance of a body temperature, consideration of transfusion, treatment of ischemia with nitroglycerin, and meticulous hemodynamic control. Patients should be well sedated with either morphine sulfate and/or diazepam at the initiation of invasive monitoring and during labor and delivery. In addition to anxiety, heart rate and myocardial oxygen demands can be increased by pain, hypotension, hypovolemia, and shivering.[40] Shivering can be decreased by warming intravenous fluids, raising the room temperature, keeping the patient well covered, and administering parenteral or intraspinal opioids.[41–45]

Minimal monitoring should include electrocardiogram, blood pressure, temperature, fetal heart rate and uterine contractions. Furthermore, pulse oximetry and direct arterial and pulmonary artery catheterization are appropriate in this high-risk population.

The method that constitutes the "safest" anesthetic will depend on particular patient characteristics and the expertise of the team caring for the patient. In the stable or minimally decompensated patient, continuous epidural anesthesia with a surgical level to the mid to high thoracic level is the anesthetic method of choice for vaginal or cesarean delivery. Its high degree of titratability ensures a gradual onset and relative hemodynamic stability with abolition of most sympathetically mediated, pain-triggered responses during the delivery period. Reports from the nonobstetric literature suggest that intraoperative blood loss and postoperative complications may be reduced.[46–49] Additional benefits provided by the high surgical level are a decrease in the surgical stress response, avoidance of tachycardia by blockade of cardiac accelerator fibers, and inhibition of sympathetically mediated vasospasm. Although not strictly a benefit, regional anesthesia avoids the problems associated with a high-dose narcotic general anesthetic such as caring for a depressed neonate or weaning and extubating the mother postoperatively.

Similar in benefits to continuous epidural anesthesia is continuous subarachnoid anesthesia. It is even more controllable and more consistently provides a reliable anesthetic. However, the possible risk of post-dural puncture headaches, the greater potential for infection, and the unfamiliarity with the technique make continuous subarachnoid anesthesia useful only in certain selected cases.

The role of high-dose narcotic general anesthesia with the necessary continued intubation postoperatively should be restricted to the decompensated patient in congestive heart failure. The complicated post-myocardial infarction patient with combined valvular lesions may also more appropriately be handled with a general anesthetic. In these unstable patients, preserving systemic vascular resistance as a variable that still can be manipulated provides greater flexibility toward achieving hemodynamic stability. Furthermore, control of ventilation removes additional constraints on pharmacologic intervention.

REFERENCES

1. Ginz B: Myocardial infarction in pregnancy. J Obstet Gynaecol Br Commonw 77:610, 1970
2. Fletcher E, Knox EW, Morton P: Acute myocardial infarction in pregnancy. Br Med J 3:586, 1967
3. Katz H: About the sudden natural death in pregnancy: during delivery and the puerperium. Arch Gynaecol 115:283, 1922
4. Hankins GDV, Wendall GD, Leveno KH, Stoneham J: Myocardia infarction during pregnancy: a review. Obstet Gynecol 65:139, 1985
5. Stokes IM, Stone M: Myocardial infarction and cardiac arrest in the second trimester followed by assisted vaginal delivery under epidural analgesia at 38 weeks gestation. Case Report. Br J Obstet Gynaecol 18:35, 1984
6. Trouton TG, Sidhu H, Adgey AJ: Myocardial infarction in pregnancy. Int J Cardiol 18:35, 1988
7. Mabie WC, Anderson GD, Addington MB, et al: The benefit of cesarean section in acute myocardial infarction complicated by premature labor. Obstet Gynecol 3:503, 1988
8. Lamb MA: Myocardial infarction during pregnancy: a team approach. Heart Lung 16:658, 1987
9. Sperry KL: Myocardial infarction in pregnancy. J Forensic Sci 32:1464, 1987
10. Cortis BS, Lee SS, Bacalla M: Acute myocardial infarction and ventricular fibrillation during pregnancy. Illinois Med J 160:17, 1981
11. Duke M. Pregnancy, myocardial infarction and normal coronary arteries. Conn Med 46:626, 1982
12. Cohen WR, Steinman T, Patsner B, et al: Acute myocardial infarction in a pregnant woman at term. JAMA 250:2179, 1983
13. Cowan NC, DeBelder MA, Rothman MT: Coronary angioplasty in pregnancy. Br Heart J 59:588, 1988
14. Hutchinson SJ, Holden RJ, Lorimer AR: Myocardial infarction in pregnancy. Scott Med J 30:116, 1985
15. Hands ME, Johnson MD, Saltzman DH, Rutherford JD: The cardiac obstetric and anesthetic management of pregnancy complicated by acute myocardial infarction. J Clin Anesth 2:258, 1990
16. Havis RB, Leuschen MP, Boyd D, Goodlin RC: Evaluation of platelet function in pregnancy. Comparative studies in non-smokers and smokers. Thromb Res 46:175, 1987
17. Lees MM, Taylor SH, Scott DB, Kerr MG: A study of cardiac output at rest throughout pregnancy. J Obstet Gynaecol Br Commonw 74:319, 1967
18. Walters WA, MacGregor WG, Hills M: Cardiac output at rest during pregnancy and the puerperium. Clin Sci 30:1, 1966
19. Ueland K, Hansen JM: Maternal cardiovascular dynamics. III. Labor and delivery under local and caudal analgesia. Am J Obstet Gynecol 103:8, 1969
20. Ueland K, Gills RE, Hansen JM: Maternal cardiovascular dynamics. I. Cesarean section under subarachnoid block anesthesia. Am J Obstet Gynecol 100:42, 1968
21. Gjonnaess H, Fagerhol MK: Studies on coagulation and fibrinolysis in pregnancy. Acta Obstet Gynaecol Scand 54:363, 1975
22. Fletcher AP, Alkjaersig NK, Burstein R: The influence of pregnancy upon blood coagulation and plasma fibrinolytic enzyme function. Am J Obstet Gynecol 134:743, 1979
23. Sasse L, Wagner R, Murray FE: Transmural myocardial infarction during pregnancy. Am J Cardiol 35:448, 1975
24. Skinner SL, Lumbers ER, Semonds EM: Renin concentration in human fetal and maternal tissues. Am J Obstet Gynecol 101:529, 1968
25. Ludmer PL, Selwyn AP, Shook TL, et al: Paradoxical vasoconstriction by aceytlcholine in atherosclerotic coronary arteries. N Engl J Med 315:1046, 1986
26. Briggs GG, Freeman RK, Yaffe SJ: Drugs in pregnancy and lactation. p. 311. Williams & Wilkins, Baltimore, 1986
27. Cottrill CM, McAllister RG, Gettes L, Noonan JA: Propranolol therapy during pregnancy, labor, and delivery: Evidence for transplacental drug transfer and impaired neonatal drug disposition. J Pediatr 912:812, 1977
28. McAnulty JH, Metcalfe J, Ueland K: Cardiovascular disease. In Burrow GH, Ferrig TF (eds): Medical Complica-

tions During Pregnancy. 3rd Ed. W.B. Saunders, Philadelphia, 1988
29. Gladstone GR, Hordof A, Gersony WM: Propranolol administration during pregnancy: effects on the fetus. J Pediatr 86:962, 1975
30. Habib A, McCarthy JS: Effects on the neonate of propranolol administration during pregnancy. J Pediatr 91:808, 1977
31. Tunstall ME: The effect of propranolol on the onset of breathing at birth. Br J Anaesth 41:792, 1969
32. Rubin PC, Butters L, Clark DM, et al: Placebo-controlled trial of atenolol in the treatment of pregnancy-associated hypertension. Lancet 1:431, 1983
33. Teramo K, Elder M, Rabinowitz B, Neufeld HN: Medical treatment of cardiovascular disorders during pregnancy. Am Heart J 104:1357, 1982
34. Duminy PC, Burger PT: Fetal abnormality associated with the use of captopril during pregnancy. S Afr Med J 60:805, 1981
35. Lewis PE, Cefalo RC, Naulty JS, Rodkey FL: Placental transfer and fetal toxicity of sodium nitroprusside. Gynecology 8:46, 1977
36. Iturbe-Alessio I, del Carmen Fonesca M, Mutchinik O, et al: Risks of anticoagulant therapy in pregnant women with artificial heart valves. N Engl J Med 27:1390, 1986
37. Villasanta U: Thromboembolic disease in pregnancy. Am J Obstet Gynecol 93:142, 1965
38. Hall JG, Pauli RM, Wilson KM: Maternal and fetal sequelae of anticoagulation during pregnancy. Am J Med 68:122, 1980
39. Moran D, et al: Phenylephrine in the prevention of hypotension following spinal anesthesia for cesarean delivery. J Clin Anesth 3:301, 1991
40. Holdcroft A, Hall GM, Cooper G: Redistribution of body heat during anaesthesia. Anaesthesia 34:758, 1979
41. Workham M: Intravenous fluid temperature, shivering and the parturient. Anesth Analg 5:496, 1986
42. Walmsberg AJ, Giesecke AH, Lipton JM: Contribution of extradural temperature to shivering during extradural anaesthesia. Br J Anaesth 58:1130, 1986
43. Casey WF, Smith CE: Intravenous meperidine for the control of shivering during emergency cesarean section under epidural anesthesia. Anesth Analg 67:s1, 1988
44. Pauca R, Savage RT, Simpson S, Roy RC: Effect of pethidine, fentanyl and morphine on post-delivery shivering in male. Acta Anaesthesiol 28:138, 1984
45. Johnson MD, Sevarino FB, Lema JM: A report of cessation of shivering and hypothermia associated with epidural sufentanil. Anesth Analg 68:70, 1988
46. Thorburn J, Louden JR, Vallance R: Spinal and general anaesthesia in total hip replacement: frequency of deep vein thrombosis. Br J Anaesth 52:1117, 1980
47. Modig J, Borg T, Karlstrom G, et al: Thromboembolism after total hip replacement: Role of epidural and general anesthesia. Anesth Analg 62:174, 1983
48. Shulman M, Sandler AN, Bradley JW, et al: Post thoracotomy pain and pulmonary function following epidural and systemic morphine. Anesthesiology 61:569, 1984
49. Rawal N, Sjostrand U, Christoffersson E, et al: Comparison of intramuscular and epidural morphine for postoperative analgesia in the grossly obese: influence on postoperative ambulation and pulmonary function. Anesth Analg 63:583, 1984

ASTHMA

Asthma affects more than 1 person out of 20 in the United States, yet it remains under-diagnosed and untreated. The number of asthma related deaths has risen in the last decade.[1]

Asthma has classically been considered a disease characterized by bronchospasm; however, asthma has an inflammatory component.[2] In many patients, a late phase inflammatory response plays an integral role in the pathogenesis of severe and chronic asthma and may precipitate bronchospasm. This finding dictates the need to re-evaluate our therapeutic approach and suggests the need for more aggressive management of the late-phase response. A step care approach to the management of asthma should be employed.[3,4]

During pregnancy, both physiologic and hormonal changes occur that affect the patient with asthma. Although there is no marked change in the total lung capacity or vital capacity, there is an upward displacement of the diaphragm that contributes to a reduction in the expiratory reserve volume and residual volume. The overall effect is a reduction in functional residual volume of about 20 percent.

With an increase in serum concentration of progesterone, which is a respiratory stimulant, respiratory rate, tidal volume, and, therefore, minute ventilation all increase. Oxygen consumption increases by approximately 20 percent. The combination of a reduction in pulmonary reserve and an increase in oxygen consumption makes exacerbations difficult for the asthmatic patient to tolerate.

Approximately 1 percent of pregnant women have asthma, and 10 to 15 percent of these women will require hospitalization for an acute attack at some time during their pregnancy. It is estimated that 50 percent of women with asthma will have no change in their condition during pregnancy; 25 percent will improve and 25 percent will worsen. A number of studies have shown that preterm delivery, low-birthweight infants, and perinatal death occur with more frequency in pregnancies complicated by asthma.[5–7] Also hemorrhage, hyperemesis, pregnancy-induced hypertension and the need to induce labor occurred more frequently in these women.

DRUGS

The goal of therapy for asthmatic pregnant women is to prevent the bronchospastic episodes that cause maternal and fetal hypoxia. Although some of the drugs used have possible teratogenic effects, the fetus is at less risk than if exposed to repeated episodes of maternal bronchospasm and hypoxia.[8]

β-Sympathomimetics

Very little data are available concerning the teratogenic effects of β-sympathomimetic drugs in humans. High-dose therapy for uterine relaxation during premature labor may cause tachycardia, hypotension, and acute pulmonary edema. Albuterol, a β_2-sympathomimetic, has been associated with uterine hemorrhage during spontaneous abortion. Despite these risks, the β_2 selective sympathomimetics for bronchodilation are extremely useful when used in conjunction with a nebulizer or a hand-held inhaler for management of the pregnant patient with asthma.

Stimulation of β-adrenergic receptors in the lung leads to the activation of adenylate cyclase, which catalyzes the breakdown of ATP to form cAMP. cAMP then activates protein kinase, leading to the phosphorylation of certain proteins within the cell. These proteins cause the uncoupling of actin-myosin in smooth muscle fibers, causing bronchial smooth muscle relaxation.

Corticosteroids

The safety of corticosteroid use during pregnancy is yet undetermined. Some studies have shown an association between steroid use and an increase in stillbirths, intrauterine growth retardation, and cleft palate, whereas others have shown no increased risk. Again, the prevention of fetal hypoxia by adequately treating the mother is the primary concern and outweighs the small likelihood of teratogenic effects. The systemic effects of inhaled steroids are markedly reduced in the nonpregnant patient, and use of inhaled steroids has now become an integral component in the step care approach to asthma. Beclomethasone by inhaler will decrease systemic absorption and limit adverse side effects in the mother. If systemic steroids are needed, the lowest effective dose should be used, preferably given every other day.

Intravenous steroids are effective but take hours to produce an effect, so, if needed in an acute asthmatic attack, they should be given early in the therapy. The mechanism of action is believed to be direct dilation of large and small bronchi and interference with the synthesis and action of biochemical mediators of asthma.

Theophylline

Although widely used and effective in treating asthmatic patients, theophylline is falling into disfavor because of the adverse systemic side effects and the concern about maintaining therapeutic levels while monitoring drug levels to prevent toxicity. The theophylline compounds appear to be free of teratogenic effects. The doses required during pregnancy should be continued. throughout parturition. Because clearance of the drug may be unchanged or decreased during pregnancy, close monitoring of blood levels for evidence of toxicity is a necessity. Theophylline is a potent relaxant of uterine musculature and, as such, may prolong labor. However, prevention of bronchospasm certainly outweighs the risk of prolonging labor. Because theophylline easily crosses the placenta, fetal heart tracings may demonstrate decreased variability. Approximately 10 percent of neonates will have transient tachycardia and jitteriness (even though maternal serum concentrations were therapeutic). The elimination half-life of theophylline is prolonged in neonates, so they should be closely monitored for signs of toxicity if exposed to the drug in utero.

Cromolyn

Cromolyn is not a bronchodilator. It works by protecting against various indirect bronchoconstrictor stimuli. It is not efficacious in all patients and it is difficult to predict which patients will respond. No significant problems have been noted when cromolyn sodium is used during pregnancy. If effective, it should be continued through the pregnancy.

Antihistamines

Antihistamines have been used during pregnancy with apparent safety. However, in premature infants, a strong association between retrolental fibroplasia and maternal antihistamine use during the last 2 weeks of pregnancy has been established. Therefore, these drugs should be avoided during the last 2 weeks of pregnancy.

ACUTE ASTHMA

As mentioned above, slight exacerbations of asthma in the pregnant patient may lead to life-threatening hypoxemia. Patients present with chest tightness, dyspnea, cough, and wheezing. In cases of severe asthma, wheezing may not be present if very little air is being expelled with ventilation. The PCO_2 in the pregnant patient normally ranges from 30 to 35 mmHg. If the PCO_2 rises above 35 mmHg, it may signify a tiring patient with impending respiratory failure. Supplemental oxygen should be the first priority in treatment. A B_2 sympathomimetic such as albuterol or metaproterenol may be administered by metered-dose inhaler or nebulizer. If prompt relief is not obtained, subcutaneous epinephrine 0.3 ml of a 1:1000 solution or terbutaline 0.25 mg should be given. Parenteral steroid administration should be considered if the patient fails to respond to the β-sympathomimetics. Hydrocortisone 100 to 200 mg may be administered intravenously every 4 to 6 hours. Aminophylline may be added if the patient is still unresponsive to the above therapies. The loading dose is 5 to 6 mg/kg over 20 minutes, to a maximum of 400 mg. If the patient has been taking theophylline but has inadequate levels, 2.5 mg/kg over 20 minutes is infused. A continuous infusion is then begun at a rate of 0.5 mg/kg/h in normal patients. If the mother is a smoker, 0.7 mg/kg/h is infused; coexisting heart or liver disease will necessitate a decrease in the dose to 0.3 mg/kg/h.

LABOR AND DELIVERY

Epidural anesthesia is the preferred method of pain relief during labor. This has the effect of decreasing stress, anxiety, and hyperventilation, which may be stimuli for bronchospasm in the asthmatic patient. Low concentrations of local anesthetics are used to prevent excessive motor block. A continuous epidural infusion of 0.125 percent bupivacaine with fentanyl 1 to 2 μg/ml is used to maintain adequate sensory anesthesia. Antiasthmatic medication can be continued throughout labor with the understanding that it will decrease uterine contractility and may retard the progress of labor.

CESAREAN DELIVERY

Regional anesthesia is the technique of choice for the parturient undergoing cesarean delivery. It is preferable to use a controlled continuous epidural or subarachnoid anesthetic to control the level of block. Subarachnoid anesthesia has the disadvantage of producing a two or three segments higher level of motor block than epidural anesthesia. This may decrease expiratory reserve volume and lessen the ability to cough. Because a less-dense block is achieved with an epidural anesthetic, patients may experience more discomfort with uterine and peritoneal traction. Fentanyl 50 μg diluted in 10 ml of preservative-free normal saline or local anesthetic injected epidurally will relieve this discomfort. Adequate hydration and supplemental oxygen are necessary as with all regional anesthetics. Sedation and other respiratory depressants should be avoided or minimized.

GENERAL ANESTHESIA

If needed, general anesthesia using a rapid-sequence induction and cricoid pressure must be performed to prevent the likelihood of regurgitation and gastric aspiration. Sodium citrate 0.3 mol/L 30 ml is administered prior to induction. Thiopental 4mg/kg pregnant bodyweight (PBW) may be used for induction; however, ketamine may prevent or reverse bronchospasm and is the induction agent of choice. When used in conjunction with aminophylline, it does not increase the incidence of arrhythmias but will lower the seizure threshold. Emergence reactions can occur but are sufficiently reduced with small amounts of a benzodiazepine. A bolus of succinylcholine 1.5 mg/kg PBW during induction to facilitate intubation and by infusion for maintenance of muscle relaxation is recommended. Curare, metocurine, and atracurium should be avoided because of their histamine-releasing properties. Potent inhaled agents (halothane, isoflurane, and enflurane) all have excellent bronchodilating effects and should be used for maintenance of anesthesia. The patient is extubated only after demonstrating the ability to protect her airway with intact reflexes.

CIGARETTE SMOKING

Women who continue to smoke are treated similarly to asthmatics in that they have very reactive airways. Regional anesthesia is preferred for labor and vaginal or cesarean delivery. If general anesthesia is necessary, the same precautions should be taken as with asthmatic patients, with special attention to the management of secretions with an antimuscarinic agent.

REFERENCES

1. Sly RM: Increase in death from asthma. Ann Allergy 53:20, 1984
2. Lemanske RF, Kaliner M: Late-phase IgE mediated reactions. J Clin Immunol 8:1, 1988
3. Bone RC: A step care strategy for asthma management. J Respir Dis 9(11):104, 1988
4. Bone RC: Step care for asthma. JAMA 260:543, 1988
5. Schaefer G, Silverman F: Pregnancy complicated by asthma. Am J Obstet Gynecol 82:182, 1961
6. Gordon M, Niswander KR, Berendes H, Kantor AG: Fetal morbidity following potentially anoxigenic obstetrical conditions. VIII. Bronchial asthma. Am J Obstet Gynecol 106:421, 1970
7. Bahna SL, Erkedalt BJ: The course and outcome of pregnancy in women with bronchial asthma. Acta Allergy 27:397, 1972
8. Sinaiko RJ, German DF: Perspective on asthma in pregnancy. West J Med 131:315, 1979

ENDOCRINE DISEASE

The anesthesiologist often is confronted with a parturient with endocrine disease who requires anesthesia for vaginal or cesarean delivery or surgical removal of an endocrine gland. It is important to be aware of the normal changes in endocrine physiology that occur during pregnancy and the specific abnormalities associated with hyposecretion or hypersecretion in disease states. This section focuses on the clinical manifestations and anesthetic considerations related to particular disease states.

THYROID DISEASE

Thyroid disease is one of the more common endocrine disorders occurring during pregnancy. The normal physiologic changes that occur during pregnancy can confuse the clinical presentation of thyroid disease and make the diagnosis of pathologic states more difficult.[1]

Nontoxic Goiter

A simple nontoxic goiter may increase in size during pregnancy because of a relative iodine deficiency that is caused by an increased glomerular filtration rate and renal excretion of iodide.[2]

Clinical Presentation. Clinical manifestations may include dyspnea, dysphagia, and changes in phonation.

Anesthetic Considerations. The potential for airway obstruction exists if the gland has extended retrosternally or has enlarged significantly. Accordingly, regional anesthesia may be a preferred technique for vaginal or cesarean delivery.[2]

Hyperthyroidism

Graves' disease, also known as diffuse toxic goiter, is the most frequent cause of thyrotoxicosis during pregnancy. Other causes include toxic nodular goiter, toxic multinodular goiter, hydatidiform moles, and choriocarcinoma.[1]

Clinical Presentation. The euthyroid pregnant patient may have many of the hyperdynamic signs and symptoms typically associated with hyperthyroidism. Common findings include amenorrhea, tachycardia, systolic flow murmur associated with increased cardiac output, heat intolerance, increased skin temperature, diarrhea, and nervousness. Weight gain as a result of pregnancy may obscure weight loss associated with hyperthyroidism. Eye changes, including exophthalmos and lid lag, are typical of Graves' disease. These changes, however, do not necessarily suggest a thyrotoxic state. Hyperemesis gravidarum may be the presenting sign of thyrotoxicosis in the parturient. The laboratory diagnosis of hyperthyroidism in pregnancy is difficult since estrogen-induced increases in thyroxine-binding globulin result in elevations of plasma thyroxine concentrations and a tri-iodothyronine resin uptake in the hypothyroid range.[1]

Anesthetic Considerations. Elective surgery should be deferred until the parturient is clinically euthyroid. If emergency surgery is necessary in the thyrotoxic patient, the anesthesiologist should avoid the administration of medications that stimulate the sympathetic nervous system and should achieve an adequate depth of anesthesia prior to surgical stimulation.[3] Plasma concentrations of catecholamines are not elevated in the hyperthyroid patient. The hyperdynamic circulatory state of hyperthyroidism was thought to result from increased sensitivity to catecholamines. However, it is generally accepted that sensitivity to catecholamines is not changed by thyroid dysfunction.[4]

Adequate premedication is important in order to decrease unnecessary catecholamine release. A benzodiazepine is a reasonable choice.[5] Generally, the use of an anticholinergic drug is contraindicated since these drugs may aggravate a tachycardia and inhibit heat loss.[2]

A thiobarbiturate is an accepted choice for induction because its thiourea structure has antithyroid properties. However, the clinical significance of the thiobarbiturate's antithyroid activity has not been demonstrated.[6] Ketamine is a poor choice because it can stimulate the sympathetic nervous system. With regard to muscle relaxants, pancuronium should be avoided because of its ability to increase the heart rate and stimulate the sympathetic nervous system. Drugs that minimally affect the cardiovascular system are the most rational choices.[5]

General anesthesia in the obstetric patient requires intubation of the trachea. Regional anesthesia is an attractive technique for the hyperthyroid parturient, because the potential for airway obstruction or inability to secure an airway due to an enlarged thyroid gland may be avoided. Historically, intraspinal anesthesia has been used in combination with general anesthesia in thyrotoxic patients to achieve a decreased heart rate and blood pressure during surgery. A sensory level of T4–T5 was achieved with the purpose of blocking the sympathetic innervation of the adrenal medulla and decreasing secretion of epinephrine.[6] The sympathetic blockade associated with a regional technique may be desirable. The potential disadvantage, however, is hypotension requiring pharmacologic support. Hyperthyroid patients may have an exaggerated response to sympathomimetic drugs. Although phenylephrine is a recommended direct-acting vasopressor, any vasopressor should be titrated to desired effect.

Superficial and deep cervical plexus block combined with local infiltration is an excellent choice for thyroid surgery in the pregnant patient. However, the addition of epinephrine to local anesthetics may precipitate unwanted hemodynamic responses associated with its systemic absorption.[5]

Hemodynamic problems in the thyrotoxic parturient in labor or undergoing surgery include tachycardia, hypertension, and increased cardiac output, which may result in cardiac decompensation and arrhythmias. β-blockers are effective in attenuating manifestations of excess sympathetic activity. Other emergency drugs include lidocaine for ventricular arrhythmias, steroids, and hypotensive agents such as sodium nitroprusside.[2]

An increased basal metabolic rate and oxygen consumption[7] in the parturient warrant continuous monitoring of oxygen saturation and arterial blood gases as needed. Capnography is essential during general anesthesia. A cooling blanket, cold intravenous fluids, and ice should be available to treat intraoperative hyperthermia.[2]

Thyroid Storm

Thyroid storm is a dangerous exacerbation of hyperthyroidism. Precipitating factors include stresses such as labor, cesarean delivery and infection.[1]

Clinical Manifestations. Clinical manifestations of thyroid storm include hyperpyrexia, severe dehydration, tachycardia, atrial fibrillation, extreme anxiety, altered consciousness, and hemodynamic instability leading to cardiovascular collapse.[2]

Anesthetic Considerations. The anesthetic considerations are the same as those described for hyperthyroidism.

Hypothyroidism

Hypothyroidism is uncommon in term pregnancy because it is associated with an increased incidence of spontaneous abortion. It is usually iatrogenic following surgery or radioactive iodine therapy.[1]

Clinical Presentation. Pregnant euthyroid women have many of the signs and symptoms associated with hypothyroidism. Mild hypothyroidism may be difficult to diagnose until the increased requirements for thyroid function during pregnancy stress the parturient.[2] Usual symptoms include fatigue, cold intolerance, cool dry skin, coarse hair, periorbital edema, hoarseness, constipation, and a decreased ability to concentrate. Delayed deep tendon reflexes, edema, cardiomegaly, and congestive heart failure secondary to decreased myocardial contractility may be present.[7] Pleural and pericardial effusions, mild anemia, and hypercholesterolemia also are consistent with the diagnosis. An electrocardiogram may demonstrate a sinus bradycardia and low-voltage complexes.[2]

Anesthetic Considerations. The hypothyroid parturient may present for emergency vaginal or cesarean delivery. These patients may be more sensitive to narcotics, sedatives, and general anesthesia. Hypoxic ventilatory drive is decreased in both hypothyroid and myxedematous patients. A decreased hypercapnic ventilatory drive has been documented in patients with myxedema; however, it is not significantly depressed in patients with hypothyroidism. Although there is little evidence that decreased ventilatory drive alone causes respiratory failure, when combined with other factors, for example, sedatives or opioids, respiratory failure may occur.[8] Metabolism of drugs, particularly opioids, may be slowed.[5] These patients demonstrate bradycardia and decreased myocardial contractility,[7] resulting in a decreased cardiac output. When cardiac output is decreased, the anesthesiologist should anticipate a delayed induction with intravenous agents as well as a more rapid induction with inhaled agents.

Hypothyroid patients typically have decreased intravascular fluid volume. Accordingly, the risks of hypotension secondary to blood loss or a sympathetic blockade from a regional anesthetic are increased. Careful preoperative hydration is recommended. Ephedrine is a useful drug to treat hypotension.[5]

When managing the hypothyroid patient, the usual doses of muscle relaxants may result in a prolonged neuromuscular block. In addition, hypoglycemia may develop secondary to thyroid hormone replacement.[5] In long-standing or severe disease, adrenal suppression may occur, requiring steroid supplementation. Moreover, these patients have an impaired clearance of free water, resulting in hyponatremia. They are also prone to develop hypothermia, which may be prevented by warming intravenous fluids, using a heating blanket, increasing the room temperature, and humidifying gases during general anesthesia.[2]

ADRENAL DISORDERS

Pheochromocytoma

The occurrence of pheochromocytoma during pregnancy is rare and coincidental. However, the associated maternal and fetal morbidity and mortality are extremely high.[1]

Clinical Presentation. The severity of symptoms is related to the amount of catecholamines released. Both α-adrenergic and β-adrenergic effects may be present. Classic symptoms include anxiety, headache, diaphoresis, palpitations with arrhythmias, blurred vision, heat intolerance, and excessive weight loss.[1] Paroxysmal hypertension is not usually associated with proteinuria or edema. The patient may present with hypotension.[9] Prolonged α-adrenergic stimulation may result in decreased plasma volume with orthostatic hypotension and a falsely elevated hematocrit.[10] Episodic attacks may be precipitated by a mechanical effect of the uterus, uterine contractions, fetal movement, or changes in posture.[2]

Anesthetic Considerations. The parturient with a pheochromocytoma that is well controlled by medical therapy may delivery vaginally at term or by elective cesarean delivery followed by excision of the tumor. The safety of adrenergic-blocking drugs during pregnancy has not been established. However, it may be assumed that fetal survival is improved with adequate control of maternal hypertension with α-blockers.[11] In the nonobstetric population, commonly used α-blockers include phentolamine, phenoxybenzamine, and prazosin.[9] Once α-adrenergic blockade is established, tachycardia and arrhythmias may be controlled with β-blockers. Suggested β-blockers include propranolol, labetalol, and esmolol. β-Blockers may decrease the fetal heart rate and increase uterine activity.[12]

It is important to avoid factors that precipitate catecholamine release, including hypoxia, hypercarbia, and hypotension. Hypotension associated with epidural or subarachnoid anesthesia may precipitate catecholamine release and a hypertensive crisis. Therefore, careful intravascular volume expansion is essential prior to initiating a regional technique. Cousins and Rubin reported the successful use of epidural sympathetic blockade combined with a light general anesthetic in a young patient for surgical removal of a pheochromocytoma. The claimed advantages include cardiovascular stability by deafferentation of the operative site, sympathetic blockade and systemic effects of local anesthetics. In contrast to deep general anesthesia, myocardial contractility is preserved and the myocardial and peripheral circulation are able to respond appropriately to catecholamines following tumor removal.[13]

It is essential to maintain uterine displacement in the obstetric patient. Prudent monitoring includes the standard intraoperative monitors, direct arterial and central venous pressure monitoring, and a Foley catheter for urinary output.[9]

It is reasonable to avoid those drugs that have been known to cause a pressor response or tachycardia. Drugs that have been implicated include droperidol, anticholinergic drugs, succinylcholine, and drugs that release histamine, pancuronium, and halothane.[9] Halothane has a greater propensity to cause arrhythmias in the presence of elevated catecholamines compared with enflurane and isoflurane. Drugs that have been used safely in the nonobstetric population include fentanyl, alfentanil, etomidate, and vecuronium.

Sodium nitroprusside, nitroglycerin, prazosin, and magnesium sulfate have all been advocated for the control of hypertension during surgery.[9]

Patients with a pre-existing cardiomyopathy may experience cardiac failure and hypotension following removal of the pheochromocytoma and source of catecholamines.[2]

Cushing's Syndrome

Excess circulating glucocorticoids secondary to adrenal adenomas, adrenal hyperplasia, or exogenous corticosteroid therapy result in Cushing's syndrome.[1] In general, ovulation and pregnancy are rare in patients with Cushing's syndrome.[2]

Clinical Presentation. Clinical manifestations of Cushing's syndrome closely resemble changes in normal pregnancy. Classic signs and symptoms include weight gain, hypertension, abdominal striae, edema, and increased pigmentation.[2] Other features include hypokalemia, hypernatremia, hyperglycemia, skeletal muscle weakness, central obesity, moon-shaped facies, "buffalo hump," hirsutism, osteoporosis, easy bruise-ability, and psychosis.

Anesthetic Considerations. General considerations for the parturient with Cushing's syndrome include appropriate management of hypertension, normalization of volume status, regulation of serum glucose concentrations with insulin therapy, and maintenance normal electrolyte balance. Hydralazine has been recommended as antihypertensive therapy. Hypokalemia can occur secondary to an increased excretion of potassium, resulting in muscular weakness and a decreased ability to cough postoperatively. Spironolactone, a potassium-sparing diuretic, is a rational choice for normalization of volume status.[2]

Preoperative steroid coverage is required in spite of increased cortisol levels because of an impaired pituitary adrenal response to stress.[2]

The potential for a difficult airway exists because the patient may be obese and have a thick stature. One should consider an awake intubation using topical anesthesia. Regional anesthesia may be technically difficult secondary to obesity and vertebral osteoporosis. Care must be taken in moving and positioning the patient to avoid pathologic fractures.[2]

The incidence of spontaneous abortion, stillbirths, and premature deliveries is increased in this patient population.[1]

Adrenocortical Insufficiency

Adrenal insufficiency, also known as Addison's disease, is the most common disorder of the adrenal gland to occur in pregnant patients.[2] Adrenal insufficiency may occur as a result of destruction of the adrenal cortex or as a result of a deficiency of adrenocorticotropic hormone (ACTH). It also commonly occurs in patients on long-term steroid therapy who are exposed to an acute stress or abruptly stop their medications.[5]

Clinical Presentation. Addison's disease may have an indolent course or present acutely with life-threatening cardiovascular collapse. Nonspecific symptoms include malaise, weight loss, nausea and vomiting, constipation, weakness, and increased skin pigmentation. These findings may be confused with changes in normal pregnancy. Other symptoms include hypotension, syncope, abdominal pain, and hypoglycemia.[2] These patients have a decreased intravascular volume, cardiac output, and decreased renal perfusion.[1] Addison's disease may be tolerated better than expected during pregnancy because of the placental transfer of corticosteroids from the fetus to the mother.[14] The diuresis and dehydration that occur postpartum may precipitate an addisonian crisis.[1] Metabolic abnormalities include hyponatremia, hyperkalemia, increased urinary excretion of sodium, and low plasma steroid levels.[5]

Anesthetic Considerations. Addisonian patients are hypovolemic.[1] Prior to inducing general anesthesia or employing a regional technique, intravascular volume expansion and steroid supplementation are essential. Dextrose-containing crystalloid solutions are a reasonable choice given patients' propensity to develop hypoglycemia.[2] These patients are also especially sensitive to drug-induced myocardial depression. Invasive monitoring of arterial and central venous pressure is reasonable to consider. An effort should be made to measure electrolyte concentrations and maintain normal electrolyte balance. Initial doses of muscle relaxants should be reduced because of these patients' baseline muscle weakness.[5]

PARATHYROID DISORDERS

Hyperparathyroidism

Parathyroid adenoma is the most common cause of hyperparathyroidism in pregnancy. Labor and delivery usually proceed uneventfully, however, the incidence of spontaneous abortions, stillbirths, premature labor, and neonatal tetany is increased.[2]

Clinical Presentation. Clinical manifestations of hyperparathyroidism include hyperemesis, generalized weakness, anorexia, lethargy, polyuria, polydypsia, hypertension, and constipation. Complications also include renal calculi, pancreatitis, and psychiatric disorders. Signs of hypercalcemic crisis include mental deterioration, coma, renal failure, arrhythmias, and congestive heart failure. In the normal parturient, serum calcium levels are decreased. The decrease in serum calcium levels has been attributed to hypoalbuminemia of pregnancy, the transfer of calcium to the fetus, and the increase in renal blood flow and glomerular filtration of calcium. Therefore, serum calcium levels may be normal in the hyperthyroid patient.[1]

Anesthetic Considerations. Anesthetic management includes maintaining adequate hydration and urine output. Electrocardiographic monitoring may detect hypercalcemia by a decreased QT interval. Patients should be carefully positioned because of osteoporosis and susceptibility to pathologic fractures. There is no evidence that specific anesthetic drugs or techniques are better than others. Patients seem to have an unpredictable response to neuromuscular blockers, therefore, monitoring with a peripheral nerve stimulator is prudent.[5]

Hypoparathyroidism

Hypoparathyroidism is uncommon in pregnancy and usually is a consequence of unintentional parathyroidectomy during thyroid surgery. Symptoms may become obvious during pregnancy because of fetal calcium demands.[2]

Clinical Presentation. Signs and symptoms include paresthesias, fatigue, muscle weakness, numbness, tetany with carpopedal spasms, convulsions, and laryngeal stridor. Other clinical features include mental status changes, dry rough skin, patchy hair distribution, and cataracts. The electrocardiogram may show a long QT interval and myocardial contractility is often depressed.[5]

Anesthetic Considerations. Anesthetic management should be directed at preventing further decreases in plasma calcium concentration. A metabolic or respiratory alkalosis can rapidly decrease plasma ionized calcium concentrations.[5] Continuous epidural anesthesia can prevent hyperventilation associated with labor, consequently decreasing the likelihood of tetany associated with alkalosis and decreased ionized calcium.[2] One should also consider small doses of intravenous sedation to decrease anxiety. Hypocalcemia accompanying blood transfusion is usually a transient phenomenon.[13] Rational calcium replacement during transfusion should be based on calcium measurements.[15]

PITUITARY DISORDERS

Hypopituitarism

Panhypopituitarism can result from necrosis of the pituitary gland following shock or hemorrhage associated with delivery. Postpartum pituitary necrosis, or Sheehan's syndrome, is the most common cause of anterior pituitary insufficiency.[1]

Clinical Presentation. The clinical picture depends on the extent of damage and is related to the deficiency of hormones secreted by the ovaries, adrenal gland, and thyroid gland.[2] The presentation may be insidious, with manifestation of disease at a time of stress. The earliest sign may be failure to lactate, with breast involution postpartum. Other signs and symptoms include abnormal menses, sparse axillary and pubic hair, pale and waxy skin, fatigue, and cold intolerance.[1]

Anesthetic Considerations. The major complications associated with hypopituitarism are adrenal insufficiency and hypothyroidism. Anesthetic management is discussed in the appropriate parts of this section.

REFERENCES

1. Burrow GN, Ferris TS: Medical Complications During Pregnancy. 3rd Ed. WB Saunders, Philadelphia, 1988
2. James FM, Wheeler AS: Obstetric Anesthesia: The Complicated Patient. FA Davis, Philadelphia, 1981
3. Stehling LC: Anesthetic management of the patient with hyperthyroidism. Anesthesiology 41:585, 1974
4. Murkin JM: Anesthesia and hypothyroidism: a review of thyroxine physiology, pharmacology and anesthetic implications. Anesth Analg 61:371, 1982
5. Stoelting RK, Dierdorf SF, McCammon RL: Anesthesia and Co-Existing Disease. 2nd Ed. Churchill Livingstone, New York, 1988
6. Knight RT: The use of spinal anesthesia to control sympathetic overactivity in hyperthyroidism. Anesthesiology 6:225, 1945
7. Amidi M, Leon DF, deGroot WJ, et al: Effect of the thyroid state on myocardial contractility and ventricular ejection in rate in man. Circulation 38:229, 1968
8. Zwilich CW, Pierson DJ, Hofeldt FD, et al: Ventilatory control in myxedema and hypothyroidism. N Engl J Med 292:662, 1975
9. Hull CJ: Phaeochromocytoma diagnosis, preoperative preparation and anesthetic management. Br J Anaesth 58:1453, 1986
10. Leak D, Carroll JJ, Robinson DC, Ashforth EJ: Management of pheochromocytoma removal. Can Med Assoc J 116(4):371, 1977
11. Barash PG, Cullen BF, Stoelting RD: Clinical Anesthesia. JB Lippincott, London, 1989
12. Langer A, et al: Adrenergic blockade: a new approach to hyperthyroidism during pregnancy. Obstet Gynecol 44:181, 1974
13. Cousins MJ, Rubin RB: The intraoperative management of pheochromocytoma with total epidural sympathetic blockade. Br J Anaesth 46:78, 1974
14. Milkovic K, et al: Maintenance of the plasma corticosterone concentration of adrenalectomized rate by the fetal adrenal glands. Endocrinology 93:115, 1973
15. Denlinger JK, Nahrwold MC, Gibbs PS, Lecky JP: Hypocalcemia during rapid blood transfuction in anesthetized man. Br J Anaesth 48:995, 1976

DIABETES MELLITUS

Diabetes is the most common medical problem faced by the maternal and neonatal care team. In this section the important pathophysiologic changes that place both the mother and the baby at high risk and the appropriate anesthetic management for labor and delivery are described.

PATHOPHYSIOLOGY

Placental insufficiency is a major problem in this disease state. Nylund et al.[1] compared uteroplacental blood flow in diabetic parturients to normal pregnant patients in the last trimester of pregnancy using indium 113. There was a 35 to 45 percent decrease in placental blood flow in diabetic subjects and this problem was further aggravated by the presence of high blood glucose (uncontrolled patients). Hemoglobin A_{1c} ($HgbA_{1c}$), a poor transporter of oxygen, is increased in diabetic parturients. Determinations of $HgbA_{1c}$ concentrations have been used clinically for some time to assess the degree of glycemic control among diabetics. Maternal oxygen saturation and oxygen tension is inversely related to $HgbA_{1c}$ concentrations.[2] There will derangement of maternal oxygen transport as well as neonatal oxygen extraction in the presence of uncontrolled diabetes associated with high $HgbA_{1c}$ concentrations. It is important to remember that hypotension following regional anesthesia will further decrease placental perfusion and fetal oxygenation, causing neonatal acidosis. Ketoacidosis has become a rare entity because of aggressive prenatal care. However, it still poses a significant threat to fetal well-being and remains the major cause of neonatal mortality. Uncontrolled diabetes-associated infection and treatment with β-mimetic drugs and dexamethasone for prematurity will increase the chance of ketoacidosis.

Besides these important pathologic changes, some important obstetric conditions are more commonly associated with the diabetic pregnancy (e.g., pregnancy-induced hypertension, premature labor, abruptio placentae, macrosomia and other major fetal congenital anomalies). The anesthesiologist should always be prepared to take care of the emergency situations that might necessitate urgent cesarean delivery.

CLASSIFICATION

In 1949, Dr. Priscilla White proposed a classification of diabetic pregnancy[3] based on criteria that could be identified at the time of the patient's first prenatal visit, including the age of onset and duration of diabetes and the presence or absence of micro- or macrovascular complications. Recently, White's classification has undergone some modifications and the present classification can be summarized as follows:

Class A: Abnormal carbohydrate tolerance in the non-pregnant state, not requiring insulin either prior to or during the pregnancy
Class B: Duration of diabetes less than 10 years
Class C: Duration of diabetes 10 to 20 years
Class D: Duration more than 20 years
Class F: Associated diabetic nephropathy
Class R: Associated retinitis proliferans
Class T: Associated renal transplant
Class H: Insulin requiring diabetes associated with coronary artery disease.

ANESTHETIC MANAGEMENT

Labor and Delivery

Early labor pain can be controlled with small doses of infusion opioids with or without a tranquilizer. Epidural anesthesia should be used for proper control of well-established labor pain and, provided there is no associated maternal hypotension, this technique has distinct advantages. Because the pain and anxiety of labor associated with increased catecholamine levels can further decrease the placental perfusion, epidural anesthesia, by decreasing catecholamine release, will increase placental perfusion.[4] Epidural anesthesia will reduce the maternal lactic acid production and, hence, fetal acidosis.[5] Epidural anesthesia will provide excellent sensory anesthesia for forceps delivery as well as appropriate anesthesia for emergent cesarean delivery for fetal distress. Subarachnoid anesthesia can also be used for forceps or cesarean delivery. A separate intravenous line for the rapid infusion of nondextrose-containing crystalloid solution to prevent hypotension may be necessary. Maternal hypotension should be treated aggressively in these patients with ephedrine.

Cesarean Delivery

Anesthetic management of the diabetic parturient requires meticulous attention to avoid anesthesia-related problems. In 1977, Datta and Brown observed a higher incidence of fetal acidosis in infants of diabetic mothers (IDM) compared to normal infants when their mothers received subarachnoid anesthesia instead of general anesthesia.[6] The effect of maternal hypotension was significantly more profound in these IDM. In a subsequent study by Datta et al. using epidural anesthesia, fetal acidosis was found to be related to both the severity of maternal diabetes and to the presence of maternal hypotension.[7] The genesis of fetal acidosis is complex; however, a number of factors may be related. An in vitro study has demonstrated increased lactic acid production from the human placenta in the presence of hypoxia, especially in the presence of higher glycogen content, which is normal in the placentas of diabetic parturients. Clinically, hypoxia can occur in association with hypotension following regional anesthesia. Hyperglycemia in the presence of hypoxia can produce lactic acidosis.

In our first two studies regarding diabetic parturients, we used acute intravascular volume expansion with 5 percent dextrose in Ringer's lactate solution, as this was the solution of choice for volume expansion at that time. Hypotension following regional anesthesia in the presence of hyperglycemia might have produced lactic acidosis and consequent fetal acidosis. An experimental study in animals has shown that infusion of insulin into the umbilical artery will increase glucose utilization, causing reduced fetal oxygenation and, ultimately, fetal acidosis.[8] This condition can exist if the diabetes of these mothers is not properly controlled, because this will increase fetal glucose concentrations and consequently fetal insulin secretion.

In 1982, Datta et al. repeated their previous study using subarachnoid anesthesia in diabetic parturients following a strict protocol that included (1) rigidly controlled diabetic parturients (80 to 120 mg/dl for fasting blood glucose), (2) non-dextrose-containing solution for volume expansion (Ringer's lactate), and (3) aggressive treatment of maternal hypotension so that none of the maternal systolic blood pressures fell below 100 mmHg.[9] In this particular study, the neonatal acid-base values in IDM were similar to infants of normal parturients.

Both subarachnoid and epidural anesthesia, if properly performed, can be used for these parturients and provide good neonatal outcome; however, epidural anesthesia might be preferable in patients with severe diabetes (class F, R, T, H) because of a higher incidence of abrupt hypotension associated with subarachnoid anesthesia. Separate intravenous lines may be necessary for acute intravascular volume expansion with non-dextrose-containing crystalloid solution. For general anesthesia, one should be aware of a number of important issues; for example, the increased gastric stasis in diabetic patients and juvenile-onset diabetic patients may be associated with "stiff joint syndrome" and the possibility of difficult intubation.

Neonatal resuscitation is very important for the IDM because of increased chances of macrosomia, respiratory distress syndrome, hypoglycemia, and other major congenital anomalies.

Finally, one should be aware of the dramatic decrease in insulin requirement immediately after delivery of the diabetic parturient.[10] Determination of blood glucose in the recovery room is mandatory.

REFERENCES

1. Nylund L, Lunell NO, Lewander R, Persson B, et al: Uteroplacental blood flow in diabetic pregnancy: measurements with indium-113m and a computer linked gamma camera. Am J Obstet Gynecol 144:298, 1976
2. Madsen H, Ditzel J: Changes in red blood cell oxygen transport in diabetic pregnancy. Am J Obstet Gynecol 143:421, 1982
3. White P: Pregnancy complicating diabetes. Am J Med 7:609, 1949
4. Shnider SM, Abboud T, Artal R: Maternal endogenous catecholamine decrease during labor after epidural anesthesia. Am J Obstet Gynecol 147:13, 1983
5. Pearson JF: The effect of continuous lumbar epidural block on maternal and fetal acid-base balance during labor and at delivery. p. 26. In Proceedings of the Symposium on Epidural Analgesia in Obstetrics. HK Lewis, London, 1968
6. Datta S, Brown WU: Acid-base status in diabetic mothers and their infants following general or spinal anesthesia for cesarean section. Anesthesiology 47:272, 1977
7. Datta S, Brown WU, Ostheimer GW, et al: Epidural anesthesia for cesarean section in diabetic parturients: maternal and neonatal acid-base status and bupivacaine concentration. Anesth Analg 60:574, 1981
8. Milley JR, Rosenberg AA, Phillips AF, et al: The effect of insulin on ovine fetal oxygen extraction. Am J Obstet Gynecol 149:673, 1984
9. Datta S, Kitzmiller JL, Naulty JS, et al: Acid-base status of diabetic mothers and their infants following spinal anesthesia for cesarean section. Anesth Anagl 61:662, 1982
10. Soler NG, Malins JM: Diabetic pregnancy: management on the day of delivery. Diabetologica 15:441, 1978

HEPATIC DISEASE

Although most of the common forms of liver disease occur during pregnancy, viral hepatitis is the most common cause of hepatic dysfunction and jaundice. It is important to be aware of the normal physiologic changes in liver function associated with pregnancy in order to recognize disease processes (see Ch. 1). This section discusses those liver disorders unique to pregnancy.

CHOLESTASIS OF PREGNANCY

Intrahepatic cholestasis of pregnancy is a syndrome most probably related to the deposition of bile acids in the skin, which causes a bothersome pruritus. It is unclear if there is an unusual sensitivity to bile acids secondary to increased estrogen production during pregnancy. An increased incidence occurs among Scandinavians and Chileans.

There is an increased risk of prematurity and fetal death. Fetal distress has been documented to occur in one-third of patients, leading to a cesarean delivery rate of 30 to 60 percent. Fifty percent of infants are born prematurely.

Clinical Presentation

Pruritus is the classic presenting feature at the beginning of the third trimester, usually involving the trunk, extremities, palms, and soles. As a consequence of the extremely bothersome pruritus, it may be associated with insomnia, fatigue, and mental disturbances. Other clinical manifestations include dark urine, mild jaundice, and light-colored stools. Interestingly, the patient usually feels well.

Anesthetic Considerations

The prothrombin time is usually normal unless there is significant vitamin K malabsorption secondary to administration of cholestyramine, a drug used to alleviate the pruritus. One should check the coagulation profile prior to instituting a regional anesthetic.

There is an increased risk of postpartum hemorrhage secondary to vitamin K deficiency. Parenteral vitamin K therapy should be considered in patients near term with a coagulopathy.

The choice of anesthesia will depend on the coagulation profile.

ACUTE FATTY LIVER OF PREGNANCY

The etiology of acute fatty liver of pregnancy is unknown, although tetracycline has been implicated. The maternal and fetal morbidity and mortality is 85 to 90 percent in the untreated patient. Immediate delivery has reduced maternal mortality to 10 to 33 percent. However, fetal mortality remains higher secondary to an increased incidence of stillbirths. If unrecognized and untreated, the disease may progress to fulminant hepatic failure, encephalopathy, disseminated intravascular coagulation (DIC), uncontrolled gastrointestinal and uterine bleeding, and death. The incidence is higher in young, primiparous women giving birth to twins or male infants.

Clinical Presentation

Acute fatty liver of pregnancy typically presents in the 36th to 40th week of gestation, however, it may present as early as the 30th week. Symptoms include headache, malaise, fatigue, severe and persistent vomiting, diffuse abdominal pain, or pain localized to right upper quadrant or back. Jaundice and fever occur in one-half of patients. Mild hypertension and peripheral edema suggest pregnancy-induced hypertension. There is usually evidence of DIC. Hepatic encephalopathy and coma are late ominous manifestations.

Anesthetic Considerations

Prompt delivery is imperative for reversal of clinical findings. Anesthetic technique depends on the stage of disease. Early in the disease, coagulation abnormalities may not be severe, permitting a regional technique. The patient with advanced disease, including encephalopathy and DIC, will require a general anesthetic. Correction of coagulation abnormalities may require transfusion of blood products. One must monitor glucose and electrolytes. The patient must be observed for signs of hemorrhage.

HEPATIC INVOLVEMENT IN PREGNANCY-INDUCED HYPERTENSION, PREECLAMPSIA, AND ECLAMPSIA

The liver may be involved in pregnancy-induced hypertension, preeclampsia, or eclampsia as an aspect of a generalized vascular disorder. An estimated 50 percent of patients have liver function abnormalities.

Clinical Presentation

Patients with preeclampsia or eclampsia usually present in the third trimester. Signs and symptoms include hypertension, proteinuria, nausea, vomiting, epigastric pain, and DIC. The combination of microangiopathic hemolytic anemia, elevation in liver enzymes, and thrombocytopenia has been called the *HELLP syndrome.* Hepatic rupture and subcapsular hematoma may occur. Clinical findings associated with hepatic rupture include severe epigastric pain or right upper quadrant pain, shock, oliguria, fever, and leukocytosis.

Anesthetic Considerations

Prompt delivery and appropriate management of preeclampsia or eclampsia with particular attention to airway and fluid management are essential. The coagulation profile should be checked prior to instituting a regional anesthetic.

SUGGESTED READINGS

1. Burrow GM, Ferris TS: Medical Complications During Pregnancy. 3rd Ed. WB Saunders, Philadelphia, 1988
2. James FM, Wheeler AS: Obstetric anesthesia: The Complicated Patient. FA Davis, Philadelphia, 1982
3. Kaplan MM: Acute fatty liver of pregnancy. N Engl J Med 313:367, 1985
4. Stoelting RK, Dierdorf SF, McCammon RL: Anesthesia and Co-Existing Disease. 2nd Ed. Churchill Livingstone, New York, 1988

RENAL DISEASE

Renal disease during pregnancy potentially poses serious risks to the parturient and fetus. Progression of renal dysfunction may occur, predisposing to both increased maternal morbidity and mortality and a suboptimal fetal environment, which results in a higher incidence of intrauterine and peripartal complications. Ideally it is important to diagnose and control preexisting renal disorders prior to conception. Renal function should be monitored closely during pregnancy, which imposes significant physiologic changes even on the normal kidney.

Renal blood flow (RBF) and the glomerular filtration rate (GFR) begin to rise early in pregnancy and remain elevated 50 percent above nonpregnant values until 4 to 6 weeks before term, when a slight decrease occurs. RBF and GFR may decrease as much as 20 percent when the patient is supine compared to the left lateral position. Etiologic factors regarding the change in RBF and GFR include a parallel increase in cardiac output, a decrease in peripheral vascular resistance, and an increase in circulating volume, all due indirectly to aortocaval compression. Blood urea nitrogen (BUN) and creatinine necessarily decrease, reflecting the change in the GFR. Normal values for BUN range between 7 and 9 mg/dl, and for creatinine, between 0.35 and 0.55 mg/dl.

Tubular resorption increases proportionately to the filtered load to maintain an almost normal sodium and water balance; however, it is not unusual to see glucosuria, aminoaciduria, and proteinuria. Serum uric acid levels decrease significantly during a normal pregnancy (mean 300 mg/dl) and are considered a sensitive indicator of tubular function.[1]

In addition to functional changes, the kidney undergoes anatomic changes. It increases in weight and size, consistent with increases in vascular and interstitial volume. Dilatation of the collecting system extends to the pelvic brim. Functionally, this represents a dead space of approximately 200 ml and must be taken into account when interpreting tests of renal function. It is difficult to find strong evidence relating baseline renal function to pregnancy outcome. Pregnancy in the presence of mild disease (creatinine less than 1.4 mg/dl) without other complications such as hypertension or proteinuria is generally not associated with adverse effects on renal function or the pregnancy.[2] Moderate renal insufficiency (creatinine greater than 2.0 mg/dl) combined with significant hypertension decreases the likelihood of conception and, should conception occur, a normal pregnancy.[2] Twenty percent of these women deliver prior to 36 weeks. There are significant increases in the number of stillbirths, the frequency of growth retardation, and the neonatal death rate, as well as deterioration in maternal renal function that may or may not be reversible after delivery. The presence or absence of concurrent hypertension in the parturient with renal disease may be the single most important determinant of maternal or fetal outcome.

Fortunately, renal disease most commonly occurs in women long after their childbearing years. However, several renal disorders encountered in younger, potentially pregnant patients occur, including glomerular disease secondary to diabetes, systemic lupus erythematosus (SLE), and hypertension; transplantation; and acute renal failure.

TYPES OF RENAL DISORDERS

Glomerular Disease

Diseases of the glomerulus can be caused by infection, inflammation, and systemic disease such as diabetes and SLE. Glomerular disease is often accompanied by proteinuria, hypertension, or both. Renal function may deteriorate as the pregnancy progresses, especially with the development of preeclampsia. In fact, the incidence of preeclampsia in patients with glomerular disease accompanied by hypertension and proteinuria is as high as 50 percent.[2]

Renal involvement may or may not be evident in the pregnant diabetic woman. Glomerular function is primarily affected but renal tubules and interstitium are also at risk. Chronic pyelonephritis is sometimes seen in diabetics as a late stage of recurrent bacterial infection. Anatomic changes resulting in dilatation of the collecting system with stasis of urine may exacerbate this problem. Proteinuria may increase during pregnancy but renal function may remain stable as long as hypertension is not severe. Chances of a poor outcome markedly increase once serum creatinine is greater than 2 mg/dl.

Fifty percent of patients with lupus nephropathy with active disease near the time of conception may experience deterioration of renal function. There may also be an increased incidence of spontaneous abortion, growth retardation, stillbirths, and neonatal lupus, including pancytopenia and complete heart block. Patients with inactive disease at the time of conception fare much better, with relatively normal pregnancies in approximately 70 percent of these women.[3] Control of the disease may require glucocorticoids, cytotoxic agents, and antihypertensives. Other systemic manifestations of SLE involving the lung, heart, central nervous system, and bone marrow may complicate obstetric and anesthetic management.

Nephrotic syndrome commonly results from glomerular disease; rarely, it may be caused by renal vein thrombosis or amyloidosis. Preeclampsia is the most common cause of nephrotic syndrome arising de novo in pregnancy. Major physiologic alterations include hypoproteinemia, which alters drug binding, and a decrease in effective circulating volume. Occasionally, IgG deficiency and/or hypothyroidism may result from loss of immunoglobulins or thyroglobulins.

Hypertension is the most common medical complication of pregnancy. Because blood pressure normally falls about 10 to 15 mmHg below baseline diastolic values, diastolic pressures greater than 85 mmHg are usually abnormal. When hypertension is discovered it is important to differentiate between essential hypertension, hypertension secondary to renal disease, and preeclampsia. This may be difficult because clinically these entities are quite similar and frequently two or three may exist simultaneously. The goal of therapy is to lower blood pressure, avoiding sudden dramatic changes. Hydralazine and methyldopa have been used safely for long-term control. β-Adrenergic blockers have also been used chronically but may have adverse fetal effects such as intrauterine growth retardation and fetal bradycardia. Calcium channel blockers are not routinely used in pregnancy. Intravenous agents such as sodium nitroprusside and trimethaphan can be used to acutely control severe blood pressure elevations. Chronic hypertension and preeclampsia can decrease renal function via their pathologic alteration of glomerular blood vessels. Renal blood flow may be diminished and frequent assessment of renal function should be performed, including urinalysis, BUN, creatinine, creatinine clearance, and 24-hour protein excretion.

Acute Renal Failure

The incidence of acute renal failure (ARF) in pregnancy is approximately 1 per 10,000,[2] and is usually related to complications occurring late in pregnancy such as abruption or other causes of hemorrhage, amniotic fluid embolus, or preeclampsia/eclampsia. However, ARF may occur as the result of the superimposition of the stress of pregnancy on patients with pre-existing renal disease. Rarely, it may be caused by postpartum hemolytic uremic syndrome.[4] Measures to treat renal failure are largely supportive, such as correcting the precipitating factors and close monitoring of fluid and electrolyte and acid-base status. Central venous pressure and/or pulmonary arterial monitoring may be necessary to adequately assess circulating volume and guide hydration. An intra-arterial catheter is helpful if vasoactive drugs are used to control hypertension and if frequent blood sampling is required. Dialysis may be needed until kidney function returns. Drug doses must be adjusted in accordance with renal function. Systemic effects of renal failure on the heart (pericardial effusion, congestive heart failure), lung (interstitial infiltrates), central nervous system (increased central nervous system depression with uremia), platelets (decreased lifespan, dysfunctional), and bone marrow (anemia) need to be considered when planning anesthetic care.

Renal Transplantation

Management of the transplant patient requires knowledge of several factors: (1) natural history of the primary renal disease, (2) current renal function, (3) time of conception relative to the time of surgery, and (4) immunosuppressive drugs used to control rejection. Maternal and fetal outcome is good in approximately 70 percent of patients who are otherwise healthy with normal renal function.[3] Potential problems include increased proteinuria (which by itself doesn't contribute significantly to morbidity), progressive decline in renal function in 25 percent of patients,[2] and the development of preeclampsia and preterm labor. The risk of prematurity may be as high as 45 percent in mothers with impaired renal function and preeclampsia. Women are advised to wait at least 1 year following surgery before becoming pregnant.[2] Immunosuppressive therapy can cause predisposition to infection in the mother, premature rupture of membranes, fetal malformation, growth retardation, adrenal insufficiency, and neonatal lymphopenia during the first few weeks of life. Azidothymidine reverses the effects of nondepolarizing neuromuscular blockers, potentiates succinylcholine, and increases excitability of skeletal muscle because it inhibits phosphodiesterase. Continuous monitoring of renal function, including BUN, creatinine, creatinine clearance, degree of proteinuria, urine cultures, and blood pressure, should be performed throughout the pregnancy with tests of fetal well-being beginning at 28 weeks. Patients may deliver vaginally, however, dystocia can occur secondary to ectopic placement of the transplanted kidney. Supplemental doses of hydrocortisone should be given at the time of delivery.

ANESTHETIC MANAGEMENT

Regional Anesthesia

Anesthetic management of the parturient with renal disease presents an additional challenge to the anesthesiologist. Usual drug doses may require adjustment, renal blood flow should be optimized, and systemic effects of altered renal function must be recognized.

Regional anesthesia has the least effect on RBF and GFR provided hemodynamic stability is maintained. Continuous epidural anesthesia (CEA), in most cases, remains the method of choice for labor and delivery. Easing the pain of labor should decrease catecholamine release, thereby reducing renovascular resistance and increasing blood flow to the kidney and uterus. The advantage of CEA over subarachnoid anesthesia is that the level of sympathetic blockade can be obtained gradually, thus usually avoiding significant hypotension, with interferes with renal and uteroplacental perfusion. Ephedrine in 5 to 10 mg increments administered intravenously can be used to treat hypotension should it occur. Acute intravenous hydration prior to the induction of anesthesia should be approached carefully in a patient with impaired renal function. Central venous pressure monitoring in addition to clinical evaluation may be helpful in judging intravenous volume replacement. Tonicity and composition of the intravenous fluid chosen will depend on specific abnormalities in blood chemistries and the degree of renal impairment.

Long-term treatment with β-adrenergic blockers are a relative contraindication to regional anesthesia. β-Adrenergic agonists such as ephedrine are less effective in correcting bradycardia and hypotension resulting from sympathetic blockade and relative hypovolemia. Clotting abnormalities may preclude use of regional anesthesia. Because it is not uncommon for coagulopathies to be associated with renal disease, bleeding time, prothrombin time, partial thromboplastin time, fibrinogen, and platelet count should be obtained to assist in the pre-anesthetic evaluation.

Amide local anesthetics are metabolized by the liver and as such as generally safe for use in patients with renal disease. Ester-type local anesthetics are degraded by plasma cholinesterases and therefore are also safe; however, some chloroprocaine solutions may contain sodium bisulfite, which can produce chronic neurologic damage. In patients with pre-existing uremic neuropathy, preparations without sodium bisulfite should be used.[5]

General Anesthesia

General anesthesia should be routinely avoided except in certain emergency circumstances or when regional techniques are specifically contraindicated. Inhaled anesthetics cause varying degrees of myocardial depression and vasodilation, which results in an increase in renovascular resistance and a decrease in RBF and GFR by as much as 30 to 50 percent. An increase in pulmonary shunt coupled with anemia (seen in both pregnancy and renal disease) may predispose the patient to severe hypoxemia. Although elimination of inhaled agents does not depend on renal excretion, enflurane and methoxyflurane are metabolized to some extent, yielding nephrotoxic fluroide ions. The metabolism of isoflurane is minimal. Halothane, in combination with electrolyte and acid-base abnormalities, can provoke myocardial irritability, leading to arrhythmias.

Intravenous induction doses of barbiturates may need to be reduced to reflect hypoalbuminemia; acid–base status, which changes the ratio of ionized to nonionized drug; and impaired biotransformation in the liver in patients who are severely debilitated.

The muscle relaxant of choice for a rapid-sequence induction in the parturient with renal disease and serum potassium exceeding 5.5 mmol/L is vecuronium 0.28 mg/kg, as only 15 percent of the drug is excreted by the kidney. It may cause muscle weakness in the neonate, which requires intervention at the time of delivery. In normokalemic patients, succinylcholine can probably be used safely. Patients receiving magnesium sulfate will be much more sensitive to neuromuscular blocking agents and will require a reduction in the usual dose.

Blood pressure control during general anesthesia, especially the response to laryngoscopy and incision, can be achieved with small doses of hydralazine, realizing that excretion is prolonged when renal dysfunction is severe. Alternatively, labetalol can be used. Methyldopa is almost exclusively excreted in the urine and, therefore, the dose must be reduced. Nitroglycerin, nitroprusside, and trimethaphan, which are not metabolized or excreted via the kidneys, may be necessary for short-term antihypertensive management. β-Adrenergic blockers may decrease patient response to β-adrenergic agonists given to treat episodes of hypotension and may diminish myocardial reserve.

REFERENCES

1. Seldin DW, Giebisch G: The Kidney: Physiology and Pathophysiology. Raven Press, New York, 1985
2. Schrier R, Gottschalk: Diseases of the Kidney. 4th Ed. Little Brown, Boston, 1987
3. Harvey G, Miller J: Renal diseases in pregnancy. Obstet Gynecol Surv 40:7, 1985
4. Hayslett J: Postpartum renal failure. N Engl J Med 312:24, 1985
5. James F, Wheeler AS, Dewan D: Obstetric Anesthesia: The Complicated Patient. 2nd Ed. p. 207. F A Davis, Philadelphia, 1988
6. Katz J, Benumof J, Kadis L: Anesthesia and Uncommon Diseases. 3rd Ed. WB Saunders, Philadelphia, 1990

HEMATOLOGIC DISEASE

Parturients who have hemoglobinopathies or coagulation disorders occasionally present themselves to the obstetric anesthesiologist. Fortunately, these patients often are aware of these conditions before pregnancy and, on the advice of their obstetrician, will often seek consultation with the anesthesiologist before delivery. The full effects of some of these conditions are often evident or are unmasked as pregnancy progresses. The obstetric anesthesiologist should be aware of the possibilities of an underlying problem, have an understanding of the cause and treatment, and be cognizant of how these conditions affect the parturient and the fetus.

In this section we consider some of the more commonly encountered problems and some of the treatment options available for these patients.

HEMOGLOBINOPATHIES

Sickle Cell Disease

Sickle cell disorders have a worldwide distribution and it is likely that the state arose as identical mutations in different parts of the world.[1] Although sickle cell disease is most common in blacks and people of Mediterranean descent, it should be noted that this distribution is not limited by skin color or race. Sickle hemoglobin is inherited following mendelian law: heterozygotes (sickle cell trait) in general are asymptomatic, whereas homozygotes will demonstrate symptoms of the disease.

Pathophysiology. A single base mutation in the DNA encoding hemoglobin β-globin chain is responsible for the substitution of valine for glutamic acid at the sixth N-terminal position. This results in the polymerization of the hemoglobin under conditions of low oxygen saturation and acidosis, leading to distortion of the red cell and shortened red cell survival time. This causes hyperbilirubinemia and anemia secondary to increased hemolysis. Vaso-occlusive events result from blood vessel occlusion by clumped sickled cells, which can cause further tissue anoxia, worsening the overall condition. A long list of complications, including splenic infarct, chest syndromes (acute episodes of chest pain, pulmonary infiltrates, and fever), sepsis, avascular necrosis, and cerebrovascular accidents, can result. Unfortunately, even though we have detailed knowledge of the cause, treatment still remains supportive in nature.

Treatment. The goal of therapy during pregnancy is to prevent factors that can precipitate a sickle cell crisis. Pregnancy in itself can increase the possibility of a sickle cell crisis even in patients who are generally asymptomatic. Decreased oxygen saturation and acidosis predispose a patient to sickle cell formation, which begins as PaO_2 decreases to below 50 mmHg. Any evidence of infection should be treated at once. Dehydration should be avoided.

During labor and delivery, the patient should be kept well oxygenated and hydrated. Supplemental oxygen, although helpful, does not ensure that sickling will be prevented. Pulse oximetry should be employed to help monitor oxygenation. Administration of at least 3 L of intravenous fluid per day is recommended, particularly in the febrile patient. The patient should be kept warm to prevent shivering and warmed intravenous fluids should be used. Regional anesthesia can be safely administered. Adequate acute intravascular volume expansion should be completed prior to the induction of anesthesia. Hypotension should be avoided and, if it occurs, rapidly corrected by rapid intravascular volume expansion rather than use of vasopressors to minimize stasis that can result from peripheral vasoconstriction. Fetal monitoring should be used throughout labor and the patient should have uterine displacement at all times.

Transfusion therapy for symptomatic crises has been reported. Prophylactic and partial exchange transfusion to lower the amount of hemoglobin (Hgb) S cells have been advocated. The use of prophylactic transfusion is controversial but many believe that is may be beneficial in multiparous patients who have had a sickle crisis with previous deliveries. Partial exchange transfusion is used in sickle cell crises, with the goal being to increase the level of HgbA to 40 percent. These patients have often received numerous transfusions during the course of their life and are likely to have multiple antibodies, making cross-matching difficult. The use of buffy coat-poor, washed packed red cells less than 5 days old, is preferred.

Hemoglobin C Anomaly

Hemoglobin C involves the substitution of a lysine for a glutamic acid at the sixth position of the β-chain. This causes crystallization of the hemoglobin at low PO_2 but not the deformation of the red cell into a sickle shape. Homozygous HgbC is usually associated with mild anemia, often with splenomegally. This disorder seldom is clinically significant in parturients but supplemental oxygen is recommended during labor.

Thalassemia

Thalassemia is a mixed disorder involving the diminished production of hemoglobin protein chains. Most common are α- and β-thalassemia, which affect the production of HgbA. The α-thalassemias (thalassemia minor) result from the full or partial deletion of HgbA genes or the reduced expression of these genes. There is a wide range of severity of symptoms. Inheritance of β-thalassemia is an autosomal codominant. There is partial or complete absence of β-globin production due most probably to a defect in the transcription of messenger RNA. Patients with β-thalassemia minor (heterozygotes) produce about half the normal amount of β-globin. Steinberg has recently reviewed the molecular pathophysiology and medical treatment.[2]

Treatment. Most patients with α-thalassemias and β-thalassemia minor require no special care but, if the anemia is of concern, patients should receive supplemental oxygen and be kept warm and comfortable to decrease oxygen requirements.

β-thalassemia major (Cooley's anemia) is a severe form of thalassemia that involves little or no production of β-globin. Most patients have hematocrits of less than 20 percent. Patients with severe symptoms have often received multiple transfusions in the past and may suffer from iron overload, which can result in cardiomyopathy with concomitant congestive heart failure and arrhythmias. In addition there is often hepatic and pancreatic dysfunction along with hepatomegaly and splenomegaly. Patients have delayed puberty and pregnancy is rare. Skeletal deformities are common as marrow expands to compensate for the anemias. These include enlarged malar bones and the resulting "chipmunk" facies, which requires careful airway assessment if general anesthesia is contemplated.[3] In addition, spinal deformities may make regional anesthesia difficult.

Epidural anesthesia can be safely administered to these patients if hemostasis is normal. Care must be taken to ensure that the cardiovascular status does not deteriorate. If there is evidence of cardiac dysfunction, hydration of these patients prior to the onset of regional anesthesia may require invasive monitoring by pulmonary artery catherization. Supplemental oxygen and warm fluids should be administered.

When cesarean delivery is performed, these parturients must be closely monitored for a change in cardiac status, which may include the use of arterial and pulmonary artery monitoring. Some authorities recommend general anesthesia for these parturients.

COAGULATION DISORDERS

Normal Coagulation

A simplified diagram of normal coagulation shown in Figure 8-5 depicts the coagulation cascade, which is usually divided into three components: the intrinsic coagulation pathway, measured by the partial thromboplastin time (PTT); the extrinsic pathway, measured by the prothrombin time (PT); and the common convergent pathway, which brings the other two pathways together and affects both the PT and the PTT. Intact and adequate platelet function is necessary for competent hemostasis, which is most often assessed by platelet number and bleeding time.

Hemostasis in Pregnancy. Normal pregnancy is characterized by the onset of a hypercoagulable state to limit the loss of blood and its oxygen-carrying capacity during delivery. As blood volume expands, there is also an elevation of factors I, VII, VIII, IX, and X. Although the platelet count remains normal, there is an increase in thromboxane A2, which stimulates platelet aggregation. There is a reduction of protein S, as well as plasminogen activators that are involved with anticoagulation.

Iatrogenic Coagulation Defects

A cause of coagulation disorders seen with increasing frequency is the induction of an anticoagulated state necessary in many patients who, for example, suffer from deep vein thrombosis or are the recipients of an artificial heart valve. These patients are often treated with warfarin (Coumadin), which crosses the placenta and can act as a teratogen. Therefore, these patients are often switched to a regimen of subcutaneous mini-dose heparin during pregnancy. Warfarin therapy will prolong the PT, and regional anesthesia should be avoided if the PT is greater then 1.5 to 2 times the control value. If major surgery such as cesarean delivery is contemplated, correction of coagulation can be accomplished in a few days by stopping the warfarin and

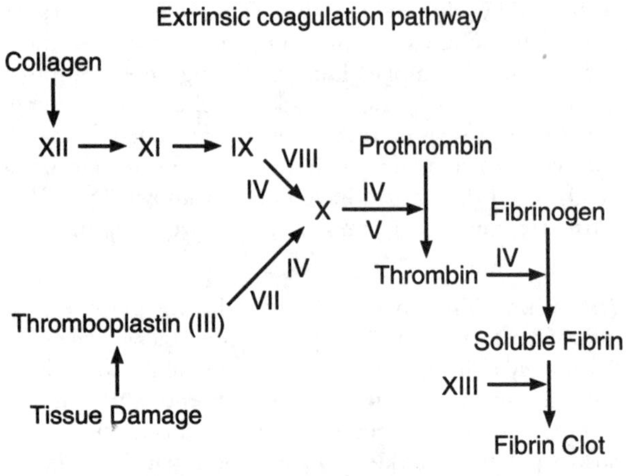

Fig. 8-5. Extrinsic coagulation pathway.

giving vitamin K. When rapid correction is required, fresh frozen plasma can be given. (It should be noted that, as a blood product, fresh frozen-plasma carries the risk of hepatitis or HIV infection).

Patients receiving minidose heparin usually have PTT values in the normal range and require no treatment. If patients are on larger doses of heparin, or if the PTT is prolonged, the effects of heparin will usually be reversed in 3 to 4 hours following its discontinuation. If the PTT remains prolonged or if heparinization needs to be corrected rapidly, it can be reversed by giving small doses of protamine (50 mg) by slow intravenous drip and following the PTT.

Idiopathic Thrombocytic Purpura

Idiopathic thrombocytic purpura (ITP) is an autoimmune disorder in which the patient generates antibodies against platelet antigens. This results in accelerated destruction of the platelets by the spleen that cannot be compensated for by bone marrow production. ITP is the most common autoimmune hematologic disorder seen during pregnancy. Normal platelet concentrations range between 200,000 and 400,000/μl, but surgical hemostasis can be maintained with platelet counts as low as 40,000 to 50,000/μl.

One complication of ITP is transplacental passage of antibodies, which may result in a platelet count of less than 100,000 in up to 50 percent of infants born to parturients with this condition. The major concern is the possibility of intercranial hemorrhage during vaginal delivery. Fetal platelet counts obtained by scalp blood sampling during labor has been suggested, with the option of cesarean delivery if the platelet count is low.[4] However, a review of 165 cases revealed one intracranial hemorrhage in 134 infants who were delivered vaginally of whom 28 had platelet counts below 30,000, and three intracranial hemorrhages in 31 infants born by cesarean delivery of whom 9 had platelet counts below 30,000. Thus, it is not clear that cesarean delivery is better therapy.

The usual treatment for these mothers has been corticosteroids. Splenectomy can improve the platelet count in over 85 percent of cases. There has been recent use of high-dose intravenous immunoglobulin in cases in which there is no response to steroids or for acute treatment at delivery.

Anesthetic management of parturients with this disorder is dictated by the integrity of the clotting process. To utilize regional anesthesia, knowledge of the platelet count is critical. In addition, bleeding time can indicate the activity of the platelets that are available. A patient with a platelet count below 100,000 or an abnormally prolonged bleeding time is not normally a candidate for subarachnoid or epidural anesthesia.[5]

Von Willebrand Disease

Von Willebrand disease is a disorder with an autosomal-dominant, variable-penetrance mode of inheritance, characterized by reduced factor VIII activity, impaired aggregation of platelets, and a prolonged bleeding time. Fortunately, factor VIII levels usually increase with pregnancy and most parturients have normal deliveries.

If factor VIII levels remain less than 25 percent of normal or the bleeding time remains prolonged, considerations should be given to giving cryoprecipitate or fresh frozen plasma to correct the problem. Subarachnoid or epidural anesthesia is counterindicated if the bleeding time is prolonged.

Factor XI Deficiency

A deficiency in factor XI is a genetic disorder whose pattern of inheritance is not completely understood. Some individuals have factor XI levels of 35 to 60 percent, whereas others have levels of 20 percent or less. However, there is poor correlation between factor levels and the severity of bleeding. Patients with low factor XI levels will demonstrate a prolonged PTT.

Most parturients do not have problems with hemostasis. If the PTT is prolonged, epidural or subarachnoid anesthesia should be avoided. Factor XI deficiency can be corrected if necessary by the use of fresh frozen plasma.

REFERENCES

1. Antoonarakis SE, et al: Origin of the beta S globin gene in blacks: the condition of recurrent mutation or gene conversion or both. Proc Natl Acad Sci USA
2. Steinberg MH: Thalassemia: molecular pathology and management. Am J Med Sci 296(5):308, 1988
3. Orr D: Difficult intubation: a hazard of thalassemia. A case report. Br J Anaesth 39:585, 1967
4. Cines DB, Dusele B, Tomaski A, et al: Immune thrombocytopenic purpura and pregnancy. N Engl J Med 306:826, 1982
5. Rolbin SH, et al: Epidural anesthesia in pregnant patients with low platelet counts. Obstet Gynecol 71(6):918, 1988

NEUROLOGIC DISEASE

Controversy surrounds the choice of anesthesia for the obstetric patient with pre-existing disease of the nervous system. If the patient's neurologic condition changes postoperatively, the cause may be unclear and the anesthetic technique or drug may be blamed. In order to develop a rational anesthetic plan, an understanding of the patient's neurologic and general medical condition is needed. Unfortunately, the anesthetic literature available on most of these conditions is limited.

CHRONIC BACK PROBLEMS

Ligamentous strain from the lumbar lordosis of pregnancy results in up to 50 percent of pregnant women reporting chronic back pain, often associated with symptoms of pain radiating down the legs.[1] Parturients may also present with a history of intervertebral disc disease. There is no evidence that regional anesthesia will exacerbate these problems. Postpartum back pain can be minimized by assuming proper placement in the lithotomy position with the hips supported and the lordotic curvature maintained but not aggravated.

In patients having undergone previous back surgery for disc disease or scoliosis, performing regional anesthesia may be difficult because of altered anatomy or adhesions. In many cases, epidural anesthesia can be performed successfully. However, the patient should be aware that the epidural block may be patchy and inadequate because of alterations in the epidural space from previous surgery. The possibility of unintentional dural puncture may be increased. For cesarean delivery, subarachnoid anesthesia may be easier to perform and have more predictable results.

MULTIPLE SCLEROSIS

Multiple sclerosis is a major cause of neurologic disability in young and middle-aged adults, with a frequency of about 0.5 per thousand,[2,3] The disease is characterized by random and multiple sites of demyelination in the brain and spinal cord. The disease does not affect the peripheral nervous system. The course consists of remissions and exacerbations of symptoms at unpredictable time intervals over years. The relapse rate during the first 3 months postpartum has been reported to be about three times as high as in the nonpregnant patient.

The literature regarding the effects of anesthesia is controversial. Several studies have implicated anesthesia in the exacerbation of multiple sclerosis during the postoperative period for the nonobstetric patient. However, the numbers of actual relapses reported in these studies are very small and the relationship of the relapses to the anesthetic technique is unclear, since other conditions in the postoperative period such as hyperpyrexia may also predispose to relapse. Later studies in both obstetric and nonobstetric patients have reported the use of both subarachnoid and epidural anesthesia in these patients without neurologic complications.

Therefore, although there is no evidence that women who receive epidural or subarachnoid anesthesia have a higher relapse rate overall, the patient should be informed that there is a higher incidence of relapse in the postpartum period, regardless of the use of anesthesia. The anesthesiologist should be aware that there is no absolute contraindication to the use of regional anesthesia for labor and delivery in these patients.

MYASTHENIA GRAVIS

Myasthenia gravis is an autoimmune disorder causing destruction of the acetylcholine receptor resulting in chronic neuromuscular fatigue.[4–6] Anticholinesterase medications are the treatment of choice. During the course of therapy, patients may present with global weakness and respiratory insufficiency due either to inadequate anticholinesterase effect or to relative anticholinesterase overdose.

Management of the pregnant myasthenic includes close surveillance of both mother and fetus. A careful history of the course of the disease, the medications taken, and an assessment of the severity of the disease should be documented. Particular attention should be paid to the patient's mother strength and respiratory function. Ideally, these patients should be referred for anesthetic consultation early in the course of the pregnancy. The anesthesiologist may wish to obtain pulmonary function tests, including spirometry and peak expiratory flow rate. Evidence of significant restrictive lung disease should be further evaluated with arterial blood gases. Anticholinesterase medications should be continued throughout pregnancy and delivery. An intramuscular or intravenous preparation of the anticholinesterase medication can be given during the time that the patient is fasting.

During the course of labor, these patients need to be continually assessed for increasing muscle weakness, which may require adjustment of their anticholinesterase dosage. The anesthesiologist may wish to perform serial spriometries to help with this evaluation. An easy way to do this is to measure three consecutive vital capacities. Increasing fatiguability is indicated by progressive reductions in the second and third vital capacity measured.

Large doses and high concentrations of local anesthetics should be avoided. If there is concern about the patient's respiratory status, slowly raising the anesthetic level with a continuous technique may be preferable to a single-dose technique. When regional anesthesia is used, it is recommended that large doses of ester-type local anesthetics such as chloroprocaine be avoided because the anticholinesterases given for treatment of the disease may prevent metabolism of the ester-type anesthetics, theoretically increasing maternal and fetal toxicity.

If general anesthesia is chosen as the anesthetic technique for a cesarean delivery, careful monitoring of neuromuscular function is critical because the effect of muscle relaxants on these patients may be unpredictable. The duration of succinylcholine used for intubation is obviously prolonged because of the anticholinesterase therapy. Usually no other muscle relaxants are required for cesarean delivery. If, at the end of anesthetic, there is any question about the patient's ventilatory capacity, the patient should remain intubated until adequacy of ventilation can be confirmed by pulmonary function testing in the recovery room.

EPILEPSY

The patient with epilepsy has an increased risk of complications such as prematurity, preeclampsia, obstetric hemorrhage, and uterine hypotonia.[7] The increased complication rate may be due to side effects of antiseizure medication or to the seizures themselves. Epileptic patients do not have an increased sensitivity to local anesthetics and regional anesthesia can be safely administered. If general anesthesia is required for cesarean delivery, agents such as enflurane and ketamine that can increase central nervous system excitability should be avoided. If anticonvulsant medications has been continued during the pregnancy, serum levels should be monitored to avoid subtherapeutic or toxic levels. Several anticonvulsants, notably phenobarbital and phenytoin, are known to interfere with vitamin K metabolism. In these cases, coagulation studies should be checked and vitamin K given if needed.

MIGRAINE HEADACHE

Seventy percent of migraine sufferers are women of childbearing age. There are no studies currently reporting an increase in the incidence or severity of migraine headaches in women who have received regional anesthesia for labor and delivery. Administration of preparations containing ergot is the common treatment for these patients. Theoretically, giving ephedrine to a patient taking a ergot preparation may cause an exaggerated rise in blood pressure. The dose of vasopressor used should be carefully titrated in these patients.

VIRAL DISEASE

Herpes

There has been concern that performing regional anesthesia in a patient with a history of herpes has the risk of contaminating the patient's cerebrospinal fluid with herpes virus particles and causing meningitis.[8] However, the patient is viremic only during the primary infection. During recurrent attacks, even when vesicles are present, patients are not viremic and subarachnoid or epidural anesthesia can be administered.

Polio

Opinions vary regarding the use of regional anesthesia in the patient with a past history of polio.[9,10] Case reports of a recrudescence of symptoms after subarachnoid anesthesia exist. However, epidural anesthesia has been used successfully for labor and delivery and epidural or subarachnoid anesthesia has been used for cesarean delivery without postpartum complications.

SPINAL CORD INJURY

Regional anesthesia can be extremely beneficial to the obstetric patient with spinal cord injury.[11,12] If the lesion is below the level of T10, patients will experience labor pain. In patients with spinal cord injuries above the level of T6, there is an increased susceptibility for the syndrome of autonomic hyperreflexia. This sympathetic response can be elicited by cutaneous or visceral stimulation below the level of spinal cord transection. Since there is no inhibition of sympathetic tone from higher centers because of the transection, patients exhibit severe hypertension, headache, and flushing above and blanching below the level of the lesion. It can also be triggered by distention of the bladder or rectum, or by uterine contractions during labor. Therefore, these patients need anesthesia for labor and delivery even though they lack sensation in these areas.

Regional anesthesia is an excellent choice for preventing autonomic hyperreflexia. Performing these blocks may be technically difficult if the spine is deformed and it may be difficult to position the patient who is paraplegic. However, there should be no fear of exacerbating neurologic damage in a patient with a complete spinal cord transection. Epidural anesthesia has been reported to be extremely reliable for preventing the autonomic hyperreflexia that may be initiated by uterine contractions. Usually, only a low concentration of local anesthetic agent or opioid is required.

If epidural anesthesia alone does not completely prevent or control the hypertension, intravenous agents such as hydralazine, trimethaphan, or nitroprusside may be used successfully. Cesarean delivery may be indicated if these methods do not satisfactorily control the hypertension during labor.

CEREBROVASCULAR ACCIDENTS

Cerebral hemorrhage can be seen in association with aneurysms, arteriovenous malformations, and preeclampsia or eclampsia.[13] Hypertension should be treated aggressively and abrupt changes in blood pressure avoided. For the parturient with a history of a cerebrovascular accident, epidural anesthesia is a good choice for labor and vaginal or cesarean delivery. If general anesthesia is required, the hypertensive response to intubation may be avoided by intravenous lidocaine; other antihypertensive medications such as labetalol, trimethaphan, or sodium nitroprusside; and adequate dosage of induction agents.

REFERENCES

1. Moir DD, Davidson S: Postpartum complications of forceps delivery performed under epidural and pudendal nerve block. Br J Anaesth 44:1197, 1972
2. Crawford JS: Epidural analgesia for patients with neurologic disease. Anesth Analg 62:671, 1983
3. Bader AM, Hunt CO, Datta S, et al: Anesthesia for the obstetric patient with multiple sclerosis. J Clin Anesth 1:21, 1988
4. Osserman KE: Pregnancy in myasthenia gravis and neonatal myasthenia gravis. Am J Med 19:718, 1955
5. Plauche WC: Myasthenia gravis in pregnancy: an update. Am J Obstet Gynecol 88:404, 1979
6. Foldes FF, McWall PG: Myasthenia gravis: a guide for anesthesiologists. Anesthesiology 23:867, 1967
7. Abouleish E: Neurologic diseases. p. 57. In James FM, Wheeler AS (eds): Obstetric Anaesthesia: The Complicated Patient. FA Davis, Philadelphia, 1982
8. Ramanathan S, Sheth R, Turndorf H: Anesthesia for cesarean section in patients with genital herpes infections: a retrospective study. Anesthesiology 64:807, 1986
9. Crawford JS, James FM, Nolte H, et al: Regional anesthesia for patients with chronic neurologic disease and similar conditions. Anaesthesia 36:821, 1981
10. Vandam LD, Dripps RD: Exacerbation of pre-existing neurologic disease after spinal anesthesia. N Engl J Med 255:843, 1956
11. Stirt JA, Marco A, Conklin KA: Obstetric anesthesia for a quadriplegic patient with autonomic hyperreflexia. Anesthesiology 51:560, 1979
12. Baraka A: Epidural meperidine for control of autonomic hyperreflexia in a paraplegic parturient. Anesthesiology 62:688, 1985
13. Minielly R, Yuzpe AA, Drake CG: Subarachnoid hemorrhage secondary to ruptured cerebral aneurysm in pregnancy. Obstet Gynecol 53:64, 1979

AUTOIMMUNE DISEASE

There are three basic types of autoimmune disease mechanisms that damage the host body. In the first type the combination of target antigen and a circulating autoantibody stimulates release of inflammation mediators, triggering the complement pathway and activating cytotoxic cells (killer T cells and macrophages), both of which cause cytolysis. This antibody-antigen complex can bind to certain cell-surface receptors, thereby stimulating, inhibiting, or destroying them. In the second type of mechanistic action this same antibody-antigen complex accumulates in various tissues; then, fixing complement, it can cause inflammation with resultant tissue damage. The final mechanism is one in which certain sensitized T cells damage tissue and/or release lymphokines, which then initiate a superinflammatory syndrome.

Although the maternal immune system in the healthy parturient seems to be intact, some immunosuppression at the level of the fetoplacental unit allows the pregnancy to continue to term in the majority of cases.[1] Progesterone inhibits the immune response of T lymphocytes.[2] A few serum proteins have been isolated in parturients and their levels seem to correlate with flare-up and remission of some of the autoimmune diseases.[3] They are pregnancy-associated globulin (2-PAG) and pregnancy zone protein (PZP). This 2-PAG (also known as pregnancy-associated plasma protein A (PAPP-A)) is an immunosuppressive glycoprotein that effects the complement system and lymphocyte transformation in normal patients and in those with autoimmune disease. 2-PAG inhibits antibody receptor function and circulating lymphocytic and monocytic human lymphocytic antigen-direct reacting (HLA-DR) antigenic expression.[1] Uromodulin is a immunosuppressive glycoprotein, isolated from normal urine, that also inhibits T-cell and macrophage activity of the parturient or the "host" organism against the fetal "graft."[4] The interplay between the maternal and fetal immune systems in patients with autoimmune disease still needs to be worked out. In this section, some of the effects of the autoimmunity on the obstetric patient are reviewed.

When informed of a pregnant patient with an autoimmune disease on the Obstetric Service, one should begin immediately to evaluate

1. The clinical presentation in pregnancy.
2. Anesthetic considerations involving the airway and cardiopulmonary system (often the chest x-ray doesn't correlate with the degree of pulmonary impairment; if low compliance and increased restrictive disease are found, a high FiO_2 is needed. If placed on intermittent positive-pressure ventilation, lower total volume and higher respiratory rates are needed. Because of the decreased compliance and other pulmonary defects, regional techniques are often preferred. Rapid-sequence induction and full stomach precautions are warranted. Also of concern are renal, vascular, central nervous system, hematologic, and neonatal syndromes; patient positioning; and preoperative laboratory tests (including preoperative pulmonary function tests and arterial blood gas data if time permits).

RHEUMATOID ARTHRITIS

Pathophysiology

Rheumatoid arthritis (RA) is a chronic, systemic, and non-organ-specific autoimmune disease of unknown etiology in which antibodies are formed against a myriad of gamma globulins and Epstein-Barr virus-related antigens. The end result of antigen-antibody complexing in RA leads to an inflammatory disorder, with its hallmark finding of ubiquitous, although not always synchronous, inflammation of synovial joints. Current dogma expresses an infectious synovitis that induces antigenic change and thus stimulates the autoimmune, body-wide havoc.

There is a female preponderance in the over five million cases in the United States. It occurs in young women three times more frequently than in young men. The disease rarely occurs during pregnancy, however, when it does, it is most serious during the puerperium. Pregnancy seems to suppress RA, perhaps by the increases in circulating adrenocorticoids, especially during the last trimester, when there is a rise in the plasma cortisol.[5] The usual scenario is for a postpartum relapse, commonly in the first 2 to 4 months.[6–10] Lactation appears to prolong remission.[11]

The most usual finding of RA is the synovitis, along with its accompanying pain and limitations to daily activities. However, many other findings are important factors in the delivery of an anesthetic to the parturient with this disease.

Anesthetic Considerations

The healthy parturient is known to have several factors that involve airway management, thus making it more difficult than in the nonpregnant patient, including an edematous airway (increasingly so toward term), as well as the fact that the patient is at risk for aspiration secondary to the relatively relaxed lower esophageal sphincter and increased intra-abdominal pressure. In the patient with RA, however, the additional factors that influence airway management include the possibility of:

1. Mandibular hypoplasia
2. Temporomandibular joint (TMJ) arthritis or growth failure in juvenile RA patients, which leads to micrognathia and hence, difficult intubation
3. Unstable/immobile cervical spine with possible fusions and/or subluxation (especially atlantoxial)
4. Cricoarytenoid arthritis
5. Laryngeal rotation

Therefore, these patients should be considered as presenting difficult intubation. Extreme sniffing positions should be avoided. A fiberoptic endoscope should be available for intubation at all times.

A pericardial effusion is quite common in the pregnant patient, however, it is usually asymptomatic. The most common form of cardiac disease in the RA patient is pericarditis, usually associated with an exudative effusion that can progress rapidly to a tamponade. Rheumatoid nodules can be found on the epicardium, myocardium, and heart valves. Less commonly found is coronary arteritis and focal interstitial myocarditis.[12]

Above and beyond the pulmonary impairments associated with normal pregnancy (decreased functional residual capacity and total volume), there are six basic forms of lung disease found in patients with RA: airway disease (with a low maximum midexpiratory flow rate and a low maximum expiratory flow rate at 50 percent forced vital capacity), pleuritis (usually subclinical), interstitial fibrosis (with a decrease in diffusing capacity of the lung of carbon monoxide, with fine, dry rales on auscultation and patchy infiltrates or a fine reticulonodular pattern on chest x-ray), nodular lung disease (Caplan's Disease), pneumonitis, pulmonary arteritis (although pulmonary hypertension is rare), and intrapulmonary rheumatoid nodules (which can rupture spontaneously, yielding a pneumothorax or a pyopneumothorax).

SYSTEMIC LUPUS ERYTHEMATOSIS

Pathophysiology

Systemic lupus erythematosis (SLE) is another devastating autoimmune disease, in which the antibody targets are intranuclear: double- and single-stranded DNA, Sm1 ribonucleoprotein, lymphocytes, erythrocytes, neurons, and gamma globulins.[11] The anticardiolipin antibody is one of many antiphospholipid antibodies present in a large percentage (20 to 65 percent) of patients with SLE. This disease incidence is on the order of 4 to 250 per 100,000 population, with an 8 to 10:1 female:male ratio. Its peak onset is in the second to fourth decade and it occurs in approximately one in 5,000 pregnancies.[13] Approximately 20 percent of cases are diagnosed at the onset of pregnancy through routine obstetric screening.[13] Usually the course of the disease is not influenced by pregnancy, however, in contrast to patients with RA, the severity and frequency of flares can approximately double in 50 percent of cases of SLE.[14–19] If a patient falls into a remission during her pregnancy, chances are that she will remain so for the duration. Pregnancy is contraindicated in patients with advanced cardiac, central nervous system, and/or renal disease. Those with active lupus nephritis often have a flare-up during pregnancy and tend to develop preeclampsia.[20] Usually the SLE parturient presents with constitutional symptoms, symmetric arthritis, myalgias, and muscle weakness. However, a preeclampsia-like syndrome can be observed in this patient population, with hypertension, edema, and proteinuria without the normal SLE symptomatology. It is usually insidious in onset, but can be abrupt and is associated with hypocomplementemia.[16,21–23]

Anesthetic Considerations

As in patients with RA, the incidence of pericardial effusions greatly increases (affecting 25% percent of patients) and the effusions can become quite symptomatic in SLE patients. In SLE, pericardial infusions are caused by an acute or a constrictive pericarditis, and can be manifest in many forms, from an asymptomatic friction rub to a pleuritic chest pain, from atrial arrhythmias to right heart failure from a tamponade.[24] Electrocardiographic changes can be anything from a persistent tachyarrhythmia to those consistent with a myocardial infarction. The valvulopathy most often seen is Libman-Sacks endocarditis, in which small vegetations form near the rings, resulting in valvular dysfunction.[11,24–27]

The lungs and pleura are involved in approximately 30 to 70 percent of SLE patients. The pulmonary manifestations include interstitial (chronic lupus) pneumonitis; fibrinous pleuritis, often with a bilateral pleural effusion; acute pulmonary vasculitis or advanced arteriosclerosis; focal alveolar hemorrhages; and bronchopneumonias. Rarely, a patient can present with a massive pulmonary hemorrhage. Pulmonary function tests usually show mixed obstructive/restrictive indices with decreased lung volumes, a decreased diffusing capacity of the lung to oxygen, and a decreased compliance. Arterial blood gas data usually display a low PaO_2 with a normal or slightly decreased $PaCO_2$.

Lupus nephritis occurs in about one-half of patients with SLE, presenting on urinalysis as hematuria and proteinuria. If the nephrotic syndrome develops, end-stage renal failure and acidosis may result. Arterial hypertension is a possible finding.[15,28]

Often one will find a slightly elevated partial thromboplastin time in the course of the preoperative hematologic evaluation. This is usually due to a circulating anticoagulant known as the lupus anticoagulant,[29–31] which in the patient with SLE, is caused by the presence of either an antiphospholipid antibody or a specific anticlotting factor antibody.

If antibody against multiple clotting factors is present, the risk of bleeding is increased. Unless the patient is transfused with the appropriate factor just prior to the administration of a regional anesthetic, this procedure should be considered contraindicated.[29] If the disease is associated with the formation of anticardiolipin antibody, there is an increased incidence of thrombocytopenia, arterial thromboses (with the possibility of cerebrovascular accident, peripheral gangrene, coronary thrombosis and myocardial necrosis, renal artery occlusion, and avascular bone necrosis), venous thromboses, and intravascular clot formation (including in the placenta).[32] The platelets in these patients exhibit increased adhesiveness and aggregation. These patients are given anticoagulation therapy with heparin and then switched over to warfarin (Coumadin).[33,34] Raynaud's phenomenon is found in approximately 15 percent of patients with SLE.[35]

Preoperatively, in addition to the routine studies for patients with SLE, one should consider obtaining an echocardiogram to rule out pericardial effusions, and valvulopathies (Libman-Sacks endocarditis); pulmonary function tests if the patient complains of dyspnea out of proportion to her pregnant state; and coagulation tests to screen for circulating lupus anticoagulant. If the patient is receiving chronic steroid maintenance, one should administer steroid coverage.[36,37]

The choice of anesthetic technique depends on the extent of the disease and the systems it involves. With a general anesthetic, there is the increased risk of aspiration pneumonitis and worsening underlying organ dysfunction, including increased mental confusion, depressed pulmonary and cardiac function, and poor renal, hepatic, and, especially, uteroplacental blood flow. Although there is an increased risk of bleeding from a regional technique, there also is a decrease in the risk of aspiration and a possible increase in the uteroplacental blood flow.

Fetal and Neonatal Considerations

In SLE patients, there is an increased incidence of premature labor, miscarriage, and stillbirth, especially in those mothers with positive antiphospholipid antibodies.[14,16,18,38–40] Patients treated with antiplatelet drugs, such as aspirin, or with subcutaneous heparin regimens have increased perinatal survival.[35,41] Transient abnormalities can be found in the offspring of mothers with SLE (the neonatal lupus syndrome). The neonatal lupus syndrome includes findings of cytopenias, a discoid rash, and cardiac conduction defects (i.e., third-degree atrioventricular block, sometimes requiring a pacemaker).

MYASTHENIA GRAVIS

Pathophysiology

Myasthenia gravis (MG) is an organ-specific autoimmune disease in which the AcH receptor and skeletal muscle are targeted. The end effect is skeletal muscle weakness had defective neuromuscular transmission. The MG patient has approximately one-fourth of the usual number of acetylcholine receptors because of an augmented rate of degradation and occupation of these receptors by the blocking. Smooth muscle (e.g., the myometrium) is unaffected by MG. The muscle weakness is progressive and increases with exertion, especially of the muscles of the face, tongue, throat, neck, arms, and respiratory system. The incidence of this disease is approximately 3 per 100,000, with a female:male ratio of 3:1. The peak prevalence is in the third decade, well within the childbearing years. It is frequently associated with thymoma or thymic hyperplasia, and occurs in patients with various connective tissue disorders.[42] Approximately 33 percent of patients improve during pregnancy, whereas another third worsen and the remainder do not change clinically. The patients usually tolerate labor well, as their muscles are already somewhat relaxed because of their disease state. They tend to have a prolonged second stage of labor and forceps deliveries are common.[43] Those patients who have already undergone a thymectomy appear to fare better during their pregnancy than those who have electively retained their thymus. The anticholinesterase therapy needs to be continued during labor. Oral doses of these agents should be converted to intramuscular dosing, which is usually one-tenth of the oral dose. Approximately 30 minutes prior to delivery, an intramuscular dose of anticholinesterase agent should be administered to maximize the patient's pushing ability.[44–47]

Anesthetic Considerations

For vaginal deliveries, regional techniques are preferred (i.e., a low subarachnoid anesthetic, (preferably with a catheter for better control, or a lumbar epidural). Because of the respiratory muscle weakness in these patients, extra care must be taken to avoid hypoventilation if a subarachnoid or epidural anesthetic is administered for a cesarean delivery. Ester local anesthetics are relatively contraindicated because chronic neostigmine or pyridostigmine therapy greatly inhibits plasma cholinesterase activity. For cesarean delivery of the patient in remission, a regional technique is also preferred, however, if the disease is in a flare state, a general anesthetic should be considered.[47] Because of the initial resistance and prolonged duration of succinylcholine, 40 percent of the usual dose is sufficient for endotracheal intubation. Hypokalemia, magnesium sulfate, scopolamine, and large doses of muscle relaxants are contraindicated. A nerve stimulator should always be used to monitor these patients. Muscle relaxants should be reversed with atropine and neostigmine. Neostigmine can be beneficial in increasing muscle strength during labor. Edrophonium can lead to forceful uterine contractions.

In MG, one can find flares during the first trimester or in the first 2 weeks postpartum, the so-called myasthenic crises, in which the need for mechanical ventilation is not unusual.

Since occasional focal myocardial necrosis is found in these patients, a preoperative 12-lead electrocardiogram is imperative for postoperative comparison.

Neonatal Considerations

Neonatal myasthenia can occur in 25 to 33 percent of babies born to MG mothers. The anesthesiologist or neonatologist must be aware of the increased possibility of neonatal emergent intubation, however, the symptoms usually occur between 12 and 48 hours postpartum.

PROGRESSIVE SYSTEMIC SCLEROSIS (SCLERODEMA)

Pathophysiology

Progressive systemic sclerosis (PSS), or scleroderma is another systemic autoimmune disease in which antibodies are formed against gamma globulins, SCL-70 protein, the centromere, and SS-A (Ro) and SS-B (La) antigens, with the end result of abnormal proliferation and overdeposition of fibrous connective tissue. The damage can be local (e.g., coup de sabre) or ubiquitous. The

CREST syndrome incorporates the findings of calcinosis, Raynaud's phenomenon, esophageal dysmotility, sclerodactyly, and telangectasias.

These related disease entities occur at all ages, however, the incidence peaks in middle-aged women (30 to 65 years of age). There are 50,000 to 100,000 known cases in the United States. Symptoms usually appear in the third to fifth decades. This disease spectrum is three to four times more common in women than in men. Usually pregnancy does not worsen the disease state, however, the gastrointestinal symptoms and cardiopulmonary dysfunction of the disease can make an already difficult pregnancy much more difficult for the patient. Pregnancy normally ends in spontaneous vaginal delivery unless the scleroderma changes produce dystocia, which requires cesarean delivery.

Anesthetic Considerations

The anesthetic considerations for patients with PSS involve several body systems.

Respiratory Tract Involvement. Respiratory tract involvement includes tight perioral skin, or "mauskopf"; TMJ involvement; and cervical arthritis. One needs to be able to perform a blind or fiberoptic intubation. Also, there exists an increased risk of aspiration, secondary to gastrointestinal tract involvement.

Cardiac Involvement. With cardiac fibrosis, one sees varying heart blocks and arrhythmias more frequently, as the fibrotic tissue replaces normal myocardium. With this cardiomyopathy, one can also see episodes of congestive heart failure, myocardial Raynaud's phenomenon (small coronary arterial vasospasm), occasional pericarditis with effusions and rarely, cardiac tamponade. The cardiac failure is also in part a result of chronic hypertension and left ventricular hypertrophic dysfunction, and usually presents as dyspnea on exertion, orthopnea, and pedal edema. On occasion, a patient presents with angina pectoris.

Pulmonary Involvement. Because of the increased incidence of fibrosis of the pulmonary arterial intima, pulmonary hypertension can be quite common. Diffuse intersitial and alveolar fibrosis may result in fine bibasilar rales, end-stage respiratory insufficiency, or cor pulmonale. The most common symptom is exertional dyspnea. Pleuritis is much less common. The diffusing capacity of the lung usually is subnormal. The chest x-ray usually shows a lineoreticular or a lineonodular density pattern. Pulmonary function testing shows a chronic restrictive disorder with decreased forced vital capacity and total lung capacity. These patients also can present with rapidly progressive respiratory failure.

Gastrointestinal Involvement. As a result of hypokinesis (severely decreased or no peristalsis) and dilation of the esophagus, there may be delayed gastric emptying, gastroesophageal reflux, esophagitis, strictures, and dysphagia. Aspiration pneumonia becomes much more common. Along with a dilated small and large intestine, all of these findings require the use of a rapid-sequence induction if general anesthesia is used, and continued surveillance during regional techniques. Nonparticulate antacids, histamine (H_2) blockers, and metoclopramide should be administered preoperatively and a 30 degree head-up position maintained. Patients often present with complaints of severe bloating, abdominal cramps, and diarrhea from bacterial overgrowth of the bowel. There is also an increased incidence of primary biliary cirrhosis in these patients.

IDIOPATHIC THROMBOCYTOPENIC PURPURA

Idiopathic thrombocytopenic purpura (ITP), or autoimmune TP (ATP), is another organ-specific autoimmune disease, one of the most common in pregnancy, wherein platelets are the antibody target of choice. This results in increased platelet destruction. In the chronic form, the female:male ratio is approximately 3:1. It exists as an incidental finding in an otherwise healthy patient or as a symptomatic thrombocytopenia with various bleeding presentations.

Central nervous system hemorrhage is the most serious complication of the disease, both for the mother and the newborn child; however, it is, fortunately, rare.

Fifty percent of ATP mothers give birth to neonates with thrombocytopenia. The antiplatelet antibody can cross the placental barrier passively, leading to varying degrees of fetal thrombocytopenia and related sequelae.[48] The fetal diagnosis is risky in itself, involving measurements of antepartum platelet counts from scalp venous or percutaneous umbilical blood specimens. Although mothers can be treated prenatally with intravenous corticosteroids or gamma globulins, their response does not correlate with that of the fetus. Approximately half of neonates born to mothers with the disease are thrombocytopenic, although usually subclinically.[49] At the other end of the spectrum of presentation is catastrophic intracranial hemorrhage. In the recent study by Samuels et al,[59] 54 percent of thrombocytopenic patients studied had a history of TIP (79 percent of whom were positive for antiplatelet antibodies), 45 percent had low platelet counts for the first time during their initial pregnancy, 23 percent had offspring born thrombocytopenic (92 percent of whom were born to mothers who carried a diagnosis of ITP), and 11 percent had children with severe thrombocytopenia (platelets less than 50,000/mm^2). These investigators concluded that mothers with a history of ITP and positive autoantibodies were likely to deliver a child with thrombocytopenia.[50]

On hematologic examination, one usually finds an increased bleeding time, thrombocytopenia, and usually iron-deficiency anemia from low-grade, chronic bleeding. Patients often take corticosteroids or intravenous gamma globulins to increase their platelet count prior to delivery. A controversy exists as to whether cesarean delivery is safer than vaginal delivery because it avoids the increased risk of intracranial neonatal hemorrhage secondary to the vaginal vault pressure on the baby's head at the time of delivery.

POLYMYOSITIS/DERMATOMYOSITIS

Polymyositis/Dermatomyositis is also a non-organ-specific disease in which the antibody targets include the nuclei; the Jo-1, Mi-2, PM-1, Ku, and PL-7 proteins; and myosin. The usual end result is that a severe, inflammatory perivasculitis causes diffuse damage to the skeletal muscles and or the skin of these patients. There are from 8 to 15 per million new cases per year, with a female: male ratio of 2:1. Patients with this disorder are most commonly found to have symmetric, proximal muscle weakness. The skin manifestations include erythematous, scaly lesions of the face, neck, shoulders, knees, elbows, ankles, metacarpophalangeal and proximal interphalangeal joints.[11] There is a high incidence of spontaneous abortion and perinatal death. Exacerbations of the disease are not uncommon during pregnancy.[51–54]

Although rare, cardiac involvement does occur in patients with polymyositis or dermatomyositis. It usually presents subclinically as electrocardiographic findings of pericarditis, arrhythmias, or conduction defects. Occasionally patients present with congestive heart failure. It is rare, however, for these patients to have respiratory muscle weakness, especially in the dermatomyocytic patient group.

REFERENCES

1. Ahmed SA, Penhale WJ, Kushner I: Sex hormones, immune responses, and autoimmune diseases: mechanism of sex hormone action. Am J Pathol 121:531, 1985
2. Beck I, Griffin JF: Lymphocyte responses in systemic lupus erythematosis in pregnancy. Am J Med 82(1):179, 1987
3. Dombrowski RA: Autoimmune disease in pregnancy. Med Clin North Am 73(3)605, 1989
4. Billingham RE, Beer AE: Reproductive immunology: past, present and future. Perspect Biol Med 27:259, 1984
5. Østenson M, Husley G: A prospective study of the effect of pregnancy on rheumatoid arthritis and ankylosing spondylitis. Arthris Rheum 26:1155, 1983
6. Stein GH, Cantor B, Panush RS: Adult Still's disease associated with pregnancy. Arthritis Rheum 23:248, 1980
7. Persellin RH: The effect of pregnancy on rheumatoid arthritis. Bull Rheumat Dis 27:922, 1977
8. Ørtensen M, Aune B, Husby G: Effect of pregnancy and hormonal changes on the activity of rheumatoid arthritis. Scand J Rheumatol 12:69, 1983
9. Bulmash JM: Rheumatoid arthritis and pregnancy. Obstet Gynecol Annu 8:276, 1978
10. Kaplan D, Diamond H: Rheumatoid arthritis and pregnancy. Clin Obstet Gynecol 8:286, 1965
11. Rodman GP, Schumacher HR (eds): Primer on the Rheumatic Diseases. 9th ed. Arthritis Foundation, Atlanta, 1989
12. Askari AD: Cardiac abnormalities. Clin Rheumat Dis 10:131, 1984
13. Zurier RB: Systemic lupus erythematosis and pregnancy. Clin Rheumatic Dis 1:613, 1975
14. Kaufman RL, Kitridou RC: Pregnancy in mixed connective tissue disease: comparison with systemic lupus erythematosis, J Rheumatol 9:549, 1982
15. Hayslett JP, Lynn RI: Effect of pregnancy in patients with lupus nephropathy. Kidney Int 18:207, 1980
16. Hayslett JP: Effect of pregnancy in patients with systemic lupus erythematosis. Am J Kidney Dis 232, 1982
17. Garsenstein M, Pollack VE, Kark RM: Systemic lupus erythematosis and pregnancy. N Engl J Med 267:165, 1962
18. Gimovsky ML, Montoso M, Paul RH: Pregnancy outcome in women with systemic lupus erythematosis. Obstet Gynecol 63:686, 1984
19. Morris WK: Pregnancy in rheumatoid arthritis and systemic lupus erythematosis. N Z J Obstet Gynecol 9:136, 1969
20. Varner MW, et al. Pregnancy in patients with systemic lupus erythematosis. Am J Obstet Gynecol 15:1025, 1983
21. Lockshin MD, Jarpel PC, Druzin ML, et al: Lupus pregnancy. II. Usual pattern of hypocomplementemia and thrombocytopenia in the pregnant patient. Arthritis Rheum 28:58, 1985
22. Buyon JP, Cronstein BN, Morris M, et al: Serum complement values (C3 and C4) to differentiate between systemic lupus activity and preeclampsia. Am J Med 81:194, 1986
23. Estes D, Larson DL: Systemic lupus erythematosis and pregnancy. Clin Obstet Gynecol 8:307, 1965
24. Knobel B, Melamud E, Kishon Y: Peripartum cardiomyopathy. Isr J Med Sci 20(11):1061, 1984
25. Gibbs PS, Kim KC: Skin and musculoskeletal diseases. p. 611. In Stoelting RK, Dierdorf SF, McCammon RL (eds): Anesthesia and Co-Existing Disease. 2nd Ed. Churchill Livingstone, New York, 1988
26. Haselby KA: The immune system. p. 695. In Stoelting RK, Dierdorf SF, McCammon RL (eds): Anesthesia and Co-Existing Disease. 2nd Ed. Churchill Livingstone, New York, 1988

27. Campbell C, Ravindran RS: The pregnant patient. p. 749. In Stoelting RK, Dierdorf SF, McCammon RL (eds): Anesthesia and Co-Existing Disease. 2nd. Ed. Churchill Livingstone, New York, 1988
28. Bear R: Pregnancy and lupus nephritis. Obstet Gynecol 47:715, 1976
29. Malinow AM, et al: Lupus anticoagulant: implications for obstetric anaesthetists. Anesthesia 42(12):1291, 1987
30. Lubbe WF, Liggins GC: Lupus anticoagulant and pregnancy. Am J Obstet Gynecol 159:322, 1985
31. Lockshin MD, Druzin ML, Goei S, et al: Antibody to cardiolipin as a predictor of fetal distress or death in patients with systemic lupus erythematosis. N Engl J Med 313:152, 1985
32. Much JR, Herbst KD, Rapaport SI: Thrombosis in patients with the lupus anticoagulant. Ann Intern Med 92:156, 1980
33. Feinstein DI: Lupus anticoagulant, thrombosis and fetal loss. N Engl J Med 313:1348, 1985
34. Harris EN, et al: Thrombocytopenia in systemic lupus erythmatosis and related autoimmune disorders: association with anticardiolipin antibody. Br J Haematol 59:231, 1985
35. Elias M, Elder A: Thromboembolism in patients with the "lupus" type circulating anticoagulant. Arch Intern Med 144:510, 1984
36. Zulman JI, Talal N, Hoffman GS, et al: Problems associated with the management of pregnancies in patients with systemic lupus erythematosis. J Rheumatol 7:37, 1980
37. Zurier RB, Argyros TG, Urman JD, et al: Systemic lupus erythematosis: management during pregnancy. Obstet Gynecol 51:178, 1978
38. Branch DW, Scott JR, Kochenour NK, et al: Obstetric complications associated with the lupus anticoagulant. N Engl J Med 313:1322, 1985
39. Lockshin MD: Lupus pregnancy. Clin Rheumat Dis 11:61, 1985
40. Tozman ECS, Urowitz MB, Goldman DD: Systemic lupus erythematosis and pregnancy. J Rheumatol 7:5, 1980
41. Stuart MJ, Gross SJ, Eliuel H, Graeber G: Effects of acetylsalicyic acid ingestion on maternal and neonatal hemostasis. N Engl J Med 307:909, 1982
42. Lisak RP: Myasthenia gravis: mechanisms and management. Hosp Pract 18(3):101, 1983
43. Fennel D, Ringel S: Myasthenia gravis and pregnancy. Obstet Gynecol Surv 41:414, 1987
44. Luz-Tobias A, Ramilo N, Yu K, Rigor B: Anesthetic management of a parturient with myasthenia gravis. J Kentucky Med Assoc Feb.78–80, 1987
45. Plauche WC: Myasthenia gravis. Clin Obstet Gynecol 26:593, 1983
46. Eden RD, Gall SA: Myasthenia gravis and pregnancy: a reappraisal of thymectomy. Obstet Gynecol 62:328, 1983
47. Rolbin SH, Levinson G, Shnider SM, Wright RG: Anesthetic considerations for myasthenia gravis and pregnancy. Anesth Analg 57:441, 1978
48. Scott JR, Rote NS, Cruikshank DP: Antiplatelet antibodies and platelet counts in pregnancies complicated by autoimmune thrombocytopenic purpura. Am J Obstet Gynecol 145(8):932, 1987
49. Burrows RF, Kelton JG: Incidentally detected thrombocytopenia in healthy mothers and their infants. N Engl J Med 319:142, 1988
50. Samuels P, Bussel JB, Braitman LE, et al: Estimation of the risk of thrombocytopenia in the offspring of pregnant women with presumed immune thrombocytopenic purpura. N Engl J Med 323(4):229, 1990
51. Bauer KA, Seigler M, Lindheimer MA: Polymyositis complicating pregnancy. Arch Intern Med 139:449, 1979
52. Baines AB, Link DA: Childhood dermatomyositis and pregnancy. Am J Obstet Gynecol 145:335, 1983
53. Tsai A, Lindheimer MD, Lamberg SI: Dermatomyositis complicating pregnancy. Obstet Gynecol 41:570, 1973
54. Gutierrez G, Dagnino R, Mintz G: Plymyositis/dermatomyositis and pregnancy. Arthritis Rheuma 27:291, 1984

TRANSPLANTATION

The transplantation of organs for various disease states has become commonplace. Replacement of kidneys, hearts, and livers are now routinely performed with excellent survival rates. Many of these procedures are performed in women of childbearing age, thus the obstetric anesthesiologist may, on occasion, encounter patients with transplanted organs presenting for anesthetic care during labor and delivery. Anesthetic implications include alterations in organ function, physiology, and pharmacology, as well as the effects of immunosuppression.

RENAL TRANSPLANTATION

Renal transplantation is now considered routine therapy for those afflicted with end-stage renal disease (ESRD). Five-year survival rates of 80 percent and 40 percent are observed in patients receiving living, related donor and cadaveric kidneys, respectively.[1] These survival rates are expected to rise as advances are made in immunosuppressive therapy and treatment of rejection episodes. Although patients with ESRD maintained on dialysis therapy are often anovulatory, a return to normal menstruation is common following a successful renal allograft. Approximately 1 in 50 women of childbearing age with a functioning renal transplant becomes pregnant.[2]

In general, pregnancy outcome in this patient population is good.[3] Approximately 10 percent of patients will experience a rejection episode during gestation; however, this rate is equal to that seen in the nonpregnant population. Permanent deterioration of allograft function during pregnancy occurs in approximately 10 percent but this also does not differ from the rate seen in the general nonpregnant renal transplant population.[3] Nevertheless, numerous factors contribute to the classification of these patients as "high risk" during pregnancy.

Infectious complications are of particular concern because of the state of immunosuppression.[1] The most common bacterial infection is in the urinary tract. Viral infections, such as herpes simplex or cytomegalovirus, are more common in renal transplant recipients and pose special problems for the pregnant patient. A general rule is that these patients often manifest infections with uncommon pathogens. Thus, appropriate cultures and aggressive therapy are mandatory whenever infection is suspected.

Premature labor and premature rupture of membranes are significantly increased in this patient population.[4,5] The reasons for this are unclear, although marginal renal function and chronic steroid therapy may be contributory. Pregnancy-induced hypertension is also more common in these patients and may account for some of the instances of premature delivery.[5] The diagnosis of preeclampsia may be difficult, as chronic hypertension, proteinuria, and edema are common in these patients.

All renal transplant recipients receive some degree of immunosuppressive therapy. The most common regimen is a combination of cyclosporine A (CyA), azathioprine (Imuran), and a corticosteroid, usually prednisone. Side effects of these agents may be of significance to the anesthesiologist. CyA is commonly associated with systemic hypertension, and most patients ultimately require antihypertensive medication. The mechanism for this effect is CyA-induced activation of the sympathetic nervous system.[6] Azathioprine may be associated with thrombocytopenia and abnormalities of liver function. Chronic steroid therapy results in a host of systemic manifestations. Glucose intolerance, avascular neurosis of bone, hypertension, poor wound healing, peptic ulcer disease, and obesity (with possible airway distortion) are all commonly seen and all have well-known implications for anesthetic care. Thin, fragile skin warrants caution with application of tape and automated blood pressure cuffs should be used with caution since high inflation pressures can result in skin abrasions. In addition, bolus ("stress") doses of parenteral steroids are recommended during labor and delivery—whether vaginal or cesarean.

Anesthetic Considerations

Renal transplant recipients with good renal function can receive virtually any type of anesthesia. The preanesthetic evaluation should include attention to current medical therapy and possible side effects. Laboratory evaluation should include white cell count, hematocrit, and renal and liver function, along with a coagulation profile. Careful assessment of bony abnormalities, joint dysfunction, and airway anatomy is important. Epidural anesthesia for labor is well tolerated, although care should be exercised with positioning after institution of the block and with taping to secure the epidural catheter. Cesarean delivery should be performed for obstetric indications and either epidural or subarachnoid anesthesia may be used. However, epidural anesthesia may be preferable, as less rapid and profound hemodynamic effects allow for more judicious fluid management, which may be an important factor if renal function is marginal or pre-eclampsia is a concern. In addition, prolonged operative time (owing to previous abdominal surgery) may also favor continuous epidural or subarachnoid anesthesia.

CARDIAC TRANSPLANTATION

Cardiac transplantation has become an accepted mode of treatment for end-stage cardiomyopathy. The most common indication for cardiac transplantation in young patients is viral cardiomyopathy, although congenital heart disease, valvular dysfunction, and peripartum cardiomyopathy may be the etiology in a small percentage of patients. (Liberalization of recipient criteria has allowed ischemic cardiomyopathy owing to coronary artery disease to become a major indication for transplantation. However, this group of patients is generally older and unlikely, although not impossible,[7] to be of concern to the obstetric anesthesiologist.) Current survival rates after cardiac transplantation average 80 to 90 percent at 1 year and 60 to 70 percent at 5 years.[8] Most patients with nonrejecting cardiac allografts are able to resume normal lifestyles, including reproductive endeavors. Childbirth, both vaginally[9] and by cesarean delivery,[10] has been reported, with a minimum of complications.

Anesthetic Considerations

The preanesthetic evaluations should include careful assessment of exercise tolerance, especially any changes noted by the patient during pregnancy. The time interval since the transplant is important, as the incidence of rejection decreases as this time interval increases. However, cardiac transplant recipients undergo accelerated coronary artery athersclerosis such that allograft coronary artery disease is detected in up to 40 percent of patients by 3 to 5 years after transplantation.[11] The current pharmacologic and immunosuppressive regimen should be noted.

Physiology and Pharmacology. The physiologic hallmark of the heart transplant recipient is the fact that the donor allograft is void of any efferent or afferent autonomic or somatic innervation.[12] The denervated state results in several anesthetic implications.

1. Any maneuver acting via reflex vagal activity (i.e., carotid sinus massage or oculocardiac reflex) will not be effective in these patients.
2. Pharmacologic agents acting via vagal pathways (e.g., atropine and neostigmine) will be free of cardiac effects. However, peripheral actions on vascular tone and peripheral cholinergic receptors will still be intact.
3. Only direct-acting vasoactive agents will reliably produce inotropic or chronotropic effects.
4. Baseline tachycardia is common, owing to absence of vagal tone.
5. Chronic denervation results in "up-regulation" of cardiac β-adrenergic receptors. Thus, extreme sensitivity to β-agonist drugs is seen.[13] (Even small amounts of epinephrine in local anesthetic solutions may have profound chronotropic effects.)[10]
6. A chronotropic response to stress (such as hypovolemia or vasodilation) is delayed, thus adequate cardiac output is dependent on maintenance of adequate preload (the Starling mechanism). Increasing preload is useful prior to anesthetic maneuvers that are likely to result in vasodilation.
7. Afferent denervation implies that myocardial ischemia will not be felt as chest pain or angina. Thus, these patients usually undergo yearly cardiac catheterization to assess the allograft for the development of coronary artery disease.

Effects of Immunosuppression. The concerns in cardiac transplantation are similar to those encountered in the renal transplant recipient. Cardiac transplant recipients are similarly likely to develop hypertension owing to chronic cyclosporine use and usually require antihypertensive therapy. To date, no fetal compromise has been noted to the offspring of cardiac transplant recipients, although only a few such cases have been reported.

Management During Labor. Successful vaginal deliveries have been accomplished both with[14] and without[9] epidural anesthesia. Primary concern should be directed toward maintenance of adequate intravascular volume as labor itself may be associated with marked degrees of dehydration. In addition to adequate hydration, careful avoidance of aortocaval compression is essential, as decreased venous return and subsequent inadequate cardiac filling will be poorly tolerated by the patient with a transplanted heart. In light of these concerns, one may argue that invasive monitoring of central venous pressures during labor is warranted. However, the nonrejecting donor allograft with documented preserved ventricular function should tolerate volume changes quite well. Moreover, a major cause of morbidity in these immunocompromised patients is infection, thus the risk of catheter-induced sepsis probably outweighs the information that would be obtained from such monitoring.

Epidural anesthesia is well tolerated during labor. Low concentrations of local anesthetic with opioid will aid in minimizing the degree of sympathectomy. If hypotension should occur, the first course of management should include uterine displacement to relieve aortocaval compression and increased fluid infusion. If vasopressors are necessary, either ephedrine or phenylphrine may be used. However, ephedrine has both direct and indirect mechanisms of action, and may thus be slightly less effective than expected. If a chronotropic agent is required, then isoproterenol (not atropine) should be utilized.

Management of Cesarean Delivery. Epidural anesthesia is the technique of choice for cesarean delivery as the sensory level can be slowly raised, allowing time for adequate intravascular volume expansion to compensate for the ensuing sympathetic blockade. Subarachnoid anesthesia may, in theory, not be as well tolerated owing to the rapidity of the sympathetic blockade. However, both intraspinal and general anesthesia have been successfully used for a wide variety of nonobstetric surgical procedures in heart transplant recipients.[15] If general anesthesia should be required, one might consider using ketamine rather than thiopental as an induction agent so as to preserve some degree of sympathetic tone.

As with renal transplant patients, appropriate attention to aseptic technique should be employed, and "stress' steroid coverage is usually required.

OTHER TRANSPLANTS

Successful pregnancies and deliveries have been reported after both bone marrow[16] and hepatic transplantation.[17] Experience in these areas, as for other organs (such as lung, pancreas, and combined heart-lung) is extremely limited and anesthetic care must be individualized to the clinical status of the patient at the time of delivery.

REFERENCES

1. Graybar GB, Tarpey M: Kidney Transplantation. p. 61. In Gelman S (ed): Anesthesia and Organ Transplantation. WB Saunders, Philadelphia, 1987

2. Penn I, Makowski EL, Harris P: Parenthood following renal transplantation. Kidney Int 18:221, 1980
3. Lau RJ, Scott J: Pregnancy following renal transplantation. Clin Obstet Gynecol 28:339, 1985
4. Davison JM, Lindheimer MD: Pregnancy in renal transplantation recipients. J Reprod Med 27:613, 1982
5. Fine RN: Pregnancy in renal allograft recipients. Am J Nephrol 2:117, 1982
6. Scherrer U, Vissing SF, Morgan BJ, et al: Cyclosporine-induced sympathetic activation and hypertension after heart transplantation. N Engl J Med 323:693, 1990
7. Curiel P, Spinelli G, Petrella A, et al: Postpartum coronary artery dissection followed by heart transplantation. Am J Obstet Gynecol 163:538, 1990
8. Fragomen LS, Kaye MP: The registry of the International Society for Heart Transplantation: Fifth official report. J Heart Trans 7:249, 1988
9. Lowenstein BR, Vain NW, Perrone SV, et al: Successful pregnancy and vaginal delivery after heart transplantation. Am J Obstet Gynecol 158:589, 1988
10. Camann WR, Goldman GA, Johnson MD, et al: Cesarean delivery in a patient with a transplanted heart. Anesthesiology 71:618, 1989
11. Renlund DG, Bristow MR, Lee HR, O'Connell JB: Medical aspects of cardiac transplantation. J Cardiothorac Anesth 2:500, 1988
12. Kent KM, Cooper T: The denervated heart—a model for studying autonomic control of the heart. N Engl J Med 291:1017, 1974
13. Yusef S, Theodoropoulos S, Mathias CJ: Increased sensitivity of the denervated transplanted human heart to isoprenaline both before and after β-adrenergic blockade. Circulation 75:696, 1987
14. Camann WR, Jarcho JA, Mintz KJ, Greene MF: Uncomplicated vaginal delivery fourteen months after cardiac transplantation. Am Heart J (In Press)
15. Bailey PL, Stanley TH: Anesthesia for patients with a prior cardiac transplant. J Cardiothroac Anesth 4 (suppl 1):38, 1990
16. Deeg HJ, Kennedy MS, Sanders JE, et al: Successful pregnancy after marrow transplantation for severe aplastic anemia and immunosuppression with cyclosporine. JAMA 250:647, 1983
17. Newton ER, Turskoy N, Kaplan M, Reinhold R: Pregnancy and liver transplantation. Obstet Gynecol 71:499, 1988

MORBID OBESITY

Obesity is the most common nutritional disorder in the United States. It is estimated that one fourth of our population is 30 percent or more over their desirable weight. The term *morbid obesity* has been coined to define a subset of obese persons who are at least twice their ideal body weight. Ideal body weight can be determined by using Broca's index, according to which ideal body weight (in kilometers) for males is equal to the height in centimeters minus 100. For females, ideal body weight (in kilograms) is equal to the height in centimeters minus 105. Another frequently used estimate of ideal body weight is the body mass index, which is equal to the weight in kilograms divided by the height in meters, squared. The normal body mass index in 25, whereas the index for the morbidly obese is considered to be greater than 30. The anesthetic management of the morbidly obese parturient requires an understanding of the physiologic changes associated with both pregnancy and obesity. Morbidly obese pregnant patients have an increased risk of perioperative respiratory failure and arrest, aspiration of gastric contents, cardiovascular failure and collapse, pulmonary embolism, infection, metabolic disturbances, and hepatic and renal dysfunction. These patients have an increased incidence of oxytocic induction and repeat cesarean deliveries. They tend to be older, to have higher parity, to have increased antepartum frequency of hypertension, diabetes mellitus, twin gestations and an increased perioperative mortality.[1]

PATHOPHYSIOLOGY

Airway management is often difficult in morbidity obese patients and therefore should be a major concern.[2] Nearly 10 percent of morbidly obese parturients can be described as having sleep apnea and have an elevated resting $PaCO_2$. Laryngoscopy is complicated by the presence of suprasternal fat pads, large breasts, compromised cervical spine extension, and redundant pharyngeal tissue. Obtaining a good mask fit often requires two hands and, on occasion, two people. These patients exhibit a restrictive pattern of pulmonary dysfunction on spirometry. They have a decreased functional residual capacity (FRC) and expiratory reserve volume (ERV) and increased closing volumes (CV). Their FRC is often less than their closing capacity, resulting in atelectasis and increased shunting.[3] These patients have an increased oxygen consumption and carbon dioxide production. They have decreased chest wall compliance and a markedly increased work of breathing. In fact, one has described breathing in the morbidly obese pregnant patient in the supine position as breathing with an 80-pound weight on one's chest. These defects are exaggerated in the supine position and amplified in the Trendelenberg position.[4] Most healthy morbidly obese patients have a residual gastric volume greater than 25 ml and a gastric pH less than 2.5.[5] Cardiac output increases proportionately with weight and total blood volume is increased in these patients. Insulin resistance and an elevation in cholesterol and triglycerides is frequently seen. Fatty infiltration of the liver associated with disturbances of liver function is common.[6] The physiologic changes of pregnancy compound the medical problems associated with obesity and further stress already minimal reserves.

Fetal monitoring may be more difficult in the morbidly obese and aortocaval compression may occur even in the left lateral position. These patients should labor in a semisitting position, receive supplemental oxygen, wear support stockings, and have an internal fetal monitoring electrode placed as soon as possible during labor.

PREANESTHETIC EVALUATION

Preoperatively, in addition to the usual preanesthetic evaluation, these patients should all have arterial air blood gas measurements on room air. Patients with an increased $PaCO_2$ are at an increased risk for postoperative apnea. A baseline electrocardiogram should be obtained and a blood sample should be sent to the blood bank for type and screen. A complete blood count, blood urea nitrogen, creatinine, serum osmolarity, and liver function tests should be obtained as well as a urinalysis with specific gravity and urine osmolarity. The status of the patient's hydration should be carefully evaluated since these patients can sequester large volumes of fluid in their interstitial spaces and can be intravascularly volume depleted while still appearing normovolemic on physical examination (skin turgor and tongue moisture). A central venous pressure (CVP) catheter should always be considered for this reason as well as the fact that intravascular access can be extremely difficult to obtain in these patients. Pulmonary function tests can be useful. If intraspinal anesthesia is a consideration or if there is a history of venous stasis or thromboembolic disease, coagulation studies should be obtained.

MATERNAL MONITORING

Maternal monitoring should consist of an electrocardiogram, pulse oximeter, and an intra-arterial catheter to monitor blood pressure and to obtain blood specimens from the patient from whom blood may be impossible to obtain in a crisis and in whom the technical difficulties of obtaining cuff pressures may be insurmountable.[7] As already mentioned, a CVP catheter should always be considered in these patients. The Trendelenberg position should be avoided in line placement because of the risk of aspiration as well as a decrease in FRC. If indicated, a pulmonary artery catheter should be used without hesitation. It must be stressed that because fetal distress could necessitate an emergency cesarean delivery at any time, all preparations for such an event should be carried out well in advance. Two large peripheral intravenous catheters or one peripheral and a CVP catheter should be placed. These patients should be NPO and should receive 30 ml of a nonparticulate antacid every 4 hours, cimetidine or ranitidine every 6 hours, and metoclopramide every 6 hours.[8] An operating room should be ready for emergency delivery. The problems and management plan should be reviewed with the patient, the anesthesia care team, the nursing staff, the obstetric team, and the recovery room staff.

ANESTHESIA FOR LABOR AND VAGINAL DELIVERY

Epidural anesthesia is the obvious choice for labor and delivery. Initiation should be carried out with the patient in the sitting position to maintain maximum respiratory function and to obtain adequate spinal flexion. If the epidural is not readily accomplished, a continuous spinal anesthetic should be considered. Continuous subarachnoid anesthesia (CSA) offers several advantages over single-dose subarachnoid or continuous epidural anesthesia (CEA).[2] The technique provides the advantages of a single-dose subarachnoid block (i.e., rapid onset, consistent effectiveness, and the ability to use low doses of local anesthetic) with the advantages of a CEA (i.e., controllable duration and controllable level). CSA should theoretically decrease complications such as a high motor block compromising respiratory function, total spinal anesthesia, and systemic toxicity from local anesthetics. However, there will be an incidence of post-dural puncture headache with this technique. This is a manageable complication and, with the introduction and further development of microcatheters, the incidence of post-dural puncture headache should decrease. With whatever technique is chosen, the local anesthetic must be administered slowly since the level obtained with a given dose is unpredictable and may vary considerably from patient to patient. In fact, we have seen the level abruptly rise following delivery of the baby. Hypotension should be aggressively treated with both crystalloid solution and ephedrine, and, if necessary, phenylephrine. The Trendelenberg position should be avoided because, although it does increase venous return, it will decrease FRC and make regurgitation likely. The anesthetic level should be kept at or below T6 since higher levels will impair the patient's ability to use her intercostal muscles for respiration. Uterine displacement should be maintained at all times, and this may be difficult to accomplish.

ANESTHESIA FOR CESAREAN DELIVERY

General Anesthesia

Many authorities would argue that anesthesia for cesarean delivery mandates the use of general anesthesia and endotracheal intubation. Cesarean delivery requires the patient to be supine with uterine displacement and involves manipulation of the abdomen. Morbidly obese pregnant patients do not tolerate intra-abdominal manipulation because of their already impaired respiratory status and their tendency to vomit and, possibly, aspirate. A high level of epidural and subarachnoid anesthesia alone will impair intercostal muscle function and further compromise respiratory status. A total spinal anesthetic can be disastrous. Thus, general endotracheal anesthesia may be necessary to support ventilation and to protect the airway. If the airway examination suggests the likelihood of a difficult intubation, an awake sedated fiberoptic intubation in the semisitting position is warranted. Another option is to use topical anesthesia on the tongue and oropharynx in order to perform direct laryngoscopy to visualize what structures can be seen before induction of general anesthesia. If direct laryngoscopy and intubation is attempted, a rapid-sequence induction with continuous cricoid pressure is mandatory. An extra (or third) person should be available to assist in the procedure. A short-handled laryngoscope can be very helpful. A large-bore suction apparatus must be available and an assortment of small endotracheal tubes (internal diameter 5, 6, and 7 mm) with stylets in place must be ready. If, after induction, the patient is found to be unintubatable and ventilation with cricoid pressure cannot be maintained, an emergency cricothyrotomy must be performed. This involves an incision through the cricothyroid membrane with the insertion of a small (5 mm) endotracheal tube and subsequent inflation of the cuff to obtain a seal. This may be very difficult to accomplish in the morbidly obese parturient. If the mother can be ventilated but not intubated, she should be allowed to awaken. A controlled awake direct or fiberoptic intubation can then be accomplished. A blind nasal intubation is an option but should usually be avoided because of the friability of the nasal mucosa in parturients and the increased difficulty accomplishing any type of intubation when the pharynx is awash in blood. Maternal safety outweighs fetal considerations at this time and surgery should not be permitted to commence until an adequate airway has been established.

Increased cardiac output and an increase in compartment size will increase the requirement for volatile agents as well. Prior to induction, these patients should be acutely oxygenated and well denitrogenated for several minutes. A rapid-sequence induction with cricoid pressure should be accomplished with thiopental and endotracheal intubation facilitated with succinylcholine. Cricoid pressure must be maintained until endotracheal tube position is verified. The endotracheal tube should be well secured and an orogastric (Salem-sump) tube inserted *orally* and gastric contents emptied. Temperature should be monitored as well. The electrocardiogram should be monitored for rhythm and ST changes. Appropriate cardiac medications should be available. Isoflurane is the volatile agent of choice because it undergoes the least biodegradation. Anesthesia is maintained with at least 50 percent oxygen supplemented with nitrous oxide and isoflurane as needed. Pulse oximetry or arterial blood gases data will help guide the required oxygen concentration. A succinylcholine infusion can be used for neuromuscular blockade, however, these patients may be predisposed to a type II block because of the large volumes of drug necessary to maintain paralysis. A better choice for neuromuscular blockade after endotracheal intubation might be an intermediate-acting nondepolarizing drug, particularly atracurium in patients with hepatic or renal impairment. The volatile agent is usually discontinued after the fetus is born because of the degree of uterine relaxation that these drugs can cause and a nitrous-narcotic-relaxant technique is used. If SaO_2 is impaired by the increase in nitrous oxide, the nitrous oxide concentration can be decreased and a volatile agent reinstituted. Narcotic supplementation is appropriate at this time. Some authorities would suggest that the amount of uterine relaxation from 0.2 to 0.4 percent isoflurane is minimal (or absent) and that this drug should be maintained for amnesia alone. Positive end-expiratory pressure (PEEP) can be used to reduce atelectasis, although high intrathoracic pressures can also reduce venous return.

There may be occasions when the risks of general anesthesia outweigh the risks of delivering the infant of a morbidly obese woman by regional anesthesia alone. In these situations a continuous epidural or continuous subarachnoid technique should be chosen. The sensory level should not be raised above T6. Epidural or subarachnoid opioids such as fentanyl can be administered to make the patient more comfortable intra- and postoperatively and to allow the surgery to proceed without impairing the patient's respiratory status, as may occur with high thoracic levels.

Intraspinal plus "light general" anesthesia offers several advantages over general anesthesia alone. It allows adequate airway protection and ventilation while reducing intravenous and volatile anesthetic requirements. It also allows for the use of the epidural or subarachnoid catheter to provide postoperative pain control.

Emergency Cesarean Delivery

If an emergency cesarean delivery is necessary, a general anesthetic with a rapid-sequence induction with cricoid pressure can be undertaken (see earlier discussion of technique). A epidural or subarachnoid catheter can be placed postoperatively for pain management. This scenario should not emerge often, however, since an elective epidural or continuous subarachnoid catheter should have already been placed during labor.

Postoperative Care

If the preoperative room air $PaCO_2$ was elevated, if there is any question of the patient's ability to protect or ensure her airway, or if there is cardiovascular instability, the patient should remain intubated overnight. The patient can be monitored in the recovery room or intensive care unit and ventilated with PEEP on an intermittent mandatory ventilation mode as necessary. She should be kept in the sitting position on an FiO_2 of 50 percent and be continuously monitored with an electrocardiograph and pulse oximeter and observed closely by the nursing staff.

The postpartum morbidly obese patient is at high risk for respiratory failure and arrest.[8] In addition to all the reasons mentioned previously, the parturient now has an abdominal incision that may cause her to splint and take shallow breaths. There may be residual anesthetic agents present. In the pregnant state, high progesterone levels cause respiratory stimulation. Postpartum, these levels fall and respiratory stimulation decreases.

Intramuscular, subcutaneous, or more frequently used "intrafat" opioid injections should be avoided. The absorption of these drugs is unreliable under optimal conditions and these patients are often cold and peripherally vasoconstricted. The obese parturient appears to have a decreased tolerance for pain and may require large doses of opioids postoperatively, which contributes to the multiple factors already described that can cause postoperative respiratory depression. Morbidly obese parturients will require large doses of pain-relieving medications; these drugs should not be given intramuscularly as they will be sequestered in adipose tissue. In the early postoperative period, if continuous epidural or subarachnoid anesthesia has been utilized, the catheter should be maintained and postoperative pain relief provided by subarachnoid or epidural opioids and/or local anesthetics. If general anesthesia has been administered, intravenous opioids must be utilized, either on demand or by patient-controlled analgesia. Change over to oral pain medications may not be feasible for 2 to 3 days. Intraspinal narcotics or a combination of narcotics and local anesthetics is the best method of pain control. Alternatively, intravenous narcotics can be titrated on an hourly basis. These patients require frequent overnight checks. All postpartum morbidly obese patients should be monitored in the recovery room or intensive care until overnight on the first postoperative night. They should be maintained in the head-up position and receive oxygen by face mask at 6–10 L/min. They should be monitored using pulse oximetry with alarms set at an SaO_2 of 90 percent. They should have continuous electrocardiographic monitoring, frequent if not continuous blood pressure monitoring, and frequent temperature checks. Urine output and osmolarity as well as hematocrit should be followed. Shivering should be avoided and treated with small doses of intravenous opioids as necessary. These patients should also be treated with minidose heparin. Once they are transferred to the floor, their arterial lines, CVP lines, and epidural or subarachnoid catheters can be removed. They should still be maintained in the head-up position and administered 50 percent oxygen by face mask. Vital signs should be checked and recorded every 2 hours for 8 hours. An intravenous line should be kept in place until discharge. Early ambulation should be vigorously encouraged.

The risks of caring for the postpartum morbidly obese patient are often not fully appreciated by nursing or medical staff members. In addition to all of the usual obstetric postoperative complications, these patients are at increased risk of respiratory failure and arrest, venous stasis and emboli, cardiovascular failure, hypertension, hypovolemia, and infection.

REFERENCES

1. Gross T, Sokol RJ, King KC: Obesity in pregnancy: risks and outcome. Obstet Gynecol 56:446, 1980
2. Malan TP, Johnson MD: The difficult airway in obstetric anesthesia: techniques for airway management and the role of regional anesthesia. J Clin Anesth 1:104, 1988
3. Luce MJ: Respiratory complications of obesity. Chest 78:626, 1980
4. Paul DR, Hoyt JL, Boutros AR: Cardiovascular and respiratory changes in response to change of posture in the very obese. Anesthesiology 45:73, 1976
5. Vaughan RW, Bauer S, Wise L: Volume and pH of gastric juice in obese patients. Anesthesiology 65:684, 1986
6. Braillon A, Capron JP, Herve MA, et al: Liver in obesity. Gut 26:133, 1985
7. Berlines K, Fujy H, Lee DH, et al: Blood pressure measurements in obese persons: comparison of intraarterial and auscultatory measurements. Am J Cardiol 8:10, 1961

8. Vaughan RW, Englehart RC, Wise L: Postoperative hypoxemia in obese patients. Ann Surg 180:877, 1974

MALIGNANT HYPERTHERMIA

Malignant hyperthermia (MH) is a rare but potentially devastating clinical syndrome triggered by exposure to certain anesthetic agents. MH can be considered an inherited subclinical myopathy that becomes manifest in the presence of potential inhalational anesthetics and/or depolarizing neuromuscular blocking agents. Exposure to these anesthetic agents sets a sequence of events into play that results in a massive increase in metabolism and production of heat, carbon dioxide, and lactic acid.[1]

MH presents as a variable and diverse constellation of signs and symptoms, each of which is itself nonspecific, but the combination of which is highly suggestive of the syndrome (Table 8-9).[2] The exact presentation in each case depends on the triggering agents employed, the presence of other drugs, and individual variation in severity of the disease. The first sign of a MH crisis may be muscle rigidity. Rigidity may first become manifest in the jaw muscles, which may make endotracheal intubation difficult or impossible. Tachycardia, often with hypertension, is a consistent early feature of MH and is often the presenting symptom. Another consistent early signs is a marked incidence in carbon dioxide production, which leads to tachypnea if the patient is not mechanically ventilated. One first will note a rise in the mixed venous carbon dioxide tension, which is then followed by changes in the arterial blood gas. In addition, marked diaphoresis, mottled cyanosis, and coagulopathy are usually evident. The combination of cyanosis and tachycardia in a well-oxygenated, previously healthy patient is highly suggestive of MH.

Early diagnosis is imperative if one is to avoid the morbidity and mortality associated with delay in treatment. MH should be suspected in an anesthetized patient who develops any of the following symptoms: tachypnea, muscle rigidity, diaphoresis, mottling, cyanosis, or hyperthermia. During anesthesia, the most rapid method of detecting MH is with capnography. If the E t CO_2 is markedly increased during constant ventilation and mechanical causes can be ruled out, the diagnosis of MH can be assumed. Confirmation of the diagnosis can be made with central venous and arterial blood gas monitoring. Under normal conditions, the difference between $PvCO_2$ and $PaCO_2$ is 5 mmHg. During an MH crisis, a difference of 15 mmHg or greater is observed. In addition, if the arterial blood gas data demonstrate either a $PaCO_2$ greater than 60 mmHg with a base deficit of at least 5 Eq/L or a pH less than 7.15, the diagnosis of MH is confirmed.

Table 8-9. Presenting Physical and Biochemical Signs of a MH Crisis

Rigidity[a]	↑ E t CO_2[a]
Tachycardia[a]	↑ Central venous CO_2[a]
Tachypnea[a]	↑ Central venous CO_2[a]
Cyanosis	↑ Metabolic and respiratory acidosis[a]
Skin mottling	↑ Creatinine phosphokinase
Diaphoresis	Hyperkalemia
Arrhythmias	Myoglobinuria
Hypertension/unstable blood pressure	
Hyperthermia	

[a] Most frequent signs of an MH crisis.

Table 8-10. Associated Diseases and Abnormalities

Associated Diseases	Associated Abnormalities
Central core disease	Ptosis
King-Denborough syndrome	Strabismus
Duchenne muscular dystrophy	Joint hypermobility
Arthrogryposis	Dislocated joints
Becker's muscular dystrophy	Kyphoscoliosis
Sudden infant death syndrome[a]	Clubfeet
Neuroleptic malignant syndrome[a]	Hernia
Osteogenesis imperfecta[a]	Intolerance to heat and exercise
Myotonia congenita[a]	Muscle cramps
	Muscle swelling
	Muscle weakness
	High fevers
	Febrile convulsions
	Blackouts
	Anxiety

[a] Controversial association.

The determination of patient risk for MH is essential prior to anesthetic induction so that adequate precautions may be taken. The clearest indication of susceptibility is a prior MH reaction, although even an uneventful prior anesthetic induction does not rule out MH susceptibility. In addition, patients with various musculoskeletal abnormalities may be at increased risk for MH (Table 8-10).[3] To evaluate susceptibility, muscle biopsy contracture studies must be performed. This test is considered the gold standard in diagnosis and is more than 95 percent reliable. Other less invasive tests have been developed but have not yet achieved validity for predicting MH susceptibility.

Triggering agents for MH include the volatile inhalational anesthetics and the depolarizing muscle relaxants. Contrary to prior reports, present evidence indicates that amide local anesthetics are safe to use in MH-susceptible patients.[4,5] Several environmental stresses have been implicated in the precipitation or potentiation of an MH crisis, including exercise, heat prostration, anoxia, apprehension, and excitement. Thus all susceptible patients should be kept as comfortable as possible before, during, and after surgical procedures. Although awake MH crisis is common in swine, it is not common in humans.

The only known therapeutic agent effective in MH is dantrolene. It must be administered early in the MH crisis while muscle perfusion is still adequate. The temporal profile of plasma concentrations of prophylactic dantrolene following an intravenous dose in a parturient suggests that pregnancy does not alter the pharmacokinetics of the drug. Placental transfer of dantrolene does occur and is dependent on placental factors such as area of transfer and diffusion distance as well as the difference in the maternal and fetal drug concentrations.[6] In MH-susceptible patients who received prophylactic dantrolene during labor and delivery, the uterine vein/maternal vein ratio was 0.29 to 0.51.[7] The infants of these mothers were vigorous and showed no adverse effects.

MANAGEMENT OF THE OBSTETRIC MH-SUSCEPTIBLE PATIENT

The MH-susceptible patient in the obstetric setting poses a unique challenge for the anesthesiologist. There have been three reported cases of MH during delivery; in each instance a cesarean delivery was performed under general anesthesia using a known triggering agent.[8–11] There have been no reported cases of MH in an obstetric patient with the use of nontriggering agents for general or regional anesthesia nor have there been any published reports of awake triggering during delivery. The fact that so few cases of MH during delivery have been published has led some investigators to speculate that pregnancy may exert some protective influence over the MH-susceptible patient. However, there are no in vitro, animal, or human studies to support this postulate. Thus, until proven otherwise, it would be prudent to consider a pregnant MH-susceptible patient to be at equal risk for the disease as any other surgical candidate.

The emotional and physical stresses of labor and delivery may act to potentiate or provoke an MH crisis, although such an event has not been documented. However, these considerations should influence the timing of anesthesia as well as the choice of monitors employed. In addition, pregnancy-induced disease such as chorioamnionitis or toxemia can add to the stresses of pregnancy and conceivably influence the onset of a MH crisis. Furthermore, the drugs used to induce, augment, or depress labor may also complicate the diagnosis and treatment of MH. It must be remembered that the child born to an MH-susceptible mother may also possess the trait and may be at risk during and after the delivery. This applies to children of MH-susceptible fathers as well.

Prophylaxis

Several cases of dantrolene prophylaxis prior to uneventful labor and delivery have been reported. However, dantrolene pretreatment is no longer considered necessary. Dantrolene is not without side effects, which may become manifest in the mother and the neonate. The neonate may experience muscle flaccidity and respiratory difficulties. In addition, uterine atony has been reported after dantrolene pretreatment.[12] Thus the routine use of dantrolene prophylaxis is not indicated, especially in the obstetric setting.[13]

Nontriggering Anesthetic Agents

All local anesthetics, with or without epinephrine, are now considered safe for use in MH-susceptible patients. For general anesthesia, a large armamentarium of agents is available. Nontriggering general anesthetic agents include barbiturates, nondepolarizing muscle relaxants, opioids, tranquilizers, nitrous oxide, and ketamine (Table 8-11).

Preoperative Preparation

All known or suspected MH-susceptible patients should have a preoperative anesthetic consultation during early pregnancy, inclusive of a complete history and physical examination. Particular emphasis should be placed on obtaining a detailed description of any previous anesthetic reactions or untoward perioperative events involving the patient or any family members. The patient should be educated about the disease and the anesthetic plan explained to her. One copy of the completed consultation form should be sent to the referring obstetrician, one copy placed in the patient's chart, and one copy placed in a department register of high-risk obstetric patients. The patient should be instructed to alert the nurse upon arrival to the labor and delivery (L&D) floor, and all involved anesthesia personnel should be notified immediately so that the appropriate preparations can be made.

A cart containing the necessary drugs and equipment for treatment of MH-susceptible patients should be made available on the floor and should be checked to ensure that the cart is fully stocked. (Table 8-12).

Table 8-11. Nontriggering Anesthetic Agents

Barbiturates	Local Anesthetics: Amides
Thiopental (Pentothal)	Lidocaine (Xylocaine)
Methohexital (Brevital)	Mepivacaine (Carbocaine)
Thiamylal (Surital)	Bupivacaine (Marcaine)
Narcotics (opioids)	Etidocaine (Duranest)
Morphine	Prilocaine (Citanest)
Meperidine (Demerol)	Local Anesthetics: Esters
Hydromorphone (Dilaudid)	Procaine (Novocaine)
Fentanyl (Sublimaze)	Chloroprocaine (Nesacaine)
Sufentanil (Sufenta)	Tetracaine (Pontocaine)
Alfentanil (Alfenta)	Muscle Relaxants
Anticholinesterases	Pancuronium (Pavulon)
Neostigmine (Prostigmine)	Atricurium (Tracrium)
Pyridostigmine (Regonol)	Vecuronium (Norcuron)
Edrophonium (Tensilon)	Tranquilizers
Other	Diazepam (Valium)
Ketamine (Ketalar)	Midazolam (Versed)
Droperidol (Inapsine)	Anticholinergics*
Nitrous oxide	Atropine
	Glycopyrrolate (Robinul)

A cesarean birth/delivery room should be designated for this patient and held for her until she delivers. The room should contain a dedicated MH "clean" machine, one free of vapor contamination. If such a special unit is not available, the standard anesthesia machine should be prepared for the patient by cleaning it of all residues of vapor anesthetic agents. The breathing circuit, reservoir bag, soda lime, and carbon dioxide absorber should be changed as should the fresh gas hose from the machine. The anesthesia machine should be flushed with oxygen at 10 L/min for 10 to 15 minutes.[14] These precautions should be instituted as soon as the patient arrives on the L&D floor, as the need for emergency cesarean delivery can arise at any time.

Anesthesia for Labor and Delivery

All patients should have a large intravenous catheter placed on admission to the L&D floor. Regional anesthesia, unless contraindicated, should be performed on all obstetric MH-susceptible patients in order to decrease the stress of labor and delivery. Epidural anesthesia instituted early in labor via a continuous infusion is the most effective means of maintaining a constant level of sensory anesthesia through all stages of labor and delivery. Perineal anesthesia should be assured at the onset of the second stage of labor, when the patient is presumably most vulnerable to MH. Subarachnoid anesthesia given prior to delivery is an alternative to epidural anesthesia, but it is less preferable since it does not protect during the early stages of labor.

Anesthesia for Cesarean Delivery

Regional anesthesia is preferred to general anesthesia for cesarean delivery. In addition to the well-recognized benefits of regional anesthesia for cesarean delivery in normal patients, awake triggering of MH has never been reported in obstetric patients. Epidural anesthesia should be administered using a continuous catheter technique. The catheter allows the regional anesthetic to be continued should surgery be prolonged and also can be used for pain relief in the postoperative period.

Table 8-12. Suggested Minimum Contents for an MH Cart

Medications
- Dantrolene—at least 50 20-mg ampules
- Procainamide—500 mg/ml and 100 mg/ml
- Furosemide—at least 200 mg
- Mannitol 25%—at least 100 ml
- Dextrose 50%—100 ml
- Chlorpromazine—250 mg
- Sodium bicarbonate—at least 10 50-ml ampules

Solutions
- Sterile water for injection—at least 2,000 ml (for reconstituting Dantrolene)
- Normal saline for injection—at least 20 1,000-ml bags (left cooled in refrigerator)
- Normal saline for irrigation—at least five 3,000-ml bags (left cooled in refrigerator)

Cooling
- Availability of continuous supply of crushed ice
- Cooling blanket and console
- Stomach and rectal tubes
- Irrigating Foley catheter with collecting bags

Monitoring
- Electronic temperature probes—2
- Extra electronic thermometer
- Oral and rectal glass thermometers
- Central venous access kits—2
- Pulmonary artery catheter
- Esophageal stethoscope
- Blood gas kits
- Blood collection tubes of all types, with appropriate labels

General
- New anesthesia breathing circuit and carbon dioxide absorber cannisters
- Syringes—all sizes, including 50 60-ml syringes specifically for dantrolene
- Intravenous catheters—all sizes
- Needles—all sizes
- Alcohol sponges, gauze, tape, instruments, needle disposal bucket, log sheets, etc.

Single-dose or continuous subarachnoid anesthesia can also be utilized. For regional anesthesia, patient monitoring during cesarean delivery should include electrocardiogram (ECG), pulse oximeter, temperature, noninvasive blood pressure, and urine output. For general anesthesia, capnography is mandated in addition to the monitors used in regional anesthesia. An arterial catheter may be placed, if desired, for continuous blood pressure and arterial blood gas monitoring.

If general anesthesia is necessary, it can be safely administered using the agents mentioned in Table 8-11. Although succinylcholine is the agent of choice for muscle relaxation during rapid-sequence induction, its use in MH-susceptible patients is contraindicated. The only alternatives are the nondepolarizing muscle relaxants. Unfortunately, in the recommended doses, these agents require 3 to 5 minutes for suitable endotracheal intubating conditions. This long onset time can be decreased by increasing the induction dose. Vecuronium when given in high doses provides rapid endotracheal intubating conditions with minimal effects on the autonomic nervous system. In doses of 0.25 to 0.4 mg/kg vecuronium has been used without significant hemodynamic changes. At these doses, vecuronium usually provides excellent intubating conditions within 1 minute without greatly increasing the duration of action.[15]

Vecuronium, because of its highly ionized state, should not cross the placenta in significant amounts if the usual doses are given. However, with high doses needed for faster onset of muscle relaxation, vecuronium may cross the placental barrier and may result in neonatal muscle weakness or paralysis.

In the recovery room, the patient should be monitored closely for any signs of an MH crisis. She should have normal laboratory tests and stable vital signs for at least 4 hours prior to discharge from the recovery room. Thereafter, vital signs, including temperature, should be monitored hourly for 24 hours. Explicit instructions should be given to notify the anesthesiologist for increases in temperature, heart rate, or respiratory rate.

Table 8-13. Suggested Treatment Protocol for an MH Crisis

1. Discontinue all triggering anesthetic agents.
2. Hyperventilate with 100% oxygen.
3. Inform the surgeon: request to expedite and terminate the procedure.
4. Call for help.
5. Have the MH cart brought to the operating room.
6. Designate people to prepare the dantrolene.
7. Administer an initial dose of 2.5 mg/kg of dantrolene as soon as possible. Response to dantrolene should occur within minutes. If not, administer dantrolene as necessary, titrating to heart rate, muscle rigidity, and temperature. Average effective dose of dantrolene is 2.5 mg/kg but occasionally 10 mg/kg or more may be necessary.
8. Change to a clean machine or replace the rubber components (breathing circuit, reservoir bag, fresh gas hose) and soda lime in the existing machine.
9. Place arterial and central venous catheters and obtain blood gases, electrolyte levels, and clotting studies STAT.
10. Institute electronic temperature monitoring.
11. Treat arrhythmias with lidocaine or procainamide.
12. Administer sodium bicarbonate guided by arterial blood gas results.
13. Control hyperthermia with surface cooling, infusion of cooled normal saline, and body cavity lavage as necessary to maintain core temperature of 38°C.
14. Maintain urine output at a minimum of 2 ml/kg/h with intravenous fluids, furosemide, and mannitol.
15. After the MH crisis is controlled, transfer the patient to the ICU and observe for recrudescence of malignant hyperthermia.
16. Follow creatinine phosphokinase, calcium, electrolytes, and clotting studies until normalized. Observe for disseminated intravascular coagulation.
17. Obtain ECG and follow postoperatively.

TREATMENT OF AN MH CRISIS (TABLE 8-13)

Effectiveness of therapy is contingent on early recognition of the MH crisis.[16] The triggering anesthetic agent should be discontinued immediately and the patient ventilated with 100 percent oxygen. The anesthesia machine should be replaced by one free of contamination from inhalational agents. If such a "clean" machine is not available, the rubber components (the breathing circuit, reservoir bag, and fresh gas hose) and the soda lime in the carbon dioxide absorber should be replaced on the machine in use. The surgeon should be informed of the patient's condition and requested to expedite and terminate the procedure. Help from additional personnel should be requested.

The MH cart should be brought immediately to the room. Several people should be designated to prepare the dantrolene. An initial dose of 2.5 mg/kg should be administered as soon as possible at a rate of 1 mg/kg/min. The dose may be repeated every 5 minutes until the symptoms are reversed (the temperature, muscle tone, and heart rate should decline) or until a total dose of 10 mg/kg is achieved. After the crisis, intravenous dantrolene should be continued at a dose of 1 mg/kg every 6 hours for 24 hours. Further dantrolene therapy should be based on clinical and laboratory findings.

Once these lifesaving measures have been instituted, appropriate monitoring of the patient should be the next priority. The ECG will already be in use and is a necessary monitor for arrhythmias. Although most arrhythmias will respond to dantrolene therapy, refractory cases can be treated with lidocaine or procainamide 10 mg/kg.

The temperature should be monitored at various sites. A Foley catheter should be inserted to monitor urine output. An arterial catheter for pressure measurement and blood gas analysis as well as a central venous catheter should be placed. Arterial and venous blood gases and serum electrolyte levels should be drawn and sent as STAT. The metabolic acidosis should be corrected with sodium bicarbonate, guided by the results of the arterial blood gas. If arterial blood gas data are not available, and initial dose of 2 mEq/kg should be administered. In a fulminant MH crisis, it may be difficult to correct the blood pH above 7.20.

Fever should be controlled using any of a variety of techniques, including surface cooling with ice and hypothermic blanket, intravenous cooling with iced saline (not lactated Ringer's solution), body cavity lavage with iced saline, or extracorporeal circulation with heat exchanger. One liter of intravenous iced saline every 10 minutes for 30 minutes is effective in lowering the core temperature. In order to avoid hypothermia, cooling should not progress below 38°C but should be restarted if the temperature rises above this level.

Urine output should be closely monitored and maintained at a minimum of 2 ml/kg/h. To achieve this high urine flow, a generous volume of saline, mannitol 12.5 mg, and furosemide 50 mg should be given intravenously. The diuretics may be repeated for a total of four doses. In addition, central venous pressure and arterial blood pressure should be maintained at adequate levels to optimize urine output. Experience has shown that with early recognition and prompt institution of treatment, recovery from an MH crisis is likely.

THE MALIGNANT HYPERTHERMIA ASSOCIATION OF THE UNITED STATES

The Malignant Hyperthermia Association of the United States was organized in 1981. Its primary goals are to educate patients and their families as well as members of the medical community about MH, its diagnosis, and treatment. The organization also raises funds to support research into the condition and has established a data bank of MH cases. A 24-hour emergency number has been established to assist physicians in the management of an MH crisis. The MH Hotline telephone number is (209) 634-4917, request Index Zero, Malignant Hyperthermia Consultant List.

ACKNOWLEDGMENT

I wish to thank Richard B. Schwartz, M.D., Ph.D., for his advice in the preparation of this manuscript.

REFERENCES

1. Gronert GA: Malignant hyperthermia. Anesthesiology 53:395, 1980
2. Rosenberg H: Clinical presentation of malignant hyperthermia. Br J Anaesth 60:268, 1988
3. Brownell AKW: Malignant hyperthermia: relationship to other diseases. Br J Anaesth 60:303, 1988
4. Harrison GG, Morrell DF: Response of MHS swine to I.V. infusion of lignocaine and bupivacaine. Br J Anaesth 52:385, 1980
5. Paasuke RT, Brownell AKW: Amide local anaesthetics and malignant hyperthermia. Can Anaesth Soc J 33:126, 1986
6. Morison DH: Placental transfer of dantrolene. (Letter) Anesthesiology 59:265, 1983
7. Glassenberg R, Cohen H: Intravenous dantrolene in a pregnant malignant hyperthermia susceptible patient. Anesthesiology 61A:404, 1984
8. Crawford JS: Hyperpyrexia during pregnancy. Lancet June: 1244, 1972
9. Cupryn JP, Kennedy A, Byrick RJ: Malignant hyperthermia in pregnancy. Am J Obstet Gynecol 150:327, 1984
10. Gibbs JM: Unexplained hyperpyrexia during labour. Anaesth Intens Care 12, No. 4:375, 1984
11. Lips FJ, Newland M, Dutton G: Malignant hyperthermia triggered by cyclopropane during cesarean section. Anesthesiology 56:144, 1982
12. Weingarten AE, Korsh JI, Neuman GC, et al: Postpartum uterine atony after intravenous dantrolene. Anesth Analg 66:269, 1987
13. Cunliff M, Lerman J, Britt BA: Is prophylactic dantrolene indicated for MHS patients undergoing elective surgery? Anesth Analg 66:S35, 1987
14. Beebe JJ, Sessler D: Preparation of anesthesia machines for patients susceptible to malignant hyperthermia. Anesthesiology 69:395, 1988
15. Lennon RL, Olson RA, Gronert GA: Atracurium or vecuronium for rapid sequence endotracheal intubation. Anesthesiology 64:510, 1986
16. Britt B (ed): Malignant Hyperthermia. Martinus Nijhoff Publishing, Boston, 1987

DRUG ADDICTION, HEPATITIS, AND ACQUIRED IMMUNODEFICIENCY SYNDROME

DRUG ADDICTION IN THE PARTURIENT

The use of illicit drugs has become endemic in our society and, as a result, anesthesiologists are now seeing a dramatic increase in the number of patients who are using so-called recreational drugs. Despite antidrug programs such as drug education in schools and the well-publicized cocaine-related deaths of several famous athletes, there is clearly an increasing incidence of drug abuse. Although substance abuse has been seen in all socioeconomic groups, it is a particularly common problem when dealing with the "inner-city" patient. Recently, there have been reports of vast increases in substance abuse during pregnancy. Recreational drugs that have been reported as being commonly abused in pregnancy include cocaine, crack (alkaloidal cocaine), amphetamines, narcotics (opioids), alcohol, marijuana, and phencyclidine. There is often evidence of multiple drug use.[1] Substance abuse in the parturients affects both mother and fetus and impacts on the care provided by the perinatologist, anesthesiologist, and neonatalogist.

Cocaine/Crack

Cocaine ($C_{17}H_{21}NO_4$, benzoylmethylecgonine) is an alkaloid obtained from the plant *Erythroxylon coca*. Cocaine use in the United States is a major problem that occurs in all segments of the population. In 1985, it was estimated that over 30 million Americans (approximately 10 percent of the population of the United States) had used cocaine at least once and over 5 million were chronic users.[2] Because of the lower cost and increased availability of cocaine when it is alkalized ("crack"), the number of cocaine/crack users is likely to be much greater today than the previous estimate. The number of pregnant patients who are using cocaine is also growing.[3] At Roosevelt Hospital (New York), which has a large indigent patient population, more than 50 percent of unregistered patients are cocaine positive on toxicologic screen. Additionally, a majority of the parturients, while testing positive, also deny drug use when asked by the anesthesiologist.[4]

Since cocaine is absorbed through all mucous membrane, there are multiple possible routes of administration. Routes of ingestion include smoking, snorting, and intravenous or subcutaneous injection. Oral and rectal administration have also been reported.[5,6] The mixing of cocaine with other drugs is quite common. Little et al. estimated that two-thirds of his patients using cocaine were also abusing other illicit drugs.[1] Oro et al. have found that combining drugs resulted in higher perinatal morbidity when compared to single-drug abuse.[7]

Effect of Cocaine on the Mother

Cocaine acts principally by inhibiting nerve conduction and preventing the reuptake of norepinephrine at the adrenergic neuron.[8] The resultant increases of circulating norepinephrine cause many of the complications seen after cocaine administration. Cocaine can have far-reaching effects on the cardiac, pulmonary, central nervous, and gastrointestinal systems (Tables 8-14 and 8-15). The increased norepinephrine levels resulting from cocaine abuse cause a reduction of cardiac electrical stability, thus predisposing these patients to malignant arrhythmias. In the pregnant patient, cocaine may also cause maternal–fetal vasoconstriction, hypertension, and tachycardia. Cocaine use has been reported as causing maternal hypertension and other symptoms of vasoconstriction that may be confused with the onset of pregnancy-induced hypertension.[9] There is a large prevalence of substance abuse, particularly cocaine, in patients admitted in preterm labor.[10,11] Cocaine has also been reported by several investigators as causing an increase in the incidence of placental abruption.[12,13] Although it is a common misconception that the placental protects the fetus from maternally ingested drugs, it does not; it has been shown that maternally administered cocaine can have adverse neonatal effects due to direct placental transfer. Woods et al.[14] have demonstrated that the administration of intravenous cocaine to pregnant ewes caused marked fetal hypoxia, hypertension, and tachycardia. These physiologic changes were due not only to placental passage of the drug but also to decreased uterine blood flow associated with cocaine-induced hemodynamic perturbations. Moore et al. found a dose-related decrease in uterine blood flow of up to 40 percent.[15] Transplacental passage of cocaine in humans has been reported.[16] Infants whose mothers

Table 8-14. Signs and Symptoms of Cocaine Use

Hypertension	Hyperpyrexia
Tachycardia	Metabolic acidosis
Convulsions	Emotional lability
Hyperreflexia	Dilated pupils
Tremors	

Table 8-15. Therapy for Cocaine Intoxication

Symptom	Therapy
Hypertension/tachycardia	Labetalol
Convulsions	Benzodiazepines; control airway
Tremors/CNS excitation	Benzodiazepines
Anginal syndromes	
Associated with hypertension	Labetalol
Associated with ECG changes	IV nitroglycerin
Ventricular fibrillation	Verapamil
Psychosis	Lithium

used cocaine just prior to delivery excreted cocaine 12 to 24 hours after delivery and continued to excrete the cocaine metabolite, benzylecgonine, for 5 days. The slow metabolism of cocaine in the neonate demonstrated by the persistence of benzylecgonine in the neonate for this lengthy period is due to low fetal plasma cholinesterase activity.[17]

Death after cocaine ingestion is most often due to cardiac abnormalities, including malignant ventricular arrhythmias, myocardial infarction, and cardiac asystole.[18–20] However, other causes of death, such as convulsions and aspiration, bronchospasm, pulmonary edema, stroke, and subarachnoid hemorrhage, have been reported.[21,22] Intestinal ischemia following ingestion of cocaine has been described.[23] Pneumomediastinum, pneumopericardium, and pneumothorax have also been reported after cocaine abuse.[24–26]

Anesthetic Implications of Cocaine Abuse

Anesthetic implications of cocaine abuse are related to the quantity and time of use and whether the abuse is chronic or acute. Chronic users may have a decrease in their anesthetic requirements due to a depletion of catecholamines; whereas the acute cocaine abuser may have increased anesthetic requirement due to increased circulating catecholamines. Sensitivity to other drugs may also occur in the cocaine abuser. Jatlow et al.[27] have reported a succinylcholine sensitivity due to cocaine use. There is also a risk associated with the administration of drugs to the cocaine abuser that sensitize the myocardium to arrhythmias (halothane) or drugs that release catecholamines. Myocardial ischemia is a common manifestation of cocaine intoxication and the anesthesiologist should be prepared to treat this as well as other complications of cocaine use. Evidence from animal studies shows that cocaine-induced ventricular arrhythmias may be prevented by the administration of the calcium channel antagonist, verapamil.[28,29] Pretreatment with verapamil prior to induction of anesthesia may protect these cocaine-abusing parturients from lethal arrhythmias, suggesting that cocaine may act by enhancing calcium influx into myocardial cells. These investigators also suggest that verapamil may antagonize the peripheral vasoconstrictive effects of norepinephrine. Treatment of the cocaine abuser with β-blockers may cause unopposed α-receptor stimulation, thus worsening hypertension.[30]

A major difficulty facing the anesthesiologist is that most cocaine-abusing parturients deny drug use. Therefore, in an inner city environment where drug addiction is prevalent, the anesthesiologist must always consider the possibility that the patient has recently used cocaine. One method that can be utilized to detect the use of cocaine prior to initiation of anesthesia is the On Trak assay for cocaine metabolites (Roche Laboratories, Nutley, NJ). This latex agglutination inhibition test provides a rapid result, which, if positive, indicates to the anesthesiologist that there is a high risk that the patient has recently abused cocaine. The On Trak assay for cocaine provides only a preliminary analytical test results. Although a more specific method, such as gas chromatography/mass spectrometry, should be used to confirm the result, this test does allow the anesthesiologist to ascertain within 4 minutes if there is an increased risk to the patient due to cocaine abuse (Roche Laboratories, personal correspondence).[31,32]

Amphetamines/Metamphetamine

Amphetamines are commonly abused both individually and in combination with other drugs. A recent study demonstrated that between 1986 and 1987, 10 percent of the toxicologic screens performed in San Diego were positive for amphetamines.[32] Acute ingestion of amphetamines causes a release of catecholamines from adrenergic nerve terminals, being both an α- and a β-adrenergic agonist. Like cocaine, amphetamines inhibit the reuptake of catecholamines. Signs and symptoms of amphetamine use resemble those of "crack" use and include confusion, tremors, hyperreflexia, fever, hypertension, tachycardia, arrhythmias, and pulmonary edema.[33] Hypertension may occur after only small doses of amphetamine and has been reported as causing cerebral hemorrhage and stroke. The combination of hypertension, convulsions, and proteinuria resulting from ingestion of amphetamines has been mistaken for eclampsia.[34] Acute amphetamine intoxication has also been reported as increasing intracranial pressure.[35] The MAC (maximal alveolar concentration) for volatile agents is increased; however, this has been shown to revert to normal during hyperventilation.[36]

Chronic use of amphetamines causes depletion of neuronal catecholamines as well as impaired response to sympathomimetics.[37] Cardiac arrest during anesthesia for cesarean delivery has been reported in patients chronically abusing amphetamines.[38] Pulmonary edema has also been reported following general anesthesia for cesarean delivery in an amphetamine abuser.[39]

Some investigators have found an association between the use of amphetamines in pregnancy and congenital anomalies.[40,41] Although Little et al. failed to find such a correlation, they did find that methamphetamine use was associated with intrauterine fetal growth retardation.[42]

Alcohol Abuse

The alcoholic parturient poses many problems to the anesthesiologist. During the preoperative evaluation, a history of the quantity and type of alcohol consumed, the duration of abuse, the time of the last consumption, and the use of other drugs should be elicited by the anesthesiologist. The medical history and review of systems should include the neurologic, cardiac, hepatic, and hematologic systems. If the patients appears intoxicated, a blood alcohol level should be obtained. A level of 100 mg/100 ml is the legal limit of intoxication. If the alcohol-abusing parturient does not present with symptoms of alcoholic peripheral neuropathy, regional anesthesia should be considered, thereby avoiding some of the potential problems associated with general anesthesia in the alcoholic patient.

Prior to initiation of regional anesthesia, the absence of peripheral neuropathies should be documented. Regional anesthesia may present other problems in the alcoholic since these patients may have a contracted blood volume and muscle wasting, and, therefore, may develop hypotension and respiratory failure after initiation of the block. In the event that a general anesthetic becomes necessary, thiobarbiturates should be used with caution since they may be potentiated by ethanol. General anesthesia presents many dangers in these patients since they may react in unexpected ways. Additionally, the alcoholic may have cardiomyopathy and hypoalbuminemia, both of which cause untoward responses to general anesthetics.[43] If the patient is intoxicated, decreased amounts of anesthetic will be needed.[44] Abnormal responses to both depolarizing and nondepolarizing muscle relaxants have also been reported. Duvaldestin et al. have demonstrated that in alcoholic cirrhosis the initial dose required to produce relaxation was higher than normal, whereas the duration of action was prolonged in these patients.[45] Because ethanol inhibits antidiuretic hormone, hypovolemia and fluid imbalance may be seen. The commonly seen manifestations of alcoholism and their anesthetic implications are reviewed in Table 8-16.

Table 8-16. Symptoms of Alcoholism and Their Anesthetic Implications

Symptom	Implications to Anesthesiologist
Peripheral neuropathy	Regional anesthesia relatively contraindicated
Cardiomyopathy	Avoid cardiodepressant anesthetics
Increased gastric acid	Give antacid/rapid-sequence induction
Decreased albumin	Neuromuscular blockade abnormalities
Coagulation defects	Regional anesthesia contraindicated (Patient may need fresh frozen plasma, platelets, vitamin K)
Esophageal varices	Caution with nasogastric tubes, esophageal stethoscope, temperature probe
Ascites	Avoid sodium solutions
Cirrhosis	Avoid halothane
Convulsions	Avoid ketamine, enflurane
V/Q mismatch	Avoid general anesthesia if possible

Narcotic (Opioid) Abuse

There are multiple problems facing the physician treating the narcotic- (opioid) abusing parturient. These problems include acquired immunodeficiency syndrome (AIDS), hepatitis, endocarditis, pulmonary emboli, pulmonary edema, anemia, renal disease, cardiac arrhythmias, and hypotension.[46] A report has described the increasing incidence of spinal/epidural abscess and disc space infection in drug-abusing patients.[47] There is an increase in the incidence of pre-eclampsia in the pregnant patient who is abusing narcotics and, therefore, the possibility of narcotic abuse should be considered in the inner-city parturient presenting with hypertension.[48] Electrocardiographic changes have also been noted in opioid abusers.[49]

Acute withdrawal syndrome begins at about 12 hours and can present as anxiety, tremors, muscle pains, nausea, vomiting, anorexia, gastrointestinal pain, mydriasis, dehydration, tachycardia, hypertension, and tachypnea.[46] These symptoms peak at 48 to 72 hours. Most opioid withdrawal symptoms are the result of sympathetic hyperactivity and may be modified by the administration of the α_2-agonist, clonidine.[50]

The anesthetic of choice in the narcotic-addicted parturient is regional anesthesia, thus avoiding the administration of narcotics. Unfortunately, regional anesthesia may be contraindicated because of coagulopathy, neuropathy, infection, and an uncooperative patient. Narcotic addicts often show a decreased pain tolerance, and a relative failure of regional anesthesia has been reported in these patients.[51] The use of pure antagonist or agonist-antagonist drugs must be avoided as they will precipitate acute withdrawal syndrome.[52] The use of epidurally administered agonist-antagonist agents are also contraindicated because of the risk of precipitating acute withdrawal.[53] If general anesthesia is needed, the anesthesiologist must take adequate precautions due to the high risk of AIDS in this patient population. Additionally, the narcotic addict has delayed gastric emptying. Therefore, to avoid the occurrence of gastric regurgitation and the development of aspiration pneumonitis

Table 8-17. Management of the Marijuana Abuser

Symptom	Treatment
Tachycardia	Propranolol
Agitation	Benzodiazepine
Hypotension	Ephedrine
Hypotension/tachycardia	Phenylephrine
Bronchoconstriction	Avoid thiopental

under general anesthesia, a rapid-sequence induction with cricoid pressure must be performed.[54,55] The anesthesiologist should also consider prophylaxis with metoclopramide and cimetidine because of the increased risk of pulmonary acid aspiration in these patients. Severe hypotension reported to have occurred in narcotic addicts under general anesthesia, has been treated with an injection of morphine.[56]

Postoperative analgesia may also present a problem in the narcotic addict. The use of epidural anesthesia in the postoperative period can provide adequate postoperative pain relief while avoiding the use of narcotics. New drugs, such as ketorolac, a parenteral nonsteroidal anti-inflammatory drug, may prove to be superior for postoperative pain relief in the narcotic addict.

Marijuana Abuse

The use of marijuana is estimated to occur in 10 to 37 percent of pregnancies.[57] Marijuana use during pregnancy may cause arrest of labor, failure of spontaneous placental delivery, increased incidence of meconium, and low birthweight.[58] Marijuana use has several implications to the anesthesiologist. Cardiac abnormalities, including tachycardia, arrhythmias, and electrocardiographic abnormalities, may be seen. MAC may be reduced in the marijuana abuser. Agitation may also be seen, and together with mental status changes may make regional anesthesia difficult to perform. Carbon monoxide levels five times greater than those of tobacco as well as major changes in bronchi may also be seen after marijuana smoking.[59] These pulmonary changes, including hypercarbia and increased carbon monoxide levels, may interfere with fetal oxygenation. Abnormal halothane metabolism due to marijuana-induced microsomal dechlorinase activity has been reported, therefore, volatile agents other than halothane should be used in these patients[60] (Table 8-17).

ANESTHESIA FOR THE PARTURIENT WITH VIRAL HEPATITIS

Viral hepatitis is a serious infectious disease that may be seen in the inner-city parturient. Five hepatitis virus causative agents have been identified. These include hepatitis A virus, hepatitis B virus, hepatitis delta virus, and two non-A, non-B hepatitis viruses, one of which is now designated as hepatitis C. These five agents, although different in structure and etiology, each cause a clinical picture marked by hepatocellular necrosis and hepatic inflammation. In addition to the above hepatotropic viruses, other viruses such as cytomegalovirus, Ebstein-Barr virus, herpes simplex virus, varicella zoster virus, rubella, and measles may also cause hepatic inflammation. Acute viral hepatitis is a common disease. According to the Centers for Disease Control (CDC), the incidence of hepatitis B has been rising. It is presently estimated that there are over 300,000 cases of hepatitis B per year in the United States. Acute viral hepatitis has a mortality of approximately 1 percent and may cause severe morbidity, including cirrhosis, chronic liver disease, hepatocellular carcinoma, and renal abnormalities. In fact, chronic viral hepatitis is thought to be one of the leading causes of cirrhosis, being surpassed only by alcohol abuse. Hepatitis B, also known as serum hepatitis, is a more serious disease and is more likely to develop into a chronic state.

Many cases of hepatitis seen on our labor floor at Roosevelt Hospital are hepatitis B secondary to intravenous drug abuse. Hepatitis B virus (HBV) may be spread via injected blood and body fluids, and during sexual intercourse (both homosexual and heterosexual). The virus can also be transmitted from mother to infant.

The diagnosis of HBV is made based on specific serologic testing. Hepatitis B surface antigen (HBsAg) is found in the serum of patients during the active phase of the disease. HBsAg appears in the blood several weeks prior to the onset of clinical symptoms, at a time when the patient is asymptomatic, but the disease contagious. HBsAg disappears from the serum as the disease resolves and is followed by the appearance of anti-HBs, the antibody to HBsAg. Anti-HBs arises during convalescence, whereas the antibody to the hepatitis B core antigen (anti-HBc) usually appears at the time that symptoms begin. Between 5 and 10 percent of hepatitis B patients will continue to exhibit the HBsAg, a sign of their being chronic carriers.

Anesthesia for the Hepatitis Patient

Anesthesiologists must deal with several problems in caring for the patient with active hepatitis. These include choice of anesthetic technique and strategies for prevention of occupational transmission of the virus.

Acute viral hepatitis may cause a decreased drug clearance secondary to both hepatocellular abnormalities and abnormal hepatic blood flow. There may be a decreased clearance of both high hepatic extraction ratio drugs such as lidocaine or low hepatic extraction ratio drugs such as benzodiazepines. General anesthesia may be safely used for surgery in the parturient with acute hepatitis, however, the doses of drugs that are cleared by the liver are reduced in these patients. The volatile agents have the added risk of decreasing hepatic blood flow. Nitrous oxide and opioids, however, do not reduce hepatic blood flow and can be safely used in these patients.

Regional anesthesia may cause hypotension and diminish further the already decreased hepatic blood flow. As long as care is taken to prevent hypotension, there is no absolute contraindication to regional anesthesia. Acute viremia, however, may dissuade the anesthesiologist from using intraspinal anesthesia to prevent "seeding" of the cerebrospinal fluid (CSF). Since there may be decreased clearance of lidocaine in patients with hepatitis, care should be taken to prevent the use of toxic doses.

ACQUIRED IMMUNODEFICIENCY SYNDROME

History

Our knowledge of acquired immunodeficiency syndrome (AIDS) began in 1980 and 1981, when opportunistic infections in homosexual men were noted in New York, San Francisco, and Los Angeles. The first report described four previously healthy homosexual men who presented with *Pneumocystis carinii* pneumonia (PCP) and were found to be immunodeficient.[61] A second paper published in 1981 suggested that drug abusers and homosexuals were at high risk for PCP.[62] It quickly became evident that this previously unrecognized disease could present with a myriad of symptoms that had devastating effects, the common denominator being an alteration in the immune system function and the subsequent development of opportunistic infections. In June 1982 the CDC named this syndrome the Acquired Immunodeficiency Syndrome[63] and defined it as the occurrence of a disease indicative of immunodeficiency in a person without a condition known to be associated with an increased incidence of diseases related to cellular immunodeficiency.[64] Although it was assumed that AIDS did not exist prior to the 1980s, a recent review of a case and frozen serum from 1968 revealed a patient with opportunistic infections and a virus related to human immunodeficiency virus. Therefore, it is now assumed that AIDS was present in the United States as early as the 1960's.

The actual virus that causes AIDS, now termed human immunodeficiency virus (HIV), was described in 1983–1984 by Barre-Sinoussi, Gallo, and Levy.[65–67] This pathogen is a retrovirus that utilizes reverse transcriptase to copy its genome into DNA. It was initially named HTLV-III (human T-cell lymphotropic virus), then renamed as HTLV-III/LAV, and finally simplified as HIV. Two variants of this virus have thus far been identified, HIV-1 and HIV-2.[68] Although both of these viruses can cause immunodeficiency, and have been identified in the United States, HIV-1 is thought to be responsible for the vast majority of cases of AIDS in the United States and Europe.

AIDS, which can be considered as the final stage of the continuum that begins with HIV infection, affects only a small portion of the patients infected with HIV. Patients who are HIV positive may be asymptomatic for a long period of time. However, they do have a progressive disease that is, in all probability, terminal. Moss followed 288 HIV-seropositive patients and estimated that the median duration of infection was 6 years.[69] The projected rate of progression to AIDS is 50 percent at 6 years. It is thought that the majority of seropositive patients will develop AIDS within 10 to 15 years after infection.[70,71]

The CDC classification of HIV infection is based on clinical manifestations. HIV infected persons are placed into one of four categories:

1. Acute infection
2. Asymptomatic but seropositive
3. Generalized lymphadenopathy
4. Symptomatic HIV disease
   (a) Constitutional disease
   (b) Neurologic disease
   (c) Secondary infectious disease

Incidence and Prevalence

As of July 1988, the World Health Organization reported over 100,000 cases of AIDS in 138 countries.[72] Although AIDS has been reported in all 50 states of the United States, it is seen mostly in several large cities, including New York, San Francisco, Los Angeles, Houston, and Washington, D.C.[73] The New York City and State departments of health have reported that 1 in every 62 children born in New York City has antibodies to AIDS. New York State is particularly hard hit, with the largest AIDS population in the United States. It is estimated that as of last year there were 10,000 AIDS-related deaths in New York. It is also estimated that over 1,000 HIV-infected infants will be born in New York this year, each carrying a major medical expense and what, at this point, amounts to a fatal disease.

The high-risk groups for the development of AIDS

are male homosexuals, intravenous drug abusers, hemophiliacs receiving transfusion therapy, Haitians, blood recipients (especially prior to the blood screening for HIV), and any person having sexual contact with someone in a high-risk group. It is estimated that by the end of 1990 nearly 10 percent of all AIDS cases will be women.[74]

Detection of anti-HIV antibodies is now routinely being performed by enzyme-linked immunosorbent assay (ELISA),[75] which although considered highly sensitive and specific, does have some deficiencies. ELISA screening for HIV-1 does not always reveal the presence of antibodies to HIV-2.[76] Additionally, false-positive results have been found to occur. Causes of false-positive ELISA include collagen vascular disease, malaria, and chronic hepatitis. Other more highly specific tests such as immunofluorescence assay (IFA) or Western blot tests are utilized if ELISA is positive.[77]

Although transfused blood is now being screened for the presence of HIV, the screening test is not foolproof. The window time (during which there is virus positivity but negativity of antibody screening) can be as long as 14 months.[78] It has been estimated that the risk of a virus-positive but antibody-negative blood transfusion is 26 per 1 million units.[79]

In addition to blood, HIV has also been isolated in seminal fluid, tears, saliva, synovial fluid, and CSF.[80,81] There is no evidence that saliva or tears act as a vector in the transmission of HIV. However, the anesthesiologist must still take precautions when dealing with any patient considered at risk. Since it is estimated that 1.5 million Americans harbor the virus, some now consider all patients as potential carriers. Discriminating behavior on the part of the anesthesiologist is, however, not warranted. Despite the large numbers of infected patients, the occupational risk of HIV transmission is very low and can be further reduced by careful adherence to simple precautions.[82] Standard sterilization and disinfection of anesthesia equipment has been shown to prevent HIV transmission. The CDC has published guidelines to decrease the risk of HIV transmission. Guidelines that may related to the practice of anesthesiology include the use of gloves for cases in which secretion contact may occur (intubation, extubation, handling of blood or other body fluids), avoidance of needle resheathing, use of puncture-resistant "sharps" containers, and use of protective eye coverings.[83]

Clinical Manifestations of HIV Infection

HIV causes a variety of clinical manifestations resulting from defects in immunologic function. The clinical condition can vary from that of asymptomatic carrier to the end stages of fatal illness. Clinical manifestations of AIDS are outlined in Table 8-18.

Table 8-18. Commonly Seen Clinical Manifestations of AIDS

Opportunistic infections, including *Pneumocystis carinii* pneumonia
Kaposi's sarcoma, Hodgkin and Non-Hodgkin lymphoma
Respiratory disease, including *Pneumocystis carinii* pneumonia and virulent mycobacterial infection
Tuberculosis
Coagulation disorders, including thrombocytopenia
Cardiac abnormalities, including myocarditis, chronic heart failure, and ventricular tachycardia
Central nervous system and psychiatric disease, including cerebral toxoplasmosis infection, encephalitis, meningitis, dementia, and schizophrenia
Peripheral nervous system, including polyneuropathy
Diffuse adenopathy, including tonsillar and adenoidal hypertrophy

AIDS and Regional Anesthesia

Anesthetic implications of HIV infection are outlined in Table 8-19.

Although it has been suggested that intraspinal anesthesia may exacerbate some of the neurologic manifestations of AIDS,[92] this has not been substantiated in the anesthesia or neurology literature. The present consensus of opinion is that regional anesthesia may be performed in the AIDS parturient if she does not have nervous system symptoms. The HIV virus has been isolated from the CSF of AIDS patients,[93] therefore

Table 8-19. Anesthetic Implications of HIV Infection

Presence of pulmonary disease may cause decreased functional residual capacity and, therefore, faster desaturation.[84]
Presence of tonsillar and adenoidal hypertrophy may make endotracheal intubation difficult.[85]
Presence of cerebral toxoplasmosis may cause increased intracranial pressure.[86]
Psychiatric disorders, including acute psychoses, may preclude regional anesthesia.[87]
Presence of cardiac manifestations of AIDS may predispose the patient to arrhythmias and chronic heart failure.[88]
Coagulation disorders (e.g., disseminated intravascular coagulation) may occur. Need to check coagulation status prior to placement of regional anesthesia.[89]
Presence of PCP may limit gas exchange during general anesthesia.[90]
Regional anesthesia may be contraindicated because of neuropathies.[91]

transdural passage during intraspinal anesthesia should not cause new CNS symptoms.

Regional anesthesia is relatively contraindicated in the AIDS parturient who has active neurologic symptoms, such as encephalitis, vacuolar degeneration of the spinal cord, meningitis, or peripheral neuropathy. Regional anesthesia is also contraindicated if the AIDS patient has a coagulopathy. Since HIV has been isolated from CSF, the anesthesiologist performing regional anesthesia must take certain precautions. An example of such a precaution would be the situation in which there may have been a dural puncture during placement of an epidural anesthetic. Allowing the unknown fluid to drop on the anesthesiogist's skin to determine its temperature should no longer be performed. Instead, the unknown fluid can be combined with sodium thiopental; the resultant precipitate will demonstrate local anesthetic rather than CSF. Since saline or diluted fentanyl can be misinterpreted, the superior method of identification would be by testing for the presence or absence of glucose.

AIDS Therapy

Since AIDS may present with a variety of symptoms there are several different drugs being used in the treatment of this disease. The immunocompromise may be treated with azidothymidine (Zidovudine, or AZT), which enhances immune function. This drug has been found to decrease the mortality from and the frequency of opportunistic infections.[94] AZT is converted to a triphosphate form that inhibits HIV reverse transcriptase. This drug does cross the placenta and blood-brain barrier and can be obtained in the CSF. AZT therapy may cause multiple side effects, which include nausea, vomiting, headache, myalgias, and meningoencephalitis. Hematologic abnormalities include anemia, leukopenia, and granulocytopenia.[95] AZT, while inhibiting HIV replication, has no activity against AIDS associated opportunistic infections, therefore, there is need for alternative therapy.

Acyclovir is being used to treat herpes zoster and ganciclovir is being used for cytomegalovirus treatment. Tuberculosis, which may be very virulent in AIDS patients, is treated with the usual triple therapy of isoniazid, rifampin, and ethambutol. Candidal infections are treated with clotrimazole or amphoteracin B. Renal function may be altered by amphoteracin B. PCP is often treated with pentamidine and cotrimoxazole, both of which are associated with severe side effects. Phenytoin (Dilantin), which is often used to treat seizure disorders associated with central nervous system disease, can cause hepatic dysfunction.

Table 8-20 describes the anesthetic implications of AIDS therapy.

AIDS in Pregnancy

Transmission of HIV from mother to child is well documented and can occur via several possible routes.[96] The mother can infect the fetus transplacentally at any time during pregnancy.[97] Since intrapartum exposure has been found to occur, cesarean delivery does not prevent fetal transmission.[98] It has also been suggested that transmission via breast milk occurs.[99,100]

Perinatal transmission of HIV cannot be prevented, although the transmission from mother to fetus is not a certainty.[101] Minkoff et al. noted that only 36 percent of children born to mothers who had previously given birth to a baby with evidence of HIV infection were HIV positive.[102]

Several retrospective studies have suggested that pregnancy may accelerate the course of HIV infection because of a pregnancy-induced immune suppression.[103] Because of the risk to both mother and fetus, the CDC have recommended that HIV-positive women postpone pregnancy until more information is available regarding the transmission and treatment of perinatal infection.

AIDS and Health Care Workers

Several reports have described health care workers who have been contaminated with HIV.[104] Hirsch et al.,[105] in an overly optimistic 1985 report, followed 30 health care workers having 31 needle sticks in whom none developed AIDS. Several other reports have found occupational transmission of HIV and as of last year more than 20 cases had been reported. In 1988, the CDC found a seroprevalence rate of 0.47 percent, a rate of seroconversion of 1:100 to 1:200 following needle stick. A recent report estimates that following exposure to blood from HIV-positive patients, the seroprevalence rate was 0.42 percent. Because of this alarmingly high risk, the CDC suggests that all patients be considered as potential hazards to health care workers. The American Society of Anesthesiologists Committee on Occupational Health has made recommendations to decrease the risk to health care workers. Suggestions include methods for decreasing accidental needle sticks, such as puncture-proof containers and policies for nonrecapping of needles. Since needle stick is the only method of transmission thus far proven to cause seroconversion in health care workers, maximal precautions must be taken to remove this hazard.

Although emphasis has been placed on the risk to health care workers who care for AIDS patients, recently

Table 8-20. Anesthetic Implications of AIDS Therapy

Drug	Implications to Anesthesiologist
AZT	Nausea/vomiting: aspiration prophylaxis needed Seizures: avoid enflurane and hyperventilation Anemia: check complete blood count preoperatively
Isoniazid	Nausea/vomiting: as above Hepatic dysfunction: avoid hepatotoxic drugs, halothane; avoid hepatically metabolized drugs Thrombocytopenia: check coagulation profile prior to use of regional anesthesia
Rifampin	Nausea/vomiting: as above Hepatitis: as above Acute renal failure: avoid drugs with renal metabolism Thrombocytopenia: as above Dyspnea: avoid respiratory depressants or secure airway
Ethambutol	Optic neuritis: opthalmology consultation Nausea/vomiting: as above Hepatic dysfunction: as above
Amphoteracin B	Nephrotoxicity: as above Hypokalemia: check potassium preoperatively; avoid hyperventilation Muscle weakness: monitor neuromuscular blockade Cardiovascular toxicity: avoid cardiodepressants
Pentamidine	Cardiotoxicity: as above ECG abnormalities: preoperative ECG Hypotension: check blood pressure frequently Hypoglycemia: monitor intraoperative glucose
Cotrimaxazole	Allergic myocarditis: avoid cardiodepressants Aplastic anemia: check complete blood count preoperatively Thrombocytopenia: check platelets before initiation of regional anesthetic
Phenytoin	Hepatic dysfunction: as above Nausea/vomiting: as above Thrombocytopenia: as above Gingival hyperplasia: care with intubation

there has been discussion about the transmission of HIV from doctor to patient. Since there have been numerous reports of the transmission of hepatitis B from infected surgeons to their patients, there is growing concern that HIV may also be transmitted from physician to patient. The CDC, in their 1987 guidelines, stated that decisions about infected health care workers performing invasive procedures should be made on a case by case basis by the infected health care worker's personal physician and hospital. These guidelines are presently being revised following the news that an HIV-infected dentist probably transmitted the virus to a patient during oral surgery. An epidemiologic study of that patient failed to reveal any AIDS risk factors or behavior that might put her at risk. Additionally, viral DNA samples from the dentist and patient showed a high degree of similarity, thereby suggesting that this actually represents a doctor to patient transmission.

REFERENCES

1. Little BB, Snell LM, Palmore MK, Gilstrap LC: Cocaine use in pregnant women in a large public hospital. Am J Perinatol 5:206, 1988
2. Abelson HI, Miller JD: A decade of trends in cocaine in the household population. Nat Inst Drug Abuse Res Mon Ser 61:35, 1985
3. Chasnoff IJ, Burns WJ, Schnoll SH, Burns KA: Cocaine use in pregnancy. N Engl J Med 313:666, 1985
4. Birnbach DJ, Grunebaum A, Weiss W: Epidural anesthesia for cesarean section in cocaine abusing parturients. Abstracts of the Society for Obstetric Anesthesia and Perinatology, May 1989
5. Gawin FH, Ellinwood EH: Cocaine and other stimulants. Actions, abuse, and treatment. N Engl J Med 318:1173, 1988
6. Van Dyke C, Jatlow P, Ungerer J: Oral cocaine: plasma concentrations and central effects. Science 200:211, 1978
7. Oro AS, Dixon SD: Perinatal cocaine and methamphetamine exposure. Maternal and neonatal correlates. Pediatrics 111:571, 1987
8. Ritchie JM, Greene NM: Local anesthesia. p. 300. In Gillman AG, Goodman LS, Gilman A: The Pharmacologic Basis of Therapeutics. 6th Ed. McMillan, New York, 1980
9. Elliot RH, Rees GB: Amphetamine ingestion presenting as eclampsia. Can J Anesth 37:130, 1990
10. New JA, Dooley SL, Keith LG: The prevalence of substance abuse in patients with suspected preterm labor. Am J Obstet Gynecol 162:1562, 1990
11. MacGregor SN, Keith LG, Chasnoff IJ, et al: Cocaine use during pregnancy: adverse perinatal outcome. Am J Obstet Gynecol 157:687, 1987
12. Keith LG, MacGregor S, Friedell S, et al: Substance abuse in pregnant women. Obstet Gynecol 73:715, 1989
13. Acker D, Sachs BP, Tracey KJ, Wise WE: Abruptio placentae associated with cocaine use. Am J Obstet Gynecol 146:220, 1983
14. Woods JR, Plessinger MA, Clark KE: Effect of cocaine on uterine blood flow and fetal oxygenation. JAMA 257:957, 1987
15. Moore TR, Sorg J, Miller L, et al: Hemodynamic effects

of intravenous cocaine on the pregnant ewe and fetus. Am J Obstet Gynecol 155:883, 1986
16. Chasnoff IJ, Bussey ME, Savich R, Stack C: Perinatal cerebral infarction and maternal cocaine use. J Pediatr 108:456, 1986
17. Stewart DJ, Inaba T, Lucassen M, et al: Cocaine metabolism: cocaine and norcocaine hydrolysis by liver and serum esterases. Clin Pharmacol Ther 25:464, 1979
18. Isner JM, Estes NAM, Thompson PD, et al: Acute cardiac events temporarily related to cocaine abuse. N Engl J Med 315:1438, 1986
19. Howard RE, Hueter DC, Davis GJ: Acute myocardial infarction following cocaine abuse in a young woman with normal coronary arteries. JAMA 254:95, 1985
20. Schachne JS, Roberts BH, Thompson PD: Coronary artery spasm and myocardial infarction associated with cocaine use. N Engl J Med 310:1665, 1984
21. Wetli CV, Wright RK: Death caused by recreational cocaine use. JAMA 241:2519, 1979
22. Lichtenfeld PJ, Rubin DB, Feldman RS: Subarachnoid hemorrhage precipitated by cocaine snorting. Arch Neurol 41:223, 1984
23. Nalbandian H, Sheth N, Dietrich R, et al: Intestinal ischemia caused by cocaine ingestion: report of 2 cases. Surgery 97:374, 1985
24. Adrouny A, Magnusson P: Pneumopericardium from cocaine inhalation. N Engl J Med 313:48, 1985
25. Bush MN, Rubenstein R, Hoffman I, et al: Spontaneous pneumomediastinum as a consequence of cocaine use. NY State J Med 84:618, 1984
26. Criegler LL, Mark H: Medical complications of cocaine abuse. N Engl J Med 315:1495, 1986
27. Jatlow P, Barash PG, Van Dyke C, et al: Cocaine and succinylcholine sensitivity: a new caution. Anesth Analg 58:235, 1979
28. Billman GE, Hoskins RS: Cocaine-induced ventricular fibrillation: protection afforded by the calcium antagonist verapamil. FASEB J 2:2990, 1988
29. Nahas G: A calcium channel blocker as antidote to the cardiac effects of cocaine intoxication. N Engl J Med 313:519, 1986
30. Ramoska E, Sacchetti A: Propranolol-induced hypertension in treatment of cocaine intoxication. Ann Emerg Med 14:112, 1985
31. Urine testing for drugs of abuse. National Inst of Drug Abuse Res Mon 73, 1986
32. Bailey DN: Amphetamine detection during toxicology screening of a university medical center population. J Clin Toxicol 25:399, 1987
33. Ong, BH: Dextroamphetamine poisoning. N Engl J Med 266:1321, 1962
34. Elliot RH, Rees GB: Amphetamine ingestion presenting as eclampsia. Can J Anaesth 37:130, 1990
35. Michel R, Adams AP: Acute amphetamine abuse. Anaesthesia 34:1016, 1979
36. Johnston RR, Way WL, Miller RD: Alteration of anesthetic requirement by amphetamine. Anesthesiology 36:357, 1972
37. Caldwell J, Seven PS: The biochemical pharmacology of abused drugs. Clin Pharmacol Ther 16:625, 1974
38. Samuels SI, Maze A, Albright A: Cardiac arrest during cesarean section in a chronic amphetamine abuser. Anesth Analg 58:528, 1979
39. Smith, DS: Amphetamine abuse and obstetrical anesthesia. Anesth Analg 59:710, 1980
40. Nelson MM, Forfar JO: Associations between drugs administered during pregnancy and congenital abnormalities of the fetus. Br Med J 1:523, 1971
41. Golbus, MD: Teratology for the obstetrician. Obstet Gynecol 55:269, 1980
42. Little BB, Snell LM, Gilstrap LC; Methamphetamine abuse during pregnancy: outcome and fetal effects. Obstet Gynecol 72:541, 1988
43. Rubin E: Alcoholic myopathy in heart and skeletal muscle. N Engl J Med 301:28, 1979
44. Bruce DL: Alcoholism and anesthesia. Anesth Analg 62:84, 1983
45. Duvaldestin P, Agoston S, Henzel D, et al: Pancuronium pharmacokinetics in patients with liver cirrhosis. Br J Anaesth 50:1131, 1978
46. Giuffrida JG: Anesthetic management of drug abusers. Anesth Analg 49:272, 1970
47. Gomar C, Luis M, Nalda MA: Sacro-ilitis in a heroin addict. A contraindication to spinal anesthesia. Anaesthesia 39:167, 1984
48. Connaughton JF: Current concepts in the management of the pregnant opiate addict. Addictive Dis 2:21, 1975
49. Lipski J, Stimmel B, Donoso E: The effect of heroin and multiple drug abuse on the electrocardiogram. Am Heart J 86:663, 1973
50. Gold MS, Pottash ALC, Extein I, Kleber HD; Clonidine in acute opiate withdrawal. N Engl J Med 302:1421, 1980
51. Scheutz F: Drug addicts and local anesthesia—effectivity and general side effects. Scand J Dental Res 90:299, 1982
52. Tornabene VW: Narcotic withdrawal syndrome caused by naltrexone. Ann Intern Med 81:785, 1974
53. Weintraub SJ, Naulty JS: Acute abstinence syndrome after epidural injection of butorphanol. Anesth Analg 64:452, 1985
54. Mendelson, CL: The aspiration of stomach contents into the lungs during obstetric anesthesia. Am J Obstet Gynecol 52:191, 1946
55. Sellick BA: Cricoid pressure to control regurgitation of stomach contents during induction of anaesthesia. Lancet 2:404, 1961
56. Mark LC, Marx G, Arkins RE, et al: Hypotension during anesthesia in narcotic addicts. NY State J Med 66:2685, 1966
57. Tennes K: Effects of marijuana on pregnancy and fetal development. Nat Inst Drug Abuse Res Monogr 44:115, 1984
58. Greenland S: The effects of marijuana use during pregnancy. Am J Obstet Gynecol 143:408, 1981
59. Wu TC, Tashkin DP, Djahed B, et al: Pulmonary hazards of smoking marijuana. N Engl J Med 318:347, 1988

60. Berman ML, Bochantin JF: Effect of delta 9 tetra hydrocanabinol on liver microsomal dechlorinase activity. Anesth Analg 51:929, 1972
61. Gottlieb MS, Schroff R, Shanker HM, et al: Pneumocystis carinii pneumonia and mucosal candidiasis in previously healthy homosexual men. N Engl J Med 305:1425, 1981
62. Masur H, Michelis MA, Greene JB, et al: An outbreak of community acquired pneumocystis carinii pneumonia. N Engl J Med 305:1431, 1981
63. CDC Update on AIDS. MMWR 31:507, 1982
64. CDC Update on AIDS. MMWR 34:245, 1985
65. Barre-Sinousi F, Chermann JC, Rey F, et al: Isolation of a T-Lymphotropic retrovirus from a patient at risk for acquired immune deficiency syndrome. Science 220:868, 1983
66. Gallo RC, Salahuddin SZ, Popovic M, et al: Frequent detection and isolation of cytopathic retroviruses (HTLV-III) from patients with AIDS. Science 224:500, 1984
67. Levy JA, Hoffman AD, Kramer SM, Landis JM: Isolation of lymphocytopathic retroviruses from San Francisco patients with AIDS. Science 225:840, 1984
68. Evans LA, Moreau J, Odeehouri K, et al: Simultaneous isolation of HIV-1 and HIV-2 from an AIDS patient. Lancet 2:1389, 1988
69. Moss AR, Bacchetti P, Osmond D, Kranpf W, et al: Seropositivity for HIV and the development of AIDS or AIDS related condition. Br Med J 296:745, 1988
70. Carne CA, Weller IV, Loveddy C, et al: From persistent generalized lymphadenopathy to AIDS. Br Med J 299:866, 1987
71. Eyster ME, Gail MH, Ballard JO: Natural history of human immunodeficiency virus infection. Ann Intern Med 107:1, 1987
72. Mann JM, Chin J: AIDS: a global perspective. N Engl J Med 319:302, 1988
73. CDC update on AIDS. MMWR 36:1, 1987
74. Public Health Service Report: Public Health Serv Rep 101:341, 1986
75. Update: Serologic testing for antibody to human immunodeficiency virus. MMWR 36:833, 1988
76. Brun-Vezinet F, Rey MA, Katlama C, et al: Lymphadenopathy-associated viral antibody in AIDS. N Engl J Med 311:1269, 1984
77. Centers for Disease Control: Interpretation and use of the Western blot assay for serodiagnosis of human immunodeficiency virus type 1 infection. MMWR: 38 (S7):1, 1989
78. Curran JW, Lawrence D, Jaffe H, et al: Acquired immunodeficiency syndrome associated with transfusions. N Engl J Med 310:69, 1984
79. Ward JW, Holmberg SD, Allen JR: Transmission of HIV by blood transfusion screened as negative for HIV antibody. N Engl J Med 318:473, 1988
80. Friedland GH, Klein RS: Transmission of the human immunodeficiency virus. N Engl J Med 317:1125, 1987
81. Seifert MH: Transmission of HIV. N Engl J Med 318:1203, 1988
82. Cantineau, JP: AIDS and implications for anesthesiologists. Cur Opin Anaesthesiol 2:349, 1989
83. Update: universal precautions for the prevention of transmission of human immunodeficiency virus, hepatitis B virus, and other bloodborne pathogens in health-care settings. MMWR 37:377, 1988
84. Varteresian-Karanful L, Josephson A, Fikrig S, et al: Pulmonary infection and cavity formation caused by mycobacterium Tb in a child with AIDS. N Engl J Med 319:1018, 1988
85. Brazan L, Carbone A, Saracchini S, et al: Nasopharyngeal lymphatic tissue hypertrophy in HIV infected patients. Lancet 1:42, 1989
86. Black PH: HTLV-III, AIDS, and the brain. N Engl J Med 313:1538, 1985
87. Atkinson JH, Grant I, Kennedy CJ, et al: Prevalence of psychiatric disorders among men infected with human immunodeficiency virus. Arch Gen Psych 45:859, 1988
88. Reilly JM, Cunnim RE, Anderson DW, et al: Frequency of myocarditis, left ventricular dysfunction and ventricular tachycardia in the acquired immunodeficiency syndrome. Am J Cardiol 62:789, 1988
89. Krilov LR, Rubin LG, Frogel M, Gloster E, et al: Disseminated adenovirus infection with hepatic necrosis in patients with human immunodeficiency virus infection and other immunodeficiency states. Rev Infect Dis 12:303, 1990
90. Gotta AW: AIDS and its implications to the anesthesiologist. In Stoelting RK (ed): Advances in Anesthesia. Vol. 7. CV Mosby, St. Louis/Year Book, Chicago 1990
91. So YT, Holtzman DM, Abrams DI, et al: Peripheral neuropathy associated with AIDS. Arch Neruol 45:945, 1988
92. Greene ER: Spinal and epidural anesthesia in patients with the acquired immunodeficiency syndrome. Anesth Analg 65:1090, 1986
93. Ho DD, Rota TR, Schooley RT, et al: Isolation of HTLV-III from cerebrospinal fluid and neural tissues of patients with neurologic syndromes related to AIDS. N Engl J Med 313:1493, 1985
94. Fischl MA, Richman DD, Grieco MH, et al: The efficacy of AZT in the treatment of patients with AIDS and AIDS-related complex. N Engl J Med 317:185, 1987
95. Richman DD, Fischl MA, Grieco MH, et al: The toxicity of azidothmidine (AZT) in the treatment of patients with AIDS and AIDS related complex. N Engl J Med 317:192, 1987
96. The European Collaborative Study—mother to child transmission of HIV infection. Lancet 2:1039, 1988
97. LaPointe N, Michaud J, Pekovic D, et al: Transplacental transmission of HTLV-III virus. N Engl J Med 312:1325, 1985
98. Jousisas E, Koch MA, Schafer, et al: LAV/HTLV-III in a 20 week fetus. Lancet 2:1129, 1982
99. Friedland GH, Klein RS: Transmission of the human immunodeficiency virus. N Engl J Med 317:1125, 1987
100. Thiry l, Sprecher-Goldberger S, Jonckheer T, Levy J:

Isolation of AIDS virus from cell free breast milk of three healthy virus carriers. Lancer 2:891, 1985
101. Ziegler JB, Cooper DA, Johnson RO, et al: Post natal transmission of AIDS: associated retrovirus from mother to infant. Lancet 1:896, 1985
102. Minkoff H, Nanda D, Monez R, et al: Pregnancies resulting in infants with acquired immunodeficiency syndrome. Obstet Gynecol 69:288, 1987
103. Scott GB, Fischl MA, Klinas N, et al: Mothers of infants with acquired immunodeficiency syndrome. Evidence for both symptomatic and asymptomatic carriers. JAMA 253:363, 1985
104. Marcus R: Surveillance of health care workers exposed to blood from patients infected with human immunodeficiency virus. N Engl J Med 319:1118, 1988
105. Hirsch MS, Wormser GP, Schooley RT, et al: Risk of nosocomial infection with HTLV-III. N Engl J Med 312:1, 1985

9

The Neonate

RESUSCITATION AND CARE OF THE NEONATE

Birth is a time of physiologic stress and change for the fetus. Usually, the asphyxial stress of birth is mild to moderate, and the neonate is able to compensate for it. When the neonate's compensatory ability is decreased or the asphyxial stress is excessive, resuscitative intervention is necessary to assist in the conversion from fetal to neonatal physiology.

Who should assume responsibility for resuscitation of the depressed neonate? Standard IV of the American Society of Anesthesiologists (ASA) "Standards for Conduction Anesthesia in Obstetrics" states: Qualified personnel, *other than the anesthesiologist attending the mother*, should be immediately available to assume responsibility for resuscitation of the depressed newborn. (The primary responsibility of the anesthesiologist is to provide care to the mother. If the anesthesiologist is also requested to provide brief assistance in the care of the neonate, the benefit to the child must be compared to the risk of temporarily leaving the mother).

The "Guidelines for Perinatal Care"[1] state: The first minutes of life may determine the quality of that life. The need for a prompt, organized, and skilled response to emergencies in this period requires institutions that provide maternal–fetal care to have written policies delineating responsibility for immediate newborn care, resuscitation, selection and maintenance of necessary equipment, and training of personnel in proper techniques. The obstetrician is responsible for providing immediate postdelivery care of the newborn and for ascertaining that the newborn adaptations to extrauterine life are proceeding normally. The hospital rules and regulations should include protocols for the transfer of medical care of the neonate in both routine and emergency circumstances. Routine care of the healthy newborn may be delegated to appropriately trained nurses.

Recognition and immediate resuscitation of the distressed neonate require an organized plan of action and the immediate availability of qualified personnel and equipment. At least one person skilled in initiating resuscitation should be present at every delivery. Everyone in the delivery area **should** be able to clear an airway, administer oxygen by positive-pressure ventilation with a mask and bag, and give closed-chest cardiac massage. Responsibility for identification and resuscitation of a distressed neonate should be assigned to a qualified individual, who may be a physician or an appropriately trained nurse-midwife, labor and delivery nurse, nurse-anesthetist, nursery nurse, or respiratory therapist. The provision of services and equipment for resuscitation should be planned jointly by the directors of the departments of obstetrics, anesthesia, and pediatrics, with the approval of the medical staff. A physician should be designated to assume primary responsibility for initiating, supervising, and reviewing the plan for management of depressed neonates in the delivery room.

However, it would seem that these guidelines are not necessarily followed. Gibbs et al.,[2] found that in small units in the United States, with less than 500 deliveries per year, personnel other than an anesthesiologist, nurse-anesthetist, pediatrician, or obstetrician perform neonatal resuscitation after vaginal delivery almost 50 percent of the time, and, for cesarean delivery, 25 percent of the time.

CARDIOVASCULAR PHYSIOLOGY (FETUS TO NEONATE)

The fetal circulation operates in parallel, in contrast to the adult circulation, which operates in series.[3,4] In the fetus, oxygenated blood returns from the placenta via the umbilical vein, largely bypassing the liver through the ductus venosus. Due to a streaming effect, this blood is preferentially shunted from the right atrium through the foramen ovale to the left atrium and via the left ventricle into the systemic circulation. This streaming of ductus venosus blood to the left side of the circulation enhances the oxygen content of the blood perfusing the organs of highest oxygen consumption—the heart and the brain.

Desaturated blood returns from the upper part of the body via the superior vena cava and streams into the right ventricle. Right ventricular output encounters high pulmonary vascular resistance due to arteriolar vasoconstriction. About 90 percent of this right-sided output passes through the ductus arteriosus and enters the aorta distal to the branches of the aortic arch; thus less well oxygenated blood perfuses the lower body, which has a lower oxygen consumption (Fig. 9-1).

At birth, two primary events initiate the conversion from fetal to adult circulatory patterns.[5] First, cessation of umbilical artery flow (by clamping the cord or exposing the cord to air) increases systemic vascular resis-

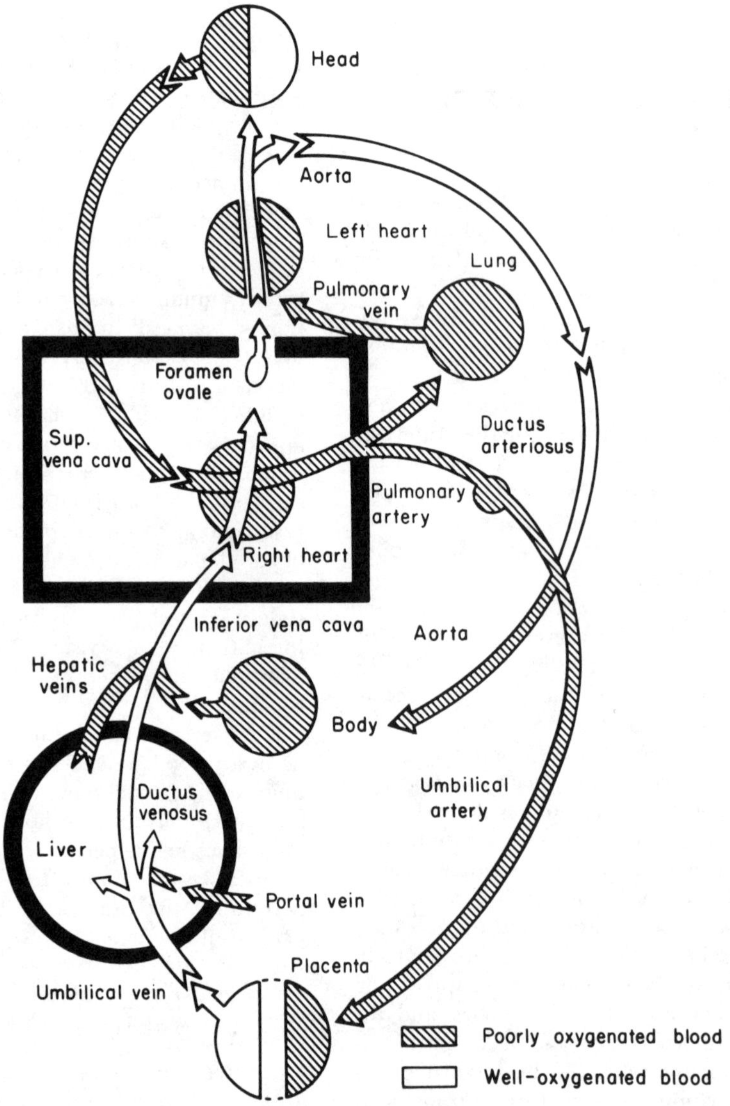

Fig. 9-1. Fetal circulation. (Modified from Ostheimer,[29] with permission.)

tance and aortic pressure, and the clamping of the umbilical vein decreases venous return and right atrial pressure. This effects a decrease in the right-to-left shunts both at the foramen ovale from the right atrium to the left and at the ductus arteriosus from the pulmonary artery to the aorta. Second, the expansion of the lungs at birth stimulates pulmonary vasodilation, with resulting falls in pulmonary vascular resistance and pulmonary arterial pressure, which helps to reduce further the right-to-left flow through the patent ductus arteriosus. Pulmonary blood flow increases, oxygenation improves, and left atrial pressure rises, further decreasing the shunt across the foramen ovale (Figs. 9-2 and 9-3).

The hallmarks of conversion to adult circulation are a rise in systemic arterial pressure, accomplished mainly by cord clamping, and a rise in pulmonary blood flow, accomplished by filling the lungs with air. Therefore, the major effort of resuscitation is usually to assist the neonate with the initiation of ventilation. More severely

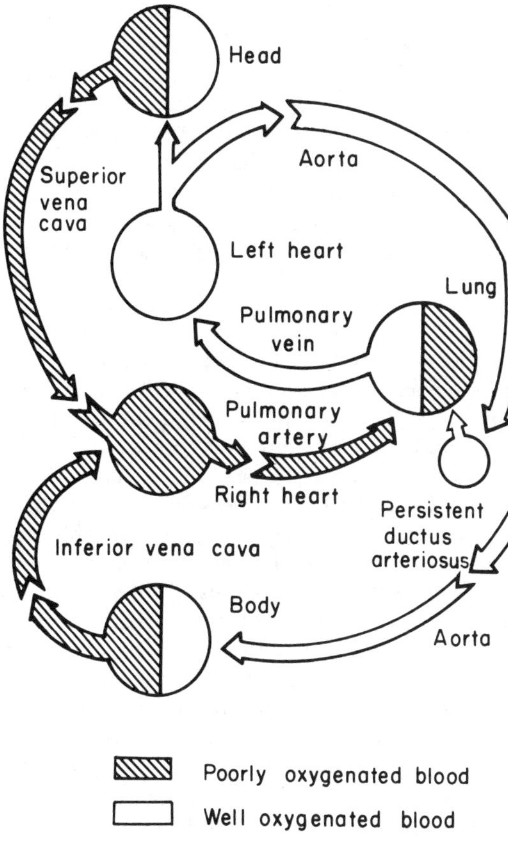

Fig. 9-2. Postdelivery circulation: intermediate phase. (Modified from Ostheimer,[29] with permission.)

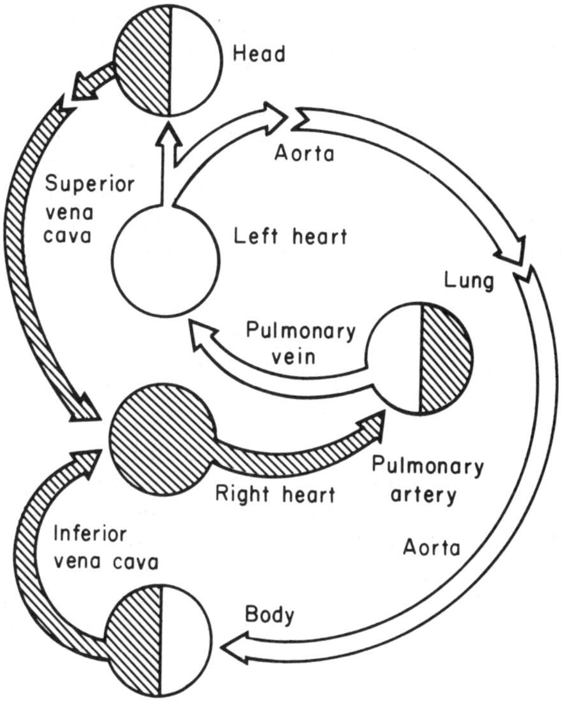

Fig. 9-3. Normal circulation: final phase. (Modified from Ostheimer,[29] with permission.)

depressed neonates may require additional forms of intervention.

The adult circulatory pattern is established rapidly in the normal, healthy neonate. However, for the first 2 weeks of life (longer in the premature neonate), the circulation can revert to the fetal pattern when the neonate is subjected to certain stresses such as hypoxemia, acidosis, hypercarbia, hypovolemia, shock, and hypothermia.[5]

RESPIRATORY SYSTEM

The fetal lung develops by a budding process from the foregut at approximately 24 days of gestation. By 20 weeks, the airways are lined with epithelium and pulmonary capillaries are developing in the mesenchyme. By 26 to 28 weeks, the capillaries are close to the developing airways so that oxygen and carbon dioxide exchange could occur making extrauterine life possible. Surfactant-like material is present in the airway epithelium between 22 and 24 weeks but is not present on the alveolar surface until 26 to 28 weeks. Steroids administered to the mother facilitate the development of the epithelial cells lining the alveoli and the production of surfactant. The onset of fetal breathing is stimulated by stress (usually hypoxia) and amniotic fluid can be drawn into the lung, as can be demonstrated by meconium aspiration in the stillborn.[6,7]

Normal neonates will begin spontaneous respirations within 30 to 60 seconds. Stimuli to breathe include rebound of the thoracic cage after vaginal birth, mild to moderate hypoxia, cord clamping, a cold environment, and tactile stimulation. (Note: only gentle stimulation is needed. Vigorous spanking, cold and hot water baths, and other excessive stimulation have no therapeutic value and may be harmful.) The volume of the first breath is from 20 to 75 ml. Subsequent tidal volume is 15 to 20 ml. When rhythmic breathing is established and the lungs are fully expanded, the normal respiratory rate is 30 to 40 breaths/min. In the first few hours of life, during the resorption of residual lung fluid, respiratory rates may be as high as 60 to 90 breath/min. Central cyanosis should clear by 5 minutes after birth. Some peripheral cyanosis may persist because of peripheral vasoconstriction. During vaginal delivery, the baby's chest is compressed with a pressure of 30 to 250 cmH_2O.[8] This "squeeze" expresses much of the fluid from the lungs, but the lungs remain collapsed and are not aerated. In order to expand the lungs against the collapsing forces of alveolar tension and elastic pulmonary recoil, the neonate exerts 40 to 80 cmH_2O negative pressure.[9,10] The resuscitator may, therefore, need to use higher than normal pressures when assisting with the initiation of ventilation, so long as the potential for pneumothorax is kept in mind (Fig. 9-4). The neonate will respond to a large rapid inflation of its lungs with a sharp inspiration of its own (Head's paradoxical reflex).

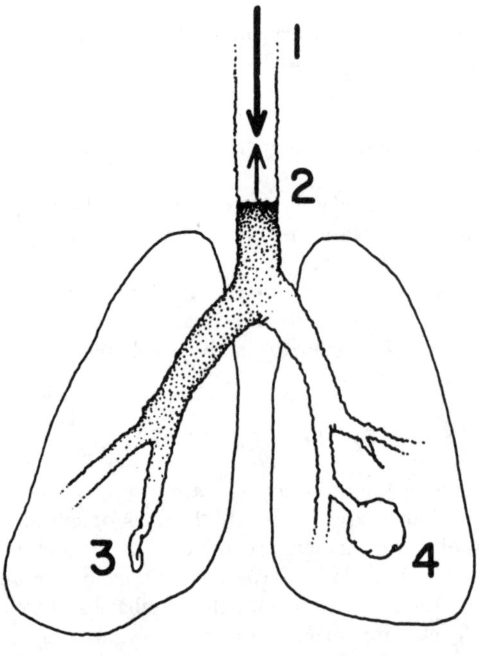

Fig. 9-4. The lung immediately after delivery. Expansion of the collapsed lung requires higher pressures than those needed to move air into the lungs (*1*) once aerated. Several forces must be overcome: outward flow of fluid in the trachea and bronchi (*2*); surface tension of the collapsed alveoli (*3*); and elastic forces of the lung (*4*). (Modified from Ostheimer,[30] with permission.)

Table 9-1. Normal Neonatal Blood Pressures

Birthweight (kg)	Pressure (mmHg) Systolic	Diastolic
<1.0	40–60	15–35
1.0–2.0	50–65	20–40
2.0–3.0	50–70	25–45
>3.0	50–80	30–50

CARDIOVASCULAR SYSTEM

The heart rate may vary from 100 to 200 beats/min (bpm) during the first 30 minutes of life, but should stabilize at 120 ± 50 bpm thereafter. Normal blood pressure varies with birthweight, as shown in Table 9-1.[11] A systolic pressure less than 50 mmHg in a term neonate is abnormally low and should be treated promptly with intravascular volume expansion. Normal intravascular volume is 85 to 100 ml/kg in the newborn.

THERMOREGULATION

Humans are homeothermic, that is, we increase our heat production when exposed to a cold environment to maintain body temperature. Poikilotherms, such as reptiles, cannot increase their heat production and their body temperature drifts to that of the environment. There are two methods of increasing heat production: a physical method of muscle contraction (shivering), used by children and adults, and a chemical method used by neonates called *nonshivering thermogenesis* (Fig. 9-5). When the neonates are cold stressed, they increase their oxygen consumption and metabolic activity. Large amounts of norepinephrine are released (in contrast to epinephrine in adults), which activates an adipose tissue lipase to break down brown fat (so called because of its rich vascular supply) into triglycerides and nonesterified fatty acids (NEFA). The NEFA may pass out of the cell, are oxidized to carbon dioxide and water in the cell—which is an exothermic (heat-producing) reaction—or are re-esterified with glycerol to form triglycerides.

Adipose tissue is not able to phosphorylate the glycerol derived from the triglycerides; therefore, re-esterification via the coenzyme A-NEFA complex requires a supply of α glycerol phosphate derived from glucose that comes from outside the cell. Resynthesis of triglycerides is also an exothermic reaction because of the utilization of adenosine triphosphate (ATP) in the formation of the coenzyme A-NEFA complex.

Nonshivering thermogenesis occurs mainly in the brown fat of the neonate, which is found in an interscapular mass (the "hibernating gland"), muscles and blood vessels entering the thoracic inlet, and the abdominal viscera, especially around the kidneys and adrenal glands. The venous drainage from the interscapular adipose tissue joins the drainage from the muscles of the back to form the external vertebral plexus, which drains to the rich venous plexus around the spinal cord, which in turn enters the jugular or azygous veins, depending on the level, thus supplying heat to the spinal cord and the heart (Fig. 9-6).

We must strive to maintain a neutral thermal environment (32 to 34°C for neonates) at which metabolism (as reflected by oxygen consumption) is minimal yet sufficient to maintain body temperature. Minimal oxygen consumption occurs when the gradient between skin and the environmental temperature is less than 1.5°C.

The infant, born into the cold environment of the delivery room, suffers an enormous heat loss, initially by evaporation since the neonate is wet from amniotic fluid and has a large surface area. Once the skin is dried, heat loss is mainly by radiation. Dahm and James[12] investigated heat loss in the first 30 minutes after delivery and found that wet infants exposed to room air lost nearly five times more heat than those who were dried and warmed.

In vigorous infants, promptly drying the skin and wrapping the baby in a warm blanket is almost as effective in decreasing heat loss as placing the baby under a radiant heater. However, in depressed or immature infants, who may be more asphyxiated or have reduced energy stores, an overhead radiant heater maintains body temperature while allowing access to the patient during resuscitation.

ROUTINE DELIVERY ROOM CARE OF THE NORMAL NEONATE

The following measures are all that is necessary in 85 to 90 percent of deliveries:

1. Aspiration of the mouth and nose by bulb syringe.

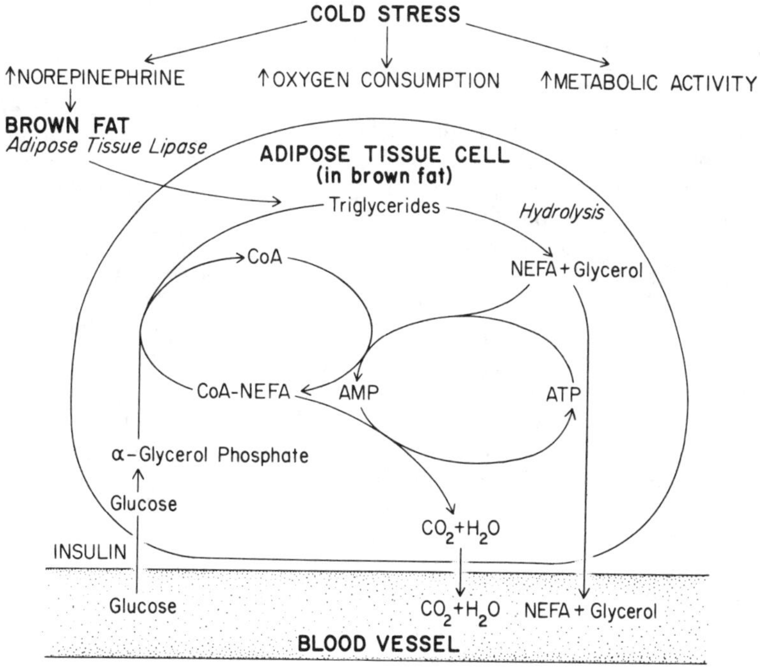

Fig. 9-5. Nonshivering thermogenesis. (From Ostheimer,[30] with permission.)

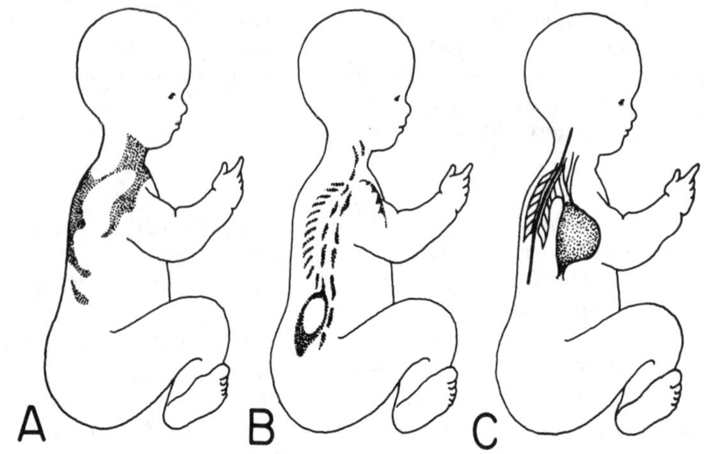

Fig. 9-6. (A&B) Sites of brown fat. **(C)** Route of venous drainage.

2. Drying the skin and maintaining normal newborn temperature.
3. Routine identification procedures.
4. Ophthalmic prophylaxis (required by law in most states).

In the remainder, in whom neonatal depression has occurred, further measures will be necessary.

PRINCIPLES OF NEWBORN RESUSCITATION

The principles of newborn resuscitation are the same as those for adult resuscitation: (1) airway management, (2) breathing, and (3) circulation or adequate cardiac output to maintain cerebral oxygenation. After birth of the baby's head, the oropharynx is suctioned with a bulb syringe before the baby's first breath and while the chest is still compressed in the vaginal canal (vaginal squeeze) to prevent aspiration of mucus and debris into the trachea with the onset of respiration (Fig. 9-7). The baby is then delivered; the umbilical cord is clamped and cut and the newborn is transferred by the obstetrician to a warmed bassinet that has been placed in a 20- to 30-degree head down position to facilitate the gravity drainage of liquid material into the oropharynx. A slight lateral tilt of the newborn concentrates the pooling of secretions into one corner of the oropharynx. Management of the airway is accomplished by gentle suction with a bulb syringe—if possible—not a plastic or rubber suction catheter. Cordero and Hon[13] investigated the effect of nasopharyngeal or oropharyngeal stimulation on heart rate and respiration. In 41 infants who received repeated nasopharyngeal suction with a bulb syringe, no decreases in heart rate or respiration were noted. However, in 46 neonates who were suctioned blindly with a catheter through the nose or mouth, 7 developed severe cardiac arrhythmias and 5 became apneic. These undesirable responses resulted from stimulation of afferent vagal fibers in the posterior pharynx of already highly vagotonic newborns.

Gentle slapping of the feet is all the stimulation needed for the healthy newborn. Spanking, cold-water showers,

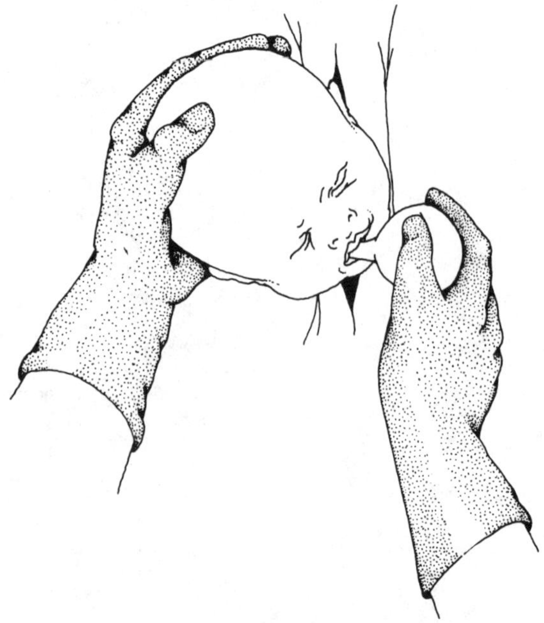

Fig. 9-7. Pharyngeal suction with the baby's head on the perineum. (Modified from Ostheimer,[30] with permission.)

jackknifing, "milking" the trachea, dilatation of the anal sphincter, alternating hot and cold baths, rocking beds, and excessive rubbing of the back are *condemned* as having no therapeutic value and are potentially harmful.

RESUSCITATION EQUIPMENT

Every delivery area should have the following equipment readily available for the resuscitation of the newborn:

1. A source of 100 percent oxygen.
2. A bag and mask for intermittent positive-pressure ventilation (IPPV). A flow-through system that requires positive pressure for oxygen delivery should be used since most neonates will not need positive pressure ventilation, just oxygen therapy.
3. A bulb syringe for suctioning the nose and oropharynx.
4. A DeLee suction catheter with mucus trap for aspiration of mucus, meconium, blood, and other secretions or stomach contents.
5. Laryngoscopes with size 0 and 1 straight blades.
6. Endotracheal tubes (Cole orotracheal tubes or straight endotracheal tubes with stylets in place in sizes 1.5 mm, 2.0 mm, 2.5 mm, 3.0 mm, and 3.5 mm). The Cole tubes are more rigid and do not require a stylet. If the neonate requires long-term ventilation, the oral tube should be changed to a straight nasotracheal tube when the infant's condition is stable.
7. Oral airways, size 00 and 0, are rarely needed but should be available.
8. A radiant heater with servomechanisms.

A neonatal "code cart" also should be available and should contain equipment for vascular access and blood sampling, intravenous infusions, drugs commonly employed in resuscitation, and charts showing typical doses and dilutions.

With the increasing concern about body fluid contaminated with hepatitis or human immunodeficiency virus (HIV), personnel participating in newborn resuscitation are using one of several devices that allows aspiration of fluids from the mouth, trachea and stomach of the newborn by vacuum suction (<80 cmH_2O). This approach should eliminate the possibility of inhaling contaminants through a mask or gauze covering while aspirating via the endotracheal tube or deLee suction apparatus.

EVALUATION AND TREATMENT OF THE DEPRESSED NEONATE

Apgar Scoring

It is easy to recognize the vigorous, healthy, normal neonate and the severely depressed neonate needing immediate cardiopulmonary resuscitation. Between these two extremes lie varying degrees of neonatal depression. While the Apgar scoring system was not meant to be used as a guide to resuscitators, it has proven useful as a means of quantifying the degree of depression (Table 9-2). The 1-minute score[14] is used here as a guide to the intervention required. However, resuscitation should not be delayed awaiting the 1-minute Apgar score. A follow-up score is determined at 5 minutes of life and will indicate the progress of the neonate. Additionally, 10-, 15-, and 20-minute scores may be assigned to document the response of the neonate to the resuscitation efforts.

Vigorous, Crying Infant (Apgar Score 7–10). No therapy is necessary beyond the routine measures mentioned above.

Moderate Depression (Apgar 4–6)

1. Administer 100 percent oxygen by mask (Fig. 9-8).
2. Stimulate by slapping the feet or by drying the skin with a soft cloth towel or blanket.

Table 9-2. The Apgar Scoring System

			Score		
Evaluation	Sign	Stimulus	0	1	2
Appearance	Color	Visual assessment	Blue, pale	Body pink, extremities blue	Completely pink
Pulse	Heart rate	Count cord pulse or auscultate heart	Absent	<100 bpm	>100 bpm
Grimace	Reflex irritability	Flick sole of foot	No response	Some motion	Cry
Activity	Muscle tone	Manipulate extremity	Limp flaccid	Some flexion of extremities	Well-flexed
Respiration	Respiratory effort	Visual assessment	Absent	Slow, irregular hypoventilation	Good strong cry

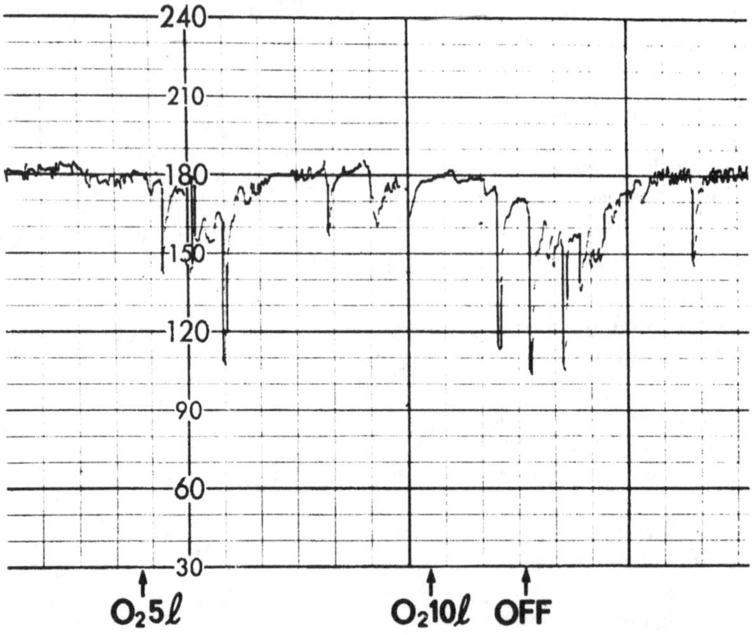

Fig. 9-8. Technique of ventilation and closed-chest cardiac massage. (From Ostheimer,[30] with permission.)

3. If the heart rate is below 100 bpm and/or respirations are inadequate, begin IPPV by bag and mask and continue it as long as necessary.
4. Monitor the heart rate and spontaneous respiratory efforts. If these deteriorate or fail to improve, treat as a severely depressed neonate.

Severe Depression (Apgar Score 0–3)

1. Administer 100 percent oxygen by bag and mask as soon as possible.
2. If there is no response (increased heart rate, respiratory effort) within a few minutes, perform laryngoscopy, suction the oropharynx and/or trachea, and intubate the trachea to facilitate ventilation (Fig. 9-9).
3. Initiate closed-chest cardiac massage (CCCM) if the heart rate remains below 100 bpm. Place both thumbs over the mid- to lower third of the sternum and the fingers behind the chest.[15,16] Compress the chest at a rate of 120 bpm, depressing the sternum two-thirds of the way to the vertebral column (see Fig. 9-8).
4. Monitor the adequacy of cardiopulmonary resuscitation. With proper intubation and ventilation, the chest should expand and breath sounds should be heard in both axillae (Fig. 9-10). Auscultate over the abdomen to rule out esophageal intubation. If ventilation and/or intubation are difficult, repositioning of the head may be necessary. Because of the relatively large head of the neonate, as well as the edema fluid (caput) that collects over the occiput during labor, the neck may be flexed enough to compress the trachea when the baby is supine. Placing a small roll under the baby's shoulders will alleviate this problem by extending the neck (Fig. 9-11). However, excessive hyperextension may also compress the soft trachea of the neonate.
5. Gastric aspiration should not be done in the first few minutes of life in order to avoid causing any arrhythmias from nasopharyngeal or oropharyngeal stimulation—unless there is massive gastric dilatation secondary to IPPV with the bag and mask or a tracheoesophageal fistula is suspected. Cordero and Hon[13] suggest that after 5 minutes of age, the neonate has become physiologically more stable and will tolerate passage of a nasogastric tube.

CONTINUED MODERATE TO SEVERE DEPRESSION

The newborn that fails to respond to adequate ventilation with oxygen and circulatory support with CCCM will require further therapy.

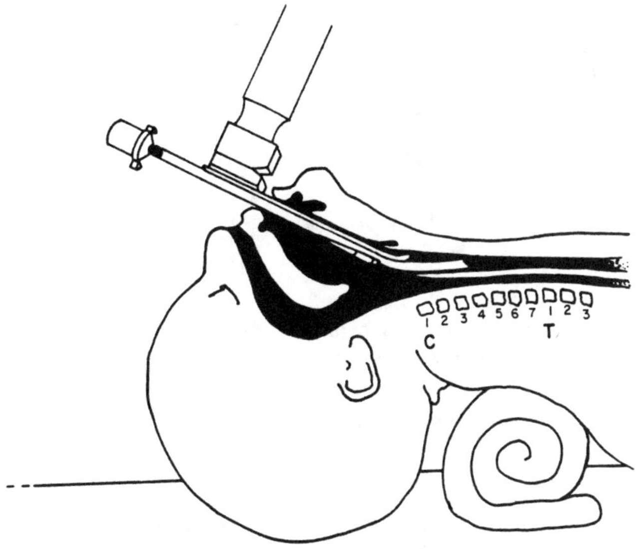

Fig. 9-9. Laryngoscopy and endotracheal intubation with a Cole tube.

Pharmacologic Intervention

Drugs commonly used in neonatal resuscitation are administered through an umbilical artery or vein catheter, although epinephrine can be given intratracheally if vascular access has not yet been established. A 5- or 8-French catheter can be threaded into the umbilical artery, although intense vasoconstriction of the artery may necessitate use of the umbilical vein in the immediate resuscitative period. In the latter case, the catheter should be threaded no more than 2 cm into the vein to avoid cannulation of a major hepatic vessel.

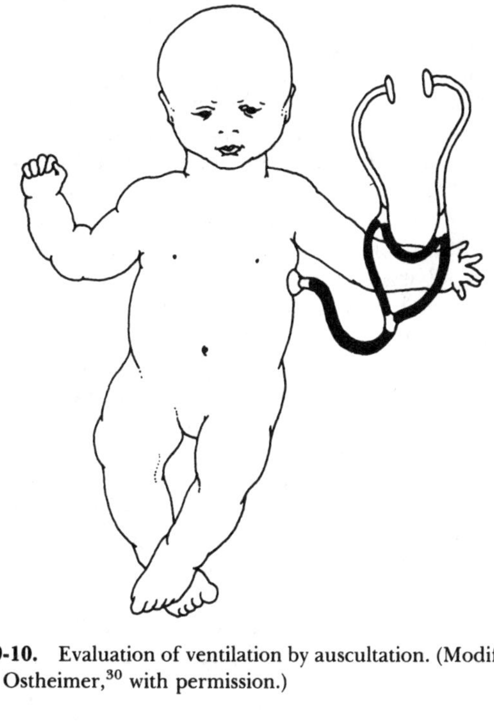

Fig. 9-10. Evaluation of ventilation by auscultation. (Modified from Ostheimer,[30] with permission.)

Drugs Used in Pharmacologic Resuscitation

Sodium Bicarbonate (2 (mEq) mmol/kg). The neonate suffering from severe birth asphyxia and not responding well to oxygen and ventilatory support probably has a respiratory and metabolic acidosis. This initial dose of sodium bicarbonate will improve the acidosis, but further doses should be administered only as indicated by the infant's pH. A sample of blood (arterial or venous) should be drawn for blood gas analysis upon insertion of the umbilical artery or vein catheter. Ventilation must be adequate to reverse the respiratory component of the acidosis.

Bicarbonate therapy has several potential complications.[17–20] It is a hyperosmolar solution, and its rapid administration in the acidotic and hypoxic newborn can lead to profound vasodilation and hypotension due to skeletal muscle vasodilation and venous pooling. Because of its lower osmolarity, a 0.22-mmol/ml solution is preferred to the 0.45 mmol/ml solution. It should be given in an intravenous infusion (5 to 10 percent dextrose or 0.45 percent saline) so that the solution can serve as a diluent to decrease the bolus effect of the sodium bicarbonate. Excessive sodium bicarbonate therapy has

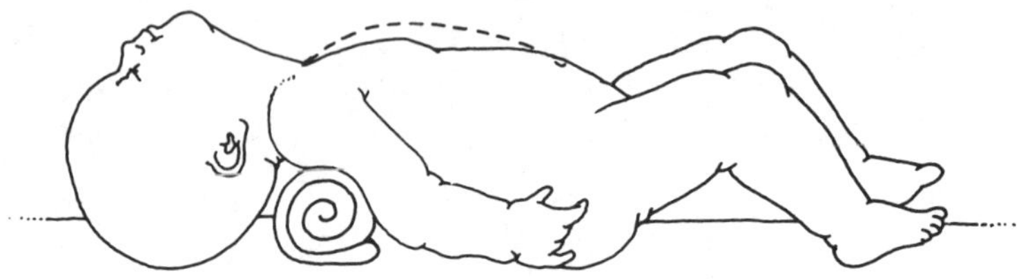

Fig. 9-11. Moderate hyperextension to relieve soft tissue obstruction. (Modified from Ostheimer,[30] with permission.)

been shown to cause hypernatremia, which has been implicated in intravascular cerebral hemorrhage in the sick neonate.[20] However, appropriate doses, guided by the infant's pH, appear to be safe in this regard.

Dextrose (2 g/kg IV push, then 5 to 8 mg/kg/min). Severely asphyxiated infants are often hypoglycemic because of their increased catecholamine levels, with initial elevation of glucose and stimulation of insulin secretion in the presence of decreased glycogen reserves and immature gluconeogenetic pathways.[5] Neonates born to diabetic mothers are at risk for hypoglycemia because of prolonged exposure to maternal hyperglycemia, with fetal islet cell hyperplasia and elevated insulin secretion. Those neonates who are small for gestational age or have suffered from uteroplacental insufficency also may develop hypoglycemia because of depleted glycogen stores. Hypoglycemia in these infants may be of later onset and they will require longer monitoring of blood glucose levels.

Epinephrine (adrenalin) (0.05 mg/kg). The hypotensive, bradycardic infant who is still acidotic may require this high dose of epinephrine for cardiac stimulation. In the nonacidotic infant, the usual dose of epinephrine is 0.01 mg/kg.

Naloxone (0.1 mg/kg IV or 0.2 mg/kg IM). Naloxone is used to reverse narcotic-related depression only. If the mother has received narcotics, the neonate may require naloxone. If this is so, the neonate should be observed for at least 4 hours after naloxone administration for evidence of recurrence of narcotic depression.

If the mother has received general anesthesia for delivery, the anesthetic can have a depressant effect on the newborn. Usually all the baby needs is oxygen, stimulation, and time to "wake up." Naloxone is not necessary in this setting, unless the mother has received narcotics as a part of the anesthetic.

Other drugs may be needed in prolonged resuscitation. The indications for and methods of their use are not discussed here in the context of the acute resuscitative effort, and their use is the prerogative of the attending pediatrician.

SPECIFIC NEONATAL PROBLEMS

Meconium Staining

Passage of meconium by the fetus is thought to occur in response to hypoxic stress in the ante- or peripartum period.[21] Meconium staining is present in 8 to 15 percent of all pregnancies, with a higher incidence occurring in the post-term pregnancy. Over half of infants born through meconium-stained fluid will have meconium in their tracheas, and if left untreated, many will develop meconium aspiration syndrome.[22–24] Since the treatment for meconium aspiration syndrome is only supportive and symptomatic, efforts have been concentrated on the prevention of the syndrome through effective airway suctioning at birth.[23–25] Immediately after the delivery of the infant's head, while the chest is still in the birth canal, the oropharynx and nasopharynx should be suctioned thoroughly by the obstetrician, using a bulb syringe or a DeLee apparatus. Immediately after delivery and, if possible, before the infant has taken his first breath, laryngoscopy and tracheal suctioning should be performed by the most experienced person present, regardless of the presence or absence of meconium in the oropharynx and nasopharynx since the obstetrician may have already completely cleared the upper airways of meconium. Tracheal suctioning should be repeated until no further meconium can be aspirated. An assistant should monitor the baby's heart rate during suctioning, since pharyngeal stimulation can cause bradycardia and other arrhythmias through vagal reflexes.[13] If the heart rate slows substantially, oxygen by mask or by clean tracheal tube should be given, with assisted ventilation if necessary. Infants who have aspirated meconium should receive chest physical therapy and postural drainage with suctioning, and should be monitored closely for the occurrence of respiratory distress. This sequence of immediate, thorough pharyngeal and tracheal suctioning has been found to be safe, and its implementation has greatly reduced the incidence and severity of meconium aspiration syndrome and its subsequent mortality.[23,24]

How often has the obstetric anesthesiologist heard that if there is thin meconium present in the airway at delivery it is not necessary to aspirate the trachea of the newborn? Chen et al. demonstrated that even small amounts of meconium in aspirated amniotic fluid can result in inactivation of surface active material from the alveolar lining of the lungs.[26] Therefore, it behooves us to be very aggressive in the management of the neonate with meconium in the amniotic fluid. However, the occurrence of in utero meconium aspiration is still a devastating problem. If we could eliminate this potentially disastrous occurrence during the later stages of pregnancy or during labor, we would virtually eliminate the meconium aspiration syndrome.

Neonatal Shock

Serious hypovolemia with secondary hypoperfusion and tissue hypoxia can occur as a result of numerous factors. Sequestration of blood in the placenta because of elevation of the infant above the mother at the time of cord clamping, prolapsed umbilical cord, abruptio placentae, placenta praevia, and rupture of the umbilical cord can significantly decrease the neonate's circulating blood volume. Low-birthweight infants may have decreased total protein concentrations, with a resultant shift of fluid out of the intravascular space because of low intravascular oncotic pressure. Also, maternal sepsis transmitted to the fetus may present as neonatal shock.

A decreasing blood pressure, tachycardia, pallor, decreased urine output, decreasing hematocrit, and metabolic acidemia all indicate that volume expansion may be needed. The preferred therapy is 20 ml/kg of fresh, uncontaminated heparinized fetal whole blood obtained from the placenta, which may be difficult to obtain.[27,28] If this is unavailable, fresh whole adult blood or packed red blood cells and fresh-frozen plasma in the same quantity may be used. Five percent albumin 1 g/kg can also serve as a volume expander. Finally, if no blood products are available, lactated Ringer's solution or 0.45 percent normal saline may be used. The neonate's blood pressure, pulse, respiration, and temperature should be monitored carefully to detect any deterioration before such a change becomes a crisis.

Constant monitoring of the hyotensive neonate is vital to proper management. Measurement of the infant's blood pressure should become a routine part of the physiologic evaluation at birth if a problem exists and all infants should have a screening blood pressure measured on admission to the nursery (Fig. 9-12). The neonate is "recovering" from the asphyxia of delivery and should have the same evaluation as a patient "recovering" from anesthesia and surgery.

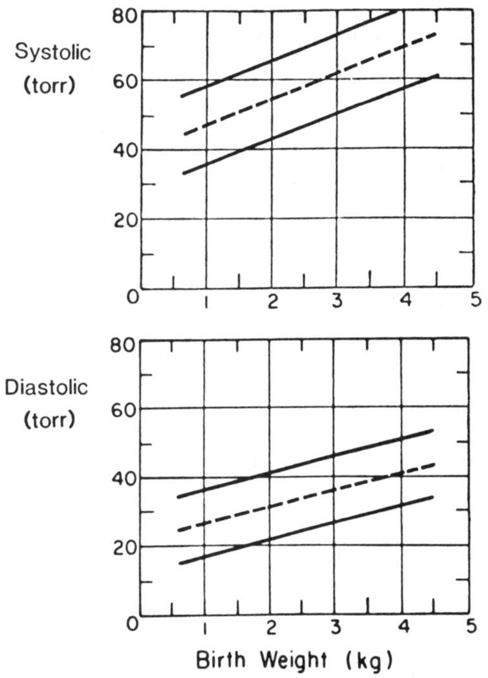

Fig. 9-12. Neonatal systolic and diastolic aortic blood pressure (From Versmold et al.,[11] with permission.)

Summary

The simple mnemonic ABCDE summarizes the five key principles of neonatal resuscitation:

1. *A*irway
2. *B*reathing
3. *C*irculation
4. *D*rugs
5. *E*valuation of concurrent and causative problems and maintenance of a neutral thermal *E*nvironment

REFERENCES

1. Frigoletto FD, Little GA: Guidelines for Perinatal Care. 2nd Ed. American Academy of Pediatrics and the American College of Obstetricians and Gynecologists, Elk Grove Village, Illinois, 1988
2. Gibbs CP, Krischer J, Peckham BM, et al: Obstetric anesthesia: a national survey. Anesthesiology 65:298, 1986
3. Behrman RE, Lees MH, Peterson EN, et al: Distribution

of the circulation in the normal and asphyxiated fetal primate. Am J Obstet Gynecol 108:956, 1970
4. Rudolph AM, Heymann MA: Fetal and neonatal circulation and respiration. Ann Rev Physiol 36:187, 1974
5. Bowen FW: Resuscitation and stabilization of the neonate. p. 445. In Bolognese RJ (ed): Perinatal Medicine: Management of the High Risk Fetus and Neonate. Williams & Wilkins, Baltimore, 1982
6. Brown BL, Gleicher N: Intrauterine meconium aspiration. Obstet Gynecol 57:26, 1981
7. Turbeville DF, McCaffress MA, Block MF, et al: In utero distal pulmonary meconium aspiration. South Med J 72:535, 1979
8. Karlberg P: The adaptive changes in the immediate postnatal period, with particular reference to respiration. J Pediatrics 56:585, 1960
9. Vyas H, Milner AD, Hopkin IE: Intrathoracic pressure and volume changes during the spontaneous onset of respiration in babies born by cesarean section and by vaginal delivery. J Pediatr 99:787, 1981
10. Milner AD, Vyas H: Lung expansion at birth. J Pediatr 101:879, 1982
11. Versmold HT, Ketterman JA, Phibbs RH, et al: Aortic blood pressure during the first 12 hours of life in infants with birth weight 610–4220 grams. Pediatrics 67:607, 1981
12. Dahm LS, James LS: Newborn temperature and calculated heat loss in the delivery room. Pediatrics 49:504, 1972
13. Cordero L, Hon EH: Neonatal bradycardia following nasopharyngeal stimulation. J Pediatr 78:441, 1971
14. Apgar V: A proposal for a new method of evaluation of the newborn infant. Curr Res Anesth Analg 32:260, 1953
15. Todres ID, Rogers MC: Methods of external cardiac massage in the newborn infant. J Pediatr 86:781, 1975
16. Fiholt DA, Kettrick RG, Wagner HR, Swedlow DB: The heart is under the lower third of the sternum. Am J Dis Child 140:646, 1986
17. Simmons MA, Adcock EW, Bard H, et al: Hypernatremia and intracranial hemorrhage in neonates. N Eng J Med 291:6, 1974
18. Volpe J: Neonatal intracranial hemorrhage—iatrogenic etiology (editorial). N Eng J Med 291:43, 1974
19. Cote CJ, Greenhow DE, Marshall BE: The hypotensive response to rapid intravenous administration of hypertonic solutions in man and in the rabbit. Anesthesiology 50:30, 1979
20. Wheeler AS, Sadri S, Gutsche BB, et al: Intracranial hemorrhage following intravenous administration of sodium bicarbonate or saline solution in the newborn lamb asphyxiated in utero. Anesthesiology 51:517, 1979
21. Walker J: Fetal anoxia. J Obstet Gynecol Br Commonw 60:162, 1953
22. Gregory GA, Gooding CA, Phibbs RH, et al: Meconium aspiration in infants: a prospective study. J Pediatr 85:848, 1974
23. Ting P, Brady JP: Tracheal suction in meconium aspiration. Am J Obstet Gynecol 122:767, 1975
24. Carson BS, Losey RW, Bowes WA, Simmons MA: Combined obstetric and pediatric approach to prevent meconium aspiration syndrome. Am J Obstet Gynecol 126:712, 1976
25. Frantz ID, Wang NS, Thach BT: Experimental meconium aspiration: effects of glucocorticoid treatment. J Pediatr 86:438, 1975
26. Chen CT, Toung TJK, Rogers MC: Effect of intra-alveolar meconium on pulmonary surface tension properties. Crit Care Med 13:233, 1985
27. Paxson CL: Collection and use of autologous fetal blood. Am J Obstet Gynecol 134:708, 1979
28. Golden SM, O'Brien WF, Metz SA: Anticoagulation of autologous cord blood for neonatal resuscitation. Am J Obstet Gynecol 144:103, 1982
29. Ostheimer GW: Resuscitating the depressed neonate. Contemp Obstet Gynecol 15:27, 1980
30. Ostheimer GW: Newborn Resuscitation. Weekly Anesthesiology Update, Inc., Princeton, NJ, 1978

DIFFERENTIAL DIAGNOSIS OF THE NEONATE IN DISTRESS

At birth, the neonate undergoes dramatic physiologic changes in the transition from intrauterine to extrauterine life. When observing the manner in which the neonate adapts to these changes, one observes three types of responses or adaptations:

1. Neonates who are adapting well (most neonates).
2. Neonates who obviously need help (i.e., no spontaneous respirations) and need the resuscitative approach to the airway, breathing, and circulation.
3. Neonates who are adapting but just "do not look quite right."

This last group of neonates will require help in adapting to their new environment. The assistance they will need must be individualized and directed at their major problems.

The previous section discussed the approach to the neonate in the first 10 minutes of life. This section will review the normal neonate's anatomy and physiology, provide a brief overview of several causes of newborn distress, and discuss several specific neonatal conditions.

THE NORMAL NEONATE

Estimated Gestational Age

A term neonate has achieved 37 to 42 weeks of gestation. This group includes approximately 80 percent of all live births. A preterm neonate is less than 37 weeks and a post-term neonate is greater than 42 weeks of gestation. By knowing the estimated gestational age (EGA), we can anticipate several of the problems the neonate may develop. For example, respiratory distress syndrome (RDS) is more common in the preterm neonate and is rare in the post-term neonate.

Anatomy

1. The average weight of the neonate based on gestational age is given below[1,2]:

Gestational Age (weeks)	Approximate Weight (g)
22	500
27	1,000
30	1,500
33	2,000
35.5	2,500
38	3,000
40	3,250
42	3,400

2. The neonate's head is relatively large. Once the head is delivered, the rest of the body usually follows easily. The average term head circumference is 35 cm.
3. The neck is short and has weak muscles.
4. The nasal passages are narrow and readily blocked by mucus, blood and secretions.
5. The tongue is relatively large, which may make intubation more difficult.
6. The cricoid cartilage is the narrowest part of the upper airway. When intubating the neonate, if the endotracheal tube meets obstruction just past the cords, the tube is too large and a smaller tube is needed. There should be a small air leak around the tube. Recommended endotracheal tube sizes are 2.5 mm internal diameter (ID) for neonates less than 2,500 g, 3.0 mm ID for neonates 2,500 to 3,500 g, and 3.5 mm ID for neonates greater than 3,500 g.
7. The tracheal length is about 4 cm. If it is necessary to intubate the neonate, the tip of the endotracheal tube should be inserted 1 to 2 cm past the vocal cords. A chest x-ray should confirm proper tube position.
8. The chest is relatively small and the ribs are more horizontal than in the adult.
9. The abdomen is protuberant.

Physiology

Respiratory System

1. The fetus initiates respiratory efforts as early as 11 weeks gestation. With increasing gestational age, these respiratory movements become more vigorous and more organized. The neonate begins extrauterine breathing within 30 seconds of birth (average time is 9 seconds).[3] This extrauterine breathing is initiated by physical stimulation such as cold and touch as well as by chemical stimulation such as mild hypoxia and acidosis. Severe hypoxia is a respiratory depressant.
2. Neonates are almost all obligate nasal breathers.[4]
3. Oxygen consumption for neonates is double that of adults (6 to 7 ml oxygen/kg/min for neonates). This relates to their high metabolic rate.
4. The respiratory rate in the newborn is 30–40 breaths/minute, about double that of adults. This rate occurs after the lungs have completely expanded and the lung fluid has been absorbed or expelled, which may take a few hours. Thus, initial respiratory rates are not uncommonly 60–90 breaths/minute decreasing with time to the normal range.[5]
5. The tidal volume is similar to the adult's: 6 to 7 ml/kg. If it is necessary to intubate and ventilate the neonate, the tidal volume needed is quite small (3,000-g neonate × 7 ml/kg = 21 ml). The approach to ventilation of the neonate is the same as the adult: watch for bilateral chest expansion and listen for breath sounds. The dead space:tidal volume ratio (VD/VT) is also similar to the adult: 0.3.
6. Slight nasal flaring, slight rales, and mild retractions are not uncommon and usually resolve in a few hours.[5] They may, however, be signs of mild respiratory difficulty and the neonate should be observed for resolution or progression of these signs.

Cardiovascular System

1. Neonates undergo a major shift in their blood circulation at birth. The intrauterine fetal circulation shifts to a transitional circulation and eventually to the adult circulation. (See Figs. 9-1 to 9-3 in the previous section.)

   The fetal circulation has a high pulmonary vascular resistance (due to the low arterial oxygen levels and the unexpanded lungs) and a low systemic vascular resistance (due to the placenta). This encourages blood flow through the two right-to-left shunts, the foramen ovale and the ductus arteriosus.

   As breathing begins and the cord is clamped, the transitional circulation begins. With breathing, the lungs fill with air, the arterial blood oxygen concentration rises, the pulmonary vascular resistance decreases, and the amount of blood entering the pulmonary circulation increases. This results in an increase in blood flow to the left atrium and an increase in left atrial pressure, which helps to functionally close the foramen ovale. When the umbilical cord is clamped, an increase in systemic vascular resistance develops, which increases systemic blood pressure and decreases blood flow across the ductus arteriosus. The ductus arteriosus may remain patent for 10 to 15 hours after birth before physiologically closing. Anatomic closure of the ductus occurs 2 weeks later in the term neonate, longer in the preterm neonate. If hypoxia or acidosis occurs before the ductus anatomically closes, the ductus may reopen. The shunt now is left-to-right because of the higher systemic pressure and the lower pulmonary pressure. The adult circulation is established when these shunts close.

2. The heart rate for the first 30 minutes is quite labile, with rates of 100 to 200 bpm commonly seen. After 30 minutes, the heart rate is about 120 to 160 bpm and varies with the neonate's activity.[5]
3. The stroke volume is fixed at about 5 ml/beat. As the heart rate decreases so does the cardiac output. Heart rates below 60 bpm require chest compressions.[6]
4. Blood pressure in newborns is less than adults[7]:

Weight (g)	Systolic (mmHg)	Diastolic (mmHg)
>3,001	70	40
2001–3,000	60	35
1001–2,000	50	30

A systolic pressure less than 50 mmHg in a term neonate is abnormal and usually needs treatment with volume expansion.

5. The blood volume in the term neonate is 85 to 100 ml/kg. If blood volume falls 10 percent, blood pressure falls 20 percent. If blood volume falls 20 percent, blood pressure falls 50 percent. When giving volume replacement, a dose of 10 ml/kg of crystalloid, colloid, or blood is given and repeated as necessary.
6. The hemoglobin level is 15 to 20 g/100 ml or a hematocrit of 45 to 60 percent. The blood is predominantly fetal hemoglobin, which has a P_{50} value of 18 mmHg, that is, hemoglobin is 50 percent saturated with oxygen at a PaO_2 of 18 mmHg. Polycythemia in the neonate is defined as a hematocrit above 70 percent.

Central Nervous System

1. The normal neonate has a 5-minute Apgar score of 7 or greater and is quite responsive to the environment for the first 10 to 150 minutes after birth. This is called the *first period of reactivity* and is followed by the *first sleep period*.[5]
2. The respiratory center is not completely mature at birth with respect to reflexes that deal with hypoxia. Severe hypoxia can act as a respiratory depressant for approximately a week in the term neonate, and longer in the preterm neonate.
3. The retinal vessels are not completely developed until 44 weeks gestational age. Before 44 weeks, excessive oxygen concentrations may lead to retrolental fibroplasia. However, in resuscitation efforts, 100 percent oxygen is often required for short periods of time.
4. Temperature regulation may not be adequate to maintain body temperature unless the neonate is dry and kept in a neutral temperature environment (32 to 34°C).
5. The CNS is still developing, as indicated by the primitive reflexes present at birth, such as Moro's and Babinski's reflexes, and by the increase in number of neurons that occurs in the first year of life.

Metabolic Factors

1. Normal neonatal blood gases are shown below[8]:

	Umbilical Cord		Arterial Blood Gases (mmHg)		
	Vein	Artery	10 min	30 min	60 min
PO_2	30	20	60	68	70
PCO_2	40	50	40	35	35
pH	7.32	7.24	7.25	7.33	7.36

2. Blood glucose is normally 40 to 60 mg/dl. Hypoglycemia is defined as a blood glucose value less than 30 mg/dl in the term neonate and less than 20 mg/dl in the preterm neonate.[9]
3. The calcium level is normally 7 to 11 mg/dl. Hypocalcemia is a calcium level of less than 7 mg/dl.
4. The magnesium level is normally 1.5 to 2.8 mEq/L. Hypomagnesemia is a magnesium level less than 1.5 mEq/L.

CAUSES OF DISTRESS

The neonate in distress may present with any number of abnormal signs, including apnea, tachypnea, chest wall retractions, cyanosis, bradycardia, and shock. Although the signs of a neonate in distress may be different from those of the adult, the approach is basically the same using the familiar ABCs mnemonic:

A = Airway

B = Breathing

C = Circulation

D = Drugs

E = Evaluate

The initial goal is to stabilize the neonate's Airway, Breathing and Circulation. The anesthesiologist should assist the neonatologist or pediatrician in diagnosing the etiology of distress in the newborn. Only after a definitive diagnosis is made can more appropriate care be administered.

In evaluating the neonate a systematic approach is needed. In this section, a common ABC approach is presented. Several conditions are presented in greater detail in the last part of this section.

Airway

A patent airway is essential for life. Because of the importance of the airway, all neonates should have their mouth and nose suctioned at birth to remove mucus, blood, or secretions that may be present. If meconium staining has occurred, depending on the presence of particulate matter, the trachea may need to be intubated and suctioned as well. Airway obstruction should be considered in all neonates. Airway obstruction can occur with foreign material (e.g., mucus, blood, meconium) or be the result of an anatomic obstruction (e.g., choanal atresia, Pierre Robin syndrome). Placement of an endotracheal tube can help establish an airway, but it must be kept in mind that these tubes can kink, become clogged, and/or slip out of proper position.

Breathing

After the airway is cleared and is patent, the adequacy of ventilation must be determined. Chest movement should be monitored to determine the respiratory rate and adequacy of chest excursion. A slow respiratory rate may have several causes, including asphyxia, sepsis, and narcotic depression. If breathing appears inadequate, ventilation is assisted by tactile stimulation (e.g., drying) or supplemental bag and mask (or endotracheal tube) ventilation. When narcotic depression is suspected (i.e., a narcotic was used for labor pain and there is a slow neonatal respiratory rate), naloxone is administered. If chronic maternal narcotic use is suspected, however, naloxone may cause acute narcotic withdrawal in the neonate and should not be administered.

Next the neonate should be observed for chest wall retractions and nasal flaring. If retractions are present, lung compliance may be reduced as seen in respiratory distress syndrome (RDS), transient tachypnea of the neonate (TTN), and pneumonia. In RDS, endotracheal intubation may be necessary to help expand the lungs.

Some neonates do not ventilate well because they are too weak to breathe. This may occur in very small premature infants whose muscles have not fully developed. These infants often need ventilatory support, especially if they also have RDS. Weakness may also result from drugs that interfere with muscular contractions such as magnesium or neuromuscular blockers. High levels of magnesium may occur in neonates whose mothers have received large doses of magnesium sulfate to prevent seizures in pregnancy-induced hypertension or as a tocolytic drug. Rarely, neuromuscular blockade has been reported in neonates whose mothers received large doses of nondepolarizing muscular blockers in the treatment of status epilepticus and in neonates with pseudocholinesterase deficiencies whose mothers received succinylcholine as part of a rapid-sequence induction to a general anesthetic. Rarely, phrenic nerve paralysis or myasthenia gravis may occur in the neonate.

Next the chest should be auscultated for bilateral breath sounds, usually using the anterior lateral chest and axillae. Decreased breath sounds on one side has several etiologies, including pneumothorax, diaphragmatic hernia, and an improperly placed endotracheal tube. It should be kept in mind that if the endotracheal tube is in the esophagus, bilateral breath sounds might be heard since the esophagus is in the midline and the chest is small. Air moving up and down the esophagus may mimic breath sounds. Reduced bilateral breath sounds may be due to small tidal volumes (e.g., in RDS), bilateral pleural effusions, or an obstructed airway.

Aspiration of meconium or amniotic fluid may lead to airway obstruction and poor gas exchange.

If the neonate has trouble breathing when feeding, a tracheoesophageal fistula may be present.

A chest x-ray can help sort out many pulmonary problems.

Circulation

Once the airway and breathing are thought to be adequate, evaluation of circulation is made. Heart rate, blood pressure, color, and perfusion are evaluated.

If the heart rate is slow, hypoxia, heart block, and drug effects should be considered. If the heart rate is less than 60 bpm, cardiopulmonary resuscitation is performed since the cardiac output may not be sufficient for survival.

If the blood pressure is low, hypovolemia, acidosis, congenital heart disease, and sepsis should be considered as possible etiologies in addition to pneumothorax and other respiratory diseases that decrease venous return and cardiac output.

If the neonate is cyanotic, 100 percent oxygen should be administered. Many etiologies can exist. In general, if improvement occurs with the administration of oxygen, respiratory diseases are more likely. Without improvement, a right-to-left shunt exists and cardiovascular diseases are more likely to be present. If the neonate is pale, hypovolemia or anemia should be considered.

If perfusion appears poor, decreased cardiac output should be considered and etiologies, including hypovolemia and acidosis, sought.

Drugs

Drugs may cause the neonate to appear in distress. The list of drugs that have adverse effects on the neonate is large. The adverse effects are often similar to the effects the drug has on an adult. The effects of analgesic and anesthetic drugs used to alleviate pain during vaginal and cesarean delivery are described in Chapter 3 (see Effects of Maternally Administered Drugs on the Fetus and Neonate). One should begin with a history of maternal drug use. A drug screen should be considered if maternal drug abuse is suspected.

Narcotic administration to the mother may cause respiratory depression in the neonate, as is shown by a low respiratory rate, but rarely produces bradycardia. Occasionally, if large doses of narcotics are given to the mother (e.g., 25 μg/kg fentanyl), the neonate may develop chest wall rigidity.[10]

β-Sympathomimetic drugs, often used as tocolytic medications, will often cause tachycardia in the neonate. This rarely requires treatment as the drug effect quickly dissipates.

Evaluate Other Etiologies

After assessing the basic ABCs and drug use, one then evaluates other body systems, including the neurologic system (for maldevelopment or asphyxia), muscular system (for weakness as with myasthenia gravis), and infectious diseases (for sepsis, group B β-hemolytic streptococcus, or herpes).

For all neonates in distress, a careful screen for metabolic disorders should be made, including glucose (especially if the mother is a diabetic) and hematocrit determinations. Other tests are done as indicated such as blood gases (looking for acidosis and respiratory failure) and calcium and magnesium levels.

Note: Although we tend to look for one cause for each neonate in distress, we must not forget that more than one cause may exist! An example is a neonate with respiratory distress syndrome who develops a pneumothorax or has hypoglycemia.

SPECIFIC CONDITIONS

Choanal Atresia

Choanal atresia is an anatomic obstruction of the nasal passages. The obstruction can be membranous and/or bony. The obstruction may be unilateral or bilateral.[4,11,12]

Signs. With unilateral choanal atresia, the neonate is often asymptomatic at birth. The diagnosis may not be made until unilateral rhinorrhea develops.

Most (but not all) neonates are unable to breathe through the mouth when resting. Neonates with bilateral choanal atresia will appear normal when the mouth is open. But when the mouth is closed, they will make inspiratory efforts without ventilation, become cyanotic, and may die if the condition is not diagnosed and treated.[4,11,12]

Diagnosis. Clinically, bilateral choanal atresia is suggested when the neonate appears pink when crying (mouth open) and blue when resting (mouth closed).

The diagnosis is further suggested when a suction catheter cannot be passed nasally. Because some nasal passages are narrow, one can place methylene blue in the nose and see whether it enters the pharynx or place a radiopaque dye in the nose and take a lateral skull roentgenogram and note whether the dye enters the pharynx.[11,12]

A computed tomography (CT) scan of the nasal area can be used to clearly outline the nature of the obstruction.[13]

Treatment. Correction of the obstruction is surgical.

With unilateral choanal atresia, the neonate has one nasal passage open and thus will have an airway when the mouth is closed. In these neonates, surgery can often be delayed several years.

With bilateral choanal atresia, the neonate is at risk of developing asphyxia when the mouth closes and thus requires the establishment of an airway. The mouth will remain open with the placement of either an oral airway or an endotracheal tube (failure to do so may risk the infant's life). After the airway is established, transfer the neonate to a neonatal intensive care (NICU) unit for further evaluation and treatment. If transport will take a few hours, hydration of the neonate must be maintained. This can be done by administration of fluid with an intravenous needle or catheter, by gavage feeding, or by bottle feeding with the use of a special McGovern nipple (an ordinary nipple with a large opening made in the tip) as swallowing and breathing at the same time are difficult. Repair may be delayed several weeks or months if the neonate can be taught to mouth breathe and feed satisfactorily.[4,11,12,14]

Congenital Heart Disease

Congenital heart disease (CHD) exists when there is an anatomic maldevelopment of the conduction system, the heart walls, valves, or major vessels leading to or going from the heart. CHD occurs at a rate of 8:1,000 live births.[15]

Classification.[16] Congenital heart disease is commonly divided into two main groups based on the ability to produce cyanosis (cyanotic heart disease and acyanotic heart disease).

Cyanotic heart disease has a predominant right-to-left shunt that decreases the amount of blood flowing through the lungs. These include:

1. Pulmonary atresia or stenosis with atrial or ventricular septal defect
2. Tetralogy of Fallot
3. Transposition of the great arteries
4. Total anomalous pulmonary venous drainage
5. Tricuspid atresia or stenosis
6. Ebstein's anomaly

Acyanotic heart disease includes all diseases that have no cardiac shunt or a predominant left-to-right shunt. These include:

1. Coarctation of the aorta
2. Aortic stenosis
3. Vascular ring anomalies
4. Atrial septal defect
5. Endocardial cushion defects (atrioventricular canal defects)
6. Ventricular septal defect
7. Patent ductus arteriosus
8. Truncus arteriosus

Signs. Signs depend on the severity and type of the cardiac lesion.

Cyanosis in the neonate may be peripheral or central. In peripheral cyanosis, the extremities are cyanotic but the mucous membranes and often the rest of the body are pink. This is due to a decrease in blood flow to the extremities and occurs in most neonates for several minutes after birth. Central cyanosis involves the entire body and is associated with a low PaO_2, often less than 40 mmHg, and is usually the result of cardiac or respiratory disease. In cardiac disease, cyanosis persists after the administration of 100 percent oxygen, signifying a right-to-left shunt and cyanotic heart disease. If cyanosis is relieved by the administration of oxygen, then respiratory disease is more likely.

If the heart rate is slow (bradycardia) and hypoxia and drug etiologies are ruled out, then congenial heart block should be considered. If the heart rate suddenly is very fast (e.g., 240 bpm), paroxysmal supraventricular tachycardia may exist.

Heart murmurs are often present but are confusing to differentiate. When murmurs are heard, an echocardiogram may be needed to better define the etiology.

In some neonates, a large left-to-right shunt develops and the initial presentation is with congestive heart failure. Signs include respiratory distress due to lung congestion and systemic venous congestion such as hepatomegaly. Because the pulmonary vascular resistance is elevated at birth, these lesions may not be diagnosed until a few weeks after birth when the pulmonary vascular resistance decreases. The earlier the presentation of congestive heart failure, the larger the defect. This most often is due to ventricular septal defect.[15]

Diagnosis. The above signs suggest heart disease but accurate diagnosis of the specific lesions often requires many tests, including an electrocardiogram, echocardiogram, chest x-rays, and sometimes a cardiac catheterization.

Treatment. Supportive care is given while the neonate is being evaluated. An intravenous infusion is established for hydration and the administration of medications. Acidosis, hypoglycemia, and hypocalcemia are treated as indicated. Oxygen is administered to neonates who are cyanotic to see if improvement occurs. In some neonates with cyanotic heart disease, the ductus arteriosus must remain open to allow blood to enter the pulmonary circulation. Administration of oxygen to these neonates may be deleterious since high arterial oxygen levels may close the ductus.

Specific treatment of the cardiac lesion will depend on the specific lesion and in particular on the symptoms, natural course, and availability of corrective or palliative surgery.

Diaphragmatic Hernia

Diaphragmatic hernia is a rare condition (occurring in 1 of 3,000 to 10,000 live births) in which part of the abdominal contents herniate through the diaphragm, usually on the left side. The lung on the side of the hernia is hypoplastic. The contralateral lung is usually also hypoplastic, but to a lesser degree. Unfortunately, even with rapid and appropriate care, including surgery, the mortality rate is 30 to 50 percent.[17–19]

Signs. These neonates often show significant respiratory compromise. Tidal volumes are markedly reduced as a result of the reduced lung tissue and elevated thoracic pressure. To compensate for the reduced tidal volumes, tachypnea must occur. Cyanosis is common and is due to poor effective ventilation and a large right-to-left shunt that develops from the elevated thoracic pressures. Sternal and intercostal retractions reflect a decrease in lung compliance.[18]

If one starts to assist breathing with bag and mask ventilation, the neonate may deteriorate further since gastric distension from air going into the stomach may compress the lungs further.

Blood gases will demonstrate hypoxia, hypercarbia, and acidosis, which can keep the ductus arteriosus open and increase the right-to-left shunt.

The heart may be displaced to the side opposite the hernia. The abdomen may appear scaphoid since part of the normal abdominal contents are in the chest.

Diagnosis. The diagnosis can be made in utero by ultrasound techniques.[17]

After birth, the diagnosis is suggested when the above signs are present and is confirmed with a chest x-ray. The chest x-ray will show air-filled loops of bowel in the chest cavity. Because these neonates also have hypoplastic lungs and require ventilatory support, a pneumothorax may also be present.

Treatment. Although this lesion is correctable with fetal surgery, many fetuses are not evaluated by ultrasound and are born with the defect. These neonates need early endotracheal intubation and oxygen supplementation. Because the lungs are small, one is tempted to try to expand their lungs. This should be avoided since their hypoplastic lungs are prone to rupture, producing a pneumothorax and further respiratory compromise. A struggling intubated neonate may also be prone to develop a pneumothorax. Paralysis with a muscle relaxant (e.g., pancuronium) and controlled ventilation have been advised.[19] Adequate ventilation can often be achieved with respiratory rates of 60 to 80 breaths/min and airway pressures less than 20 cmH_2O.

Elevating the neonate's head and tilting the neonate toward the side of the hernia may help reduce the size of the hernia and may make ventilation easier.[18]

A nasogastric tube should be placed to decompress the stomach and an umbilical or intravenous catheter should be placed to prevent dehydration and prepare the neonate for surgery. Once the intravenous infusion is established, a dose of sodium bicarbonate should be considered since these neonates invariably have a pH less than 7.20.[19]

The neonate's ventilation should be monitored with blood gases and metabolic acidosis treated. It should be kept in mind that hypoxia and acidosis may increase pulmonary vascular resistance and increase an already present right-to-left cardiac shunts.

Arrangements should be made to transport the neonate to a pediatric surgical center as soon as possible, as corrective surgery is indicated.

Hypoglycemia

For the first 72 hours of life, hypoglycemia is defined as a blood glucose level of less than 30 mg/dl in term neonates and less than 20 mg/dl in the preterm neonate. After 72 hours, blood glucose levels should be above 40 mg/dl. (Plasma levels are 5 mg/dl higher.)[9]

Signs. Often there are no obvious signs of hypoglycemia. Decreases in muscle tone, apnea, or irregular respirations may be seen and are thought to be due to a lack of fuel for muscle contractions. Cyanosis can also be present. Tremors and seizures may occur as a result of extremely low blood glucose levels.

Diagnosis. The diagnosis is made by laboratory tests.

Because signs may not always be apparent and untreated hypoglycemia may lead to brain damage, blood glucose levels should be measured in all neonates in distress as well as in all neonates of diabetic mothers, as they are prone to develop hypoglycemia.

Treatment. Prevention of hypoglycemia is best achieved by early feedings with 10 percent dextrose in water (D10W) in infants of diabetic mothers or by intravenous hydration with glucose in any infant in distress.

If hypoglycemia develops in otherwise healthy neonates, oral feedings with D5W or D10W may be sufficient.

If hypoglycemia is present in neonates who are distressed, the intravenous administration of 200 mg/kg of dextrose (D10W 2 ml/kg) is infused over 1 to 2 minutes followed by a dextrose infusion of 8 mg/kg/min (D10W 4.8 ml/kg/h).[20]

Blood glucose levels are rechecked every 30 minutes until stable.

Hypovolemia (Shock)

Hypovolemia occurs when the intravascular volume is decreased. It should be considered in any neonate who requires resuscitation, since blood loss is frequently not obvious.[6] Occasionally, blood loss is obvious and rapid, as in a vasa previa with a ruptured fetal vessel, which can result in rapid fetal demise.

Signs. Signs relate to the decrease in circulating blood volume and hemoglobin concentration and may not be obvious if less than 15 percent blood volume is lost. If greater than 20 percent blood volume is lost, signs are common and include pallor with decreased capillary refill, tachycardia with decreased pulse *volume*, hypotension, tachypnea, and a poor response to resuscitation.[6] If enough time transpires, a decrease in urine output may be measurable.

Diagnosis. History is important, especially if an obvious cause of bleeding exists. Otherwise, the signs above are suggestive.

Treatment. Treatment begins as in all cases of shock: establishment of an intravenous infusion and administration of volume. Treatment is started with a bolus over 5 to 10 minutes of 10 ml/kg of crystalloid, colloid (e.g., 5 percent albumin), or whole blood (O negative cytomegalovirus-negative blood cross-matched with the mother's blood, if time permits).[6]

The blood pressure and heart rate are rechecked. Volume expansion is repeated as needed with doses of 10 ml/kg.

Arterial or venous blood is checked for hemoglobin content and for the presence of a metabolic acidosis, which may develop after previously poorly perfused tissue beds become better perfused. Acidosis can produce cardiovascular depression and may require treatment with sodium bicarbonate. The standard solution of sodium bicarbonate is 1 mEq/ml. This standard solution should be diluted with sterile water to decrease the osmolarity (rapid infusion of a hyperosmolar solution has been implicated in causing hypotension and intracranial bleeding).

With systemic hypotension, a right-to-left shunt may exist so it must be ascertained that the intravenous infusion is bubble free.

A hematocrit above 40 percent must be maintained.

Immature Respiratory Center (Apnea and Bradycardia)

In the neonate, two types of arrested respiratory patterns can be observed. Periodic breathing consists of pauses in respiration of less than 15 seconds (this is of little concern and is sometimes seen in normal term neonates). Apnea and bradycardia (A and B spells) result in pauses in respiration of greater than 20 seconds with a resultant slowing of the heart rate and, often, cyanosis. If untreated, A and B spells could lead to death. The heart rate usually starts to fall by about 15 seconds and by 30 seconds is below 100 bpm.[21]

Hypoxia and hypercarbia should stimulate a response in the respiratory center. Absence of stimulation may be related to an immature respiratory center. Hypoxia in the neonate can not only be a respiratory depressant, but also a cardiac depressant, as seen by the bradycardia.

Incidence. Apnea is common in the neonatal period, with spells occurring in about 25 percent of infants less than 2,500 g.[21]

Diagnosis. Diagnosis is made by observation and by an apnea and bradycardia monitor.

Treatment. For periodic breathing, the only treatment needed is observation.

Because the first apnea and bradycardia spell could cause death, all premature infants should be monitored for a few days to see if these spells develop. In 80 to 90 percent of apnea and bradycardia spells, simple tactile stimulation will start breathing. The rest will need a few breaths of oxygen by bag and mask. Theophylline is sometimes used as a respiratory stimulant in doses of 3 mg/kg every 6 hours.[22]

This condition is mainly one of recognition for anesthesiologists. Small neonates have pauses of respiration that resolve as they mature. These infants need observation in NICU and work-up as required by a neonatologist. An increase in the frequency of A and B spells may be an early sign of sepsis.

Periodic breathing is a potential problem in the premature or prior premature neonate who requires surgery since an increased number of spells may occur in the postoperative period.

Meconium Aspiration

Meconium consists of the contents of the fetal gastrointestinal (GI) tract and includes swallowed amniotic fluid, desquamated cutaneous cells, and GI secretions such as bile salts, which give meconium its green color.

Meconium is sterile and is rarely formed to any great extent before 34 weeks gestation.[23] Although the passage of meconium may be a normal physiologic event related to increasing maturity of the fetus, it may also be a sign of fetal distress. When the fetus is stressed (i.e., hypoxic), an increase in GI motility and relaxation of the anal sphincter may permit meconium to be passed.[24,25] When this occurs, the normally clear amniotic fluid becomes green stained.

Meconium aspiration occurs when the stained amniotic fluid is aspirated into the trachea. This can occur in utero[26] or at the time of delivery when the neonate starts to breathe.[27]

Incidence. Staining occurs in about 10 percent of all live births (one-third will have thick, particulate, "pea soup"-appearing amniotic fluid; the rest will have thin, watery amniotic fluid).[28,29] Staining is more common in neonates who weigh more than 3,500 g.[28] This is to be expected as these infants are older and have had more time to accumulate meconium. The average length of gestation in which meconium staining is present is 10 days past the estimated date of confinement.

About 60 percent of neonates stained at birth have meconium in their tracheas but only 10 to 30 percent will develop respiratory difficulty.[29] Thus, signs of meconium aspiration syndrome occur in 1 to 3 percent of all live births.[29,30] Although meconium may not be found in the pharynx with laryngoscopy, about 20 percent will have meconium in their tracheas.[29] In these infants, the meconium in the pharynx was removed through suction (with a Delee suction catheter or bulb syringe) by the obstetrician or swallowed by the neonate before laryngoscopy and intubation was performed.

Signs. Clinical signs of meconium aspiration are respiratory in nature and relate to obstruction of the airways and the shunting of blood that develops. The severity of respiratory compromise parallels the amount and thickness of meconium aspirated. When a small amount is aspirated, tachypnea and mild cyanosis are common, resulting from peripheral airway obstruction with atelectasis and ventilation : perfusion abnormalities. When a large amount of meconium is aspirated, the neonate is often severely depressed with profound cyanosis and irregular and gasping respirations. Occasionally, complete airway obstruction and death occurs. Inspissated meconium can also create a ball-valve effect, resulting in a pneumothorax.[30]

A chest x-ray can suggest outcome.[29,31] If the chest x-ray is normal, the neonates do well. Neonates with air leaks, consolidation, or atelectasis have a higher incidence of respiratory failure and death.[31] Coarse infiltrates, if seen, will usually clear within 12 to 36 hours.[29,31] Clinical judgment should dictate which neonates should have a chest x-ray.

Some infants with meconium aspiration and respiratory distress develop a condition called *persistent fetal circulation* (pulmonary hypertension with a right-to-left shunt through a patent foramen ovale and ductus arteriosus). These infants generally do very poorly.

In utero meconium aspiration may cause severe respiratory distress at birth. Even the most aggressive attempts at pulmonary ventilation may be unsuccessful. The use of extracorporeal membrane oxygenation may give these neonates a chance to survive by allowing the resolution of the meconium aspiration.

Overall, the mortality for meconium-stained neonates is 3.3 percent versus 1.7 percent in unstained neonates.[28]

Treatment. When the head is delivered and prior to delivery of the shoulders, the obstetrician suctions the mouth and nose with a Delee suction catheter or, preferably, with a bulb syringe.[32,33] The bulb syringe is as effective, is easier to use, is more cost-effective, and may be safer than the DeLee catheter.[33]

Immediately following delivery, the mouth is suctioned again and the trachea is intubated and suctioned, preferably before the infant takes a breath (each breath may move tracheal meconium distally).[27] The resuscitator applies suction with a device attached to the endotracheal tube connector. The negative pressure generated by the suction device should be less than the usual pressure of wall suction at 400 mmHg. Usually 80 to 100 mmHg will suffice. If meconium is aspirated from the neonate's trachea, intubation and suctioning of the trachea may need to be repeated a few times in order to clear the trachea of meconium.

Although laryngoscopy and endotracheal intubation are important in the management of these neonates, one must keep in mind the adverse effects of intubation, including bradycardia and, rarely, esophageal perforation. The fetal heart rate may decrease during laryngoscopy or be low as a result of fetal asyphxia. The heart rate should be monitored during intubation. If the fetal heart rate is below 80 bpm, consideration must be given to the administration of oxygen by positive-pressure ventilation even though positive-pressure ventilation may push some meconium distally. Neonates who develop esophageal perforations from intubation present with excessive oropharyngeal secretions, feeding difficulties, and sometimes respiratory distress. Perforations often respond to conservative medical therapy but may require surgery.[34]

Recently, the need to intubate all neonates with meconium staining has been questioned. Some investigators think that after suctioning the mouth and nose, the infant, if vigorous, does not benefit from intubation.[35] Others recommend only intubating the tracheas of neonates with thick meconium staining.[6] However, the thickness of the meconium may be difficult to determine, and if any question exists the trachea should be intubated and suctioned.

Neonates with mild aspiration usually have a benign clinical course with resolution of signs within 24 to 72 hours.[30] If mild respiratory distress develops, supplemental oxygen by hood is administered to keep the PaO_2 between 50 and 100 mmHg. A pulse oximeter and/or an umbilical artery catheter are used to guide therapy. With massive aspiration, tracheal suctioning, and ventilatory support may be needed. Despite appropriate airway management, some of these infants will die![30,36]

The development of a pneumothorax should be anticipated and treated as indicated.

A Delee suction catheter is passed in the stomach by the nasal or oral route when the infant is stabilized to suction stomach contents and help prevent aspiration of any meconium the infant may have swallowed.

Chest physical therapy may prove helpful in loosening secretions that cannot be reached by tracheal suction. Tracheobronchial lavage with saline has not been shown to be of any benefit and in some cases may increase respiratory distress.[32]

If persistent fetal circulation develops, mechanical hyperventilation producing mild respiratory alkalosis combined with a pulmonary vasodilator, such as tolazoline, may be required. Hypotension that may accompany tolazoline therapy is treated with volume expansion and, if necessary, with dopamine. Hypoxia, acidosis, and/or hypothermia can lead to an increase in pulmonary artery pressure and an increase in the right-to-left shunt.

Myasthenia Gravis

Myasthenia gravis (MG) is an autoimmune neuromuscular disease in which antibodies (IgG class) are directed against the acetylcholine receptor (AchR) in skeletal muscle. It is associated with muscle weakness, which can become profound with exercise and relieved with rest or with the administration of anticholinesterase agents.[37,38]

Incidence and Types. Two types of MG are seen in the neonate.

Neonatal MG (transient MG) occurs in about 10 to 20 percent of infants born to mothers with MG.[37] The development of neonatal MG is unrelated to the severity of the mother's disease or to the level of her AchR antibody.[38]

Congenital MG (persistent MG) may appear in infants of unaffected mothers.[38]

Signs. Hypotonia with respiratory weakness and arrest may be present at birth or appear within the first 72 hours of birth. These infants usually have a decreased ability to feed due to a poor sucking response.

Diagnosis. The diagnosis can be made by identifying antibodies to AchR in the serum; however, detectable levels are not always present in patients with MG. Increased muscle tone will develop with the administration of anticholinesterase agents such as neostigmine 0.1 to 0.2 mg, which is considered diagnostic. This increase in muscle tone develops in a few minutes.

Treatment. Untreated infants may die. For those with transient neonatal MG, neostigmine 0.2 mg should be given every 6 hours until strength returns. This may take several weeks. However, the average duration of treatment is 18 days.[37] Infants with persistent neonatal MG need anticholinesterase agents for life.

Persistent Fetal Circulation (Primary Pulmonary Hypertension)

Persistent fetal circulation (PFC) is a condition of the neonate in which the pulmonary vasculature is in vasospasm, producing pulmonary hypertension. As a result of the high pulmonary vascular resistance, the foramen ovale and the ductus arteriosus remain open, producing a large right-to-left shunt and cyanosis. This syndrome is more common in term infants and is associated with an increase in muscle mass of the pulmonary arterioles.

Signs. Although the neonates can be pink at rest, they often are cyanotic, especially when crying. The cyanosis may not be relieved with oxygen. Tachypnea and retractions can be seen as the neonate is struggling to oxygenate. Hypoxemia, acidosis, and hypercarbia are present and are partially due to right-to-left shunting. Hypoglycemia often occurs in these stressed infants, whose glycogen stores are rapidly depleted. PFC is not uncommonly associated with severe meconium aspiration, sepsis, asphyxia, and diaphragmatic hernia.[39]

Diagnosis. Diagnosis is difficult and often considered only after exclusion of other causes of cyanosis. The echocardiogram shows a normal heart and the chest x-ray shows hypoperfusion of the lung fields. Hypoxemia is usually unrelieved with 100 percent oxygen but the PaO_2 may be greater than 40 mmHg. If the infant is hyperventilated with 100 percent oxygen, infants with pulmonary hypertension usually show a rise in PaO_2 to above 100 mmHg. This does not occur in neonates with cyanotic heart disease. Cardiac catheterization can confirm the diagnosis and demonstrates pulmonary artery pressures that are usually higher than systemic artery pressures.[40]

Treatment. Treatment is aimed at preventing a further rise and, preferably, producing a fall in pulmonary vascular resistance. High concentrations of oxygen are used initially since hypoxia can increase pulmonary vascular resistance. Even with 100 percent oxygen, blood oxygen saturation is often low, making the risk of retrolental fibroplasia small. If further treatment improves oxygen saturation the oxygen concentration may be slowly reduced. An acceptable oxygen saturation is 80 to 85 percent.[39]

A respiratory alkalosis ($PaCO_2$ in the range of 25 to 30 mmHg and occasionally lower) may decrease pulmonary resistance and pulmonary blood pressures to the point where the right-to-left shunting ceases.[39,40] A metabolic alkalosis produced by the administration of sodium bicarbonate may also be of benefit.[39]

To further reduce pulmonary resistance the administration of a vasodilator such as tolazoline (Priscoline) has been suggested.[40] The dose is 1 to 2 mg/kg as a bolus followed by an infusion of 1 to 2 mg/kg/h.[41] The infusion is given into a scalp vein to get preferential blood flow into the pulmonary circulation. Because tolazoline may also dilate the systemic vasculature as well, it is important to maintain an adequate circulating blood volume.

The combination of arterial hypoxemia and a large right ventricular afterload may lead to myocardial dysfunction. The use of an inotrope such as dopamine (starting at 5 to 7 μg/kg/min) has also been recommended.[39]

These infants often require intensive therapy, and should be transferred to a NICU as soon as possible. Even with the best care, mortality can be as high as 20 percent.[40]

Pneumothorax

A pneumothorax occurs when air is present in the pleural cavity. It may occur spontaneously with or without apparent underlying lung disease. It may also occur as a result of excessive airway pressures that sometimes occur with mechanical ventilation.

Lungs of infants with RDS often need elevated airway pressures to distend the alveoli. Pneumothoraces are more likely to occur in these infants.[42–44] Neonates who have aspirated meconium are also at increased risk for pneumothorax. This is believed to be secondary to localized increases in airway pressures that occur with the ball-valve effect of meconium in the airways.[27,29,44]

Pneumothorax should be included in the differential diagnosis of any infant who suddenly develops a deterioration of respiratory function.

Incidence. Asymptomatic pneumothorax occurs in 1 to 2 percent of all live births. Symptomatic pneumothorax in "normal neonates" is much less common. Because it is usually not diagnosed and treated in time, the mortality approaches 20 percent.

Signs. Signs of a pneumothorax relate to the mechanical effect of the pneumothorax and depend on the size of the pneumothorax and the amount of pressure in the chest.

Decreased breath sounds may be heard on the side of the pneumothorax; however, this may be difficult to distinguish as the room in which auscultation is carried out is often noisy and lungs sounds are easily transmitted through the chest wall. The heart may be displaced to the side opposite the pneumothorax. Displacement of the heart to the right is often easier to pick up than displacement to the left.

Because of the smaller lung volumes that result, the neonate may try to compensate by increasing the respiratory rate. Tachypnea with rates above 60 breaths/min are often seen.

Cyanosis may result because of shunting of pulmonary blood flow into the smaller, less well-expanded lungs. It may also be due to shunting of blood from right-to-left through the foramen ovale, which may open secondary to the elevated pulmonary artery resistance seen with elevated lung pressures.

Hypotension can also develop secondary to a decrease in venous return and a decrease in cardiac output.

Diagnosis. The diagnosis is made clinically when respiratory distress is relieved by the evacuation of air from the chest.

Transillumination of light across the chest wall can be helpful. A light pressed on the chest wall normally will be transmitted for about 1 cm around the light source because the underlying lung prevents further transmission. Over a pneumothorax, the light is transmitted further because the lung does not block the light. When seen, it is often dramatic. Occasionally, the entire chest lights up and the heart can be seen beating as well.

A chest x-ray will demonstrate the pneumothorax and differentiate it from other space-occupying lesions such as a congenital lung cyst or a diaphragmatic hernia.

Treatment. If the pneumothorax is small and asymptomatic, only observation is needed. If the pneumothorax causes compromise, the air must be removed by a chest tube or a catheter. The chest tube is placed in the midaxillary line just above the seventh rib. Midaxillary line placement keeps the chest tube away from the pectoralis and the latissimus dorsi muscles. Following placement, the tube is connected to a vacuum with 10 to 12 cmH_2O negative pressure. If a chest tube is not readily available, a 16-gauge intravenous catheter over a needle, a three-way stopcock, and a syringe are needed. The needle and catheter are placed; the needle is withdrawn, leaving the catheter in the pleural space. The three-way stopcock and syringe are then attached to the catheter. Air is aspirated with the syringe. The three-way stopcock closes the catheter when the syringe needs to be emptied of air. This technique can also be used to drain large pleural effusions.

A chest x-ray is used to confirm chest tube placement and the resultant success of therapy.

Respiratory Distress Syndrome (Hyaline Membrane Disease)

Respiratory distress syndrome (RDS) is a disease of the neonate associated with prematurity and low levels of pulmonary surfactant. The low concentrations of surfactant produce a decrease in lung compliance due to the collapse of alveoli. Typically, RDS gets worse over the first 24 to 72 hours and then improves unless complications such as a pneumothorax or a patent ductus arteriosus develop. In uncomplicated cases, RDS may resolve within a week.[45,46]

Incidence. The incidence varies inversely with the gestational age of the infant and is more common with cesarean deliveries than vaginal deliveries. For vaginally delivered neonates, the incidence of RDS is 65 percent at 25 to 28 weeks gestation; 35 percent at 31 to 32 weeks; 5 percent at 35 to 36 weeks; and less than 1 percent after 39 weeks.[45] RDS is more common in males and in infants of diabetic mothers, and often is more severe in the second of twins. Occasionally, the second twin develops RDS while the first twin does not.[45]

Twenty to thirty percent of infants with RDS die. Of those who survive, many have little or no measurable lung disease when tested several years after birth.[47] Some, however, develop bronchopulmonary dysplasia.[48] Retrolental fibroplasia may develop in the course of treatment and, in some mild cases, may be reversible.

Signs. Most signs of RDS are related to the decrease in lung compliance that results from the low levels of pulmonary surfactant.[43,45,46]

About one-half of affected neonates have difficulty initiating breathing. Many of these infants are too weak to expand their noncompliant lungs. For the rest, breathing starts promptly but within minutes to a few hours signs of respiratory difficulty develop.

Chest wall retractions (suprasternal, intercostal, subcostal) are one of the more obvious common signs and are due to the chest wall expanding in an attempt to expand the noncompliant lungs. The severity of the retractions depends on the respiratory effort of the infant and the severity of the lung disease. Grunting may occur in an attempt to expand the lungs during exhalation. Nasal flaring can also be seen.

To overcome the decrease in tidal volume that occurs with noncompliant lungs, the infant increases its respiratory rate. Tachypnea (respiratory rate above 60 breaths/min) is common.

Depending on the severity of the disease, cyanosis can be seen and blood gas reports will confirm respiratory failure (hypoxemia, hypercarbia, and acidosis). Hypoxemia and acidosis can reopen the ductus arteriosus. Hypotension may also be present.

Pathology. If the infant dies from RDS, gross findings include firm, collapsed lungs. Microscopically, alveoli are collapsed and hyaline membranes are seen on the alveolar walls and ducts. Biochemically, a low concentration of surfactant (mainly lecithin) will be measured. Surfactant production begins about 23 weeks gestation.

Diagnosis. The diagnosis is suspected clinically in any preterm neonate with progression of the above signs. Many normal infants have tachypnea and nasal flaring at birth but improve over several minutes.[5] In RDS, these respiratory signs are progressive and reflect more airway closure. Arterial blood gases can quantitate the compromise in oxygenation and ventilation and can guide therapy. A chest x-ray will show a diffuse reticulogranular or "ground-glass" appearance and air bronchograms (a diffuse disease gives a diffuse appearance).[43–46]

Treatment. Prevention of premature delivery is the aim in obstetric care. If premature delivery is likely, delaying delivery for 48 hours after the administration of glucocorticoids may reduce the incidence of RDS.[49–51]

Treatment begins in the delivery room or pediatric resuscitation area and usually will require transfer to a NICU. These preterm infants often need to be transferred not only for respiratory care but because of the other problems of prematurity as well (apnea and bradycardia, feeding problems, etc.).

Respiratory care is the primary factor in resuscitation. The goal is to maintain the PaO_2 at 50 to 80 mmHg, $PaCO_2$ below 55 mmHg, and pH above 7.25. Methods to maintain these parameters will vary. If the $PaCO_2$ and pH are acceptable and the PaO_2 is low, use of an oxygen hood (up to a FIO_2 of 0.60) to maintain a PaO_2 of 50 to 80 mmHg should be considered. If the FIO_2 is more than 0.60, the infant should be intubated and continuous positive airway pressure or CPAP initiated. CPAP should be started at 8 cmH_2O of pressure and increased by 2 cmH_2O as needed until a desirable PaO_2 is obtained (usually pressures are 8 to 15 cmH_2O). Once CPAP is added, the FIO_2 can often be substantially decreased while maintaining an adequate PaO_2. The CPAP may open collapsed alveoli even in the absence of surfactant. If the $PaCO_2$ is above 55 mmHg on CPAP, mechanical ventilation is needed. With pressure-cycled ventilators, ventilation is begun with pressures of 25–50 cmH_2O. For adequate gas exchange it may be necessary to adjust the inspiratory:expiratory ratio to allow more time for inspiration (normal I:E ratio, 1:2).[46]

Apnea and bradycardia monitors are placed on all infants not on mechanical ventilation.

Because group B β-hemolytic streptococcal infections may present with signs and symptoms similar to RDS, all neonates are treated with antibiotics after cultures are obtained.[52,53] Therapy is directed by the pediatrician.

Recently, surfactant (artificial or synthetic) has been administered into the trachea of neonates at risk for RDS immediately after birth as well as in infants with established RDS. The dose is 3 to 5 ml of surfactant per kilogram of neonatal weight. This is followed by a few manual inflations of the lungs. One must remember that the normal tidal volume is 6 to 7 ml/kg and the dose must be given slowly or else a fall in oxygen saturation occurs. I have found that if the FIO_2 is increased for a few breaths before administering the surfactant, the fall in oxygen saturation is attenuated. Presumably this relates to increasing the oxygen reserve in the lung before administering the drug. Early results show improvement in gas exchange.[42]

Consider the use of a pulse oximeter to guide oxygen therapy.[54] Too high of a PaO_2 may increase the chance of retrolental fibroplasia.

Tracheoesophageal Fistula

Tracheoesophageal fistula (TE fistula) is an abnormality in the development of the esophagus in which there is atresia of the esophagus, usually with a fistula between the trachea and the esophagus. The incidence is 1:3,000 to 4,500 live births. Five main types of TE fistula exist:[55–57]

1. Atresia of the upper esophagus and a fistula between the trachea and lower esophagus (86 percent).
2. Atresia of the upper esophagus and a fistula between the trachea and upper esophagus (1 percent).
3. Atresia of the esophagus and no fistula (8 percent).
4. Atresia of the esophagus and two fistulas, one from the trachea to the upper esophagus, one from the trachea to the lower esophagus (1 percent).
5. The H-type fistula, a fistula from the esophagus to the trachea. The esophagus is patent (4 percent).

The fistula is usually 3 to 5 mm in cross-sectional diameter and can easily allow air or gastric contents to pass through it.[57]

In addition to the TE fistula, many of these neonates have other problems as well, including congenital heart lesions (20 percent) and prematurity (35 percent).[55,57]

Signs. In the delivery room, the possibility of a TE fistula (except the H type) can be suspected when a suction catheter fails to enter the stomach.

Since passage of a suction catheter into the stomach is not always performed, most often signs relate to the consequences of esophageal atresia. These include drooling and vomiting of food as well as coughing, cyanosis, and sometimes brochospasm if the food gets into the trachea. Respiratory distress can also occur secondary to pulmonary aspiration of gastric contents. Abdominal distension can occur from air going from the trachea into the lower esophagus and stomach. In some cases, gastric distension is so great that it impedes movement of the diaphragm and hypoventilation occurs.[56]

Dehydration may occur because of the decreased GI absorption.

Diagnosis. The diagnosis of esophageal atresia is made by the inability to pass a rigid radiopaque 10- to 14-French suction catheter (more-flexible catheters can coil) into the stomach. Obstruction will commonly occur 9 to 13 cm from the nares.[55] Esophageal atresia can also be diagnosed with a chest x-ray when the esophagus is filled with a radiopaque contrast dye. The chest x-ray can rule out significant pulmonary (e.g., aspiration, RDS) and some congenital heart problems. If there is no air in the lower GI tract, a fistula between the trachea and lower esophagus is absent. If air is present, a fistula is present between the trachea and the lower esophagus.

The H type is diagnosed by observing aspiration of a radiopaque solution during feeding under fluoroscopy.

Treatment. Without surgery these infants will die.

Early diagnosis and preoperative preparation is important before the infant's condition deteriorates as a result of dehydration and pulmonary complications such as aspiration or regurgitation. Oral feedings should be withheld and suctioning (intermittent or continuous) of the upper esophageal pouch should be performed. An intravenous infusion should be established to prevent dehydration. The infant should be placed in a semisitting position to decrease the chance of gastric content aspiration and to make breathing easier. The placement of a gastrostomy tube under local anesthesia to decompress the stomach and remove gastric contents has been suggested.[55,57] Arrangements for transport of the infant to a pediatric surgical center should be made promptly.

Dr. C. E. Koop[58] reported on a series of 134 neonates operated on with TE fistulas. Overall survival was 66 percent (70 percent term neonates, 52 percent preterm neonates). If the term neonate did not have a major associated congenital anomaly and did not have pneumonia, 100 percent survived.

Transient Tachypnea of the Neonate

Transient tachypnea of the neonate (TTN) may present similarly to RDS in that these infants have tachypnea, retractions, grunting, and occasionally, mild cyanosis. Although these signs are similar to RDS, infants with transient tachypnea may be term and have faster respiratory rates (80 to 140 breaths/min), fewer retractions, less grunting, and less cyanosis. A chest x-ray shows mild cardiomegaly, prominent central-vascular markings, and hyperaeration. This disease is believed to be due to slow resorption of lung fluid. Treatment is supportive and usually requires only oxygen by hood (commonly only 35 percent oxygen). This disease resolves in a few days.[59]

REFERENCES

1. Brenner WE, Edelman DA, Hendricks CH: A standard of fetal growth for the United States of America. Am J Obstet Gynecol 126:555, 1976
2. Lubchenco LO, Searls DT, Brazie JV: Neonatal mortality rate: relationship to birth weight and gestational age. J Pediatr 81:814, 1972
3. Milner AD, Vyas H: Lung expansion at birth. J Pediatr 101:879, 1982
4. Fearon B, Dickson J: Bilateral choanal atresia in the newborn—plan of action. Laryngoscope 78:1487, 1968
5. Desmond MM, Franklin RR, Vallbona C, et al: The clinical behavior of the newly born. I. The term baby. J Pediatr 62:307, 1963
6. American Heart Association-American Academy of Pediatrics Textbook of Neonatal Resuscitation. American Heart Association, New York, 1987
7. Versmold HT, Kitterman JA, Phibbs RH, et al: Aortic blood pressure during the first 12 hours of life in infants with birth weight 610 to 4,220 grams. Pediatrics 67:607, 1981
8. Modanlou H, Yeh S-Y, Hon EH: Fetal and neonatal acid-base balance in normal and high-risk pregnancies. Obstet Gynecol 43:347, 1974
9. Pildes RS, Pyati SP: Hypoglycemia and hyperglycemia in tiny infants. Clin Perinatol 13:351, 1986
10. Jarvis AP, Arancibia CU: A case of difficult neonatal ventilation. Anesth Analg 66:196, 1987
11. Flake CG, Ferguson CF: Congenital choanal atresia in infants and children. Ann Otol Rhinol Laryngol 73:458, 1964
12. McGovern FH, Fitz-Hugh GS: Surgical management of congenital choanal atresia. Arch Otolaryngol 73:627, 1961
13. Harner SG, McDonald TJ, Reese DF: The anatomy of congenital choanal aresia. Otolaryngol Head Neck Surg 89:7, 1981
14. McGovern FH: Bilateral choanal atresia in the newborn—a new method of medical management. Laryngoscope 71:480, 1961
15. Mitchell SC, Korones SB, Berendes HW: Congenital heart disease in 56,109 births: incidence and natural history 43:323, 1971
16. Beynen FM, Tarhan S: Anesthesia for the surgical repair of congenital heart defects in children. In Tarhan S (ed): Cardiovascular Anesthesia and Postoperative Care. 2nd Ed. Year Book Medical Publishers, Chicago, 1989
17. Benacerraf BR, Adzick NS: Fetal diaphragmatic hernia—ultrasound diagnosis and clinical outcome in 19 cases. Am J Obstet Gynecol 156:573, 1987
18. Bray RJ: Congenital diaphragmatic hernia. Anaesthesia 34:567, 1979
19. Ein SH, Barker G, Olley P, et al: The pharmacologic treatment of newborn diaphragmatic hernia—a 2 year evaluation. J Pediatr Surg 15:384, 1980
20. Lilien LD, Pildes RS, Srinivasan G, et al: Treatment of neonatal hypoglycemia with minibolus and intravenous glucose infusion. J Pediatr 97:295, 1980
21. Daily WJR, Klaus M, Meyer HBP: Apnea in premature infants: monitoring, incidence, heart rate changes, and an effect of environmental temperature. Pediatrics 43:510, 1969
22. Davi MJ, Sankaran K, Simons KJ, et al: Physiologic changes induced by theophylline in the treatment of apnea in preterm infants. J Pediatr 92:91, 1972
23. Matthews TG, Warshaw JB: Relevance of the gestational

age distribution of meconium passage in utero. Pediatrics 64:30, 1979
24. Fenton AN, Steer CM: Fetal distress. Am J Obstet Gynecol 83:354, 1962
25. Walker J: Foetal anoxia. J Obstet Gynaecol Br Emp 61:162, 1954
26. Brown BL, Gleicher N: Intrauterine meconium aspiration. Obstet Gynecol 57:26, 1981
27. Ting P, Brady JP: Tracheal suction in meconium aspiration. Am J Obstet Gynecol 122:767, 1975
28. Fujikura T, Klionsky B: The significance of meconium staining. Am J Obstet Gynecol 121:45, 1975
29. Gregory GA, Gooding CA, Phibbs RH, et al. Meconium aspiration in infants—a prospective study. J Pediatr 85:848, 1974
30. Bacsik RD: Meconium aspiration syndrome. Pediatr Clin North Am 24:463, 1977
31. Yeh TF, Harris V, Srinivasan G, et al: Roentgenographic findings in infants with meconium aspiration syndrome. JAMA 242:60, 1979
32. Carson BS, Losey RW, Bowes WA Jr, et al: Combined obstetric and pediatric approach to prevent meconium aspiration syndrome. Am J Obstet Gynecol 126:712, 1976
33. Cohen-Addad N, Chatterjee M, Bautista A: Intrapartum suctioning of meconium: comparative efficacy of bulb syringe and DeLee catheter. J Perinatol 7:111, 1987
34. Topsis J, Kinas HY, Kandall SR: Esophageal perforation—a complication of neonatal resuscitation. Anesth Analg 69:532, 1989
35. Linder N, Aranda JV, Tsur M, et al: Need for endotracheal intubation and suction in meconium-stained neonates. J Pediatr 112:613, 1988
36. Davis RO, Philips JB III, Harris BA Jr, et al: Fatal meconium aspiration syndrome occurring despite airway management considered appropriate. Am J Obstet Gynecol 151:731, 1985
37. Scheife RT, Hills JR, Munsat TL: Myasthenia gravis—signs, symptoms, diagnosis, immunology, and current therapy. Pharmacotherapy 1:39, 1981
38. Seybold ME: Myasthenia gravis—a clinical and basic science review. JAMA 250:2516, 1983
39. Clarke WR: Anesthetic care of the infant with abnormal transitional circulation. Probl Anesth 2:477, 1988
40. Peckham GJ, Fox WW: Physiologic factors affecting pulmonary artery pressures in infants with persistent pulmonary hypertension. J Pediatr 93:1005, 1978
41. Physicians' Desk Reference. 44th Ed. Medical Economics, Oradell, NJ, 1990, p. 863
42. Enhorning G, Shennan A, Possmayer F, et al: Prevention of neonatal respiratory distress syndrome by tracheal instillation of surfactant: a randomized clinical trial. Pediatrics 76:145, 1985
43. Inselman LS: Respiratory distress syndrome. Pediatr Ann 7:243, 1978
44. Miller LK, Calenoff L, Boehm JJ, et al: Topics in radiology/diagnosis—respiratory distress in the newborn. JAMA 243:1176, 1980
45. Auld P, Hodson A, Usher R: Hyaline membrane disease—a discussion. J Pediatr 80:129, 1972
46. Kleinberg F: The management of respiratory distress syndrome. Chest 70:643, 1976
47. Driscoll DJ, Kleinberg F, Heise CT, et al: Cardiorespiratory function in asymptomatic survivors of neonatal respiratory distress syndrome. Mayo Clin Proc 62:695, 1987
48. Northway WH Jr: Observations on broncopulmonary dysplasia. J Pediatr 95:815, 1979
49. Ballard PL, Ballard RA: Glucocorticoids in prevention of respiratory distress syndrome. Hosp Pract 81, Sept. 1980
50. Collaborative Group on Antenatal Steroid Therapy: Effect of antenatal dexamethasone administration on the prevention of respiratory distress syndrome. Am J Obstet Gynecol 141:276, 1981
51. Morales WJ, Diebel ND, Lazar AJ, et al: The effect of antenatal dexamethasone administration on the prevention of respiratory distress syndrome in preterm gestations with premature rupture of membranes. Am J Obstet Gynecol 154:591, 1986
52. Ablow RC, Driscoll SG, Effmann EL, et al: A comparison of early-onset group B streptococcal neonatal infection and the respiratory distress syndrome of the newborn. N Engl J Med 294:65, 1976
53. Vollman JH, Smith WL, Ballard ET, et al: Early onset group B streptococcal disease: clinical, roentgenographic, and pathologic features. J Pediatr 89:199, 1976
54. Ramanathan R, Durand M, Larrazabal C: Pulse oximetry in very low birth weight infants with acute and chronic lung disease. Pediatrics 79:612, 1987
55. Ashcraft KW, Holder TM: Esophageal atresia and tracheoesophageal fistula malformations. Surg Clin North Am 56:299, 1976
56. Calverley RK, Johnston AE: The anaesthetic management of tracheo-oesophageal fistula: a review of ten years experience. Can Anaesth Soc J 19:270, 1972
57. Randolph JG: Esophageal atresia with tracheo-esophageal fistula—results at Children's Hospital, 1965–1981. Clin Proc CHNMC (Children's Hospital National Medical Center) 38:84, 1982
58. Koop CE, Schnaufer L, Broennie AM: Esophageal atresia and tracheoesophageal fistula—supportive measures that affect survival. Pediatrics 54:558, 1974
59. Avery ME, Gatewood OB, Brumley G: Transient tachypnea of newborn—possible delayed resorption of fluid at birth. Am J Dis Child 111:380, 1966

10 Special Considerations

EFFECT OF LUMBAR EPIDURAL ANESTHESIA ON THE PROGRESS OF LABOR AND THE INCIDENCE OF OPERATIVE DELIVERIES

Epidural anesthesia is currently a common technique of pain relief used during labor. In 1981, Gibbs et al.[1] surveyed approximately 1,200 U.S. hospitals about the type of analgesia used in obstetrics and found that 16 percent of women received epidural anesthesia during labor. The frequency of epidural anesthesia use depended on the size of the obstetric service. In hospitals reporting over 1,500 births, the epidural rate was 22 percent; in hospitals with 500 to 1,499 deliveries, the epidural rate was 13 percent; in hospitals with fewer than 500 deliveries, the rate was 9 percent. In 21 percent of the hospitals surveyed, epidural anesthesia for labor was not available.

In hospitals where epidural anesthesia is available, the frequency of epidural anesthesia administration is commonly between 20 and 80 percent. At the Mayo Clinic from 1986 to 1988, the epidural rate for all women who delivered (vaginal and cesarean) was 47 percent and for women who delivered vaginally was 43 percent.

With its widespread use, concern has been raised as to whether epidural anesthesia may lead to an increase in maternal and/or fetal morbidity or mortality. Several aspects must be considered in order to address this concern. Do the pharmacologic (direct drug effect) or physiologic effects (maternal blood pressure and uterine blood flow) of epidural anesthesia adversely affect the mother or fetus? (See the discussion of maternally administered drugs on the fetus and newborn in Ch. 3). Does the epidural anesthetic affect the mechanism of labor? Does the use of epidural anesthesia lead to more operative deliveries? If epidural anesthesia does affect labor or the mode of delivery, does this lead to an adverse maternal or fetal outcome?

This section reviews the available data as they relate to the effects of epidural anesthesia on the progress of labor and the incidence of operative deliveries. (Instrumental deliveries refer to vaginal deliveries in which obstetric forceps or vacuum extraction is employed, whereas operative deliveries include instrumental as well as cesarean deliveries.)

EFFECT OF LUMBAR EPIDURAL ANESTHESIA ON THE PROGRESS OF LABOR

The progress of labor is affected by several factors, including the frequency and strength of the uterine contractions, the size and position of the fetus, and the size and shape of the pelvis. Commonly, these are referred to as the "3 P's": Power, Passenger, and Pelvis. *If* epidural (peridural) anesthesia has an effect, perhaps one could refer to the 4 P's: Power, Passenger, Pelvis, and Peridural.

Forces in Labor

Two forces are involved in the progress of labor and both must be evaluated. The primary force is produced by the uterine muscle (involuntary) and the secondary force is produced by an increase in intra-abdominal pressure (voluntary).

The uterus is composed of smooth muscle and, like all smooth muscle, has the intrinsic capacity to contract and relax. This intrinsic activity may be modified by many factors. Estrogen, oxytocin, α-adrenergic drugs, prostaglandins, and mechanical manipulation of the cervix (e.g., by digitally stripping the membranes from the lower uterine segment or by the insertion of internal fetal monitors) stimulate uterine contractions. Progesterone, magnesium sulfate, calcium channel blockers (e.g., nifedipine), prostaglandin synthetase inhibitors (e.g., indomethacin), alcohol, aminophylline, and β-adrenergic drugs inhibit uterine contractions. In addition, a decrease in uterine blood flow that may occur with hypotension can decrease uterine contractions. This primary force is important in both the first and second stages of labor.

Intra-abdominal pressure can be increased by two sets of muscles, the abdominal wall muscles and the diaphragm. This secondary force is important during the second stage of labor.

First Stage of Labor

Effects of Epidural Anesthesia on Uterine Contractions. In 1961, Vasicka and Kretchmer[2] looked at the effects of regional anesthesia (23 subarachnoid anesthetics and 12 lidocaine epidural anesthetics) on uterine contractions. In the absence of hypotension, regional anesthesia did not interfere with uterine contractions. In some patients, the intensity of the contractions decreased about 10 to 20 mmHg for up to 30 minutes, then the intensity of the contractions resumed to preanesthetic levels. One patient developed hypotension, which was associated with a marked drop in uterine activity. They noted no inhibition of the effects of exogenously administered oxytocin. Whether this temporary inhibition of uterine contractility was an effect of the epidural anesthesia or the effect of the fluid bolus given at the start of epidural anesthesia is unclear.

In 1970, Sala et al.[3] saw no changes in spontaneous uterine contractions (Montevideo units) in five women in spontaneous labor when epidural anesthesia (lidocaine without epinephrine) was started. These women had previously received meperidine, promazine, and promethazine intravenously for analgesia. In addition, they did not see any changes in uterine contractions in the same women when artificial cervical dilatation was performed after the epidural anesthesia had been established.

In 1976, Raabe and Belfrage[4] noted a decrease in uterine contraction pressure but not frequency after the administration of epidural anesthesia using bupivacaine with epinephrine. The depression in pressures lasted about 30 minutes, and then the pressures resumed to preanesthetic levels.

Also in 1976, Matadial and Cibils[5] noted no significant changes in uterine activity when 1.0 to 1.5 percent lidocaine without epinephrine was administered epidurally (activity increased in 14 cases, decreased in 16 cases). However, when 1.0 to 1.5 percent lidocaine with epinephrine was used, a decrease in uterine activity was noted (activity increased in 12 cases, decreased in 39 cases). The decrease in activity was a decrease in pressure generated with no decrease in the frequency of the contractions.

In 1977, Schellenberg[6] failed to show a decrease in uterine activity with epidural 0.25 to 0.5 percent bupivacaine without epinephrine. He stressed the avoidance of aortocaval compression during labor when evaluating the effect of an epidural anesthetic on uterine activity; this was not consistently done in previous studies.

In 1977, Jouppila et al.[7] saw a mild increase in uterine activity when 0.5 percent bupivacaine was administered; when 0.5 percent bupivacaine with 1:200,000 epinephrine was administered, a mild fall in uterine activity was seen. All patients had left uterine displacement to avoid aortocaval compression. Although these changes were not significant when comparing the uterine activity before and after epidural administration within each group, the change in uterine activity between the two groups (bupivacaine without and bupivacaine with epinephrine) was significant. Clinically, this was reflected in longer induction-to-delivery times in the epinephrine group. They recommended avoiding the addition of epinephrine to the local anesthetic solutions used for epidural anesthesia during labor since it decreases uterine activity.

In several studies, Abboud et al. failed to see any significant changes in uterine activity after establishing epidural anesthesia with bupivacaine, lidocaine, or chloroprocaine without epinephrine,[8] lidocaine with epinephrine,[9] or bupivacaine with epinephrine.[10]

Clinical Studies on the Duration of the First Stage of Labor (see Table 10-1). In 1972, Crawford[11] reported shorter first stages of labor in multiparous women compared to primiparous women. This observation held true when spontaneous labors were compared to induced labors. He also demonstrated slightly shorter duration of the first stage of labor in primiparous women and a slightly longer duration of the first stage of labor in the multiparous women who received epidural anesthesia compared to those who did not. The local anesthetic was bupivacaine.

In 1979, Jouppila et al.[7] reported poor progress of labor prior to establishing epidural anesthesia in women who elected to have epidural anesthesia when compared to a control group. After the block was established, the subsequent course of labor was similar. This suggests that women with longer latent phases of labor are more likely to receive epidural anesthesia.

In 1980, Robinson et al.[12] reported similar durations of the first stage of labor for primiparous and multiparous women in their epidural group when compared respectively to primiparous and multiparous women in the control group. Women in the control group received meperidine and perphenazine intramuscularly and/or inhalational analgesia (50 percent nitrous oxide and 50 percent or 0.35 percent methoxyflurane).

In 1980, Studd et al.[13] noted that epidural anesthesia did not affect the rate of cervical dilatation in women with spontaneous labors or with labors augmented with oxytocin. However, the overall duration of the first stage of labor was longer in women who received epidural anesthesia compared to the control group. This may be explained by the fact that women who later received epidural anesthesia has less cervical dilatation on admission (2.7 cm for primiparas and 3.3 cm for multiparas) than women in the control group (3.8 cm for primiparas and 4.6 cm for multiparas). In women with augmented labors, the duration of labor was similar in the epidural and control groups.

Second Stage of Labor

Effects of Epidural Anesthesia on Voluntary Expulsive Forces. In 1972, Johnson et al.[14] looked at the effects of regional anesthesia on the intrauterine pressure developed during the second stage of labor. They found an increase in voluntary or "pushing" effort (pressure produced above the peak of a uterine contraction) as the second stage of labor progressed in women with no or local anesthesia. Women who received pudendal nerve blocks pushed better after the block was estab-

Table 10-1. Mean Duration of the First Stage of Labor (Hours)

	Primpara		Multipara	
	Epidural	No Epidural	Epidural	No Epidural
Crawford[11]				
Spontaneous labor	8.7	8.9	6.4	5.7
Induced labor	10.3	12.1	7.1	6.5
Joupilla et al.[7]				
Entire first stage	9.6	7.8	5.3	5.0
I-D interval[a]	3.5	3.7	2.1	2.3
Robinson et al.[12]	8.2	8.3	6.0	6.4
Studd et al.[13]				
Spontaneous labor	8.4	5.7	5.2	3.5
Augmented labor	12.4	11.9	9.2	10.0

[a] The I-D interval is the time interval from the induction of epidural anesthesia to delivery. For women without epidural anesthesia, an equivalent time from similar cervical dilation was used.

lished. With epidural anesthesia (1 percent lidocaine), a slight decrease in voluntary effort was noted overall (46 mmHg produced after the block compared to 55 mmHg before the block). A closer look demonstrated that one-third of patients pushed better after the epidural was started, and two-thirds pushed less effectively. When looking at the voluntary effort and the level of anesthesia produced, two-thirds of patients with an anesthetic level of T10 or lower pushed better, whereas all patients pushed less effectively when the level was T9 or higher.

Clinical Studies on the Duration of the Second Stage of Labor (See Table 10-2). In 1972, Crawford[11] reported longer durations of the second stage in primiparous women compared to multiparous women, and in women who received epidural anesthesia (0.25 and/or 0.5 percent bupivacaine) compared to those who did not. Because of the longer second stage of labor seen with epidural anesthesia, more instrumental deliveries were performed for a diagnosis of failure to progress or prolonged second stage.

In 1979, Bleyaert et al.[15] achieved short second stages with 0.125 percent bupivacaine with 1:800,000 epinephrine in 3,000 women (1,496 primiparas and 1,504 multiparas). The second stage lasted 21 minutes for primiparous and 14 minutes for multiparous women. Note that 61 percent of the primiparous and 27 percent of the multiparous women had instrumental deliveries.

In 1979, Jouppila et al.[7] looked at the duration of the second stage in women with or without epidural anesthesia in a prospective, nonrandomized study of 200 women (77 primiparas and 23 multiparous in the epidural group, and 77 primiparas and 23 multiparas in the control group). They used a low-dose epidural technique consisting of 4 ml of 0.5 percent bupivacaine per dose repeated as needed. In the control group, meperidine (50 to 150 mg) was administered intramuscularly for first stage analgesia in 58 percent of the primiparous and in 30 percent of the multiparous women. They did not find a significant difference in the duration of the second stage in women with or without epidural anesthesia.

In 1980, Robinson et al.[12] found a significant increase in the duration of the second stage of labor in patients receiving epidural anesthesia (0.5 percent bupivacaine) compared to their control group (meperidine with perphenazine and/or inhalational analgesia consisting of nitrous oxide or methoxyflurane).

In 1980, Studd et al.[13] also found a significant increase in the duration of the second stage of labor in women who had epidural anesthesia compared to those without. They observed this in women with spontaneous labors as well as in women whose labors were augmented with oxytocin.

Clinical Studies on the duration of the Second Stage of Labor. How long should the second stage be?

The first time limit placed on the duration of the second stage was made in 1817 by Denman.[16] "The use of forceps is not indicated until the second stage of labor has lasted six hours and all other means of delivery have been tried." In 1861, Hamilton recommended a shorter duration of the second stage, 2 hours.[16]

Table 10-2. Mean Duration of the Second Stage of Labor (Minutes)

	Primiparas		Multiparas	
	Epidural	No Epidural	Epidural	No Epidural
Crawford[11]				
Spontaneous labor	58	46	39	19
Induced labor	59	47	37	20
Bleyaert et al.[15]	21		14	
Joupilla et al.[7]	17	15	7	8
Robinson et al.[12]	54	42	30	18
Studd et al.[13]				
Spontaneous labor	64	44	46	18
Augmented labor	58	46	33	20

In 1952, Hellman and Prystowsky[16] looked at 13,377 deliveries performed for the years 1937 to 1949. For primiparous women, 40 percent delivered spontaneously, and 60 percent by forceps. For multiparous women 80 percent delivered spontaneously, and 20 percent by forceps. Overall, 77 percent delivered within 1 hour and 92 percent delivered within 2 hours. An increase in fetal mortality was noted when the second stage of labor was greater than 150 minutes. They also noted an increase in maternal postpartum hemorrhage and puerperal febrile reactions when the second stage of labor was greater than 150 minutes.

In 1974, Pearson and Davies,[17] looked at fetal acid-base values during the second stage of labor in a control group of 13 patients who received meperidine and/or promazine, and in two epidural groups, one group of eight women who pushed and a group of seven women who did not push during the second stage. They noted progressive fetal acidosis in all three groups. The fall in pH was fastest in the control group, less in the epidural group who pushed, and the least in the epidural group whose mothers did not push. All women labored in the supine position.

In 1977, Cohen[18] looked at 4,403 nulliparous women to determine the effects of the duration of the second stage of labor on neonatal outcome and maternal morbidity. He noted no increase in perinatal mortality or poor 5-minute Apgar scores with a progressive lengthening of the second stage. A significant increase in postpartum hemorrhage was noted after a second stage of 3 hours. This was thought to be related to the increase in midforceps and cesarean deliveries that were performed. If only normal spontaneous vaginal deliveries and low forceps were reviewed, no increase in hemorrhage was seen. He concluded, "It would thus appear that the elective termination of labor simply because an arbitrary period of time has elapsed in the second stage is clearly not warranted."

In 1983, Maresh and Choong[19] compared women who pushed early in the second stage with women who pushed late in the second stage. (A top-up dose of local anesthetic was administered if they had the urge to push early in the second stage). The top-up dose delayed the start of pushing by a mean of 96 minutes. In both groups, the women pushed for an average of 50 minutes. In the early pushing group, the spontaneous delivery rate was 35 percent, whereas in the late pushing group, the spontaneous delivery rate was 50 percent. There was no increase in abnormal fetal heart rate abnormalities and there was no decrease in umbilical cord pH or Apgar scores.

In 1990, Moon et al.[20] noted that neonates born after a prolonged second stage (at least 2 hours) did not have an increase in newborn acidosis —umbilical artery pH less than 7.20), or low 5-minute Apgar scores (< 7), nor did they need neonatal intensive care unit admission more often when compared to neonates born after a normal second stage (less than 2 hours).

The American College of Obstetrics and Gynecology (ACOG)[21] recently revised the guideline for the approximate duration of the second stage of labor. For the nulliparous woman, the diagnosis of a prolonged second stage is made when more than 3 hours with a regional anesthetic or more than 2 hours without a regional anesthetic has elapsed. For the parous women, more than 2 hours with a regional anesthetic or more than 1 hour without a regional anesthetic is considered a prolonged second stage.

Although a time limit can be a helpful guideline, it remains that: a guideline. With the current technology available for monitoring the fetus and the mother, assessment on a case-by-case basis can allow continuation of the second stage unless intervention is indicated.

Conclusions

There is a wide variation in the reported duration of the first and second stages of labor. The optimal duration of the second stage of labor is still controversial. However, in most of the studies describing the duration of the second stage, neonates have been delivered well within the ACOG guidelines.

In the very early stages of labor (latent phase), any analgesic may slow labor; confounding conclusions could be drawn regarding the length of the first stage if studies include patients who have received epidural anesthesia in the latent phase. Most recent studies reviewing the effects of epidural anesthesia on the duration of the first stage of labor or the rate of cervical dilation look primarily at the active phase of the first stage of labor.

Epidural anesthesia appears to have little effect on the rate of cervical dilation or the duration of the first stage of labor (active phase). If hypotension is avoided, epidural anesthesia has minimal effect on uterine contractions. In several studies, a short term (< 30 to 60 minutes) and probably insignificant depression in uterine intensity develops mainly when epinephrine-containing local anesthetics are used. Perhaps a slight β-adrenergic effect of absorbed epinephrine causes this observed decrease. After 30 minutes, uterine activity returns to normal.

The second stage of labor may be prolonged in women who have epidural anesthesia compared to women who do not receive epidural anesthesia. Several reasons for the longer second stage of labor in women who receive epidural anesthesia have been suggested, including loss of the bearing-down reflex (urge to push), and the generation of lower intra-abdominal pressures with expulsive efforts (too weak to push, too exhausted from a long labor to push). How the patient is managed may have an effect of the duration of the second stage. The level and density of anesthesia can be adjusted to allow better sensations and better expulsive efforts. Appropriate coaching on the timing, direction, and duration of the "pushing" efforts is important.

EFFECT ON THE INCIDENCE OF OPERATIVE DELIVERIES

Controversy abounds regarding the question, "Does epidural anesthesia given during labor have an effect on the incidence of operative deliveries (forceps deliveries, vacuum extractions, or cesarean deliveries)?"

This section reviews the concerns surrounding the performance of operative deliveries, the studies that look at the association of epidural anesthesia with the frequency of operative deliveries, observations that support as well as observations that oppose the view that epidural anesthesia increases the incidence of operative deliveries, factors associated with the performance of operative deliveries, and ways to achieve a low incidence of operative deliveries.

Concerns about Operative Deliveries

Cesarean Delivery. Cesarean delivery has been associated with a two- to fourfold increase in maternal mortality when compared to vaginal deliveries.[22–24] The incidence of maternal mortality for women delivered by cesarean delivery ranges from 1 per 2,500[25] to none reported in 10,231 consecutive deliveries.[26] Approximately half of the maternal deaths associated with cesarean delivery are attributed to the operative procedure and the rest attributed to the obstetric complications leading to the cesarean delivery.[22]

Cesarean delivery has a greater frequency of maternal morbidity than vaginal delivery. The incidence ranges from 10 to 80 percent! In 1981, Amirikia et al.[27] reviewed 9,718 patients who underwent cesarean delivery. They reported a maternal morbidity of 28 percent, with endometritis, urinary tract infection, anemia, wound infections, and fever being the five most common etiologies. In 1976, Jones[28] reported an overall maternal morbidity of 49 percent, with significant morbidity in 12 percent of 2,563 patients delivered by cesarean delivery.

Though infrequent, neonatal complications due to cesarean delivery can occur. These include traumatic delivery, blood loss (e.g., cutting through the placenta), and iatrogenic prematurity.[22]

Instrumental Deliveries. Over the course of the past several decades, the trends and theories behind the use of forceps, and later vacuum extractors, have varied. Initially, they were instruments of last resort, used to achieve delivery when all other means had been exhausted. Later, maternal exhaustion and a prolonged second stage (≥ 2 hours) became indications for intervention.

In 1920, Delee[29] promoted the concept of "prophylactic forceps operations" to shorten painful labors, to help preserve the integrity of the birth canal, and to decrease the stress of labor and delivery on the fetus. Since that time, concerns about the safety of forceps deliveries have led to several conflicting reports.[30–35]

In 1973, Niswander and Gordon[33] reviewed the neonatal outcome in a collaborative project of nearly 30,000 neonates. They looked at several neonatal factors, including the neonatal death rate, 1- and 5-minute Apgar scores, Bayley Scales of Mental and Motor Development at 8 months of age, and the Stanford-Binet Intelligence Quotient at 4 years of age. They found the "prophylactic forceps operation" to be a safe method of delivery. It did not increase the chance of neonatal death or neurologic impairment of the neonate. "Whether the operation is 'protective' to the infant is less certain, although the data suggest this possibility."[33]

In 1983, Richardson et al.[35] did an extensive review of the literature concerning the safety of midforceps delivery. They believed that "the bulk of evidence suggests that it [midforceps] can be a useful and safe tool in the armamentarium of the obstetrician, *when properly indicated and skillfully applied.*"

In 1984, Friedman et al.[31] looked at the effects of midforceps and low-forceps deliveries on 7-year intelligence quotient data (Stanford-Binet Intelligence Scale) with matched controls. Outcome for low-forceps cases were similar to the controls. However, midforceps delivery cases were associated with nearly a 6-point reduction in scores compared to the control cases. They concluded, "unless one can provide justification in the form of documentable benefit on a case-by-case basis to counterbalance the potential risk, midforceps procedures should no longer be done."

In 1984, Gilstrap et al.[32] studied 704 women who underwent forceps delivery compared to 303 spontaneous vaginal deliveries and 111 cesarean deliveries. No significant differences in acidosis were seen in infants delivered by low forceps, midforceps or cesarean delivery when performed for similar reasons. Significantly more neonates delivered by cesarean delivery had Apgar scores ≤ 6 at 1 and 5 minutes. Infants delivered spontaneously compared to those delivered by low forceps had no significant difference in acidosis or low Apgar scores. Vaginal wall lacerations and lower postdelivery hematocrits were more common with midforceps than low-forceps delivery.

In 1986, Dierker et al.[30] compared neurologic outcome of 110 infants delivered by midforceps with a matched group of 110 infants delivered by cesarean delivery at 2 years of age or older unless death occurred earlier. Their match included the indication for operative delivery (dystocia or fetal distress), something not consistently done in previous studies, as well as birthweight, gestational age, sex, and race. They found no difference in abnormal neurologic outcomes between the two groups.

Even in the absence of physical morbidity to the mother or neonate, emotional and psychological trauma in the mother can occur. As stated by Morgan et al.[36], "The mother's satisfaction with her experience of childbirth is lessened in forceps delivery even when it is not traumatic."

Outlet and low-forceps deliveries as well as vacuum deliveries are considered by most to be relatively safe modes of delivery. Although the safety of midforceps deliveries is controversial, most studies[30,32,35] support the judicious use of midforceps deliveries in select circumstances by skilled operators.

Epidural Anesthesia and Operative Deliveries

When one looks at studies (Tables 10-3 and 10-4) that report the incidence of operative deliveries in women with and without epidural anesthesia, three trends are noted.

First, there is a large difference between studies in the incidence of operative deliveries in women who have received epidural anesthesia (6 percent to 93 percent).

Second, in most studies, women who received epidural anesthesia have about a 2 to 10 times greater frequency of operative deliveries when compared to women who deliver without epidural anesthesia.

Third, primiparous women have a higher frequency of operative deliveries compared to multiparous women in both the epidural groups and in the control groups. This is important since more primiparous women receive epidural anesthesia than multiparous women, making studies that do not differentiate the primiparous from the multiparous patients more difficult to interpret.

Does epidural anesthesia directly cause an increase in operative deliveries? Are there other factors that result in operative deliveries that are also associated with an increased use of epidural anesthesia? If so, this may lead to the erroneous conclusion that it is the epidural anesthetic causing the increased rate of operative delivery.

Observations Supporting the View that Epidural Anesthesia Increases the Incidence of Operative Deliveries

Many women who have epidural anesthesia do not push effectively. This may be due to the inability to feel the contractions, the loss of the urge to "push" or the bearing-down reflex, not knowing when, how long, or in what direction to focus the "pushing efforts." Some women are too weak to push (muscle weakness from the local anesthetic) or are too exhausted to push. These factors can lead to a prolonged second stage, which may

Table 10-3. Frequency of Operative Deliveries (%): Retrospective and Prospective Nonrandomized Studies

Author	Primipara		Multipara		All	
	Epidural	No Epidural	Epidural	No Epidural	Epidural	No Epidural
Vaginal and Cesarean Deliveries						
Duthie et al. (1968)[37]					93	
DeVere (1969)[38]					91	
Browne & Catton (1971)[39]					90	
Brown & Vass (1977)[40]	75		40		70	
Graffagnino & Seyler (1938)[41]					68	
Brownridge 91982)[42]					65	
Thorburn & Moir (1981)[43]					58	14
Crawford (1972)[44]	70		27		55	
Studd (1980)[13]	64	23	32	7	53	14
Raabe & Belfrage (1976)[45]	48		16		44	
Rudick et al. (1983)[46]					33	
Abboud et al. (1984)[8]					31	
Matouskova et al. (1975)[47]					19	15
Hanson & Hanson (1985)[48]					19	
Maltau & Andersen (1975)[49]	22		7		17	
Hollmen et al. (1977)[50]	15		6		12	
Jouppila et al. (1977)[51]					11	
Vaginal Deliveries Only						
Mastroianni et al. (1956)[52]					65	
Hoult et al. (1977)[53]	71	22	42	6	58	11
Kaminski et al. (1987)[54]	52	23	43	7	50	20
Morgan et al. (1980)[36]	55		35		47	
Bleyaert et al. (1979)[15]	61		27		44	
Walton & Reynolds (1984)[55]	52	14	26	2	43	6
Doughty (1969)[56]	51	42	17	16	33	26
Chestnut et al. (1990)[57]	18				18	
Jouppila let al. (1979)[7]	8	3	0	0	6	2

be considered an indication for an instrumental or operative delivery.

Patients with epidural anesthesia are comfortable and have better perineal and pelvic relaxation; they will tolerate an operative delivery better than patients without such anesthesia. Instrumental deliveries are then easier to perform or to teach, and may increase the likelihood of an instrumental delivery.

Epidural anesthesia may increase the frequency of fetal malpresentations (e.g., occiput posterior) because of relaxation of the muscles of the pelvic sling.

Hoult et al.[53] in a prospective nonrandomized study reported a more than threefold increase in fetal malpresentations in women who received mainly 0.5 percent bupivacaine epidural anesthesia (21 percent) compared to a control group (6 percent). The incidence of malpresentations was not affected by the timing of induction of anesthesia (less than or greater than 4 cm cervical dilation).

Kaminski et al.[54] reported a 27 percent incidence of occiput posterior (OP) presentation in the epidural group and 8 percent in the control group. Raabe et al.[45] reported a 9 percent incidence of OP presentation in the epidural group. Their control group had a 3 percent

Table 10-4. Frequency of Operative Deliveries (%): Prospective Randomized Studies

Author	Primipara		Multipara		All	
	Epidural	No Epidural	Epidural	No Epidural	Epidural	No Epidural
Vaginal and Cesarean Deliveries						
Robinson et al. (1980)[12]	61	27	30	6	49	19
Philipsen & Jensen (1989)[58]					42	37
Noble et al. (1971)[59]					31	9

incidence of OP presentations. Both groups of investigators thought that the increase in OP presentations in the epidural group could be related to either (1) pelvic floor relaxation, or (2) selection bias (e.g., more patients with OP presentations request epidural anesthesia because of more painful and longer labors).

Studd et al.[13] reported a 20-fold increase in rotational forceps deliveries, but no increase in cesarean delivery in women who received epidural anesthesia compared to their control group.

This increase in malpresentation was not seen in the studies by Jouppila et al.[7] or by Maltau and Anderson[49] and Matouskova et al.[47] who stressed lower doses of local anesthetics.

Some prospective randomized studies seem to indicate an increase in the incidence of instrumental deliveries in patients with epidural anesthesia.

In 1971, Nobel et al.[59] looked at the incidence of instrumental deliveries in women with and without epidural anesthesia. They initially had 245 patients in the study but deleted 43 patients (18 percent). Most of the deleted patients in the epidural group delivered before the epidural anesthetic could be performed, whereas most of the patients in the nonepidural group were deleted because inadequate analgesia was obtained, leading to the request for epidural anesthesia. In the remaining 202 patients (100 with epidurals, 102 controls), 30 forceps deliveries occurred in the epidural group and only six in the control group. There was also one cesarean delivery in the epidural group and three in the control group. Although they showed a higher incidence of operative deliveries in the epidural group, they noted better neonatal outcome in the epidural group as noted by the Apgar scores and the umbilical cord artery blood pH.

In 1980, Robinson et al.[12] noted an increase in instrumental deliveries in their epidural group compared to their control group (meperidine and inhalational analgesia). This was significant only for the primiparous patients, in which the epidural group had two times the number of instrumental deliveries. They deleted a large number of patients because they did not complete the interview process, the clinical considerations dictated a deviation of analgesic plan, or labor was too advanced when they were admitted.

Observations Opposing the View That Epidural Anesthesia Increases the Incidence of Operative Deliveries

Some women experience severe pelvic and perineal pain and cannot push effectively. Establishing epidural anesthesia can allow the patient to push more effectively and shorten the second stage of labor.

The likelihood may be greater when an epidural anesthetic is placed in women who are having an abnormally prolonged and painful labor than in those who are experiencing a normal labor. In these cases, the epidural anesthetic will allow the mother to rest free of pain, allowing time for further progression of labor and culminating in a vaginal delivery. In these cases, an instrumental delivery may be implemented to end the long and exhausting labor, not because of a direct effect of the epidural anesthetic.[60–62]

Epidural anesthesia may be placed more often in women who are destined to have an operative delivery as a result of other factors, whether or not an epidural anesthetic is used. This question may be looked at indirectly in two ways.

In 1969, Doughty[56] reported a decrease in the incidence of operative deliveries over a time span of 13 years as the frequency of epidural anesthesia increased. They suspected the epidurals were initially placed in patients with difficult or abnormal labors, but as time continued, epidurals were being placed in more women with normal labors. Note the trend of decreasing instrumental deliveries (100 to 24 percent) as the frequency of epidural anesthesia increased from 2 to 82 percent over the three time periods (1957 to 1962; 1963 to 1965; 1966 to 1969) (see Table 10-5).

In 1983, Bailey and Howard[63] looked at the effect of starting an epidural service on the incidence of operative deliveries. The first 2 years of their study were before epidural anesthesia was available and served as their control. The following 3 years were after epidural anesthesia was introduced. They reported a very small increase in the incidence of instrumental deliveries (14 to 15 percent) and cesarean deliveries (7 to 9 percent) despite a dramatic increase in the incidence of epidural anesthesia performed (0 to 43 percent) (see Table 10-6).

In 1983, Rudick et al.[46] did a similar study over a 2-

Table 10-5. Frequency of Operative Vaginal Deliveries under Epidural Anesthesia over Several Years

Years	% Epidurals[a]	% Instrumental Deliveries: Primipara	Multipara	All
1957–1962	2	100	100	100
1963–1965	37	87	56	75
1966–1969	82	42	11	24
All years (1957–1969)	52	51	17	33

[a] Percentage of all vaginal deliveries under epidural anesthesia.

(From Doughty,[56] with permission.)

Table 10-6. Frequency of Obstetric Deliveries (%) for 2 Years before and 3 Years after an Epidural Anesthesia Service Became Established

	Before		After		
	1976	1977	1978	1979	1980
All patients					
NSVD	74	74	69	71	71
Instrumental	14	14	17	15	15
Cesarean	8	7	9	9	9
Epidural rate	—	—	27	37	43
Primipara					
NSVD	63	63	54	56	58
Instrumental	24	24	29	28	27
Cesarean	7	8	11	9	10
Epidural rate	—	—	49	67	72
Multipara					
NSVD	81	81	77	78	79
Instrumental	8	8	10	8	9
Cesarean	8	7	8	9	7
Epidural rate	—	—	14	21	26

NSVD, normal spontaneous vaginal delivery.
Note: Breech and twin deliveries were excluded.
(From Bailey and Howard,[63] with permission.)

year period. They noted a slight increase in instrumental deliveries (9 to 11 percent) when the epidural anesthesia rate rose from 0.1 to 37 percent.

A prospective randomized study suggests no effect of epidural anesthesia on the incidence of instrumental deliveries.

In 1989, Philipsen and Jensen[58] compared epidural anesthesia with meperidine analgesia during labor. They found no significant difference between the groups with respect to the duration of the first stage or second stage of labor or the incidence of instrumental deliveries. Epidural analgesia did provide better pain relief than meperidine.

Factors Associated with the Selection of Operative Deliveries

As mentioned previously, the trends in the use of forceps have varied over the past decades. In 1968, in a study by Duthie et al.,[37] the instrumental rate was 93 percent for vaginal deliveries; it would have been 100 percent but a few women requested delivery without forceps. As cesarean delivery became safer, as the use of "prophylactic forceps" fell out of favor and with the development of the silastic vacuum cup, forceps deliveries are currently performed less often.

In 1990, Notzon[34] looked at the rate of operative cesarean deliveries (21 countries) and operative vaginal deliveries (14 countries) for the years 1975 through 1986. The cesarean rates varied from 7 to 32 percent and for operative vaginal deliveries, from 2 to 16 percent. For most countries that reported both cesarean and operative vaginal rates, cesarean delivery rates rose as operative vaginal delivery rates fell.

Thus, studies done on the incidence of instrumental deliveries may be affected by the "trend of the times."

Some physicians tend to perform instrumental deliveries more often than others.[64] At the Mayo Clinic for the years 1987 and 1988, the incidence of instrumental vaginal deliveries was 15 percent for all deliveries. When uncomplicated primiparous patients who delivered vaginally at the Mayo Clinic were reviewed, the incidence of instrumental deliveries for women was 21 percent for the family physicians and 33 percent for the obstetricians. Furthermore, incidence of instrumental deliveries for the obstetricians ranged from 20 to 74 percent! The training and skill of the individual may influence the frequency with which instruments will be used.

Unresolved fetal distress is an indication for prompt delivery. If the second stage of labor has been achieved and the fetal presentation is favorable, an instrumental vaginal delivery may be attempted.

In women with a prolonged second stage, ineffective pushing, or "maternal exhaustion," an instrumental delivery can end the long labor.

Although not commonly admitted, an instrumental delivery may be performed as a matter of convenience to shorten the stay of the physician at the obstetric suite.

Academic programs usually involve resident training. It is easier to teach proper instrument placement and maintain patient satisfaction when patients are comfortable (i.e., have epidural anesthesia).

Achieving a Lower Incidence of Operative Deliveries

1. Use operative deliveries only when obstetrically indicated and not when obstetrically convenient or for teaching purposes.
2. Allow the second stage to be longer.

   In many of the studies in this section a short second stage was decreased further by use of instruments. The ACOG guidelines[21] reflect a view allowing the second stage to be longer. (See the section on duration of the second stage.)
3. Adjust the epidural block to allow a greater chance for a spontaneous delivery.
   a) Decrease the density of the epidural block (by using a lower concentration and/or smaller volumes of local anesthetic) to allow mild sensation of contractions or perineal pressure. This may allow the parturient to retain the urge to push

and may increase the efficacy of the expulsive efforts.

Crawford[11] noted that about 50 percent of patients who delivered spontaneously under epidural anesthesia lost the urge to push, whereas about 70 percent of patients who had instrumental deliveries lost the urge to push. He also noted the concentration of bupivacaine made a difference. When 0.25 percent bupivacaine was used, 50 percent of women lost the urge to push, whereas 75 percent of women lost the urge to push when 0.5 percent bupivacaine was used.[44]

Thorburn and Moir[43] compared 0.5 percent bupivacaine (group A, 6 to 8 ml/dose) with 0.25 percent bupivacaine (group B, 10 to 14 ml/dose; group C, 6 to 8 ml/dose). They noted a higher frequency of spontaneous deliveries when a lower concentration or smaller volume was used; group A had 32 percent, group B had 39 percent, and group C had 53 percent spontaneous deliveries. They also noted less motor block and less sensory anesthesia in group C as well.

Some investigators use a low concentration of local anesthetics to retain the urge to push in the parturient, whereas others use a low volume of a high concentration (i.e., 0.5 percent bupivacaine), producing a more segmental block.[50]

Although the concentration of local anesthetic may be important, other factors such as total dose may also be important. Jouppila et al.[7] achieved a 6 percent instrumental rate with 0.5 percent bupivacaine (4 ml/dose), whereas Bleyaert et al[15] had a 44 percent instrumental rate with 0.125 percent bupivacaine (10 ml/dose).

It has been suggested the epidural anesthetic should be turned off during the second stage so that the parturient can push better. Theoretically this is because the parturient is either too weak to push or too comfortable (and thus not motivated) to push. However, the data in Table 10-7 do not consistently support this approach.

A better approach would be to individualize the epidural block. If the patient is comfortable and pushing well, maintain the epidural block at its current level. For some women, if it hurts to push, they will not push effectively. Thus, anesthesia should be maintained. For others, mild sensation will increase the effectiveness of their expulsive efforts, in which case the epidural block may be adjusted to allow some return of sensation.

b) High concentrations and large volumes of some local anesthetics may cause muscle weakness. If this is the problem, a local anesthetic with a good differential blockade such as bupivacaine at a low concentration (0.125 percent or less) may be tried. If pain relief is not sufficient, the addition of an epidural narcotic, such as fentanyl, may help as this produces no motor blockade.

c) Consider using a lower concentration of local anesthetic (such as 0.25 percent bupivacaine or 1 percent lidocaine or lower concentrations) for sensory anesthesia during the first stage of labor. This may decrease the incidence of abnormal fetal presentations.[47,49]

If the fetus is in the OP position, consider the use of epidural anesthesia with a higher concentration of local anesthetic (such as 0.5 percent bupivacaine or 2 percent lidocaine); this may relax the pelvic floor and allow spontaneous rotation during the first stage or can enable the physician to more easily turn the fetus to an occiput anterior position in the second stage of labor. Less trauma may result to the mother and the fetus.[38,52] The approach of making the block more dense should be fully discussed with the obstetrician or family physician prior to its use.

d) Perhaps the choice of local anesthetic makes a

Table 10-7. Letting the Epidural Wear Off: Frequency of Instrumental Deliveries (%)

	Epidural Wear Off	Epidural Continued	Significance
Phillips & Thomas (1983)[65] Bupivacaine, intermittent	43	25	N.S.
Chestnut et al. (1987)[66] 0.75% Lidocaine, continuous	35	31	N.S.
Chestnut et al. (1987)[67] 0.125% Bupivacaine, continuous	28	53	$P < 0.05$
Chestnut et al. (1990)[57] 0.0625% Bupivacaine + 0.0002% fentanyl, continuous	15	21	N.S.

N.S., not significant.

Table 10-8. Continuous Infusion Epidural Anesthesia; Three Different Local Anesthetics

	Group I: Bupivacaine (23 Pts.)	Group II: Chloroprocaine (19 Pts.)	Group III: Lidocaine (19 Pts.)
First stage	286 min.	301 min.	390 min.
Second stage	171 min.	113 min.	67 min.
NSVD	10 (43%)	16 (84%)	16 (84%)
Forceps & vacuum delivery[a]	6 (26%)	1 (5%)	2 (11%)
Cesarean	7 (30%)	2 (11%)	1 (5%)

[a] Only one of the cesarean deliveries was for fetal distress.
(From Abboud et al.,[8] with permission.)

difference. Abboud et al.[8] reported a higher rate of instrumental deliveries with bupivacaine compared to lidocaine and chloroprocaine (see Table 10-8). Further work in this area is needed.

e) Over the past few years, the continuous infusion of local anesthetic into the epidural space has become widely used. The level of anesthesia is better maintained than with the bolus-injection technique. Once the level of anesthesia is established, fine tuning of the epidural block is possible during the entire labor.

4. In some cases, the patient is exhausted from her long labor. Permitting her to rest before pushing may be helpful.
5. The assistance of a good labor coach can overcome the parturient's lack of sensation by directing the timing and direction of the expulsive efforts.[52]

REFERENCES

1. Gibbs CP, Krischer J, Peckham BM, et al: Obstetric anesthesia—a national survey. Anesthesiology 65:298, 1986
2. Vasicka A, Kretchmer H: Effect of conduction and inhalation anesthesia on uterine contractions. Experimental study of the influence of anesthesia on intra-amniotic pressures. Am J Obstet Gynecol 82:600, 1961
3. Sala NL, Schwarcz RL Jr, Althabe O Jr, et al: Effect of epidural anesthesia upon uterine contracility induced by artificial cervical dilatation in human pregnancy. Am J Obstet Gynecol 106:26, 1970
4. Raabe N, Belfrage P: Epidural analgesia in labour. IV. Influence on uterine activity and fetal heart rate. Acta Obstet Gynecol Scand 55:305, 1976
5. Matadial L, Cibils LA: The effect of epidural anesthesia on uterine activity and blood pressure. Am J Obstet Gynecol 125: 846, 1976
6. Schellenberg JC: Uterine activity during lumbar epidural analgesia with bupivacaine. Am J Obstet Gynecol 127:26, 1977
7. Jouppila R, Jouppila P, Karinen JM, Hollmen A: Segmental epidural analgesia in labour—related to the progress of labour, fetal malposition and instrumental delivery. Acta Obstet Gynecol Scand 58:135, 1979
8. Abboud TK, Afrasiabi A, Sarkis F, et al: Continuous infusion epidural analgesia in parturients receiving bupivacaine, chloroprocaine, or lidocaine—maternal, fetal, and neonatal effects. Anesth Analg 63:421, 1984
9. Abboud TK, David S, Nagappala S, et al: Maternal, fetal, and neonatal effects of lidocaine with and without epinephrine for epidural anesthesia in obstetrics. Anesth Analg 63:973, 1984
10. Abboud TK, Sheik-ol-Eslam A, Yanagi T, et al: Safety and efficacy of epinephrine needed to bupivacaine for lumbar epidural analgesia in obstetrics. Anesth Analg 64:585, 1985
11. Crawford JS: The second thousand epidural blocks in an obstetric hospital practice. Br J Anaesth 44:1277, 1972
12. Robinson JO, Rosen M, Evans JM, et al: Maternal opinion about analgesia for labour—a controlled trial between epidural block and intramuscular pethidine combined with inhalation. Anaesthesia 35:1173, 1980
13. Studd JWW, Crawford JS, Duignan NM, et al: The effect of lumbar epidural analgesia on the rate of cervical dilatation and the outcome of labour of spontaneous onset. Br J Obstet Gynaecol 87:1015, 1980
14. Johnson WL, Winter WW, Eng M, et al: Effect of pudendal, spinal, and peridural block anesthesia on the second stage of labor. Am J Obstet Gynecol 113:166, 1972
15. Bleyaert A, Soetens M, Vaes L, et al: Bupivacaine, 0.125 per cent, in obstetric epidural analgesia—experience in three thousand cases. Anesthesiology 51:435, 1979
16. Hellman LM, Prystowsky H: The duration of the second stage of labor. Am J Obstet Gynecol 63:1223, 1952
17. Pearson JF, Davies P: The effect of continuous lumbar epidural analgesia upon fetal acid-base status during the second stage of labour. J Obstet Gynaecol Br Common 81:975, 1974
18. Cohen WR: Influence of the duration of second stage labor on perinatal outcome and puerperal morbidity. Obstet Gynecol 49:266, 1977
19. Maresh M, Choong KH: Delayed pushing with lumbar epidural analgesia in labour. Br J Obstet Gynaecol 90:623, 1983

20. Moon JM, Smith CV, Rayburn WF: Perinatal outcome after a prolonged second stage of labor. J Reprod Med 35:229, 1990
21. American College Obstetricians Gynecologists Committee Opinion: Obstetric forceps. No. 71:1 August 1989
22. Hibbard LT: Cesarean section and other surgical procedures. Ch. 17. p. 518. In Gabbe SG, Niebyl JR, Simpson JL (eds): Obstetrics: Normal and Problem Pregnancies. Churchill Livingstone, New York, 1986
23. NIH—The cesarean birth task force: NIH consensus development statement on cesarean childbirth. Obstet Gynecol 57:537, 1981
24. Zuspan FP, Quilligan EJ: Cesarean childbirth. Ch. 16. p. 483. In Zuspan FP, Quilligan EJ (Eds): Douglas–Stromme Operative Obstetrics. 5th Ed. Appleton & Lange, East Norwalk, CT, 1988
25. Sachs BJ, Brown DAJ, Driscoll SG, et al: Maternal mortality in Massachusetts: trends and prevention. N Engl J Med 316:667, 1987
26. Frigoletto FD Jr, Ryan KJ, Phillippe M: Maternal mortality rate associated with cesarean section: an appraisal. Am J Obstet Gynecol 136:969, 1986
27. Amirikia H, Zarewych B, Evans TN: Cesarean section: a 15-year review of changing incidence, indications and risks. Am J Obstet Gynecol 140:81, 1981
28. Jones OH: Cesarean section in present-day obstetrics: presidential address. Am J Obstet Gynecol 521, 1976
29. DeLee JB: The prophylactic forceps operation. Am J Obstet Gynecol 1:34, 1920
30. Dierker Jr LJ, Rosen MG, Thompson K, Lynn P: Midforceps deliveries: long-term outcome of infants. Am J Obstet Gynecol 154:764, 1986
31. Friedman EA, Sachtleben-Murray MR, Dahrouge D, Neff RK: Long-term effects of labor and delivery on offspring: a matched-pair analysis. Am J Obstet Gynecol 150:941, 1984
32. Gilstrap LC III, Hauth JC, Schiano S, Connor KD: Neonatal acidosis and method of delivery. Obstet Gynecol 63:681, 1984
33. Niswander KR, Gordon M: Safety of the low-forceps operation. Am J Obstet Gynecol 117:619, 1973
34. Notzon FC: International differences in the use of obstetric interventions. JAMA 263:3286, 1990
35. Richardson DA, Evans MI, Cibils LA: Midforceps delivery—a critical review. Am J Obstet Gynecol 145:621, 1983
36. Morgan BM, Rehor S, Lewis PJ: Epidural analgesia for uneventful labour. Anaesthesia 35:57, 1980
37. Duthie AM, Wyman JB, Lewis GA: Bupivacaine in labour—its use in lumbar extradural analgesia. Anaesthesia 23:20, 1968
38. DeVere RD: Epidural analgesia. Proc R Soc Med 62:186, 1969
39. Browne RA, Catton DV: The use of bupivacaine in labour. Can Anaesth Soc J 18:23, 1971
40. Brown SE, Vass ACR: An extradural service in a district general hospital. Br J Anaesth 49:243, 1977
41. Graffagnino P, Seyler LW: Epidural anesthesia in obstetrics. Am J Obstet Gynecol 35:597, 1938
42. Brownridge P: A three year survey of an obstetric epidural service with top-up doses administered by midwives. Anaesth Intens Care 10:298, 1982
43. Thorburn J, Moir DD: Extradural analgesia—the influence of volume and concentration of bupivacaine on the mode of delivery, analgesic efficacy and motor block. Br J Anaesth 53:933, 1981
44. Crawford JS: Lumbar epidural block in labour—a clinical analysis. Br J Anaesth 44:66, 1972
45. Raabe N, Belfrage P: Lumbar epidural analgesia in labour—a clinical analysis. Acta Obstet Gynecol Scand 55:125, 1976
46. Rudick V, Niv D, Golan A, et al: Epidural analgesia during labor in 1,200 monitored parturients. Isr J Med Sci 19:20, 1983
47. Matouskova A, Dottori O, Forssman L, Victorin L: An improved method of epidural analgesia with reduced instrumental delivery rate. Acta Obstet Gynecol Scand 54:231, 1975
48. Hanson AL, Hanson B: Continuous mini-infusion of bupivacaine into the epidural space during labor—experience from 1000 deliveries. Reg Anesth 10:139, 1985
49. Maltau JM, Andersen HT: Continuous epidural anaesthesia with a low frequency of instrumental deliveries. Acta Obstet Gynecol Scand 54:401, 1975
50. Hollmen A, Jouppila R, Pihlajaniemi R, et al: Selective lumbar epidural block in labour. A clinical analysis. Acta Anaesth Scand 21:174, 1977
51. Jouppila P, Jouppila R, Kaar K, Merila M: Fetal heart rate patterns and uterine activity after segmental epidural analgesia. Br J Obstet Gynaecol 84:481, 1977
52. Mastroianni L Jr, Kelly JV, Lavietes S, Carbone P: The use of continuous epidural combined with continuous caudal anesthesia for labor and delivery. Am J Obstet Gynecol 71:300, 1956
53. Hoult IJ, MacLennan AH, Carrie LES: Lumbar epidural analgesia in labour—relation to fetal malposition and instrumental delivery. Br Med J 1:14, 1977
54. Kaminski HM, Stafl A, Aiman J: The effect of epidural analgesia on the frequency of instrumental obstetric delivery. Obstet Gynecol 69:770, 1987
55. Walton P, Reynolds F: Epidural analgesia and instrumental delivery. Anaesthesia 39:218, 1984
56. Doughty A: Selective epidural analgesia and the forceps rate. Br J Anaesth 41:1058, 1969
57. Chestnut DH, Laszewski LJ, Pollack KL, et al: Continuous epidural infusion of 0.0625% bupivacaine—0.0002% fentanyl during the second stage of labor. Anesthesiology 72:613, 1990
58. Philipsen T, Jensen N-H: Epidural block or parenteral pethidine as analgesic in labour; a randomized study concerning progress in labour and instrumental deliveries. Eur J Obstet Gynecol Reprod Biol 30:27, 1989
59. Noble AD, Craft IL, Bootes JAH, et al: Continuous lumbar epidural analgesia using bupivacaine—a study of the fetus and newborn child. J Obstet Gynaecol Br Common 78:559, 1971
60. Climie CR: The place of continuous lumbar epidural

analgesia in the management of abnormally prolonged labour. Med J Austral 2:447, 1964
61. Maltau JM, Andersen HT: Epidural anaesthesia as an alternative to caesarean section in the treatment of prolonged, exhaustive labour. Acta Anaesth Scand 19:349, 1975
62. Moir DD, Willocks J: Management of incoordinate uterine action under continuous epidural analgesia. Br Med J 111:396, 1967
63. Bailey PW, Howard FA: Epidural analgesia and forceps delivery—laying a bogey. Anaesthesia 38:282, 1983
64. Doughty A: Epidural analgesia in labour—the past, the present and the future. J R Soc Med 71:879, 1978
65. Phillips KC, Thomas TA: Second stage of labour with or without extradural analgesia. Anaesthesia 38:972, 1983
66. Chestnut DH, Bates JN, Choi WW: Continuous infusion epidural analgesia with lidocaine: efficacy and influence during the second stage of labor. Obstet Gynecol 69:323, 1987
67. Chestnut DH, Vandewalker GE, Owen CL, Bates JN, Choi WW: The influence of continuous epidural bupivacaine analgesia on the second stage of labor and method of delivery in nulliparous women. Anesthesiology 66:774, 1987

ANESTHESIA FOR IN VITRO FERTILIZATION PROCEDURES

The first live birth produced by an externally fertilized human egg was reported in England in 1978.

In vitro fertilization (IVF) involves four steps: (1) exogenous hormonal stimulation of multiple ovarian follicles, (2) collection of the oocytes, (3) fertilization of the oocyte and growth of the embryo outside the body, and (4) replacement of the embryo back into the uterus.

On day 3 of the menstrual cycle, menotropins (a combination of leutinizing hormones and follicle-stimulating hormones) are administered to promote ovarian follicular growth and maturation. Follicular growth is monitored with ultrasonography and serial estrogen levels. When the follicles reach an average diameter of 1.5 cm, human chorionic gonadotropin is administered to stimulate ovulation. Oocytes are aspirated from the follicles 34 to 36 hours later, transferred to culture media, incubated, and then fertilized. The oocytes are collected either by transabdominal laparoscopy or by transvaginal ultrasound-directed needle aspiration. A transvesical approach, in which needle is guided transurethrally through the posterior wall of the bladder to the ovarian follicle, may also be used. After fertilization, the embryo is transferred to the uterus via a fine catheter inserted through the cervix. The harvest of oocytes requires some form of analgesia or anesthesia, whereas the replacement of the embryo is relatively painless.

A newer technique, gamete intrafallopian transfer (GIFT), allows fertilization to take place in the fallopian tube rather than in culture media. As the name implies, oocytes and sperm are injected directly into the fallopian tubes and fertilization and implantation of the embryo in the uterine wall occurs naturally. The GIFT procedure is usually performed by laparoscopy or minilaparotomy.

PREANESTHETIC EVALUATION

The IVF patient population can be very challenging from an anesthetic standpoint. These patients are generally older than most obstetric patients, and frustrated from months to years of unsuccessful attempts at pregnancy. Hormonal therapy prescribed to hasten oocyte maturation may contribute to emotional lability. Anxiety can increase gastric acidity and decrease gastric emptying, thus the incidence of nausea and risk of aspiration is increased. To offset the increased risk of aspiration, the "full stomach" protocol used in obstetric patients should be the standard approach to these patients. This is a completely elective, but urgent, procedure. Very real time constraints exist because the oocytes must be harvested within a small window of time.

ANESTHETIC OPTIONS

An optimal anesthetic for IVF will provide safety and comfort with a brief recovery period, as this is an ambulatory patient population. Benzodiazepines are useful as premedicants. Midazolam is preferable to diazepam because of its shorter half-life. Also, because midazolam is water soluble, it is not associated with the venous irritation often produced by diazepam. In early pregnancy, diazepam is considered to be teratogenic. This a potential but unproven risk with midazolam. However, oocyte harvest occurs before conception, so this problem should not be an issue. Sodium citrate (0.3 mol/L) should be routinely considered as a premedicant along with metoclopramide and histamine-2 (H_2) receptor antagonists.

General anesthesia is commonly administered for laparoscopy. The use of the Trendelenberg position and the insufflation of the abdomen with carbon dioxide may lead to difficulties with spontaneous respiration plus nausea and vomiting when major regional anesthesia is used. The anesthetic options for transvaginal or transvesical ultrasound needle aspiration include local, general, and regional (subarachnoid, epidural, continuous spinal) anesthesia.

ANESTHETIC TECHNIQUES

Local/Monitored Anesthesia Care

The nature of this procedure is one of multiple exposures to brief, but intense stimulation. Most of the discomfort is generally from passage of the needle through the posterior vaginal wall and peritoneum. Local anesthesia is frequently inadequate and patients typically require heavy sedation, which increases recovery room stay.

General Anesthesia

General anesthesia has its drawbacks, which include postoperative somnolence and long recovery room stays. In addition to the inherent risk of aspiration with general anesthesia, volatile agents, nitrous oxide, and narcotics all may increase the incidence of nausea and vomiting in the postoperative period.

Subarachnoid Anesthesia

Subarachnoid anesthesia is frequently used because the onset time is rapid and the duration of the procedure is usually predictable (1 to 1.5 hours). These benefits must be weighed against the possibility of a post-dural puncture headache, which is 3 to 8 percent with a 26-gauge spinal needle. The use of 27-gauge or conical point spinal needles may decrease the risk of post-dural puncture headache, though actual statistics are not yet available. The sedation requirements are significantly reduced as compared to monitored anesthetic care. This is helpful in decreasing the incidence of postoperative nausea and vomiting. In addition to anxiety and opioids, nausea may be due to peritoneal traction and bleeding. At least a T6 level is necessary with subarachnoid anesthesia to minimize discomfort from peritoneal traction. Nausea can also occur from either hypotension or the addition of epidural or subarachnoid narcotics. The addition of fentanyl improves the quality of a subarachnoid block and relieves some discomfort from peritoneal manipulation as well as provides 2 to 3 hours of postoperative analgesia.[1] We commonly add fentanyl 10 to 25 μg to 10 to 15 mg of 0.75 percent hyperbaric bupivacaine or 50 to 75 mg of 5 percent hyperbaric lidocaine for this procedure.

Continuous Spinal Anesthesia

Small-gauge catheters for continuous spinal anesthesia are presently under investigation for use in IVF. These 24 to 32-gauge microcatheters offer the advantages of a titratable level with reduced local anesthetic requirements. Using various concentrations of lidocaine, including the 5 percent hyperbaric formulation, these microcatheters allow rapid onset with a controllable duration and level of anesthesia; this reduces recovery room stay, which is important in these ambulatory patients. Unfortunately, at present, these microcatheters are technically more difficult to use and multiple attempts at placement may be necessary until one is successfully inserted. This increases cost as well as preparation time. In preliminary reports, the incidence of post-dural puncture headache is similar to that seen with 26-gauge needles, as these microcatheters are placed through a 26-gauge spinal needle. As facility with continuous subarachnoid catheters increases, this technique may play an important role in anesthesia for IVF.

Epidural Anesthesia

Epidural anesthesia offers the advantage of decreased risk of post-dural puncture headache as compared to subarachnoid anesthesia. An epidural anesthetic may be preferable when the duration of the case is expected to take longer, such as with aspiration of many follicles. A T6 level is desirable to minimize peritoneal discomfort. The disadvantages of epidural anesthesia are the increased doses of local anesthetic required, the longer onset time compared to subarachnoid anesthesia, and the higher failure rate.

Despite adequate levels of anesthesia, some patients still experience uncomfortable peritoneal symptoms. Epidural (and subarachnoid) fentanyl has been shown to relieve intraoperative discomfort due to intra-abdominal manipulations.[2] Usually epidural administration of 2 percent lidocaine 10 to 15 ml is sufficient to achieve a T6 level and adding fentanyl 50 μg will improve the quality of the block as well as provide 2 to 3 hours of postoperative analgesia.[2]

Diluting the fentanyl in at least 10 ml of preservative-free normal saline or local anesthetic has been shown to shorten the onset time and increase the duration of analgesia as compared to use of less diluent.[3]

Fentanyl is most commonly used, because although morphine gives longer analgesia (12 to 24 hours), the risk of respiratory depression, while low, is still present. Highly lipid-soluble opioids such as fentanyl may produce a more segmental block and have not been associated with respiratory depression. The side effects of epidural (or subarachnoid) fentanyl are nausea, vomiting, pruritis, and urinary retention. These symptoms are usually transient and mild, and do not require treatment. Small doses of naloxone or diphenhydramine may be useful in treating these side effects.

REFERENCES

1. Hunt CO, et al: Perioperative analgesia with subarachnoid fentanyl–bupivacaine for cesarean delivery. Anesthesiology 71d:535, 1989
2. Naulty SJ, Datta S, Ostheimer GW, et al: Epidural fentanyl for postcesarean delivery pain management. Anesthesiology 63:694, 1985
3. Birnbach DJ, Johnson MD, et al: Effect of diluent volume on analgesia produced by epidural fentanyl. Anesth Analg 68:808, 1989

ANESTHETIC MANAGEMENT OF THE PREGNANT SURGICAL PATIENT

Anesthetic management of the pregnant surgical patient must address the well-being of both the mother and fetus. The patient's surgical condition, pregnancy-induced physiologic changes, and possible adverse effects (both direct and indirect) of anesthesia all have a bearing on anesthetic management. Attention must be paid to the duration of the planned surgical procedure, possible sequelae from anesthesia and surgical intervention, the condition of the pregnancy, and the gestational age and viability of the fetus.

Nonobstetric surgery is required in about 1 percent of pregnancies.[1–4] Surgery may be directly related to pregnancy (e.g., cerclage procedures), associated with pregnancy (e.g., torsion of an ovarian pedicle), or incidental to pregnancy (e.g., trauma or appendicitis).[5] The consultant anesthesiologist must be patient and understanding in answering difficult questions from both the patient and surgeon about "what is best." Decreasing the psychological stress of the patient and surgeon will help optimize operating room conditions.

FETAL CONSIDERATIONS

Teratogenicity

Teratogenic susceptibility/resistance differs among species, making any correlation between animal data and humans difficult. Retrospective epidemiologic studies of anesthetic exposure provide the only human data available; direct control of the experimental conditions has been lost. For a teratogenic effect to occur, a fetus must be exposed to a teratogenic dose of drug for a particular duration and during a susceptible period of embryonal development. In humans, the susceptible period of organogenesis is days 14 through 56. Development of the central nervous system and peripheral nervous system continues into the neonatal period. Results of multiple surveys reveal that *there is no increase in the incidence* of congenital abnormalities in pregnant patients who have undergone surgery during this period.[1–4,6,7] These thoughts must be tempered with the fact that the number of anesthetic exposures during pregnancy reported in the world literature is insufficient to detect possible human teratogenesis. Matching of gestational age, duration of anesthetic exposure, dose of drug, and surgical stress can best be accomplished in animal models. The only controlled experimental data are all from animal studies.

Inhaled Agents. Halothane, isoflurane, enflurane, and nitrous oxide have not been shown to be associated with congenital malformation in rats repeatedly exposed to anesthetic concentrations of inhaled agent.[8]

Nitrous Oxide Controversies. The use of nitrous oxide during early pregnancy presents a difficult problem. Nitrous oxide inhibits methionine synthetase activity through the inactivation of vitamin B_{12}, interfering with thymidine and, therefore, DNA synthesis.[9] Twenty-four-hour exposure of pregnant rats to 50 percent or greater inspired nitrous oxide concentrations will produce teratogenic effects.[10]

In humans, only significant exposures (approximately 2 hours or more) to nitrous oxide have resulted in altered enzyme activity.[9] Additionally, epidemiologic studies have presented evidence, albeit weak, that early nitrous oxide exposure in clinically administered anesthetic concentrations does not produce teratogenic effects.[11] Some animal data report a degree of protection conferred by supplemental (intramuscular) folinic acid,[12] although this is controversial.[10] Administration of supplemental folinic acid to pregnant surgical patients is routinely practiced at some major obstetric anesthesia centers.[13]

Effect on Gestational Viability. Surgery and/or anesthesia in early pregnancy lead to an increased risk of spontaneous abortion.[6] Traditionally, surgical procedures anatomically distant to the pregnant, and therefore irritable, uterus were thought to carry a lower risk of premature labor and possible pregnancy loss. However, recent large epidemiologic surveys present conflicting evidence.[6,7] Pregnancy loss is increased particularly when associated with gynecologic procedures[2,6] and general anesthesia for nonabdominal procedures.[6] More low-birthweight infants (due to both prematurity and intrauterine growth retardation) are born to mothers that have had surgery and anesthesia during pregnancy.[7] This increased incidence was not associated with a specific type of anesthesia or surgery. While the results of these studies are statistically significant, the authors admit that the causative factors are still unknown.[6,7] Nitrous oxide has been associated with increased reproductive loss in the pregnant rat model.[8,10] Interestingly, the use of low-concentration isoflurane in combination with 50 percent nitrous oxide has adverse reproductive effects similar to nonexposed rats.[14]

Indirect Effects. Volatile inhaled agents in concentrations of greater than 0.5 MAC (minimum alveolar concentration) will decrease uterine tone. Up to 1 MAC, inhaled agents will produce uterine artery vasodilation and increased blood flow; above 1 MAC the decrease in maternal cardiac output will offset this vasodilation, decreasing uterine artery flow.[15]

Direct and Indirect Effects of Other Agents

The maternal administration of 100 percent *oxygen* will not raise the fetal oxygen much above 60 mmHg[16] and will not predispose the fetus to the adverse effects of hyperoxia. Maternal hyperventilation may decrease fetal oxygen levels because of effects on uterine blood flow[17] and a left-shift of the maternal oxyhemoglobin dissociation curve.

Certain *narcotics* (morphine, meperidine, and hydromorphone) have been associated with animal fetal abnormalities,[18] although never in humans. Fentanyl, alfentanil, and sufentanil have been shown not to be teratogenic.[19] Fentanyl has shown no deleterious effects on uterine blood flow.

Barbiturates in a single dose have not been shown to be teratogenic. However, barbiturates may further decrease uterine blood flow in an already hypoperfused placenta.

Diazepam has been associated with different fetal abnormalities, notably cleft lip,[20] although this relationship is controversial.[21] The fetal half-life of diazepam is about 30 hours, which might cause delayed neurobehavioral effects in the fetus if premature delivery is necessary.

Antisialagogues seem to have little, if any, effect on the fetus.

Muscle relaxants do not readily cross the placenta, yet can be measured in the fetal circulation after very large maternal doses. This may necessitate the need for ventilatory support in infants delivered in the perioperative period.

Ketamine in doses greater than 1.5 mg/kg will increase uterine tone and, therefore, decrease uterine blood flow. This tonic effect is seen throughout the second and third trimesters of pregnancy.[22]

Vasopressors have predominantly indirect fetal effects, affecting uterine blood flow. Predominantly β-adrenergic agonists are preferred,[23] yet there may be a place for α-adrenergic agents in *severely hypotensive patients*.[24]

Drugs used for prophylaxis against acid aspiration (e.g., histamine-2 (H_2) antagonists) have not been shown to have significant fetal effect in the dosage regimens commonly employed.

Local anesthetics have well-known indirect effects on the fetus. Although presumably cytotoxic, they have not been shown to be teratogenic.[25] The effects of local anesthetics on neurobehavioral scores is discussed in Chapter 3.

Sodium nitroprusside (*SNP*) has caused fetal cyanide toxicity in laboratory animals when doses far exceeding safe clinical anesthetic practice have been administered.[26] SNP has been used without harm for induced hypotension.[27,28]

Nitroglycerin and trimethaphan are used often during the management of pre-eclampsia and have proven human safety records.

Mannitol will cause bulk flow of water from the fetus across the placenta, but has been used without apparent harm in low doses.[29]

Chronic administration of *β-adrenergic blocking agents* has been associated with intrauterine growth retardation as well as expected fetal β-adrenergic blockade. Acute intravenous administration of labetalol in the gravid ewe model has produced insignificant fetal β-adrenergic blockade.[30] Clinical observation of infants born to mothers chronically treated with oral labetalol did not demonstrate significant adrenergic blockade.[31] Acute intravenous administration of esmolol in nonhypertensive gravid ewes has produced fetal hypoxemia.[32]

MATERNAL CONSIDERATIONS

Safeguarding the pregnant patient during surgery requires knowledge of the anesthetic implications of the altered physiology of pregnancy.

Hematologic System

Hematocrit values less than 35 percent are considered abnormal, although may pregnant women with a lower hematocrit carry to term and deliver without adverse outcome. Intraoperative blood loss should be replaced keeping this level in mind. Pregnancy is a hypercoagulable state. Early ambulation or the use of minidose heparin should be considered when appropriate in patients who are confined to bed for extended periods of recovery.

Cardiovascular System

Cardiac output is 40 percent above prepregnant values by the early third trimester. Increased plasma volume, venous capacitance, and cardiac output keep systemic arterial and central venous pressures at essentially non-pregnant values. Aortocaval compression will decrease cardiac output or uterine blood flow or both. Uterine displacement is required at all times during the second half of pregnancy.

Respiratory System

Renal excretion of bicarbonate offsets the respiratory alkalosis produced by normal maternal hyperventilation ($PaCO_2$ = 32 mmHg). Pregnancy-associated increase in minute ventilation as well as decrease in dead space significantly decrease the arterial-to-alveolar carbon dioxide gradient toward zero.[33] End-tidal capnography is, therefore, additionally helpful in intraoperative monitoring. Pulse oximetry is invaluable. Increased oxygen demand, increased cardiac output, and decreased functional residual capacity lower apneic blood oxygen tensions faster in the pregnant woman. Denitrogenation before induction along with facile laryngoscopy and intubation of the trachea are obligatory. The possible anatomically difficult airway in the pregnant patient requires extra attention to be given to preinduction positioning of the patient. Immediate availability of endotracheal tubes in a wide selection of internal diameters as well as a short-handled laryngoscope is prudent. Vascular, friable nasopharyngeal muscosa may make passage of gastric tubes a bloody mess. Gentle insertion of well-lubricated gastric tubes is necessary. If the gastric tube is used only during the operative procedure, oral placement is an easier and safer choice. Finally, mucosal vasoconstrictors may have negative effects on uterine blood flow.[34]

Renal System

Blood urea nitrogen and serum creatinine are decreased to 5 to 10 mg/dl and 0.5 mg/dl, respectively. These values should be considered when interpreting laboratory data. The possibility of urinary stasis due to ureteral compression by the gravid uterus makes meticulous fluid management necessary in an attempt to minimize the need for bladder catheterization.

Gastrointestinal System

Pharmacologic means to alter gastric acidity and volume should be an integral part of acid aspiration prophylaxis. When appropriate, regional anesthesia with intact airway reflexes is preferable to general anesthesia. If general anesthesia is selected, rapid-sequence induction of general anesthesia is routinely advised. If the surgical condition warrants a more deliberate induction of general anesthesia (e.g., severely increased intracranial pressure), experienced personnel should be available to maintain cricoid pressure and otherwise assist the anesthesiologist from induction of anesthesia through endotracheal intubation.

Central Nervous System

The MAC of inhaled agents decreases.[35] This is especially important if inhalational analgesia is contemplated. Loss of protective airway reflexes in a possibly anesthetized patient demands careful titration of agent to effect, and then, only in the most experienced hands. A fasting pregnant patient presenting electively for surgery in the first trimester would possible (but rarely) be a candidate for inhalational analgesia. The gravida presenting for surgery in the second trimester and beyond should be treated with the same precautions as the nonfasting patient presenting emergently for surgery. Neural sensitivity to local anesthetics increases during pregnancy.[36] The induction of surgical epidural or subarachnoid anesthesia will require less anesthetic in the pregnant patient. Use of continuous epidural or subarachnoid catheters allows the anesthesiologist to titrate the dose of local anesthetic to desired effect.

GENERAL RECOMMENDATIONS

First Trimester

Possible teratogenic effects should be kept in mind but there is no reason to avoid general anesthesia if appropriate for the planned surgical procedure or if requested by the patient. The use of nitrous oxide in the first trimester as well as in the entire pregnancy is controversial. Maintenance of general anesthesia can easily be accomplished while avoiding the use of nitrous oxide.

Second and Third Trimester

Support of uteroplacental perfusion is of prime importance. Uterine displacement is essential in the supine pregnant patient, especially after 20 weeks gestation. Intermittent comparison of brachial blood pressure to blood pressure distal to the uterus (e.g., popliteal area) is helpful in detecting occult supine hypotension. Fetal heart rate should be monitored throughout the perioperative period by personnel familiar with its interpretation in all pregnancies that are thought to be viable.

Obstetric consultation should be readily available to evaluate fetal well-being before, during, and after the procedure as well as to treat obstetric complications such as premature labor. Gastrointestinal changes demand acid aspiration prophylaxis. Rapid-sequence induction of general anesthesia is indicated.

Remember: **Meticulous care of the mother will help ensure fetal well-being.**

REFERENCES

1. Smith BE: Fetal prognosis after anesthesia during gestation. Anesth Analg 42:521, 1963
2. Shnider SM, Webster GM: Maternal and fetal hazards of surgery during pregnancy. Am J Obstet Gynecol 92:891, 1965
3. Brodsky JB, Cohen EN, Brown BW, et al: Surgery during pregnancy and fetal outcome. Am J Obstet Gynecol 138:1165, 1980
4. Konieczko KM, Chapk JC, Nunn JF: Fetotoxic potential of general anaesthesia in relation to pregnancy. Br J Anaesth 59:449, 1987
5. Weingold AB (ed): Surgical diseases in pregnancy. Clin Obstet Gynecol 24(4):793, 1983
6. Duncan PG, Pope WDB, Cohen MM, et al: Fetal risk of anesthesia and surgery during pregnancy. Anesthesiology 64:790, 1986
7. Mazze RI, Kallen B: Reproductive outcome after anesthesia and operation during pregnancy: a registry study of 5405 cases. Am J Obstet Gynecol 161:1178, 1989
8. Mazze RI, Fujinaga M, Rice SA, et al: Reproductive and teratogenic effects of nitrous oxide, halothane, isoflurane and enflurane in Sprague-Dawley rats. Anesthesiology 64:339, 1986
9. Nunn JF: Clinical aspects of the interaction between nitrous oxide and vitamin B12. Br J Anaesth 59:3, 1987
10. Fujinaga M, Mazze RI, Baden JM: Reconsiderations of the mechanisms of nitrous oxide teratogenicity. Anesthesiology 69: A658, 1988
11. Crawford JS, Lewis M: Nitrous oxide in early human pregnancy. Anaesthesia 41:900, 1986
12. Keeling PA, Rocke DA, Nunn JF, et al: Folinic acid as protection against nitrous oxide teratogenicity in the rat. Br J Anaesth 58:528, 1986
13. Marx GF: The N_2O dilemma. Obstet Anesth Dig 5:126, 1985
14. Fujinaga M, Baden JM, Yhap EO, et al: Reproductive and teratogenic effects of nitrous oxide, isoflurane, and their combination in Sprague-Dawley rats. Anesthesiology 67:960, 1987
15. Biehl DR, Yarnell R, Wide JG, et al: The uptake of isoflurane by the foetal lamb in utero: effect on regional blood flow. Can Anaesth Soc J 30:581, 1983
16. Baraka A: Correlation between maternal and foetal pO2 and pCO2 during cesarean delivery. Br J Anaesth 42:434, 1972
17. Levinsohn GL, Shnider SM, deLorimier AA, et al: Effects of maternal hyperventilation on uterine blood flow and fetal oxygenation and acid-base status. Anesthesiology 40:340, 1974
18. Geber WF, Schramm LC; Congenital malformations of the central nervous system produced by narcotic analgesics in the hamster. AM J Obstet Gynecol 123:705, 1975
19. Fujinaga M, Mazze RI, Jackson EC, et al: Reproductive and teratogenic effects of sufentanil and alfentanil in Sprague-Dawley rats. Anesthesiology 67:166, 1988
20. Safra MJ, Oakley GP: Association between cleft lip with and without cleft palate and prenatal exposure to diazepam. Lancet ii:478, 1975
21. Rosenberg L, Mitchell AA, Parsells JL, et al: Lack of relation of oral clefts to diazepam use during pregnancy. N Engl J Med 309:1282, 1983
22. Galloon S: Ketamine for obstetric delivery. Anesthesiology 44:522, 1976
23. Ralston DH, Shnider SM, deLorimier AA: Effects of equipotent metaraminol, mephenteramine and methoxamine on uterine blood flow in the pregnant ewe. Anesthesiology 40:354, 1974
24. Ramanathan S, Friedman S, Moss P, et al: Phenylephrine for the treatment of maternal hypotension due to epidural anesthesia. Anesth Analg 63:262, 1984
25. Fujinaga M, Mazze RI: Reproductive and teratogenic effects of lidocaine in Sprague-Dawley rats. Anesthesiology 65:626, 1986
26. Naulty JS, Cefalo RC, Lewis PE: Fetal toxicity of nitroprusside in the pregnant ewe. Am J Obstet Gynecol 139:708, 1981
27. Kofke WA, Wuest HP, McGinnis CA: Cesarean section following ruptured cerebral aneurysm and neuroresuscitation. Anesthesiology 60:242, 1984
28. Rigg D, McDonogh A: Use of sodium nitroprusside for deliberate hypotension during pregnancy. Br J Anaesth 53:985, 1981
29. Neuman B, Lam AM: Induced hypotension for clipping of a cerebral aneurysm during pregnancy: a case report and brief review. Anesth Analg 65:675, 1986
30. Eisenach JC: Maternally administered labetalol produces less adrenergic blockade in fetus than in mother. Anesthesiology 71:A915, 1989
31. MacPherson M, Broughton Pipkin F, Rutter N: The effect of maternal labetalol in the newborn infant. Br J Obstet Gynecol 93:539, 1986
32. Eisenach JC, Castro MI: Maternally administered esmolol produces fetal beta adrenergic blockade and hypoxemia. Anesthesiology 71:718, 1989
33. Shankar KB, Moseley H, Kumar Y, et al: Arterial to end-tidal carbon dioxide tension difference during caesarean section. Anaesthesia 41:698, 1986
34. Woods JR, Plessinger MA, Clark KE: Effect of cocaine on uterine blood flow and fetal oxygenation. JAMA 257:957, 1987
35. Palahniuk RJ, Shnider SM, Eger EI II: Pregnancy decreases the requirements of inhaled anesthetic agents. Anesthesiology 41:82, 1987

36. Datta S, Lambert DH, Gregus J, et al: Differential sensitivity of mammalian nerve fibers during pregnancy. Anesth Analg 62:1070, 1983

ANESTHESIA FOR FETAL SURGERY

Anesthesia for fetal surgery is a provocative possibility. In the most basic sense, it is the merging of the management of two distinct, yet joined, organisms. The most fundamental principles of obstetric anesthetic care must apply. In addition, perinatal (actually *antenatal*) considerations apply.

Fetal intervention was first described by Liley in 1963 for treatment of infants with erythroblastosis fetalis.[1] Until recently, few therapeutic options existed when serious fetal anomalies were present. If pregnancy was not medically terminated, many of these infants would die in utero or shortly after birth.

In the subsequent 25 years, the potential for fetal surgery improved dramatically. Today, surgical intervention early in fetal development (for conditions such as diaphragmatic hernia, hydronephrosis, and obstructive hydrocephalus) is a viable option because of improvements of intrauterine diagnostic capabilities and new surgical techniques.[2–4]

Anesthesia can have a profound effects on both the mother and fetus. Minimal clinical data are available upon which to base decisions regarding the management of anesthesia for fetal surgery.[1–4]

PHYSIOLOGIC CHANGES OF PREGNANCY

The physiologic changes of pregnancy influence the conduct of anesthesia. Aortocaval compression can become clinically important as early as the 10th week of gestation. At term, the maternal cardiac output has increased by 25 percent, the plasma volume by 50 percent, and the red cell mass by 30 percent (resulting in the physiologic anemia of pregnancy).[5] Pregnancy is associated with alterations in the levels of several coagulation factors (plasma fibrinogen is increased by 50 percent; factors VIII and XII are increased, whereas factors XI and XIII are usually decreased). The fibrinolytic system may be depressed, especially plasminogen activator and antithrombin III. Venous stasis in the lower extremities, due to the enlarged gravid uterus and compression of the inferior vena cava, may be associated with an increased risk of thrombophlebitis. As the uterus increases in size, maternal oxygen consumption and minute alveolar ventilation increase and the functional residual capacity declines. The pregnant patient compensates for the increases in minute ventilation by renal excretion of bicarbonate to maintain a normal acid–base balance. Thus, with reduced cardiopulmonary reserve, the pregnant patient rapidly becomes hypoxic when apneic. She has less ability to buffer the acidotic state.

PHARMACOKINETIC CONSIDERATIONS

Uptake, distribution, metabolism, and excretion of anesthetic agents are altered in pregnancy.[6] These alterations are secondary to an increased cardiac output, increased volume of distribution, altered plasma protein levels and enzyme activity, increased glomerular filtration rate, altered hepatic function, and increased minute ventilation. Pregnant patients are more sensitive to the effects of general and local anesthetic agents. Thus, the mean alveolar concentration of volatile agents needs to be reduced by approximately 25 to 50 percent and the dosage of local anesthesics diminished by about one-third. This reduction in anesthetic requirement may be due in part to an altered hormonal state, particularly increased levels of progesterone.[7]

Pregnant patients are at increased risk for aspiration of gastric contents. Nonparticulate antacids, metoclopramide, and cimetidine may be given preanesthetically.[8] Induction of general anesthesia should be performed in a "rapid-sequence" fashion with cricoid pressure (Sellick's maneuver).

Considerations in maintenance of uteroplacental perfusion include avoidance of aortocaval compression and maintenance of adequate maternal blood pressure and cardiac output with intravenous volume expansion and ephedrine. Pure α-agonists should be avoided because of the reported deleterious effect of these agents on placental perfusion.[9] Supplemental oxygen should be administered. Pure oxygen administration to the mother for extended periods does not cause retinopathy of prematurity in the fetus unless hyperbaric pressures are used.[10] Maternal $PaCO_2$ should be kept in the normal range. Maternal stress and drugs that increase uterine tone (ketamine in doses greater than 1 mg/kg and neostigmine) should be avoided.

REGIONAL VERSUS GENERAL ANESTHESIA

For surgical procedures on the fetus, regional anesthesia is intuitively appealing because it may limit the amount of fetal drug exposure, thereby reducing the risk of exposure to possible toxic or teratogenic effects of anesthetic agents. Regional approaches may also reduce the risk of maternal aspiration associated with general anesthesia.[11] However, regional anesthesia does not completely prevent the maternal stress response to anxiety nor does it provide fetal anesthesia or block the response of the fetus to surgery-induced stress. Anand et al.[12] demonstrated that preterm infants undergoing surgery had a substantial hormonal response indicative of stress if not given adequate anesthesia. Regional anesthesia cannot provide uterine relaxation or fetal neuromuscular block. Fetal movement may occur and disrupt the operative field. In such situations, intramuscular injections of muscle relaxants into the fetus have been reported to maintain a motionless surgical field.[13] Therefore, general anesthesia offers several advantages for fetal surgery.[14]

In a recent case report of fetal surgery, the author and his associates chose general anesthesia for several reasons. With general anesthesia, there is maternal skeletal muscle relaxation, uterine smooth muscle relaxation, fetal immobility, fetal anesthesia, maintenance of normal uteroplacental perfusion and a block of maternal awareness.[15–18] To minimize toxic drug effects on the fetus, agents with minimal biodegradation and long safety records in pregnant humans should be used. The reduction of the maternal stress response and the maintenance of placental perfusion of equal importance. Isoflurane has some merits that may make it the volatile anesthetic of choice. It undergoes the least biodegradation, has an excellent safety record in obstetric anesthesia, and provides a good uterine and skeletal muscle relaxation.

Nitrous oxide should be avoided because of its inhibitory effect on the activity of vitamin B_{12}-dependent enzymes (methionine synthetase and thymidylate synthetase).[19] Methionine synthetase catalyzes the conversion of homocystine to methionine, a precursor of myelin. Interference with either of these enzymatic processes could theoretically compromise normal fetal development. Vanucci and Wolf observed that nitrous oxide in conjunction with muscle relaxation led to profound metabolic alterations in fetal rat brains, suggestive of inhibition of aerobic metabolism.[20] The combination of mild hypoxia and nitrous oxide produced more anomalies than hypoxia alone.[21] Nitrous oxide, when given to rats for 1 or 2 days, caused a high incidence of fetal death and malformations.[22] For these reasons, many authors recommend avoiding fetal exposure to nitrous oxide during the first and second trimesters. Theoretically, intravenous alfentanil may be a useful adjunct for general anesthesia in fetal surgery. Its rapid redistribution and metabolism allow it to be used as a continuous intravenous infusion. Alfentanil can be used to maintain a profound maternal narcotic effect that will rapidly dissipate when discontinued. It does tend to accumulate on the fetal side of the placenta, and this accumulation may provide a prolonged level of stress reduction in the fetus after surgery. Alfentanil has not been correlated with any teratogenic effects to date.

NEUROMUSCULAR BLOCKADE

Succinylcholine, because of its highly ionized state at normal body pH, minimizes fetal exposure and is rapidly metabolized by maternal and fetal plasma cholinesterase. Although the levels and activity of fetal cholinesterase at 20 weeks gestation are not well documented, succinylcholine has been reported to be rapidly metabolized by premature infants.[23] Nondepolarizing agents such as pancuronium and d-tubocuraine are highly ionized compounds that are slow to cross the placenta.[24,25] The amount of these drugs that reaches the fetus after maternal administration is small. Adequate fetal skeletal muscle relaxation cannot be ensured when conventional doses are administered only to the mother. Direct fetal intramuscular injections of 3 mg/kg of d-tubocurarine to immobilize the fetus during surgery have been reported.[13] Fetal cardiac output is heart rate dependent. Pancuronium may be preferred over d-tubocurarine for intrauterine fetal surgery because it has been shown to maintain a higher fetal heart rate and mean arterial pressure.[26–28] Fetal movement did not occur in a case when 1.5 percent isoflurane in oxygen was used, and no additional fetal muscle relaxants were required.[15]

The use of a sterile neonatal pulse oximeter for monitoring of the fetus is a consideration. However, a technical problem may be encountered. The pulse oximeter probe is attached to the fetus with an adhesive band. The risk of denuding the immature dermal layers with this adhesive is of concern, since the manipulation of the fetus by surgeons caused a noticeable sloughing of the dermis in one case.[15] A sterile probe without adhesive would be advantageous. Seeds et al.[26] have used fetal heart rate monitoring, utilizing the standard scalp electrode, with a reference electrode on the maternal abdomen.

A QUESTION OF ETHICS

The question arises as to what could be done therapeutically in the event that the monitors suggest fetal compromise. Ensuring stable maternal hemodynamics and ventilation and the avoidance of aortocaval compression is the fundamental doctrine for preservation of fetal homeostasis.

Although fetal surgery is at its inception, it is clear that as technology improves, these procedures will become more widely used. Early animal and human studies indicate that these surgical procedures can correct what would otherwise be fatal abnormalities. As technology becomes more sophisticated, ethical conflicts become unavoidable. Most fetal malformations do not pose a threat to maternal health, whereas general anesthesia and laparotomy do. Ethical guidelines need to be developed for fetal surgery.

REFERENCES

1. Liley AW: Intrauterine transfusion of foetus in haemolytic disease. Br Med J 2:1107, 1963
2. Frigoletto FD, Birholz JC, Greene MF: Antenatal treatment of hydrocephalus by ventriculoamniotic shunting. JAMA 248:2496, 1982
3. Golbus MS, Harrison MR, Filly RA, et al: *In utero* treatment of urinary tract obstruction. Am J Obstet Gynecol 142:383, 1982
4. Berkowitz RI, Glickman MG, Smith GW, et al: Fetal urinary tract obstruction: what is the role of surgical intervention *in utero*? Am J Obstet Gynecol 144:367, 1982
5. Bonica JJ: Obstetric analgesia and anesthesia. World Federation of Societies of Anesthesiologists. p. 2, 1980
6. Davis AG, Moir DD: Anaesthesia during pregnancy. Clin Anaesthesiol 4:233, 1986
7. Flanagan JL, Datta S, Lambert D, et al: Effect of pregnancy on bupivacaine-induced conduction blockade in the isolated rabbit vagus nerve. Anesth Analg 66:123, 1987
8. Solanki DR, Suresh M, Ethridge HC: The effects of intravenous cimetidine and metoclopramide on gastric volume and pH. Anesth Analg 63:599, 1984
9. Shnider SM, Levinson G: Anesthesia for Obstetrics. 2d Ed. p. 32. Williams &Wilkins, Baltimore, 1987
10. Ricci B, Calagero G: Oxygen induced retinopathy in newborn rats: effects of prolonged normobaric and hyperbaric oxygen supplementation. Pediatrics 83:193, 1988
11. Spielman FJ, Seeds JW, Corke BC: Anaesthesia for fetal surgery. Anaesthesia 39:756, 1984
12. Anand KJS, Sippel WG, Green A: A randomized trial of fentanyl anesthesia in preterm babies undergoing surgery. Lancet 1:243, 1987.
13. De Crespigny LC, Robinson HP, Ross AW, Quinn M: Curarization of fetus for intrauterine procedures. Lancet 1:1164, 1985
14. Levine MD, McNeil DE, Kabuck MM, et al: Second trimester fetoscopy and fetal blood sampling: current limitations and problems. Am J Obstet Gynecol 120:937, 1974
15. Johnson MJ, Birnbach DJ, Burchman CA et al: Fetal surgery and general anesthesia: a case report and review. J Clin Anesth 1:363, 1989
16. Delany AG: Anesthesia in the pregnant women. Clin Obstet Gynecol 20:795, 1983
17. Duncan PG, Pope WD, Cohen MM, Greer N: Fetal risk of anesthesia and surgery during pregnancy. Anesthesiology 20:795, 1986
18. Warren TW, Datta S, Ostheimer GW, et al: Comparison of the maternal and neonatal effects of halothane, enflurane, and isoflurane for cesarean deliveries. Anesth Analg 62:516, 1983
19. Nunn JF, Chanarin I: Nitrous oxide inactivates methionine synthetase. p. 211. In Eger EI (ed): Nitrous Oxide. Elsevier, New York; 1985
20. Vanucci RC, Wolf JW: Oxidative metabolism in fetal rat brain during maternal anesthesia. Anesthesiology 48:238, 1978
21. Smith BE, Gaub MI, Moya F: Teratogenic effects of anesthetic agents. Anesth Analg 44:726, 1965
22. Fink BR, Shepard TH, Blendau RJ: Teratogenic activity of nitrous oxide. Nature 214:146, 1967
23. Escobichon PJ, Stephens DS: Perinatal development of human esterases. Clin Pharmacol Ther 14:41, 1973
24. Abouleish E, Wingard LB, de la Vega S, Uy N: Pancuronium in cesarean section and its plancental transfer. Br J Anaesth 52:531, 1980
25. Kivalo I, Saarikoski S: Placental transmission and foetal uptake of 14C-dimethyl-tubocurarine. Br J Anaesth 44:557, 1972
26. Seeds JW, Corke BC, Spielman FJ: Prevention of fetal movement during invasive procedure with pancuronium bromide. Am J Obstet Gynecol 155:818, 1986
27. Chestnut DH, Weiner CP, Thompson CS, McLaughlin GL: Intravenous administration of d-tubocuraine and pancuronium in fetal lambs (abstract). Anesthesiology 69:A652, 1988
28. Harrison MR, Anderson J, Rosen MA, et al: Fetal surgery in the primate. Anesthetic, surgical and tocolytic management to maximize fetal-neonatal survival. J Pediatr Surg 17:115, 1982

ANESTHESIA FOR POSTPARTUM SURGERY

Surgery in the postpartum period may be required for a variety of elective or emergent conditions. Elective postpartum sterilization procedures are relatively benign when compared to an emergency obstetric hysterectomy in a patient with a coagulopathy. A brief review of the physiologic changes of the postpartum period precedes a discussion of obstetric situations that may require surgical intervention and their anesthetic management.

PHYSIOLOGY OF THE PUERPERIUM

The maternal physiology as altered by pregnancy does not immediately revert to the nonpregnant state at delivery. The exact time course of reversal is unknown. Some changes are exaggerated in the immediate postpartum period; others gradually reverse, while some do so dramatically. The highest level of cardiac output occurs immediately after delivery, which is attributed to the autotransfusion and increased venous return associated with uterine involution.[1] The increased blood volume returns to prepregnant levels within several days. This conservation of red cells allows the mother to tolerate the blood loss of delivery with minimal decrease in hemoglobin or hematocrit.[2]

While the mechanical reasons for the increased gastric volume in pregnancy are at least partially mitigated after delivery, hormonal and pharmacologic reasons for delayed gastric emptying may persist for days. Labor itself and the use of narcotics during labor can also delay emptying.[3] In the postpartum patient, the volume and pH of gastric contents have been reported to be independent of the length of time from delivery.[4] In one study, patients more than 9 hours and less than 23 hours after delivery had the smallest gastric volumes. Nonetheless, a significant number of patients (40 to 73 percent) were still considered "at risk" for aspiration pneumonitis.[5] Another study confirms that a high percentage of postpartum patients (33 percent) are "at risk" for aspiration.[6] Thus, postpartum patients should be considered at high risk for aspiration pneumonitis and, in this regard, should be managed as if the patient were still pregnant. The increased sensitivity to anesthetic agents may rapidly dissipate after delivery. The requirements for local anesthetics are higher 8 to 24 hours postpartum than in the parturient.[7]

Pseudocholinesterase activity is decreased for 2 to 3 days postpartum. However, the action of succinylcholine in a 1-mg/kg dose is only prolonged by 3 minutes in the postpartum patient.[8]

ELECTIVE POSTPARTUM SURGERY

The only elective procedure routinely performed in the postpartum period is sterilization.

Timing of Surgery

The Committee on Obstetrics: Maternal and Fetal Medicine of the American College of Obstetrics and Gynecology (ACOG) has stated:

> The decision as to when to proceed with anesthesia and surgery should be based on the anesthesiologist's assessment of the patient and judgment of the relative risks and benefits for that patient.[9]

The anesthesiologist must be aware of the risks and benefits of various choices in timing. Technically, the surgery is a simple procedure when the uterine fundus is near the umbilicus. The fundus remains so for at least 2 days postpartum, allowing ample time to perform the procedure.

Certain elements of maternal risk may decrease with a delay of 8 to 24 hours. Postpartum hemorrhage, which occurs in about 5 percent of parturients, can occur without warning and be life-threatening even after an apparently uneventful vaginal delivery.[10] The incidence decreases dramatically after 10 hours in multiparous women.[11] Postpartum hemorrhage presenting during a tubal ligation might be difficult to diagnose initially and would clearly increase maternal risk during postpartum sterilization.

The prognosis of any infant can better be predicted several hours than minutes after delivery. Immediate postpartum tubal ligation carries the risk of sterilization prior to a full evaluation of the neonate. However, immediate postpartum tubal ligation may avoid the need for an additional anesthetic in a patient who already has anesthesia for labor and/or delivery. Continuous epidural or spinal techniques can easily be extended to provide surgical anesthesia for a tubal ligation. Therefore, the patient with a continuous technique may incur the least additional risk if an immediate sterilization is performed. Exceptions should be made when there have been complications of the labor and/or delivery, for example, major blood loss or cardiac compromise.

In contrast, a patient who delivers without anesthesia is probably best served by a tubal ligation 8 to 24 hours later. That is, women delivering before midnight would have their procedure the next day and those delivering after midnight, the next day after that. With the demands of decreasing hospital stay, spinal anesthesia can be used for immediate post partum sterilization. We believe general anesthesia should not be induced in the immediate postpartum period solely for a tubal ligation.

These guidelines assume that patient load and staffing can accommodate what is fundamentally an elective procedure. Other activities in the labor and delivery suite should not be compromised.

Anesthetic Management

The considerations of acid aspiration prophylaxis, difficult intubation, and fluid requirements to avoid hypotension are the same for postpartum surgery as for cesarean delivery. Recent and/or ongoing blood loss may modify the choice of anesthetic technique and raise the question of postponement to 6 week postpartum.

Table 10-9. Recommended Anesthetic Agents for Postpartum Sterilization

Regional Anesthesia
Epidural
Lidocaine 2 percent with 1:200,000 epinephrine
Chloroprocaine 3 percent
Subarachnoid[a]
Hyperbaric lidocaine 5 percent[b]
Hyperbaric bupivacaine 0.75 percent[b]

[a] More dilute solutions may be used with a continuous subarachnoid technique.
[b] Epinephrine may be added, if desired.

An in situ continuous lumbar epidural (or subarachnoid) catheter may be used to provide anesthesia for an immediate postpartum tubal ligation. If immediate surgery is not to be done, the catheter should be removed. Catheter tip migration (and subsequent inadequate surgical anesthesia) is common in ambulatory patients. Local anesthetic agents may be chosen, as in Table 10-9. Subarachnoid anesthesia is most frequently used for the tubal ligation in the postpartum period and is preferable to epidural anesthesia because of its speed of onset and reliability of block. Drug dosage may need to be increased by the second day after delivery. Epidural anesthesia induced only for tubal ligation is more time consuming and is not usually considered unless specifically indicated for other reasons.

The decreased likelihood of problems with intubation and/or aspiration makes regional anesthesia preferable to general anesthesia. General anesthesia may be used for surgery the next day after delivery at the patient's request. A rapid sequence induction should be followed by endotracheal intubation. Routinely, intravenous thiamylal 5 mg/kg or thiopental 4 mg/kg and succinylcholine 1 to 1.5 mg/kg are used to induce anesthesia. Anesthesia is maintained with 70 percent nitrous oxide in oxygen and intravenous narcotic supplementation using a succinylcholine infusion for muscle relaxation. Volatile anesthetic agents are usually avoided, as the risk of uterine relaxation may still exist.

EMERGENCY POSTPARTUM SURGERY

Obstetric Considerations

Postpartum hemorrhage is the most frequent reason for emergency surgery in the immediate postpartum period.

Causes of postpartum hemorrhage include:

1. Uterine atony (failure of the uterus to contract and adequately compress vessels at the placental implantation site). Predisposing factors include:
   a) An over distended uterus prior to delivery (multiple gestations, polyhydramnios, macrosomia)
   b) Prolonged labor
   c) Rapid labor
   d) Vigorous use of oxytocin stimulation during labor
   e) Multiparity
   f) Hypotension
   g) Uterine infection
   h) Amniotic fluid embolism
2. Laceration/injury to the perineum, vagina, cervix, or uterus. Predisposing events include:
   a) Delivery of a large infant
   b) Midforceps delivery
   c) Forceps rotation
   d) Delivery through an incompletely dilated cervix
   e) Intrauterine manipulation
   f) Vaginal birth after cesarean delivery
   g) Dührssen's incisions
3. Retained placental tissue, which may be due to an abnormally adherent placenta (placenta accreta, increta, or percreta) or a normal placenta incompletely removed.
4. Uterine inversion, which is a rare cause of hemorrhage that should be immediately recognized in order to prevent life-threatening consequences. Blood loss in this situation is frequently underestimated.

Anesthetic Considerations

Hypovolemia is a major risk factor in emergency postpartum surgery. Estimating blood loss is notoriously unreliable in determining blood loss.[2] Cardiovascular changes of hypovolemia should be evaluated in every patient. The presence of hypotension, tachycardia, or orthostatic changes may be the first clues of hypovolemia. Its presence should directly affect the choice of anesthetic technique.

Anesthetic Management

If a regional anesthetic is elected, subarachnoid anesthesia is frequently chosen for its speed of onset and reliability. The intraspinal anesthetic technique is similar to that for vaginal delivery. Intravenous hydration is extremely important because of the possibility of unrecognized hypovolemia. However, regional anesthesia with its sympathetic blockade often exaggerate hypotension, possibly increasing maternal morbidity and mortality. Therefore, general anesthesia usually is used in the hypovolemic patient.

For emergency postpartum surgery, optimal care would include:

1. Availability of compatible blood products
2. Determination of maternal hemoglobin/hematocrit
3. Placement of large intravenous catheters (two catheters required for major hemorrhage)
4. Use of a blood and fluid warmer
5. Colloid or blood infusion
6. Capacity to directly measure maternal systemic blood pressure and central venous pressures

After premedication and denitrogenation, general anesthesia is induced, in a rapid-sequence fashion, with thiamylal or thiopental (up to 4 mg/kg), ketamine (up to 1 mg/kg) or etomidate (up to 0.2 mg/kg), depending on the degree of hypovolemia. Endotracheal intubation is facilitated with succinylcholine (1 to 1.5 mg/kg). Muscle relaxation is maintained with a succinylcholine infusion or a nondepolarizing relaxant, depending on the anticipated duration of the procedure. Volatile agents are avoided unless they are specifically indicated for their uterine relaxant properties (e.g., in the initial management of uterine inversion). Nitrous oxide, narcotics and/or benzodiazepines are used to maintain anesthesia as tolerated.

Blood Replacement

A postpartum patient hemorrhaging in the delivery room encompasses all the indications for a potential disaster. Obstetric hemorrhage is still one of the major causes of maternal mortality.[12] Seemingly minor hemorrhage can progress to major blood loss within minutes. Transfusion will not be necessary in all patients. In fact, hemorrhage is rare enough that autologous blood donation is not encouraged for pregnant patients not at high risk for complications (e.g., placenta previa).[13] Yet, every patient having emergency surgery for postpartum hemorrhage should have compatible blood products available. The risks of transfusion warrant an initial attempt to correct hypovolemia with crystalloid or colloid, although packed red cells, platelets, and fresh frozen plasma may be necessary in certain patients. Uncrossmatched O negative blood or, preferably, type-specific blood can be used in the emergency situation. Dilutional coagulopathy and thrombocytopenia are common and should be treated when they occur. Early determination of platelet count may be helpful.

Table 10-10. Laboratory Findings in DIC

Early
Decreased fibrinogen
Decreased platelet count
Increased fibrin degradation products
Abnormal red cell morphology
Late
Prolongation of prothrombin time
Prolongation of partial thromboplastin time
Prolongation of thrombin time

Massive hemorrhage and transfusion can lead to disseminated intravascular coagulation (DIC). Additionally, DIC is associated with the following obstetric conditions:

1. Placental abruption
2. Fetal death
3. Severe preeclampsia/eclampsia
4. Amniotic fluid embolism
5. Saline abortion
6. Septicemia and intravascular hemolysis

Diagnosis of acute DIC does not generally require laboratory evaluation. Hemorrhage associated with any of the above conditions with supporting laboratory abnormalities (Table 10-10) should be considered DIC.

The management of DIC focuses on treatment of the underlying disease (i.e., removal of the source of thromboplastin or bacterial endotoxin) as soon as possible. Administration of procoagulant factors and/or platelets is frequently necessary. The use of heparin is controversial and not recommended.

REFERENCES

1. Hansen JM, Ueland K: The influence of caudal analgesia on cardiovascular dynamics during normal labor and delivery. Acta Anaesthesiol Scand Suppl 23:449, 1966
2. Pritchard JA: Changes in the blood volume during pregnancy and delivery. Anesthesiology 26:395, 1965
3. O'Sullivan GM, Sutton AJ, Thompson SA, et al: Noninvasive measurement of gastric emptying in obstetric patients. Anesth Analg 66:505, 1987
4. Rennie AL, Richard JA, Milne MK, et al: Post-partum sterilisation—an anaesthetic hazard? Anaesthesia 34:267, 1979
5. James CF, Gibbs CP, Banner T: Postpartum perioperative risk of aspiration pneumonia. Anesthesiology 61:756, 1984
6. Blouw R, Scatliff J, Craig DB, et al: Gastric volume and pH in postpartum patients. Anesthesiology 45:456, 1976
7. Abouleish EI: Postpartum tubal ligation requires more bupivacaine for spinal anesthesia than does cesarean section. Anesth Analg 65:897, 1986

8. Leighton BL, Cheek TG, Gross JB, et al: Succinylcholine pharmacodynamics in peripartum patients. Anesthesiology 64:202, 1986
9. Committee on Obstetrics: Maternal and Fetal Medicine: Postpartum tubal sterilization: Appropriate timing of surgery after vaginal delivery. ACOG Committee Opinion #50, 1987
10. Lewis JM, Fontrier T: Near Misses in Anesthesia: Lessons Learned. Butterworths, Boston, 1988
11. Pritchard JA, MacDonald PC, Gant NF: Williams Obstetrics. 17Ed. Appleton-Century-Crofts, East Norwalk, CT, 1985
12. Rochat RW, Koonin LM, Atrash HK, et al: Maternal mortality in the United States: report from the maternal mortality collaborative. Obstet Gynecol 72:91, 1988
13. The National Blood Resource Education Program Expert Panel: The use of autologous blood. JAMA 263:414, 1990

ALLERGIC REACTIONS TO LOCAL ANESTHETICS

Local anesthetics are an invaluable tool in the practice of obstetric anesthesia. Unfortunately, it is not uncommon for a patient to report that she is allergic to Novacaine, lidocaine, or even worse, all "caines." Frequently, this diagnosis has come from a prior exposure to one of the local anesthetics during a dental procedure or a regional nerve block. If taken at face value, this patient may be denied regional anesthesia for labor or cesarean delivery and would require general anesthesia for any surgical intervention.

Before proceeding, it is necessary to obtain a complete history from the patient about her reaction to the local anesthetic. Ideally, the patient should be referred to the anesthesiologist by her obstetrician in a timely manner before any anesthetic intervention is required. An attempt should be made to obtain any records detailing the incident in question.

CLASSIFICATION OF ADVERSE REACTION TO LOCAL ANESTHETICS

Adverse reactions to local anesthetics may fall into one of four categories[1]: vasovagal reactions, epinephrine reactions, toxic reactions, and allergic reactions.

Vasovagal reactions may occur in particularly anxious patients. These patients, commonly with "needle phobias," may complain of light-headedness or nausea at the time an anesthetic is administered. Signs include bradycardia, hypotension, pallor, diaphoresis, tachypnea, and syncope. Placement of the patient in a supine position with left uterine displacement and legs elevated may be all that is needed to reverse this episode. Pharmacologic treatment is rarely needed.

Epinephrine reactions occur when a significant portion of an epinephrine-containing local anesthetic solution is absorbed systemically. Toxic effects of the local anesthetic itself may not be noticed and the patient may complain of symptoms related to the epinephrine. These include nervousness and palpitations. Elevated blood pressure, tachycardia, and extrasystoles may be present. Because of the short serum half-life of epinephrine, the episode usually subsides without intervention. Appropriate treatment is needed if conditions become life-threatening.

Toxic reactions to local anesthetics are due to an excess plasma concentrations of the drug. The toxicity of these drugs involves primarily the central nervous system (CNS) and the cardiovascular system. Early CNS effects include restlessness, tinnitus, vertigo, difficulty focusing, light-headedness, and a bitter taste in the mouth. As concentrations of the drug increase, slurred speech and skeletal muscle twitching occur. Higher blood levels result in seizures followed by CNS depression. Cardiovascular effects of local anesthetics include hypotension, arrhythmias, and atrioventricular heart block. Management of both CNS and cardiovascular system toxicity is reviewed elsewhere[2] and in chapter 7.

The last category of reactions to local anesthetics, true allergic reactions, is extremely rare,[3] estimated at less than 1 percent of all adverse reactions.[4] An allergic reaction is defined as an immune response that is exaggerated and leads to gross tissue damage.[5] The terms *allergy*, *hypersensitivity*, and *sensitivity* are often used interchangeably in the anesthesia literature.[6]

Hypersensitivity reactions are classified according to the immune system's response. Gell and Coombs[7] defined four different types of reactions as follows: type 1, anaphylactic sensitivity; type 2, antibody-dependent, cytotoxic hypersensitivity; type 3, complex-mediated hypersensitivity; and type 4, cell-mediated or delayed-type hypersensitivity. For purposes of this review, type 2 and type 3 reactions will not be discussed in further detail since there are virtually no known occurrences of local anesthetic-induced type 2 or type 3 responses.[8]

Anaphylactic reactions (type 1) are mediated by antibodies from the immunoglobulin E (IgE) class. This is the most serious reaction and requires previous exposure to the drug or a chemically similar substance. On initial exposure to the antigenic substance, the individual's B lymphocytes are stimulated to produce IgE. The IgE antibodies then attach to receptor sites on the cell membranes of mast cells present in tissues and basophils circulating in plasma.[9] When stimulated, these "sensitized" mast cells and basophils are capable of participating in an anaphylactic reaction. On re-exposure to the antigen, two cell-bound IgE antibodies may become cross-linked, leading to conformational changes in the cell membrane and release of granules (degranulation) from the mast cells and basophils.

Degranulation of these cells leads to release of several chemical mediators, the most prominent of which is histamine. Histamine dilates terminal arterioles and increases capillary permeability, leading to extravasation of intravascular fluid. Histamine also causes bronchospasm as a result of its role in constriction of bronchial smooth muscle. Additional chemical mediators that are released include heparin, slow-reacting substance of anaphylaxis, prostaglandins, and platelet-activating factor, among others.

The anaphylactic syndrome may include pruritis, erythema, flushing, urticaria, angioedema, nausea with diarrhea and vomiting, laryngeal edema, bronchospasm, hypotension, cardiovascular collapse, and death, all occurring within minutes. Anaphylaxis has been reported after the raising of an intradermal wheal, injection of a milliliter of solution for a minor surgical procedure, the topical application of a small quantity of drug, or the instillation of a drop or two in the conjunctival sac of the eye.[10]

Nonimmunologic stimulation of mast cells and basophils leading to the release of histamine has been termed *anaphylactoid*.[11] The magnitude of histamine released in this reaction is usually related to the dose of the drug and its rate of administration. In the extreme, a shock-like state may result which is indistinguishable from that of a true anaphylactic reaction.

Type 4, cell-mediated or delayed-type hypersensitivity, accounts for 90 percent of allergic reactions to local anesthetics.[12] This reaction involves interaction of an antigen with a primed T-cell lymphocyte, causing tissue damage characterized by inflammation, pruritis, burning, erythematous macules, and papules. No circulating antibodies are involved and the damage is due to localized release of chemical mediators. The term *delayed-type hypersensitivity* is used because the symptoms may not occur for hours. Antihistamines and other such antagonistic substances are not helpful in treatment of this reaction since histamine and other circulating vasoactive substances are not involved. This type of sensitization can be detected by skin patch testing and occurs most often in individuals repeatedly exposed to a drug, for example, physicians, nurses, and dentists. Contact dermatitis is the most common example.

CAUSATIVE AGENTS

Commonly used local anesthetics fall into two distinct chemical groups, the aminoesters and the aminoamides. Aminoesters include procaine, chloroprocaine, and tetracaine. Aminoamides include lidocaine, prilocaine, bupivacaine, mepivacaine, and etidocaine.

Aminoester local anesthetics are capable of producing metabolites related to para-aminobenzoic acid (PABA), which is a highly allergic substance. Most of the cell-mediated hypersensitivity reactions that were experienced by members of the dental profession were due to aminoesters.[3] These drugs may cross-sensitize and cross-react immunologically but do not cross-react with aminoamides.

Allergic reactions to aminoamide local anesthetics have been reported (Arens J: Personal communication),[13–14] but only one case[15] has had serial immunologic confirmation of its nature. Other reports, which have taken into account the role of preservatives,[16,17] seem to present a relatively convincing picture of true allergic reactions. Interestingly, most investigators suggest that aminoamide local anesthetics may not be substantially cross-reactive with each other.[18]

Allergic reactions may also be due to other chemicals or contaminants present in the local anesthetic solution. Methylparaben, a preservative for multiple-dose vials or ampules, is structurally similar to PABA. Other allergenic preservatives include methylhydroxybenzoate and bisulfites. Bisulfites are used to stabilize vasoconstrictors that are in solution. The Food and Drug Administration estimates that 5 percent of the nine million people with asthma in the United States may be hypersensitive to sulfites.[19] Patients with chronic atropy (allergies to foods or inhalants; bronchial asthma) are at higher risk to develop sensitization to drugs.

APPROACH TO THE PATIENT

A thorough history is essential in approaching the patient with a presumed allergy to a local anesthetic. Other types of adverse reactions, as previously discussed, should be ruled out. If the patient's history points toward a true allergic reaction, the simplest alternative may be to use a local anesthetic that is chemically unrelated to the one that is implicated. There is *no* simple, satisfactory, and reliable method for testing for allergies to local anesthetics that a clinician may use for identifying susceptible individuals,[12] but allergy testing may be helpful.

A more complete evaluation of a patient is sometimes warranted, and this involves referral to an allergist or others who are familiar with allergy testing. The most commonly available in vivo tests for local anesthetic allergy are skin testing, incremental challenge, and patch testing. A unique in vitro test, the leukocyte histamine release test, will also be discussed.

Skin testing involves various dilutions of the preservative-free local anesthetic, applied initially to a scratch or prick in the skin and later injected in intradermal wheals. Protocols for this are well-described elsewhere.[8,18] There are literature reports of at least 257 subjects in whom a negative skin test to a local anesthetic was followed by challenge to that drug without reaction.[20] False-negative tests have been reported in only five subjects undergoing local anesthetic testing.

Incremental challenge is used to confirm a negative skin test and should be used before a clinical trial of the drug is recommended.[20] This test involves subcutaneous injection of increasing dilutions and volumes of the local anesthetic. One study concluded that local anesthetics can be safely used despite the history of previous reactions if skin tests are negative and incremental challenge is used.[21]

Patch testing is the accepted method for identifying the cell-mediated hypersensitivity reaction. The drug is applied directly to the skin to detect local hypersensitivity.[22] The appearance of erythema, swelling, papules, and vesicles within 24 to 48 hours implies a positive reaction. Patch testing does not detect the types of reactions due to circulating IgE antibodies.

The leukocyte histamine release test (LHRT) is an in vitro correlate of IgE mediated allergy.[23] The test involves incubation of washed leukocytes from the patient with and without the implicated local anesthetic. Histamine released is measured and is expressed as the percentage of total leukocyte histamine (in basophils) released into the resultant supernatant. In one study,[24] the LHRT was thought to be useful in confirming skin testing, especially negative or inconclusive skin tests. The authors believed that if both skin testing and the LHRT are negative, the likelihood of an anaphylactic reaction is small. They went on to state, though, that direct challenge in vivo, starting with low dosage and with proper monitoring and preparation for resuscitation, is the final resort in unresolved cases.

Although anaphylactic reactions to local anesthetics, especially the aminoamides, are relatively rare, prompt and aggressive treatment is necessary when this condition occurs. Many standard internal medicine or emergency medicine textbooks discuss detailed treatment protocols.[25,26] Some highlights of therapy will be discussed.

All parturients should have a large intravenous line established before a conduction anesthetic is administered. Clinical manifestations of an anaphylactic reaction may vary from mild to severe and the chosen therapy should vary accordingly. Early recognition is critical since irreversible anoxic organ damage or death can occur rapidly. Initial pharmacologic therapy for a mild reaction is the subcutaneous injection of epinephrine 0.2 to 0.5 mg repeated every 20 to 30 minutes as necessary. If generalized urticaria or hypotension occurs, subcutaneous absorption may be unpredictable and the epinephrine should be given by the intramuscular route. In the more severe reaction, the immediate goals of therapy include correction of hypoxemia, inhibition of further chemical mediator release, and restoration of intravascular volume and blood pressure. Supplemental oxygen should be given and intravenous epinephrine (5 μg/kg) should be administered immediately, but cautiously.[27] Aortocaval compression should be avoided by using left uterine displacement in the pregnant woman. In extreme circumstances, endotracheal intubation and controlled ventilation may be necessary. A crystalloid or colloid infusion should accompany the other therapeutic measures in order to replace intravascular volume. Diphenhydramine 0.5 to 1.0 mg/kg is useful in reducing the likelihood that circulating histamine will bind to unoccupied receptors. Aminophylline 6 mg/kg (loading dose) over 20 to 30 minutes followed by an infusion of 0.5 to 1.0 mg/kg/h may be used to relieve bronchospasm. In the parturient, ephedrine is still the vasopressor of choice, but other emergency drugs, including dopamine, norepinephrine, metaraminol, or phenylephrine, may be required to maintain adequate arterial pressure. Steroids may be useful in preventing late sequelae.[28]

A full-blown anaphylactic reaction can have devastating effects. Because of this, appropriate resuscitative equipment, including the necessary medications, should be available whenever a local conduction anesthetic is administered.

REFERENCES

1. Baker JD, Blackman BB: Local anesthesia. Clin Plastic Surg 12:25, 1985
2. Moore DC: Toxicity of local anesthetics in obstetrics. Clin Anaesthesiol 4:113, 1986
3. Covino BG, Vassollo HG: Local anesthetics: Mechanisms of Action and Clinical Use. p. 123. Grune & Stratton, Orlando, FL, 1976.
4. Giovannetti JA, Bennett CR: Assessment of allergy to local anesthetics. JAMA 98:701, 1979
5. VanArsdel PP: Diagnosing drug allergy. JAMA 247:2576, 1982
6. Adriana J, Naraghi M: Etiology and management of ad-

verse reactions to local anesthetics. J Am Med Wom Assoc 33:365, 1978
7. Gell DG, Coombs RRA: Classification of allergic reactions responsible for clinical hypersensitivity and disease. In Clinical Aspects of Immunology. 2nd Ed. Blackwell Scientific Publications, Oxford/Longon, 1962
8. Canfield DW, Gage TW: A guideline to local anesthetic allergy testing. Anesth Prog 34:157, 1987
9. Altman LC: Basic immune mechanisms in immediate hypersensitivity. Med Clin North Am 65:941, 1981
10. Adriani J, Zepernick R: Allergic reactions to local anesthetics. South Med J 74:669, 1981
11. Stoelting R: Allergic reactions during anesthesia. Anesth Analg 62:341, 1983
12. Adriani J: Labatt's Regional Anesthesia: Techniques and Clinical Applications. p. 78. Warren H. Green, Inc., St. Louis, 1985
13. Lynas RFA: A suspected allergic reaction to lidocaine. Anesthesiology 31:380, 1969
14. Morrisset LM: Fatal anaphylactic reaction to lidocaine. Armed Forces Med J 8:740, 1957
15. Brown DT, Beamish D, Wildsmith JAW: Allergic reaction to an amide local anesthetic. Br J Anaesth 53:435, 1981
16. Falace DA, Hill JS: Allergy to lidocaine and mepivacaine: report of a case. Compend Continuing Educ Dentist 6:280, 1985
17. Kennedy KS, Cave RH: Anaphylactic reaction to lidocaine. Arch Otolaryngeal Head Neck Surg 112:671, 1986
18. Schatz M: Skin testing and incremental challenge in the evaluation of adverse reactions to local anesthetics. J Allergy Clin Immunol 74:606, 1984
19. Seng GF, Gay BJ: Dangers of sulfites in dental local anesthetic solutions: warning and recommendations. JADA 113:769, 1986
20. Schatz M, Fung DL: Anaphylactic and anaphylactoid reactions due to anesthetic agents. Clin Rev Allergy 4:215, 1986
21. Chandler MJ, Grammer LC, Patterson R: Provocative challenge with local anesthetics in patients with a prior history of reaction. J Allergy Clin Immunol 79:883, 1987
22. Shelley WB: The patch test. JAMA 200:874, 1967
23. Assem ESK, Vickers MR: Investigation of the response to some haptenic determinants in penicillin allergy by skin and in vitro allergy tests. Clin Allergy 5:43, 1975
24. Assem ESK, Punnia-Moorthy A: Allergy to local anaesthetics: an approach to definitive diagnosis. Br Dent J 164:44, 1988
25. Lichtenstein L: Anaphylaxis. p. 1950. In Wyngaarden JB, Smith LH (eds): Cecil Textbook of Medicine. 18th ed. WB Saunders, Philadelphia, 1988.
26. Lindzon RD, Silvers WS: Anaphylaxis. p. 203. In Rosen P (ed): Emergency Medicine: Concepts and Clinical Practice. 2nd ed. CV Mosby, St. Louis, 1988
27. Kelley JF, Patterson R: Anaphylaxis: course, mechanisms, and treatment. JAMA 227:1431, 1974
28. Wasserman SI: Anaphylaxis. p. 689. In Middleton E (ed): Allergy. 2nd Ed. CV Mosby, St. Louis, 1983

ANESTHETIC CONSIDERATIONS FOR PARTURIENTS WITH HERPES SIMPLEX OR CHORIOAMNIONITIS

HERPES SIMPLEX VIRUS TYPE II

Over the past decade, the incidence and prevalence of infection with genital herpes simplex virus (HSV) has dramatically increased, especially in the reproductive-age group.[1] The herpes simplex virus causes a chronically recurring disease process that is characterized by asymptomatic periods with episodes of viral reactivation from its latent phase in sensory ganglia and postganglionic nerve fibers. Approximately 1 percent of obstetric patients have a history of HSV infection. Many controversies and concerns surround the anesthetic care of the parturient with HSV.

The Virus

The herpesviruses are double-stranded DNA viruses and include cytomegalovirus, Epstein-Barr virus, varicella-zoster virus, and the herpes simplex virus. Two different subtypes of viruses, HSV-I and HSV-II are responsible for genital herpes infection. The HSV-II subtype leads to 93 percent of primary infection and 98 percent of recurrent infections. The remainder of the infections are caused by HSV-I.

The Disease

Primary maternal HSV infections are associated with viremia, and symptoms include fever, headache, and lymphadenopathy. Approximately 8 percent of these patients have aseptic meningitis.[2] During the first 20 weeks of gestation, there is an associated increase in frequency of stillbirths, spontaneous abortions, and congenital malformations.[3] Transplacental transmission may occur during the primary infection.

Recurrent episodes, on the other hand, are manifested by localized outbreaks and, since viremia is absent, the occurrence of systemic symptoms and meningitis are rare. Viral shedding in the birth canal, however, can occur for up to 2 weeks after healing of the lesion. Asymptomatic shedding can also occur.[4] Of women with a confirmed history of recurrent infection, 1.4 percent will have virus in the lower genital tract at the time of labor.[5]

Neonatal Infection

The incidence of HSV infection in the neonate is estimated to be between 1:2500 to 1:10,000 deliveries per year.[3] The consequences of this infection can be heartbreaking. The virus is usually transmitted to the neonate during delivery by passage through an infected maternal genital tract. Ascending infection, especially with prolonged rupture of membranes, or transplacental virus transmission can occur.

Clinical evidence of infection is usually present between 5 to 17 days of life. It can be limited to the skin, eyes, and mouth or it can affect the central nervous system and visceral organs to cause hepatitis, pneumonitis, disseminated intravascular coagulopathy, and encephalitis.[6] Death can occur in up to 50 percent of infants with disseminated disease, even with antiviral therapy.

Women with active genital lesions or positive cultures at term are advised to avoid neonatal exposure by undergoing cesarean delivery.

Anesthesia

The use of regional anesthesia in obstetric patients with HSV infections is a controversial topic. Two major issues arise. The first issue centers around the possibility of introducing the virus into the central nervous system during the placement of a subarachnoid or epidural anesthetic, resulting in meninigitis or encephalitis, especially in primary infection when viremia is present. Second, if postoperative headache or neurologic sequelae occur, it may be difficult to exclude the regional anesthetic from the differential diagnosis in a patient with HSV infection.

The literature on this topic has been limited to date. Ranvindran et al., in 1982, reported a study in which 30 patients with HSV infection who received epidural anesthesia had no complications related to anesthesia.[7] The authors, however, did not indicate if any patient had a primary infection.

In 1986, Ramanathan et al. reported a retrospective series of patients with recurrent genital herpes infection who underwent cesarean delivery. None of the patients who received general (28 patients) or epidural (48 patients) anesthesia developed any neurologic or anesthetic complications.[8] Indeed, 75 percent of patients who received epidural anesthesia had lesions at the time of delivery. Crosby et al., in 1989, presented the results of a 6-year retrospective analysis of 89 patients with active recurrent HSV infections who received epidural anesthesia and had no septic or neurologic complications related to anesthesia.[9]

Most recently, Bader, Camann, and Datta performed a 6-year retrospective study of the anesthetics of 169 patients who underwent cesarean delivery because of both primary and recurrent HSV infection (awaiting publication).[10] None of the 164 patients with recurrent infection had anesthetic-related complications with either subarachnoid or epidural anesthesia. Of the five patients with no previous history of HSV infection, three received spinal anesthesia and two received general anesthesia. The only postoperative complication was a transient leg weakness, which spontaneously resolved in a patient with the diagnosis of primary HSV infection who received a spinal anesthetic.

These studies demonstrate that both subarachnoid and epidural anesthetics are safe choices for a parturient with recurrent HSV infection. The safety of regional anesthesia for parturients with primary infection remains unclear.

CHORIOAMNIONITIS

Chorioamnionitis is present in approximately 1 percent of all parturients and is one of the most common infectious processes to occur in the pregnant woman.[11] It is usually accompanied by fever, chills, elevated white cell count, and fetal tachycardia, and is a frequent cause of both maternal and fetal sepsis as well as congenital pneumonia. Both aerobic and anaerobic bacteria found in the lower genital tract may be responsible for chorioamnionitis. The most common organisms are group B streptococci *Escherichia coli*.[12]

The complex mechanism of this process includes direct placental transport of maternal blood-borne infectious agents to the fetus and amniotic fluid as well as ascending infection through ruptured membranes into the intrauterine cavity. Amniotic fluid generally protects against infection with specific antibacterial substances, including lysozymes and immunoglobulins. Rupture of the amniotic membrane has a potential to lead to infection, especially with prolonged duration. Delivery of the fetus is the only definitive cure.

Anesthesia

Although epidural anesthesia is desired by many pregnant women, it may be denied by the anesthesiologist to the febrile patient for fear of seeding bacteria into the epidural or subarachnoid space. To date, no clear relationship has been demonstrated between the febrile parturient and the possibility of bacteremia. Blanco et al., in 1981, reported the incidence of bacteremia in febrile pregnant women as 9 percent. Therefore, approximately 90 percent of these patients had negative cultures.[11] In another study, these investigators reported that there is an 8 percent incidence of bacteremia in chorioamnionitis and that approximately half of these patients with positive blood cultures were not febrile.[13] Absence of fever does not mean absence of bacteremia.

There have been no reports of epidural abscess or meningitis following regional anesthesia in patients with chorioamnionitis. A recent retrospective study by Vaddadi et al. assessed the use of epidural anesthesia in parturients with chorioamnionitis.[14] Of the 115 patients who received regional anesthesia, none developed signs or symptoms of epidural abscess or meningitis. The authors did not include blood cultures in their study, so the incidence of actual bacteremia was not available.

Recently, Carp and Bailey attempted to further delineate the relationship between bacteremia and the risk of developing meningitis after dural puncture.[15] Forty chronically bacteremic rats were studied 24 hours after undergoing cisternal puncture. Bacteremic rats after cisternal puncture showed evidence of central nervous system infection, whereas bacteremic animals not having cisternal puncture had sterile spinal fluid. In addition, in the absence of bacteremia, the cisternal puncture did not result in infection. While this study suggests the possibility that bacteremia is a risk factor in developing meningitis, the extrapolation to humans undergoing intraspinal anesthesia is not clear.

REFERENCES

1. Brown ZA, Berry S, Vontver LA: Genital herpes simplex virus infections complicating pregnancy. J Reprod Med 31:440, 1986
2. Corey L, Adams HG, Brown ZA, et al: Genital herpes simplex virus infections: clinical manifestations, course and complications. Ann Intern Med 98:958, 1983
3. Stagno S, Whitley RJ: Herpes virus infections in pregnancy. N Engl J Med 313:1327, 1985
4. Brock B, Selke S, Benedetti J, et al: Frequency of asymptomatic shedding of herpes simplex virus in women with genital herpes. JAMA 203:418, 1990
5. Arvin A, Hensleigh PA, Prober CG, et al: Failure of antepartum maternal cultures to predict the infants risk of exposure to herpes simplex virus at delivery. N Engl J Med 315:796, 1986
6. Kibrick S: Herpes simplex infection at term. What to do with mother, newborn, and nursery personnel. JAMA 243:157, 1980
7. Ravindran RS, Gupta CD, Stoops CA: Epidural analgesia in the presence of patients with herpes simplex virus (type 2) infection. Anesth Analg 62:714, 1982
8. Ramanathan S, Sheth R, Turndorf H: Anesthesia for cesarean section in patients with genital herpes infection: a retrospective study. Anesthesiology 64:807, 1986
9. Crosby ET, Halpern SH, Rolbin SH: Epidural anesthesia for cesarean section in patients with active recurrent genital herpes simplex infections: a retrospective review. Can J Anesth 36:701, 1989
10. Bader AM, Camann WR, Datta S: Anesthesia for cesarean section in patients with herpes simplex virus type 2 infections. Reg Anesth 15:261, 1990
11. Blanco JD, Gibbs RS, Castaneda YS: Bacteremia in obstetrics: Clinical course. Obstet Gynecol 58:621, 1981
12. Schnider S, Levinson G: Anesthesia for Obstetrics. 2nd ed. Williams & Wilkins, Baltimore, 1987
13. Gibbs RS, Castillo MS, Rodgers PJ: Management of acute chorioamnionitis. Am J Obstet Gynecol 136:709, 1980
14. Vaddadi A, Ramanathan J, Angel J, et al: Epidural anesthesia in women with chorioamnionitis (a retrospective study). Anesthesiology 71(Suppl): A 863, 1989
15. Carp H, Bailey S: Meningitis after dural puncture in bacteremic rats. Anesthesiology 71(Suppl): A 862, 1989

SEPTIC SHOCK IN OBSTETRICS

Septic shock is a clinical syndrome of hypotension and hypoperfusion induced by an infective agent and mediated by host defense systems. It is the most frequent cause of death in the intensive care unit in the United States and its incidence is increasing, in part because of increased use of immunosuppressive drugs, broad-spectrum antibiotics, and invasive monitoring devices.

Obstetric patients seem to have much lower mortality from septic shock compared with the general population (0 to 3 percent versus 40 to 90 percent).[1] However, because the overall mortality in parturients is very low, septic shock contributes a significant percentage of the deaths occurring in obstetric patients.

The sources of septic infection in obstetrics are premature rupture of membranes with subsequent chorioamnionitis, endometritis, pyelonephritis, wound infections, and septic abortions.[2] Common pathogens in the septic parturient are *Escherichia coli*, *Klebsiella* sp., *Enterobacter* sp., *Proteus* sp., *Pseudomonas* sp., *Streptococci* sp., and *Bacteroides* sp.[3]

The mainstay of therapy for sepsis and septic shock is eradication of the nidus of infection. In obstetrics, this often equates with delivery, such as in the case of chorioamnionitis, but other problems may involve surgical procedures, such as drainage of abcesses. Appropriate antibiotic therapy is essential but does not replace the need for surgical drainage or debridement if a pus collection can be located.

Concomitant supportive therapy is essential to minimize morbidity or mortality from septic shock. Support of the circulation with volume, vasopressors, and ino-

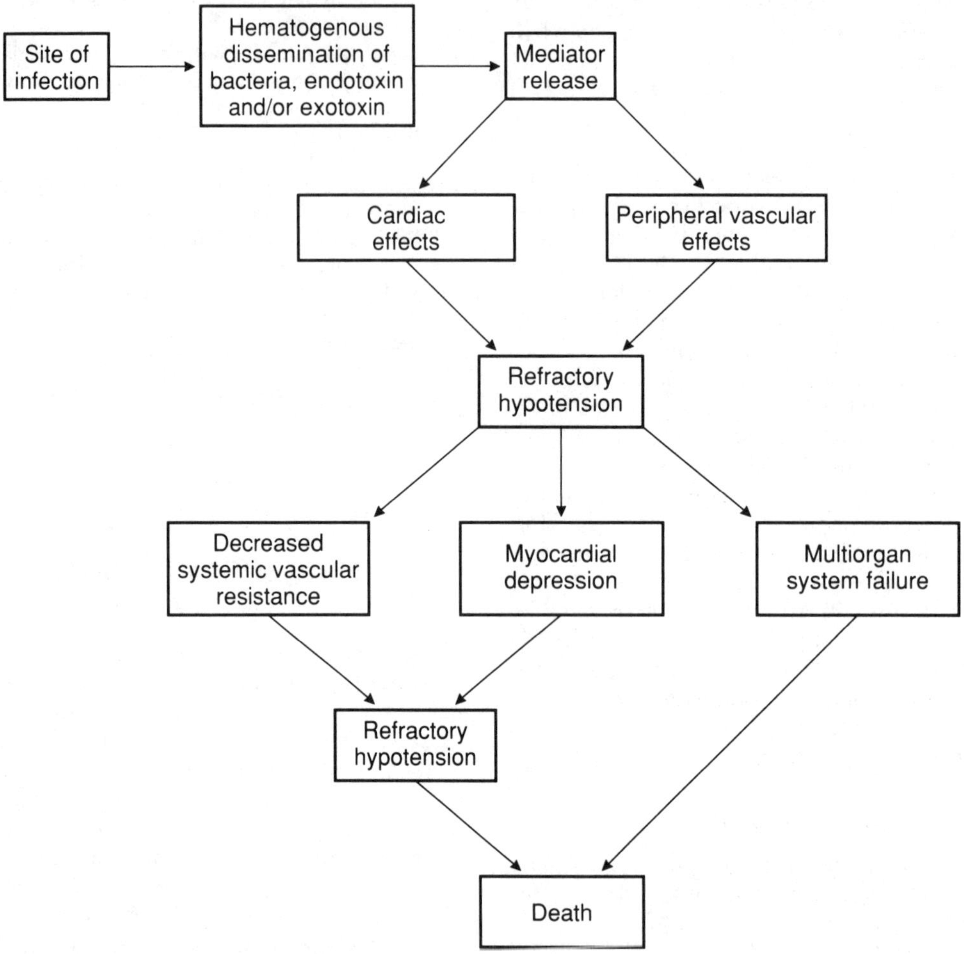

Fig. 10-1. The pathophysiology of septic shock. (Adapted from Hoffman and Natanson,[4] with permission.)

tropes as indicated is crucial (Fig. 10-2), as death is usually the sequela of severe hypoperfusion of vital organs. Careful attention must also be paid to avoiding and/or treating complications such as acute respiratory distress syndrome (ARDS), disseminated intravascular coagulation, acute tubular necrosis, and hepatic failure, which occur frequently in this setting. Any treatment of the pregnant patient must include consideration of the effects of therapy on the fetus if the fetus is likely to survive (e.g., the effects of vasopressors on uteroplacental perfusion).

Certain therapies directed toward neutralizing the mediators of septic shock (i.e., naloxone, monoclonal antibodies, prostaglandin inhibitors, etc.) are in experimental stages of development and cannot be uniformly recommended.[4]

Anesthesiologists may be called on to assist in the management of these critically ill patients either pre- or postpartum, to assist in managing delivery of the patient, or often in the postpartum period to anesthetize a patient for a procedure such as dilatation and curettage or hysterectomy.

The basic principles of caring for parturients apply to these patients as well. These include prophylaxis against aspiration of gastric contents (nonparticulate antacid, metoclopramide, and rapid-sequence induction of general anesthesia utilizing cricoid pressure), prevention of aortocaval compression by left uterine displacement, and a thorough understanding of the physiologic changes occurring during pregnancy.

Attention to ventilation and oxygenation is of prime importance because of the additional stress of the hy-

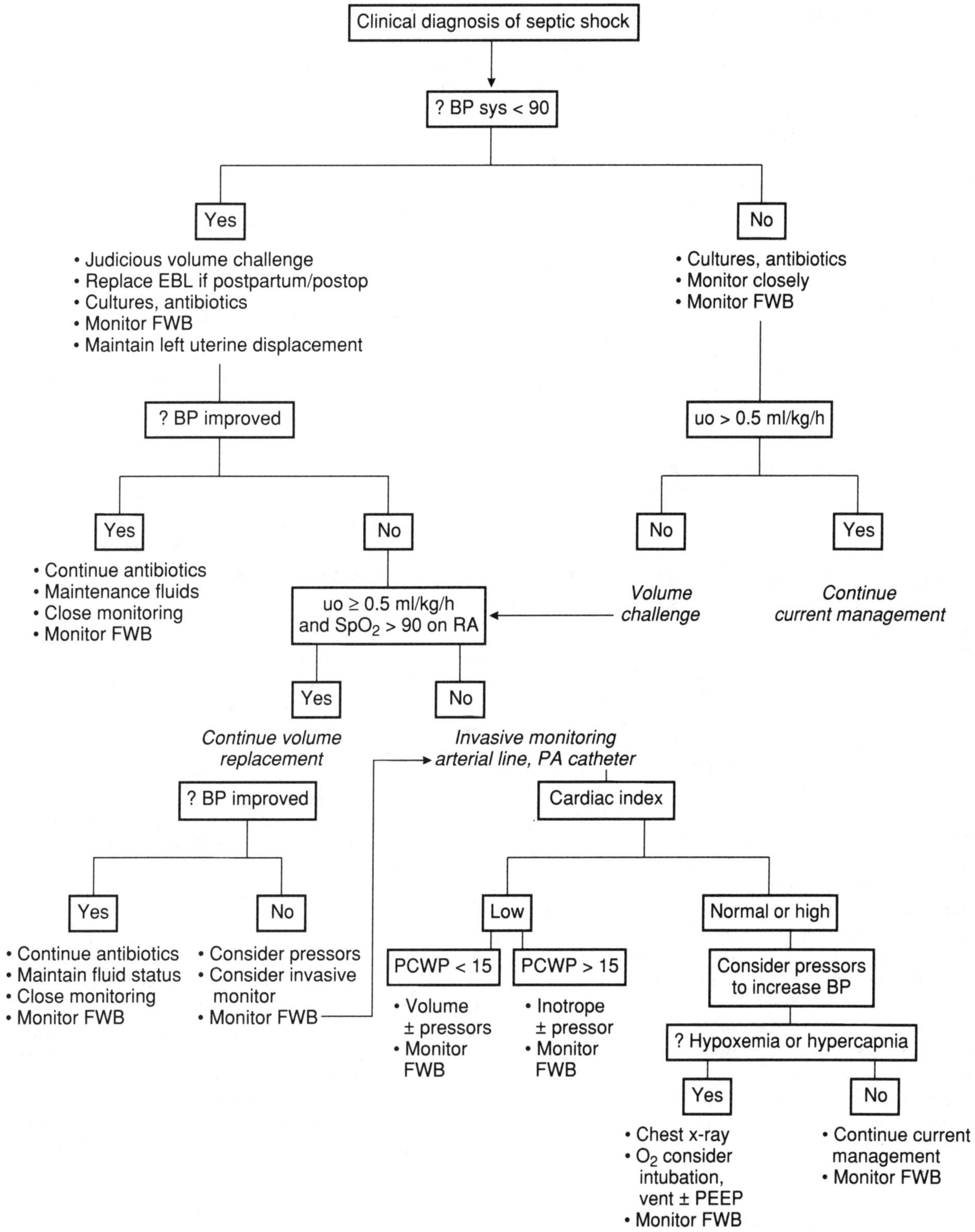

Fig. 10-2. A decision tree for the treatment of the septic obstetric patient. EBL, estimated blood loss; FWB, fetal well-being; BP, blood pressure.

permetabolic state of sepsis superimposed on that of pregnancy, which is complicated by decreased lung volumes and functional residual capacity. Supplemental oxygen should be provided and oxygen saturation monitored continuously with a pulse oximeter. Arterial catheterization should be considered early in the course of the disease to allow frequent arterial blood gas determinations and close monitoring of blood pressure. The development of ARDS is a ominous complication of sepsis and should be treated with intubation, mechanical ventilation, and positive end-expiratory pressure as necessary.

Another primary goal of anesthetic management in these patients is to optimize perfusion and cardiac performance (see Fig. 10-2). Initial attempts should be directed toward ensuring adequate preload. This consists of preventing aortocaval compression and providing volume replacement. Further therapy with inotropes and vasopressors should, in general, be guided by information derived from pulmonary artery catheterization (i.e., cardiac index, stroke volume, and systemic vascular resistance).

Choices of anesthetic technique may be limited by the patient's condition. Although each case requires careful consideration, and exceptions may exist, regional anesthesia is contraindicated in the setting of systemic sepsis, usually for one or more of the following reasons. First, it would be undesirable to inoculate the cerebrospinal fluid or central nervous system of a bacteremic patient by use of a spinal or epidural needle. Second, the patient may have developed a coagulopathy, which would prohibit the use of regional anesthesia. Lastly, patients who are hypotensive, volume depleted, and with limited myocardial reserve may tolerate a subarachnoid or epidural-induced sympathectomy very poorly.

General anesthesia may be undertaken safely, utilizing a rapid-sequence induction, with ketamine 1 to 2 mg/kg and succinylcholine 1.5 mg/kg. Alternatively, patients who have had adequate intravascular volume replacement may tolerate small doses of thiopental, although caution must be exercised. Continuous monitoring of fetal heart rate should be employed to help prevent detrimental decreases in uteroplacental perfusion, particularly if vasopressors are utilized.

Postoperatively, provisions must be made to continue the aggressive care and monitoring initiated in the labor suite or operating room. An intensive care setting may be necessary to provide the optimum care for these patients, who are susceptible to developing further complications postoperatively or postpartum. Close monitoring or cardiorespiratory, renal, and metabolic function must be provided, with rapid institution of support if necessary. Consultation with subspecialists such as infectious disease, renal, and gastroenterology experts may be required if significant improvement does not occur rapidly once the infectious source is eradicated.

REFERENCES

1. Creasy RK, Resnick R (eds): Material and Fetal Medicine: Principles and Practice. p. 457 WB Saunders, Philadelphia, 1989
2. Camann WR, Tuomala R: Infectious disease. p. 557. In Datta S (ed): Management of High-Risk Pregnancy. Mosby-Yearbook Medical Publishers, St. Louis, Chicago, 1991.
3. Lee WL, Clark SL, Cotton DB, et al: Septic shock during pregnancy. Am J Obstet Gynecol 159:410, 1988
4. Hoffman WD, Natanson C: Bacterial septic shock. Anesth Clin North Am 7:845, 1989

REGIONAL ANESTHESIA IN OBSTETRIC PATIENTS WITH PREVIOUS SPINAL SURGERY

A history of previous major spinal surgery is considered by some anesthesiologists to be a relative contraindication to intraspinal anesthesia because of questions regarding its safety and efficacy. The guidelines are unclear because the available literature concerning this topic is very limited.

In the North American population, the incidence of scoliosis is approximately 0.4 percent. Spinal curves of less than 10 degrees are equally common in males and females, whereas curves of greater than 20 degrees, which require treatment, are seven times more frequent in females.[1] Idiopathic scoliosis is more common than other causes, which include neurologic diseases (poliomyelitis, neurofibromatosis, cerebral palsy), myopathic disorders (muscular dystrophy, myotonic dystrophy), connective tissue disorders (rheumatoid arthritis, Marfan's syndrome), vertebral anomalies, and infection (particularly tuberculosis).[2] Thoracolumbar curves are more common than isolated thoracic or lumbar curvature. The severity of the disease is determined by measuring the degree of spinal curvature. Curves of greater than 60 degrees, if untreated, can lead to cardiopulmonary compromise, progressive deformity, and early death due to cardiorespiratory failure.

In female parturients with untreated scoliosis, pregnancy may exacerbate both the degree of spinal curvature and the extent of cardiopulmonary compromise. Maternal morbidity and mortality correlate well with the severity of functional impairment that existed in the prepregnant state. Patients who have undergone corrective surgery for scoliosis tolerate pregnancy, labor, and delivery well, although the incidence of operative delivery in these patients is 2.4 times greater than that for normal parturients.[2]

Treatment for scoliosis is most frequently sought because of symptoms of back pain, but also for curve progression, poor body image, and deterioration of pulmonary function.[10] In a skeletally immature patient, spinal curves of less than 40 to 45 degrees are usually best treated with an orthotic device, whereas curves of greater than 45 to 50 degrees are usually managed by spinal fusion with internal fixation.[3] The object of spinal fusion is to create a bony fusion of the spinal curve that should include all rotated vertebrae.

In 1947, Paul R. Harrington began to develop his surgical treatment for scoliosis while working with poliomyelitis patients, among whom he saw a high prevalence of spinal deformities and pulmonary compromise. He developed the Harrington instrumentation as a means of halting progression and gaining correction of the spinal deformity. This technique consists of decortication of the laminae and transverse processes followed by removal of the spinous processes together with the interspinous soft tissue. Next, a distraction and compression system is applied. This system is comprised of a smooth distraction rod with ratchets at its upper end, a threaded compression rod with hooks locked into position by twisting nuts on the threaded rod, and a selection of hooks. Afterward, facets are fused in the thoracic area and lateral transverse processes are fused in the lumbar region; then an autogenous iliac bone graft is added. Newer methods of spinal fusion include the Lugue and Cotrel-Dubousset techniques.[3]

Spinal fusion should not be extended caudally to L4, because fusion to L5 is associated with a high incidence of low back pain at long-term follow-up. Harrington fusion to L5 or S1 also produces an unacceptable loss of lumbar lordosis and increases stress on the lower back. Idiopathic scoliosis does not involve L5 or S1, so fusion to these levels is not necessary.[3]

Early surgical correction (prior to adulthood) results in significant increases in lung volume postoperatively and prevents the cardiopulmonary complications. The degree of curvature is reduced by 50 percent, and 85 to 90 percent of back pain is relieved. There may be a long-term increased incidence of degenerative disease due to a reduction in the number of mobile lumbar spinal segments, which leads to increased mechanical stress on those segments below the level of fusion.[2] Other complications are most commonly perioperative, due to anesthetic complications or to cord injury (less than 0.5 percent of cases), direct trauma, vascular compromise or overdistraction with neurologic impairment. Early postoperative complications include wound infection; pulmonary, gastrointestinal, and urinary problems, and hook dislodgment. Late postoperative problems include failure to produce a solid spinal arthrodesis, which results in increased stress on the rod, metal fatigue and rod breakage, and bursitis.[3]

EPIDURAL ANESTHESIA

Epidural anesthesia after major spinal surgery has been considered as relatively contraindicated because of a number of potential complications. The epidural space may be difficult to identify because of surgical and degenerative changes. Insertion of a needle through a midline or lateral approach in the fused region may not be possible because of presence of scar tissue and bone graft. Ideally, the needle should be inserted below the lowest fused segment, however, this area often undergoes retrolisthesis and spondylolisthesis; furthermore, 20 percent of patients have fusions involving L4-L5.[2] Multiple attempts may be necessary for successful epidural placement. Surgical obliteration of the epidural space may lead to unintentional dural puncture. An epidural blood patch may be difficult to perform if a significant post-dural puncture headache results. Blood vessel trauma may also be more likely to occur. There is a possibility of introducing infection during the procedure, which is of particular concern in these patients because of the present of a foreign body. There may be unpredictable spread of local anesthetic, resulting in a "patchy" block. This is attributed to injury to the ligamentum flavum during surgery, which causes adhesions or obliteration of the epidural space in some areas. An increased volume or concentration of local anesthetic may be required to achieve an adequate block.[2] Patients with idiopathic scoliosis or neuromyopathic syndromes that predispose to scoliosis may have an increased incidence of malignant hyperthermia. Significant respiratory compromise may occur if intercostal muscles are paralyzed as a result of a high level of anesthesia. Persistent back pain may exist even after surgical correction of scoliosis and pregnancy may exacerbate this problem. Coincidental exacerbation of musculoskeletal or neurologic symptoms secondary to the underlying disorder may be attributed to the epidural anesthetic, which may pose a medicolegal issue. Finally, these patients have a high degree of anxiety regarding their backs and they may be reluctant to consent to epidural anesthesia.

The significance of most of these potential complications of epidural anesthesia is *not* supported by the limited literature that exists. In 1985, Hubbert discussed his experience with attempted epidural anesthesia in 17 obstetric patients with Harrington rod spinal fusion. Nine attempts resulted in epidural anesthesia, whereas two resulted in unintentional dural puncture. Numerous "false" losses of resistance were encountered and 11 patients underwent multiple attempts at various interspaces, using both midline and lateral approaches. In one patient, blood was encountered in each of three attempts. The volume and concentration of local anesthetic required to produce an adequate epidural block did not differ from patients without spinal fusion, and no patients reported postpartum back pain or other complications.[4]

In 1989, Crosby and Halpern reported a retrospective study of 16 patients with previous Harrington rod instrumentation for correction of idiopathic scoliosis who requested epidural anesthesia for labor. Of the nine epidural procedures, four required multiple attempts and two never received adequate anesthesia. Complications included failure to identify the epidural space despite attempts at two interspaces, blood vessel trauma, and dural puncture. Thirty-eight percent of their patients required operative delivery.[2]

Daley et al., in 1990, reviewed their experience with 18 patients who had a history of previous major spinal surgery and who requested epidural anesthesia for labor. Fifteen of 21 attempts produced satisfactory anesthesia; however, four patients required larger than usual doses of local anesthetic. No correlation was seen between the ease of insertion or quality of anesthesia and the surgical level.[5]

Feldstein and Ramanathan, in 1985, reported successful lumbar epidural anesthesia for labor and cesarean delivery in three patients with a history of extensive spinal surgery. They found no difference in onset of action, spread, dose requirement, highest sensory level achieved, or duration of action of local anesthetic from that expected for normal parturients.[1]

In 1978, Carlson reported a successful epidural anesthetic for cesarean delivery in a 25-year-old woman with severe, uncorrected idiopathic kyphoscoliosis.[6] As Carlson discussed, lesions of the lumbar spine may cause changes in the pelvic architecture severe enough to lead to dystocia. Thoracic spinal lesions may cause disorders of normal cardiac and pulmonary function that are exacerbated as a result of the normal rise in cardiac output during pregnancy and labor as well as the encroachment of the enlarging uterus on the nondistensible thorax; which does not allow the normal increase in maternal alveolar ventilation to occur. Carlson suggested several advantages of epidural anesthesia for patients with scoliosis: avoidance of the use of respiratory depressants such as narcotics during labor; minimization of the undesirable rise in cardiac output during labor; and a means of providing postoperative analgesia, which attenuates the reduction in vital capacity that normally follows abdominal surgery because of pain-induced limitation of respiratory excursion.[6]

Few large studies involve epidural anesthesia for obstetric patients after major spinal surgery. However, the existing literature fails to show any long-term complications due to the procedure. Despite the potential short-term complications, the available reports indicate that epidural anesthesia is safe and usually effective for these patients.[7–11]

An antepartum anesthetic consultation is necessary in order to discuss anesthetic and analgesic options with the patient in a relatively stress-free environment. The patient must be advised of the potential difficulties of epidural needle insertion as well as the lack of evidence for long-term adverse sequelae. Furthermore, the prelabor consultation affords the anesthesiologist an opportunity to obtain a complete history and physical examination, which should include documentation of existing low back pain, or cardiopulmonary or neurologic dysfunction. Spine roentgenograms and operative reports should be obtained to determine the lowest level of fused vertebrae. If these are not available, the lower extent of spinal surgery must be estimated based on patient history (which is often unreliable) and physical examination. No spinous processes will be palpable in the fused region, and the incisional scar usually extends to one level below the lowest level of the fusion.

Many spinal fusions have the appearance of Swiss cheese on x-ray examination. The midline approach to the epidural space may not be possible with an appliance in place. However, it is a reasonable approach in the patient with a long fusion, particularly in the lower lumbar area, even when no spinous processes are palpable.

Patients with a history of major spinal surgery should *not* be automatically denied epidural anesthesia for labor and delivery. Insertion of the epidural needle and catheter may be attempted, providing that the patient and anesthesiologist are both aware of the increased incidence of short-term complications and of the possibility of failure to obtain satisfactory anesthesia.

SUBARACHNOID ANESTHESIA

Although some anesthesiologists avoid subarachnoid anesthesia in obstetric patients who have undergone previous spinal surgery, the limited available literature suggests that subarachnoid anesthesia is a safe and effective alternative to general anesthesia for these patients. In 1980, Berkowitz and Gold performed 42 successful subarachnoid anesthetics in patients with previous lumbar laminectomies without complications. Interestingly, they pointed out that while some anesthesiologists are reluctant to perform subarachnoid anesthesia in patients with previous spinal surgery, radiologists routinely perform myelograms in patients with laminectomies or spinal fusions, injecting a radiopaque dye into the subarachnoid space.[12] In Hubbert's 1985 report on epidural anesthesia for patients with spinal fusions, 2 out of 17 patients received adequate subarachnoid anesthesia (after unintentional dural puncture or unsuccessful epidural placement) without complications.[13]

Subarachnoid anesthesia is a useful alternative for obstetric patients with previous spinal surgery after an unintentional dural puncture occurs or when epidural placement is unsuccessful. Furthermore, subarachnoid blocks may have some advantages over epidural anesthesia. Subarachnoid injection may be technically easier in these patients, due to disruption of the epidural space by surgery or degenerative changes. A subarachnoid anesthetic may also provide a more reliable and complete spread of local anesthetic solution with less likelihood of obtaining a "patchy" block, as is sometimes seen with epidural anesthesia (thought to be secondary to adhesions and obliteration of areas of the epidural space). In 1990, Johnson and Moran, while administering continuous spinal anesthesia for an obstetric patient with severe kyphoscoliosis and congenital heart disease, found that a distortion of the spinal column may cause an alteration in the normal gravity-directed distribution of hyperbaric local anesthetic solution in the cerebrospinal fluid. They suggested that the local anesthetic layers in the dependent areas of the spinal column, causing a unilateral block that they were able to raise by the addition of an isobaric local anesthetic solution.[14] Bozeman and Chandra, in 1980, explained this phenomenon on the basis of Valentino's myelography, which showed a unilateral distribution of contrast in patients with severe scoliosis. He proposed that the dura on the convex side of the spine stretches, which presses the spinal cord against the opposite surface of the spinal canal, squeezing the subarachnoid space between the spinal canal wall and the cord. This would hinder movement of local anesthetic in the subarachnoid space.[15] The editor has also found discrepancies in the height of the block that can be achieved with both epidural and subarachnoid anesthesia despite utilization of a number of maneuvers to raise the level of the block.

Subarachnoid and epidural anesthesia carry similar risks of complications, such as blood vessel trauma (possibly less for subarachnoid anesthesia because of the smaller needle size), subdural catheter placement (particularly after multiple attempts or dural puncture),[16] introduction of infection, respiratory compromise due to intercostal muscle paralysis, coincident exacerbation of low back pain during labor and delivery, and patient anxiety. An additional disadvantage to subarachnoid anesthesia may be the difficulty in performing an epidural blood patch on these patients, should a significant postdural puncture headache occur. For this reason, the smallest possible spinal needle or a 32-gauge spinal microcatheter should be used.[17] Such a catheter may actually reduce the incidence of post-dural puncture headache by creating an inflammatory reaction, which seals the hole in the dura after the catheter is removed, thus preventing cerebrospinal fluid leakage into the epidural space. Because of the greater ease of insertion and more reliable anesthesia, subarachnoid anesthesia may be preferable to epidural anesthesia for cesarean delivery, and may be used for labor as well (with a subarachnoid catheter and low concentrations of hyperbaric local anesthetic) in obstetric patients with previous major spinal surgery.

REFERENCES

1. Feldstein G, Ramanathan S: Obstetric lumbar epidural anesthesia in patients with previous posterior spinal fusion for kyphoscoliosis. Anesth Analg 64:83, 1985
2. Crosby ET, Halpern SH: Obstetric epidural anaesthesia in patients with Harrington instrumentation. Can J Anaesth 36:693, 1989
3. Renshaw TS: The role of Harrington instrumentation and posterior spine fusion in the management of adolescent idiopathic scoliosis. Orthop Clin North Am 19:257, 1988
4. Hubbert CH: Epidural anesthesia in patients with spinal fusion. Anesth Analg 64:843, 1985
5. Daley MD, Rolbin S, Hew E, Morningstar B: Continuous epidural anaesthesia for obstetrics after major spinal surgery. Can J Anaesth 37:S112, 1990
6. Carlson W, Engelman DR, Bart J: Epidural anesthesia for cesarean section in kyphoscoliosis. Anesth Analg 57:125, 1978
7. Crawford JS, James FM, Nolte H, et al: Regional analgesia for patients with chronic neurological disease and similar conditions. Anaesthesia 36:821, 1981
8. King HA: Selection of fusion levels for posterior instrumentation and fusion in idiopathic scoliosis. Orthop Clin North Am 19:247, 1988
9. Vaagenes P, Fjaerestad I: Epidural block during labour in a patient with spina bifida cystica. Anaesthesia 36:299, 1981
10. VanDam BE: Operative treatment of adult scoliosis with posterior fusion and instrumentation. Orthop Clin North Am 19:353, 1988
11. Walpole JB: Continuous lumbar epidural block in labour in the presence of a Meurig Williams plate from L1-L4. Br J Anaesth 46:163, 1974

12. Berkowitz S, Gold MI: Spinal anesthesia for surgery in patients with previous lumbar laminectomy. Anesth Analg 59:881, 1980
13. Hubbert CH: Epidural anesthesia in patients with spinal fusion. Anesth Analg 64:843, 1985
14. Moran DH, Johnson MD: Continuous spinal anesthesia with combined hyperbaric and isobaric bupivacaine in a patient with scoliosis. Anesth Analg 70:445, 1990
15. Bozeman PM, Chandra P: Unilateral analgesia following epidural and subarachnoid block. Anesthesiology 52:356, 1980
16. Howard R, Anderson W: Subdural catheterization and opiate administration in a patient with Harrington rods. Can J Anaesth 37:712, 1990
17. Hurley RJ, Lambert DH: Continuous spinal anesthesia with a microcatheter technique: preliminary experience. Anesth Analg 70:97, 1990

MATERNAL MORTALITY

Investigation of maternal mortality is an important form of audit. It identifies major causes of mortality and indicates where further teaching and research may minimize preventable deaths.

Maternal mortality rates (MMR) have fallen dramatically in developed countries during this century. Since 1937, in England and Wales, MMR has fallen from around 400 to 8.6 per 100,000 pregnancies (Fig. 10-3), and United States statistics show similar trends. Several factors have led to this reduction in mortality rate, including the introduction of blood banks, antibiotics, improving maternal health, and better training of midwives and obstetricians. The continuing fall in MMR appears to reflect improved obstetric care. However, a high proportion of the deaths that still occur are associated with avoidable factors or substandard care, indicating that there is further room for improvement.[1]

Although total MMR has fallen, it is distressing for anesthesiologists that the percentage of maternal deaths due to anesthesia appears to be increasing, according to United Kingdom data. Anesthesia is now the third commonest cause of maternal death in England and Wales. The administration of anesthesia, including epidural anesthesia, has increased dramatically over the last two decades, so it is likely that the number of deaths per total number of anesthetics has fallen dramatically.[2] This section concentrates on causes of deaths related to anesthesia before looking at other major causes of maternal death.

DEFINITIONS

1. Maternal mortality rate (MMR): Number of maternal deaths per 100,000 live births. In the U.K. reports, maternal deaths are related to the number of pregnancies, rather than the number of births. Therefore the denominator will be somewhat lower because of twin and other multiple births.
2. Maternal death: "Death of a woman while pregnant, or within 42 days of termination of pregnancy, irrespective of the duration and site of the pregnancy, from any cause related to or aggravated by pregnancy or its management, but not from accidental or incidental causes." (From the International Classification of diseases—9th Revision [ICD 9].)
3. Direct causes: "Those resulting from obstetric complications of the pregnant state (pregnancy, labor and puerperium) from interventions, omissions, incorrect treatment or from a chain of events resulting from any of the above." (ICD-9)
4. Indirect causes: "Those resulting from previous existing disease or disease that developed during pregnancy and which was not due to direct obstetric causes, but which was aggravated by physiological effects of pregnancy." (ICD 9)
5. Nonobstetric–fortuitous causes: Accidental or incidental causes unrelated to pregnancy or its treatment.

Although the International Classification of Disease, 9th Revision, defines a maternal death as occurring within 42 days of the end of pregnancy, recent reports from the United States and the United Kingdom have included deaths up to 1 year, as the shorter time interval may exclude a significant number of deaths.[3–5]

MATERNAL MORTALITY DATA COLLECTION

United States

Registration of maternal deaths has been mandatory in the United States since 1915. Most data have been collected by individual states based on information available on the subject's death certificate. Recent work has demonstrated that data produced by the National Center for Health Statistics seriously underestimates the incidence of maternal deaths.[3–5]

Kaunitz et al. performed a nationwide analysis of maternal deaths from 1974 to 1978, and reported an MMR of 15.3.[6] The maternal mortality collaborative, a special interest group of the American College of Obstetricians and Gynecologists, established voluntary surveillance of maternal deaths in 1983. Nineteen reporting areas of the United States voluntarily contributed reports of deaths for the years 1980 to 1985, representing 20.7 percent of U.S. maternal deaths.[7] They reported an MMR of 14.3, but emphasized this could not be gener-

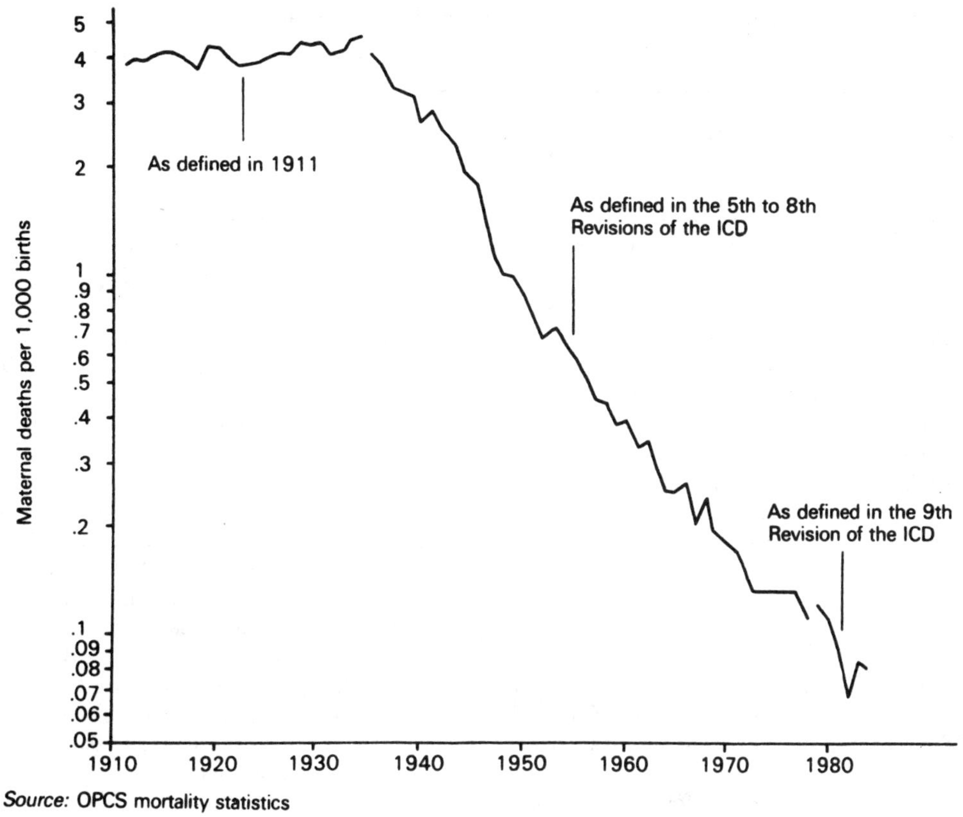

Fig. 10-3. Maternal mortality in England and Wales (1911–1984), plotted on a logarithmic scale. (From Report on Confidential Enquiries into Maternal Deaths in England and Wales in 1982–1984,[1] with permission.)

alized for the whole U.S. population. In both these reports, although deaths related to anesthesia are classified, there is little further information available on them. Sachs and co-workers have reviewed anesthetic-related maternal mortality in Massachusetts over a 30-year period,[8] and this will be discussed later.

United Kingdom

The confidential inquiries into maternal deaths in England and Wales began in 1952, and 11 triennial reports have been produced. The District Medical Officer, who receives all death certificates, institutes the inquiry by sending forms to all the relevant staff. Replies are reviewed by obstetric assessors and, where appropriate, anesthetic assessors. All replies are confidential; names of mothers are deleted from all forms, which are destroyed after the report is published.[2] The retrieval rate is almost 100 percent. From 1952 to 1984, MMR has fallen from 98.9 to 8.6 per 100,000 pregnancies in England and Wales.[1]

These studies provide comprehensive data on causes of maternal death. The section devoted to maternal deaths associated with anesthesia is of major interest to anesthesiologists as it classifies the causes of death and makes recommendations for further improvements.

DEATHS RELATED TO ANESTHESIA

Data from U.K. Confidential Inquiries

The most detailed information regarding anesthesia-related deaths is available in these reports. Since 1973, all cases in which the mother received an anesthetic are reviewed by an anesthetic assessor, thus improving the classification of these deaths. In the latest report, covering the 3-year period from 1982 to 1984, there were 18 deaths directly associated with anesthesia and one further death to which anesthesia contributed.[1] Anesthesia was the third commonest cause of death and there were 7.2 anesthetic-related deaths per million pregnancies (Table 10-11).

Although the number of deaths associated with anes-

Table 10-11. Deaths Associated with Anesthesia: Estimated Rate per Million Pregnancies and Percentage of Direct Maternal Deaths 1970–1984

	1970–1972	1973–1975	1976–1978	1979–1981	1982–1984	1970–1984
Number of deaths directly associated with anaesthesia	37	27	27	22	18	131
Rate per million pregnancies	12.8	10.5	12.1	8.7	7.2	10.2
Percentage of direct maternal deaths	10.8	11.9	12.4	12.4	13.0	11.9

(From Report on Confidential Enquiry into Maternal Deaths in England and Wales, 1982–1984,[1] with permission.)

thesia has fallen continuously over successive trial reports—since 1970 it has fallen from 37 to 18—in all of these deaths, it was ascertained that anesthetic care was substandard. The term *substandard care* takes into account not only poor clinical care, but also includes other factors that might lead to a low standard of care, including inadequate resources for staffing and administrative failures leading to inadequate numbers of anesthesiologists, for example.[9]

The major causes of deaths in this report are as follows:

1. *Inhalation of Gastric Contents.* This occurred in 7 of the 19 patients and was associated with difficulty in endotracheal intubation in 2, with poor postoperative care in 3, and with hemorrhage in 1.
2. *Difficulty with Endotracheal Intubation.* Ten deaths in this report were due to problems with endotracheal intubation and there was one additional late death. Two of these patients also inhaled gastric contents.
3. *Substandard Postoperative Care.* In five patients who died, postoperative care was substandard; three inhaled gastric contents, in one there was unskilled management of artificial ventilation postoperatively, and one patient died of cardiac arrest, probably related to hypoxia, consequent to inadequate reversal of muscle relaxants at the end of general anesthesia.
4. *Hemorrhage.* Hemorrhage was implicated in four patients' deaths.
5. *Miscellaneous.* Other deaths were related to misuse of drugs, including muscle relaxants and sedatives, and to misuse of anesthetic apparatus. There was one death associated with the use of epidural anesthesia. An epidural catheter was injected by a midwife, when an anesthesiologist was not immediately available; a total spinal anesthetic occurred.

Data from U.S. Studies

Anesthesia was implicated in 98 of 247 maternal deaths in Kaunitz' study. Of these, 28 were reportedly due to aspiration of gastric contents.[6] The Maternal Mortality Collaborative reported 42 anesthesia-related deaths in 712 cases investigated.[7] In neither study was there an anesthetic assessor.

Sachs' review of anesthesia-related deaths over three decades in Massachusetts provides more detailed information. Thirty-seven anesthesia-related deaths were recorded between 1954 and 1985—4.2 percent of all maternal deaths; deaths up to 90 days after termination of pregnancy were included. Deaths from aspiration were common during the first decade, when mask anesthesia was commonplace. Cardiorespiratory problems were commoner in the second decade, when regional techniques were used more frequently, but monitoring was insufficient. Only three deaths occurred in the last decade,[8] and all were associated with general endotracheal anesthesia.

Comment

In the conclusion of the section on deaths related to anesthesia in the most recent U.K. triennial report, it was noted that although deaths related to anesthesia continued to fall, there remained problem areas:

1. Insufficient supervision of inexperienced junior anesthesiologists.
2. Poor communication between obstetric and anesthetic teams, with anesthesiologists often being presented with difficult cases as emergencies, with no prior warning.
3. Continuing administrative problems, with too few anesthesiologists for the number of obstetric units.

Inhalation of gastric contents continues to be a common problem in the United Kingdom and the United States; seven patients died in the most recent U.K. report and the Kaunitz study reported 28 of 98 anesthetic deaths had been due to gastric aspiration.[1,6] In the U.K. report, six of seven women who died from gastric aspiration had received magnesium trisilicate mixture during labor in an attempt to raise the pH of gastric contents above 2.5. The safety of administering particulate antacid has already been questioned[10,11];

sodium citrate seems a safer alternative. In U.K. practice it is routine to attempt to reduce the volume of gastric contents using histamine-2 (H_2) receptor antagonists; Thorburn and Moir's regimen of administering cimetidine 200 mg intramuscularly when the decision to proceed to cesarean delivery is made, and sodium citrate 30 ml before induction of anesthesia, seems a reasonable alternative to treating all patients in labor.[12]

Metoclopramide will hasten gastric emptying and has the advantage of raising intraesophageal pressure, but the effect is antagonized by opioid analgesics, which also delay gastric emptying.[13]

Problems with endotracheal intubation remain a common cause of death. Patients most at risk are short in stature and obese, with short, fat necks. Morgan has reviewed the factors that lead to problems during induction of general anesthesia in pregnant patients[2]:

1. Full dentition
2. Thorax lifted into an unusual position by wedge
3. Degree of laryngeal edema possible—particularly if pregnancy induced hypertension is present
4. Incorrect placement of cricoid pressure, which may distort larynx
5. Combination of large breasts and applying cricoid pressure by hand, which leads to difficulty in introducing the laryngoscope blade. (The editor recommends the use of a short-handled laryngoscope [see Ch. 1].)
6. "Anesthesiologist anxiety," which may lead to premature attempts at performing laryngoscopy

Some attempt to anticipate difficult intubation should be made, and Malampatti et al. have suggested a useful bedside technique.[14] When the subject opens her mouth and protrudes her tongue, the visibility of the faucial pillars, the soft palate, and the base of the uvula are noted; if the faucial pillars and uvula are obscured by the base of the tongue, endotracheal intubation is likely to be difficult.

Skilled assistance and a variety of laryngoscope blades, handles, and stylets must be available. Scott has pointed out that patients die as a result of *the failure to stop trying to intubate*.[15] All anesthesiologists must be capable of ventilating the lungs using a mask, airway, and reservoir bag, and a failed-intubation drill should be familiar to all anesthesiologists and their assistants.[16] Endotracheal intubation should be verified by an end-tidal carbon dioxide monitor to avoid undiagnosed esophageal intubation. As in previous studies, death were more frequently associated with emergency than elective procedures, with a ratio of 14:4 (Table 10-12).

The correct application of cricoid pressure is essential to prevent acid aspiration, and Morgan's observation of various operating room personnel has shown that many fail to apply it correctly.[2] Sellick described the technique in 1961[17] and recommended that before induction the cricoid be palpated and lightly held between the thumb and second finger; as anesthesia is induced, pressure should be exerted onto the cricoid cartilage, mainly by the index finger (Fig. 10-4). Cricoid pressure should be initiated as consciousness is lost (not before!) in order to avoid tracheal stimulation, which may result in cough-

Table 10-12. Deaths Associated with Anesthesia: Procedures for Which Anesthetic Was Given

Operation	Indication	Number of Deaths
Laparotomy	Ruptured ectopic pregnancy	3
Dilatation and curettage with tubal ligation	Legal termination with sterilization	1
Proposed evacuation of retained products of conception (died during inducation of anaesthetic)	Incomplete abortion	1
Forceps delivery	Delay in second stage of labour	1
Proposed emergency cesarean section–vaginal delivery	Fetal distress	1
Proposed elective cesarean section (died during induction of anaesthetic	Fetal growth retardation	1
Elective cesarean section (died during inducation of anaesthetic)	Failed forceps delivery	1
Emergency cesarean section	Pre-eclampsia	1
	Failed forceps delivery	1
	Breech presentation	
	Fetal distress	1
	Prolonged labour	1
		3
		7
Manual removal of placenta	Retained placenta	1

(From Report on Confidential Enquiries into Maternal Deaths in England and Wales, 1982–1984,[1] with permission.)

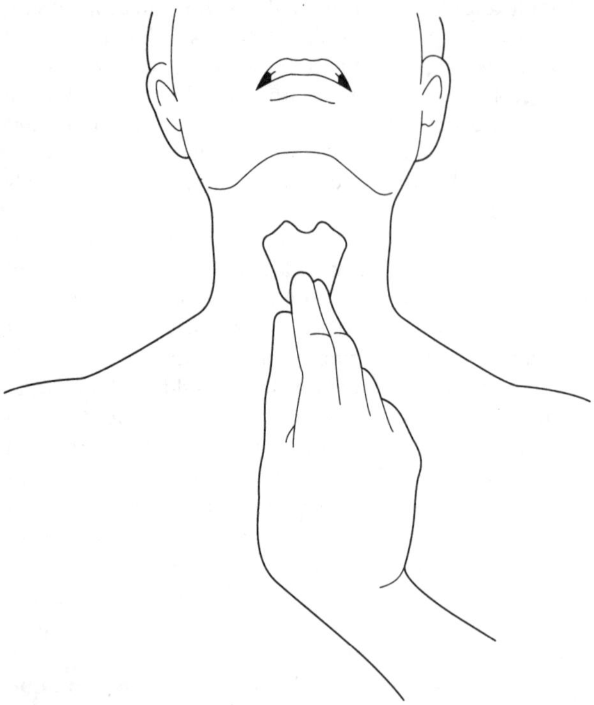

Fig. 10-4. Diagram of the correct application of cricoid pressure. The cricoid cartilage is held between the thumb and second finger and backward pressure is exerted on the cricoid cartilage mainly by the index finger. (From Sellick,[17] with permission.)

ing, retching, or active vomiting. Succinylcholine should be administered immediately after the induction agent and must be allowed to circulate for at least 30 seconds to produce relaxation. Because fasciculations may *not* be observed, a neuromuscular stimulator will be a valuable aid in demonstrating the onset and intensity of neuromuscular block. Cricoid pressure should be maintained until intubation and inflation of the cuff of the endotracheal tube is complete and its position confirmed by auscultation and end-tidal carbon dioxide monitoring. Up to 47 percent of anesthetic and paramedical staff failed to apply cricoid pressure correctly in a recent study.[18]

OVERVIEW OF OTHER CAUSES OF MATERNAL MORTALITY

The Maternal Mortality Collaborative[7] identified embolism, hypertensive disease of pregnancy, ectopic pregnancy, cerebrovascular accident, and obstetric hemorrhage as the commonest causes of maternal death (Table 10-13); in the United Kingdom, hypertensive disease, pregnancy, pulmonary embolism, and anesthesia were most frequently responsible.[1]

In the U.S. study, 45 percent of deaths were associated with cesarean delivery. MMR for women of black and other races was higher than rates for white women. This report also suggests that obese women may have an increased risk of maternal death; women over 30 years of age have a higher rate of mortality from most causes. Kaunitz has suggested there may be over-reporting of embolism on death certificates[6]; emboli are seen as nonpreventable and therefore medicolegal repercussions may be less likely. The diagnosis of embolism should be confirmed by autopsy.

The U.K. survey shows similar findings; maternal deaths were commoner among women born outside the United Kingdom and maternal death rates rose from the age of 20, particularly for mothers aged 35 or older. The ratio of direct deaths related to emergency and elective cesarean delivery is 4.5:1. There were no deaths at cesarean delivery related to epidural anesthesia, although eight deaths in this section of the report were related to general anesthesia, suggesting that perhaps regional techniques are the methods of choice.[1]

CONCLUSIONS

In 1987 the Safe Motherhood Conference, sponsored by the World Health Organization, convened in Nairobi. The Safe Motherhood Initiative, calling for action to reduce maternal deaths on a global scale, was produced.[19] Audits of maternal deaths, as performed in the Maternal Mortality Collaborative and U.K. confidential inquiries, facilitate the reduction of deaths in developed countries, and should be strongly encouraged. Reductions in MMR reflect improvement in both obstetric and anesthetic care.

Other extraneous factors influence the trend in maternal death rates. Introduction of antibiotics and improved maternal health were instrumental in reducing MMR earlier. Improved antenatal care and education have, and will, play a role. Despite improvements in MMR in developed countries, substandard care at delivery is an important cause of anesthesia related mortality, and was associated with all 19 anesthesia-related deaths in the 1982 to 1984 U.K. report. Crawford, in 1970, suggested that the major blame for substandard care remains with consultant anesthesiologists, who should ensure appropriate standards are met.[20] In addition, there are administrative problems with insufficient anesthesiologists available for the number of obstetric units. Small units are unlikely to receive full 24-hour anesthetic coverage and regionalization of units may lead to safer care.[21] Gibbs' survey of obstetric anesthesia in the United States indicates that obstetric units with fewer than 500 deliveries per annum were considerably

Table 10-13. Maternal and Nonmaternal Deaths, Deaths Occurring More Than 42 Days after Pregnancy Ended, U.S., 1980–1985[a]

Cause of Death	All Deaths	No. Died after Pregnancy Ended	Died More Than 42 Days after Pregnancy Ended No.	%
Maternal—direct				
Embolism	102	80	7	9
Hypertensive disease	74	63	1	2
Ectopic pregnancy	60	53	2	4
Hemorrhage	55	47	2	4
Cerebrovascular accident	51	35	2	6
Anesthesia complications	52	40	4	10
Abortions (all types)	31	24	3	13
Cardiomyopathy	25	19	11	58
Obstetric infection	21	19	1	5
Hydatidiform mole	3	3	2	67
Other direct causes	43	31	3	10
TOTAL DIRECT	507	414	38	9
Maternal—indirect				
Infectious conditions	34	22	3	14
Cardiovascular	31	22	6	27
Other	29	14	3	21
TOTAL INDIRECT	94	58	12	21
TOTAL MATERNAL	601	472	50	11
Nonmaternal				
Injury	90	16	5	31
Other	21	13	2	15
TOTAL NONMATERNAL	111	29	7	24
ALL DEATHS[b]	712	501	57	11

[a] Excludes women who died with an undelivered infant or whose outcome of pregnancy was unknown.

[b] Excludes two deaths of unknown cause.

(From Rochat et al.,[7] with permission.)

understaffed when compared with larger units[22]; an anesthesiologist provided general anesthesia for cesarean delivery in fewer than 50 percent of cases in these hospitals.

In contrast with women in developed countries, women who live in developing countries have MMR estimated at 50 to 800 per 100,000; 99 percent of maternal deaths occur in these countries.[19] It is estimated that 50 percent of women in the world receive no assistance from trained personnel during childbirth. The lifetime risk of dying in pregnancy in a developing country may be up to 2 per 100, and even more women are permanently disabled and may be ostracized from their families. Illegal abortion is responsible for up to 25 to 50 percent of deaths.[23] U.S. and U.K. statistics show a dramatic fall in abortion-related mortality when abortion was legalized; in countries where access to abortion remains restricted, deaths associated with abortion remain high.[24]

At the Nairobi conference, urgent action was recommended, including reallocation of resources to improve maternal health care, improve education to women and their careers, expand family planning, and upgrade existing health care services. Modest resources, compared with developed countries, could greatly reduce the MMR. One of the Safe Motherhood Initiative's objectives was a 50 percent reduction in worldwide MMR in one decade.[19]

Developed countries have taken the lead with their progress in reducing MMR. Complacency should be avoided, as many deaths could still be prevented. However, maternal mortality remains a global issue, and priority should be given to allocation of resources dedicated to reducing it.

REFERENCES

1. Report on Confidential Enquiries into Maternal Deaths in England and Wales in 1982 to 1984: DHSS, 1989. Her Majesty's Statistics Office, London, 1989

2. Morgan M: Anaesthetist's contribution to maternal mortality. Br J Anaesth 59:842, 1987
3. Rubin GL, McCarthy B, Shelton J, et al: The risk of childbearing re-evaluated. Am J Public Health 71:712, 1981
4. Smith JC, Hughes JM, Pekow PS, Rochat RW: An assessment of the incidence of maternal mortality in the United States. Am J Public Health 74:780, 1984
5. Benedetti TJ, Starzyk P, Frost F: Maternal deaths in Washington State. Obstet Gynecol 66:99, 1985
6. Kaunitz AM, Hughes JM, Grimes DA, et al: Causes of maternal mortality in the United States. Obstet Gynecol 65:605, 1985
7. Rochat RW, Koonin LM, Koonin PH, et al: Maternal mortality in the United States: report from the Maternal Mortality Collaborative. Obstet Gynecol 72:91, 1988
8. Sachs BP, Oriol NE, Ostheimer GW, et al: Anesthetic related maternal mortality, 1954 to 1985. J Clin Anesthesiol 1:333, 1989
9. Report on Confidential Enquiries into Maternal Deaths in England and Wales 1979–1981: DHSS, 1986. Her Majesty's Statistics Office, London, 1986
10. Morgan M: Confidential enquiry into maternal deaths (editorial). Anaesthesia 41:689, 1986
11. Gibbs CP, Schwartz DJ, Wynne JW, et al: Antacid pulmonary aspiration in the dog. Anesthesiology 51:380, 1979
12. Thorburn J, Moir DD: Antacid therapy for emergency cesarean section. Anaesthesia 42:352, 1987
13. Todd JG, Nimmo WS: Effects of premedication on drug absorption and gastric emptying. Br J Anaesth 55:1189, 1983
14. Malampatti SR, Gatt SP, Gugino LD, et al: A Clinical sign to predict difficult tracheal intubation: a prospective study. Can Anesth Soc J 32:429, 1985
15. Scott DB: Endotracheal intubation: friend or foe? Br Med J 292:157, 1986
16. Tunstall ME: Failed intubation drill. Anaesthesia 31:850, 1976
17. Sellick BA: Cricoid pressure to control regurgitation of stomach contents during induction of anaesthesia. Lancet 2:404, 1961
18. Wraight WJ, Chamney AR, Howells TH: The determination of an effective cricoid pressure. Anaesthesia 38:461, 1983
19. Mahler H: The Safe Motherhood Initiative: a call to action. Lancet 1:668, 1987
20. Crawford JS: The anaesthetist's contribution to maternal mortality. Br J Anaesth 42:70, 1970
21. Rosen M, Fujimora M: Maternal mortality and manpower. Comparison in relation to anaesthetists, obstetricians and paediatricians in England and Whales, and in Japan. Anaesthesia 40:892, 1985
22. Gibbs CP, Krischer J, Peckham BM, et al: Obstetric anesthesia: a national survey. Anesthesiology 65:298, 1986
23. Kwast BE: Maternal mortality: levels, causes and promising interventions. J Biosoc Sci Suppl 10:51, 1989
24. Laguardia KD, Rotholz MV, Belfort P: A 10-year review of maternal mortality in a municipal hospital in Rio de Janeiro: a cause for concern. Obstet Gynecol 75:27, 1989

PERINATAL MORTALITY

OVERVIEW

Natality and mortality statistics are determined from birth and death certificates from each state. These statistics are compiled by the National Center for Health Statistics and provide a variety of useful data such as evaluation of health care systems as well as the health of the population studied. The usefulness of these statistics is limited by differences in defining specific terminology and reporting requirements at the state, national, and international levels.[1]

An example of this problem concerns the definition of stillbirth or fetal death (synonomous terms). Some states report a stillbirth according to weight (from 350 to 500 g); others report by gestational age (from 16 to 20 weeks) and some utilize both weight and age.[2]

Uniformity in statistical reporting is essential to correctly evaluate the quality of perinatal health care, to identify a particular area for improvement and to establish criteria to achieve the desired solution.[3]

DEFINITIONS

To attain uniformity in reporting, the World Health Organization[4] recommends: "National perinatal statistics should include all fetuses and infants delivered weighing at least 500 grams or, when birth weight is unavailable, the corresponding gestational age (22 weeks) or body length (25 cm crown to heel), whether alive or dead." Further recommendations concerning countries reporting statistics include: "Countries should present, solely for international comparisons, standard perinatal statistics in which both the numerator and denominator of all rates are restricted to fetuses and infants weighing 1000 grams or more or, when birth weight is unavailable, the corresponding gestational age (28 weeks) or body length (35 cm crown to heel)."

The American Academy of Pediatrics and the American College of Obstetrics and Gynecology as well as six other prominent national health organizations prepared, reviewed, and approved the following definition of fetal death: "death prior to the complete expulsion or extraction from the mother of a product of human conception, fetus and placenta, irrespective of the duration of pregnancy; death is indicated by the fact that, after such expulsion or extraction, the fetus does not breathe or show any other evidence of life, such as beating of the heart, pulsation of the umbilical cord, or definite movement of voluntary muscles. Heartbeats are to be distinguished from transient cardiac contractions; respirations are to be distinguished from fleeting respiratory efforts or gasps. This definition excludes induced terminations of pregnancy."[5]

Perinatal mortality comprises the total number of stillbirths or fetal deaths and neonatal deaths. Neonatal death is defined as death of an infant within the first 28 days after birth and may be subdivided into early and late neonatal death. Early neonatal death refers to a liveborn infant that expires within the first 7 days of life. Late neonatal death is defined as death of a liveborn infant after the 7th day but not later than the 28th day after birth. The neonatal mortality rate is calculated per 1,000 live births. The perinatal mortality rate is determined by the sum of stillbirths and neonatal deaths per 1,000 total births.[6]

STATISTICAL INFORMATION

Fetal death or stillbirth amounts to an estimated 15 to 20 percent of overall perinatal mortality in clinically diagnosed pregnancies.[2] According to the World Health Organization,[4] the probability of fetal death by gestational age is greatest postconception and drops rapidly until 16 weeks gestation. Fetal death is said to occur in less than 1 percent of pregnancies after 20 weeks gestation.[3,7]

Causes of fetal death vary, however, approximately one-third of all stillbirths are unexplained by either fetal or maternal pathologic conditions. This failure is most likely due to not having appropriate studies performed on the fetus and placenta. Most investigators report that chromosomal aberrations are responsible for first-trimester abortions, with the type of abnormality varying according to gestational age, parental age, and reproductive history. According to Warburton,[8] 55 percent of fetal deaths up to 28 weeks gestation are due to trisomies. Other causes of stillbirth are related to single or multiple anomalies such as heart defects, neural tube defects, and urinary tract anomalies.[9] Stillbirth of an infant may occur without warning in an apparently normal pregnancy.

Chronic or acute states of fetal anoxia are most commonly due to placental abruption secondary to a maternal pathologic condition or event and is responsible for about 20 percent of all stillbirths.[4] The second most common cause of fetal anoxia is cord accident. The most significant maternal conditions adversely affecting fetal oxygenation are diabetes and pregnancy-induced hypertension.

By studying statistical data related to maternal mortality and altering maternal care, the medical community has been able to effect a decrease in the maternal mortality rate. Improvement in maternal mortality has caused the perinatal mortality rate to decline. In support of this statement, Davidson[10] recommends using maternal mortality reviews as an historic model. He proposes a process that will encourage cities and states on a national level and hospitals on a local level to develop specific guidelines for in-depth reviews of fetal and infant mortality and to seriously and comprehensively examine the reasons for each death.

Since the 1950s, the mortality rates for neonates and infants have been gradually decreasing.[7] In 1976, the neonatal mortality rate was 10.9 percent and in 1985, the rate had dropped to 7.0 percent. Within the United States, the District of Columbia has the highest rate (15.9 percent), followed by Delaware (10.6 percent). The states reporting the lowest neonatal mortality rates are Montana (5.0 percent) and Alaska (5.1 percent).[7]

Analysis of infants mortality rates shows that very low birthweight (less than 1,500 g) is the principal predictor of mortality in the neonatal period.[2] Concerns have been raised about variables affecting the collection of these weight data and recognizing the importance of birthweight to infant mortality. Variation in state-reported rates of births of infants weighing less than 500 g does appear. There is a twofold difference between the neonatal mortality rate of Montana, the state with the lowest rate, and Delaware, the state with the highest rate. National statistics were examined in an attempt to estimate the incidence of underreporting.[1] In their analyses, it was concluded there may be approximately 1.1 neonates with weights of less than 500 g who were underreported for every 1,000 live births.

POSSIBLE CAUSES OF UNDERREPORTING

Part of the problem of underreporting may be attributed to the individual state's definition of terms. Other factors that must be considered may be perceptual problems in the clinical setting. For instance, if a baby is declared to weigh more than an arbitrary amount, and thus considered live at the time of birth, the family would then be faced with the expense of a funeral. Monetary reimbursement for medical or hospital care for delivery as opposed to a spontaneous abortion may be another issue to consider in the reporting of live births. How a birth is described may also affect the use of reimbursement codes.

HISTORY OF NEONATAL INTENSIVE CARE

In the 1920s and 1930s, specially designed centers for the care of premature neonates were established in the United States. Many centers trace their origin in part to the work of Dr. Julius Hays Hess from Chicago,[11] who became intrigued by the fetal specimens at various stages of gestation that were on exhibition at fairs and expositions in the United States and Europe in the early 1900s. During the 1940s and 1950s, the study of academic neonatology evolved with the establishment of uniform standards of care for the neonate, recognizing their need for isolation, thermal stability, proper nutrition, and specialized nursing care.

The establishment of these specialized centers was the forerunner of the neonatal intensive care unit, which began to develop in the late 1950s and through the 1960s. It was also during this time frame that the concept of intensive care for adults and children evolved. During the 1960s, the rapid expansion of neonatal care resulted in more aggressive medical and surgical care of neonates, with the focus primarily on the low-birthweight infant.

With improved knowledge to identify high-risk factors for both the mother and fetus, a new era of obstetric and neonatal care has evolved. Advanced technology has enabled physicians to assess fetal health, including fetal maturation, and diagnose congenital anomalies, and has permitted aggressive management of preterm birth. Utilization of the multidisciplinary approach is essential to assess, intervene, and manage the neonate.[12] In substantiation of the effectiveness of the multidisciplinary approach, intrauterine fetal surgery has been undertaken in a few instances, although this treatment is still in experimental stages. Harrison and colleagues[13] successfully performed intrauterine fetal surgery to correct congenital diaphragmatic hernia. Other procedures such as fetal blood exchange for hematologic disease have also been successfully performed. Thus, ongoing research and advancing technology have enabled neonatal practitioners to improve the survivability of the preterm or ill neonate, thereby reducing mortality and long-term morbidity. Immediate aggressive resuscitation is a key factor in decreasing neonatal mortality and morbidity with these infants.[14]

Avery and Mead[15] demonstrated in 1959 that respiratory distress syndrome (RDS) was due to a deficiency in pulmonary surfactant. For over 30 years, researchers have looked for methods to prevent or more successfully treat RDS in premature infants. Artificial surfactant therapy for prevention and treatment of RDS has recently become a reality.

Clinical trials using artificial pulmonary surfactant have shown promising initial results by reducing the duration and severity of RDS and chronic lung disease in the infants affected by RDS at birth. Artificial surfactant therapy can be initiated in the delivery room or in the first few hours of life. The therapy involves the installation of the surfactant preparation directly into the trachea through an endotracheal tube. Positive-pressure ventilation may or may not be utilized in the acute phase of therapy.

PREDISPOSING FACTORS TO PERINATAL MORTALITY

Prevention of preterm birth remains the most important unresolved issue currently confronting obstetricians and neonatologists. Immaturity (weight of less than 1,000 g) accounts for up to 50 percent of all perinatal deaths as well as increases long-term morbidity.

In a study by Amon et al.,[16] maternal diagnoses responsible for preterm birth were found to include the following factors, listed according to their frequency of occurrence:

1. Idiopathic preterm labor
2. Chorioamnionitis
3. Premature rupture of membranes
4. Pregnancy-induced hypertension
5. Incompetent cervix

Their study encompassed three variables: maternal diagnosis primarily responsible for delivery, past obstetric outcome, and antepartum and intrapartum factors.

Of interest, their study showed that of the patients with idiopathic preterm labor, the majority had received no prenatal care. In addition, after their admittance to the hospital, most were in advanced stages of labor with little or no opportunity to try to arrest labor.[16]

METHODS TO DECREASE PERINATAL MORTALITY

Prenatal care must begin early so that those parturients who are at high risk can be identified as soon as possible and effective therapy against preventable maternal factors instituted, thereby prolonging pregnancy. Maternal characteristics that relate to the increased incidence of preterm delivery such as idiopathic preterm labor and incompetent cervix may be identified and managed more aggressively.

Factors responsible for predisposing the fetus to premature delivery or intrauterine growth retardation may be identified and altered through patient education. One of the most devastating problems in the United States today concerns maternal drug abuse, specifically "crack" cocaine. Not only is maternal health affected, but the fetus is exposed to the barrage of chemical assault each time the mother uses the drug. Intervention for addicted mothers has proven most successful in programs designed to manage all the mother's needs rather than just those relating to her pregnancy.[17] Prevention of perinatal complications through patient and community education is vital in fighting this growing problem as well as other alterable behavioral problems.[18] (See Chapter 8.)

Miller and Merritt[19] identified the following behavioral factors that strongly relate to low-birthweight delivery:

1. Low maternal weight for height
2. Lack of adequate weight gain in pregnancy
3. No prenatal care
4. Delivery before age 17 or after age 35
5. Smoking during pregnancy
6. Use of alcohol and addicting drugs

Traditionally, obstetric approaches have been primarily focused on treatment rather than timely identification of those women at risk. Creasy and co-workers, in 1980,[20] modified a risk scoring system initially devised by Papiernik and Kaminski,[21] that identifies women at increased risk for preterm delivery. Included in their criteria are a variety of factors relating to pregnancy, such as socioeconomic status, reproductive history, daily habits, and any current complication of pregnancy.

Recommendations to improve the perinatal mortality rate include:

1. Availability of prenatal care
2. Early prenatal care
3. Identification of those parturients at high risk
4. Education in hopes of altering behavioral characteristics
5. Early maternal transport to a tertiary care center if delivery is inevitable
6. Aggressive resuscitation of the preterm infant[14]
7. Medical/surgical intervention, if indicated, incorporating a multidisciplinary approach
8. Uniformity regarding definitions of terms and criteria

Eisner et al.[22] noted that, within the United States, the greatest risk factor for low birthweight is no prenatal care.

In a desire to learn from experiences of countries whose infant mortality rates have decreased more quickly than those of the United States, the National Center for Health Statistics established an International Collaborative Effort on Perinatal and Infant Mortality (ICE). Research has been carried out with scientists from Denmark, the Federal Republic of Germany, United Kingdom, Israel, Japan, Norway, and Sweden. Two symposia have been held, the first in August 1984 and the next in March 1990. Reports at the latter symposium made one point of special interest: in the Scandinavian countries, almost every pregnant woman receives high-quality prenatal care early. This is a goal that must be emphasized in the United States, with every effort made to increase the quality and quantity of prenatal care available to all women and thereby more favorably affect perinatal mortality.

REFERENCES

1. Wilson AL, Fenton LJ, Munson DP: State reporting of live births of newborns weighing less than 500 grams: impact on neonatal mortality rates. Pediatrics 78:850, 1986
2. Final Mortality Statistics, 1983, advance report: Monthly Vital Statistics Report. National Center for Health Statistics, 34(6 suppl 2):Sept 26, 1985
3. Block BS: Evaluating the quality of perinatal health care. Am J Perinatol 7:146, 1990
4. World Health Organization: Manual of the International Statistical Classification of Diseases, Injuries and Causes of Death. p. 763. World Health Organization, 1977
5. Guidelines for Perinatal Care. 2nd Ed. p. 308. American College of Obstetrics and Gynecology, Washington D.C., 1988
6. Cunningham FG, MacDonald PC, Gant NF: Williams Obstetrics. 18th Ed. p. 1. Appleton & Lange, East Norwalk CT, 1989
7. Infant and Perinatal Mortality Rates by Age and Race, United States, Each State and County. 1976–1980, 1981–1985. p. 1. Maternal and Child Health Studies Project, Information Science Research Institute, Vienna, VA, 1988
8. Warburton D: Chromosomal malformations and syndromes associated with stillbirth. Clin Obstet Gynecol 30:268, 1987
9. Hall BD: Nonchromosomal malformations and syndromes associated with stillbirth. Clin Obstet Gynecol 30:278, 1987
10. Davidson EC: A strategy to reduce infant mortality. Obstet Gynecol 77:2, 1991
11. Guidelines for Perinatal Care. 2nd Ed. p. 2. American College of Obstetrics and Gynecology, Washington D.C., 1988
12. Lorenz RP, Kuhn MH: Multidisciplinary team counseling for fetal anomalies. Am J Obstet Gynecol 161:263, 1989
13. Harrison MR, Adzick NS, Longaker MT, et al: Successful repair in utero of a fetal diaphragmatic hernia after removal of herniated viscera from the left thorax. N Engl J Med 322:1582, 1990
14. Hack M, Fanaroff AA: Special report: changes in the delivery room care of the extremely small infant (< 750 gm). N Engl J Med 314:660, 1986
15. Avery ME, Mead J: Surface properties in relation to atelectasis and hyaline membrane disease. Am J Dis Child 97:517, 1959
16. Amon E, Anderson GD, Sibai BM, et al: Factors responsible

for preterm delivery of the immature newborn infant (< 1000 gm). Am J Obstet Gynecol 156:1143, 1987
17. Marsh JC, Miller NA: Female clients in substance abuse treatment. Int J Addict 20:995, 1985
18. Herron MA, Katz M, Creasy RK: Evaluation of a preterm birth prevention program: preliminary report. Obstet Gynecol 59:452, 1982
19. Miller HC, Merritt TA: Fetal Growth in Humans. Year Book Medical Publishers, Chicago, 1977
20. Creasy RK, Gummer BA, Liggins GC: System for predicting spontaneous preterm birth. Obstet Gynecol 55:692, 1980
21. Papiernik E, Kaminski M: Multifactorial study of the risk of prematurity at 32 weeks of gestation: a study for the frequency of 30 predictive characteristics. J Perinat Med 2:30, 1974
22. Eisner V, Brazie JV, Pratt MW, et al: The risk of low birthweight. Am J Public Health 69:887, 1979

MEDICOLEGAL ASPECTS OF OBSTETRIC ANESTHESIA

The overlap between clinical and legal issues in obstetric anesthesia is more extensive than most anesthesiologists realize. A variety of legal questions besides those of malpractice and informed consent can have an impact on obstetric anesthetic practice.

For most anesthesiologists, however, malpractice is the major legal issue of obstetric anesthesia—and with good reason. A recent study found that among anesthetic malpractice claims, those relating to obstetric anesthesia cost almost three times as much to settle as the nonobstetric claims.[1]

Therefore, it is reasonable that the topic of negligence should begin the legal discussion concerning obstetric anesthesia.

NEGLIGENCE

Negligence is the legal theory that supports almost all claims against anesthesiologists. Under the theory of negligence, a court will award damages if certain conditions can be demonstrated. First, there must be some actual and measurable damage. Merely feeling wronged, or even suffering a provable wrongdoing but not suffering a loss, will not entitle a person to an award. Second, the anesthesiologist must have been under a duty to act in the interest of the injured patient. Third, the duty to the patient must not have been fully met. Fourth, the failure of the anesthesiologist to meet the duty must have caused the injury at issue. To prevail in court, the attorney for the plaintiff must show that all four of these conditions occurred, whereas the defendant's attorney need only show that one did not.

Evidence

The Expert Witness. Most cases revolve around the issue of whether or not the anesthesiologist fulfilled his duty to the patient. This is another way of saying that the issue is whether anesthesiology was correctly practiced. Since few laws, if any, dictate how anesthesiology must be practiced, the courts must ask other anesthesiologists to answer this question.

The answers of "expert" anesthesiologists are often the best evidence a court has on which to make its decision. The importance of these answers is seen in the latitude of expression granted by courts to medical experts. It is underscored by the high regard in which courts hold the expert physician's opinion.

As a rule, expert opinions on anesthetic care are given by physicians—but not always anesthesiologists! This is partly a matter of witness credibility and partly a matter of who the court is likely to recognize as an expert. For example, in one case a court was asked to decide whether an epidural catheter should have been left in a parturient for several days following a cesarean delivery. The testimony of a registered nurse concerning the propriety of this act was given no standing by the court, which noted that the nurse's opinion pertained to ". . . the exercise of medical judgment or involves decisions and treatment exclusively within the scope of a physician."[2] Since nothing indicated that the nurse was qualified to express an expert opinion on anesthesiology, the court concluded that the testimony of the physicians would stand unrebutted on that issue.

Another sign of the court's regard for the expert physician is the fact that an expert need not agree with all, most, or even many other experts in his field. In fact, his opinion may be a minority view or it may simply be a theory that he happens to hold (unfortunately)!

An example of this was demonstrated in a case involving the possibly cardiotoxic nature of bupivacaine. Two obstetric anesthesiologists were allowed to testify to the existence of this property (of cardiotoxicity) even though their theories were not widely accepted.[3] In allowing their views into evidence, the court pointed out that peer acceptance affected only how much weight the injury might give to their theory. The degree of peer acceptance should not determine whether a jury should hear the theory in the first place, particularly when the theory was contradicted by other testimony.

Given the deference and the latitude accorded to the expert anesthesiologist by the court, it is essential that the expert show a corresponding respect for the court's needs. A witness should be familiar with, and should truthfully describe, current practice and opinion in his area of expertise. He should be ready to substantiate his opinion when he agrees with a widely held practice and to distinguish it when he does not. In short, an expert anesthesiologist should, when asked, ably represent both his own opinions and those of his peers. Neither justice nor the profession are served when these principles are disregarded.

Standards. In recent years the American Society of Anesthesiologists (ASA) and other organizations have supported practice guidelines and standards that address issues in obstetric anesthesia.[4] Standards may serve several purposes but, from a liability standpoint, they seem to provide irrefutable evidence of what constitutes acceptable care. In fact, to the anesthesiologist, standards may appear to dictate the *legally* acceptable response to a given clinical situation. It turns out, however, that the courts have quite a different view.

Several courts have been asked to rule on the admissibility of standards to answer questions about specific episodes of anesthetic care. Each court found that the standards could be properly admitted, but only as *evidence*. The different courts variously described standards as evidence of accepted practice, guides for measuring care, and a substitute for expert testimony; but each court refused them any more deference than would be shown a human witness. This gives standards the weight of expert testimony but it also gives the jury the freedom to disregard any standard it finds unhelpful.

The specific point, which was emphasized by each court, is that standards are not conclusive in determining negligence. In other words, a standard cannot by itself *dictate* the applicable standard of care to which a physician should be held.

This position reflects the court's understanding that standards are generally based on what is customary to an industry or profession. Custom is by definition rooted in the past and so the custom of a profession or an industry may well lag in the adoption of new practices. For this reason, the courts reserve to themselves the right to determine negligence based on all the currently available evidence.[5]

This is a philosophy that anesthesiologists should encourage. Even where a standard may appear to reflect the correct response to a clinical situation, all the relevant evidence should be examined before a judgment is made. The label of "negligent" is too stigmatizing and too emotionally devastating to apply solely on the basis of some single, though simple, rule.

Duty

Good Samaritan Statutes and the Newborn Infant. Establishing the anesthesiologist's duty to the parturient is seldom difficult. Duty will arise out of either an explicit or implicit agreement to provide coverage for obstetric anesthesia and it will be confirmed by the act of providing care.

The newborn infant, however, can raise an entirely separate question of duty. This is because the anesthesiologist's commitment to the mother does not imply an equal commitment to the infant after delivery occurs. At delivery, the infant becomes a second patient, separate from its mother.

At some time after delivery, an infant usually becomes the patient of a pediatrician, who then owes a duty of care to that infant. At the moment of delivery, however, the pediatrician is often absent. This leaves the obstetrician, the anesthesiologist, and the nurse to jointly decide how to manage, and who has responsibility for, any complications concerning the infant. In the absence of a pediatrician, the anesthesiologist is frequently *assumed* to have that responsibility.

In law, there is no reason to assume that a patient–physician relationship exists between the newborn infant and the anesthesiologist. In fact, several states have statutes that have been used to deny both the relationship and duty that goes with it. These statutes are often called "Good Samaritan" statutes, because they protect people who voluntarily render emergency assistance to an injured person.

As a rule, a Good Samaritan statute prevents a person from being liable for negligent acts or omissions committed while *voluntarily* providing emergency care. Such a statute may even relieve a physician of the duty to take reasonable care when volunteering assistance in a medical emergency.

In consideration of this principle, an appellate court was asked to determine if a Good Samaritan statute provided immunity to an anesthesiologist asked to resuscitate an infant.[6] The court found that in general there is *no* immunity for the anesthesiologist where either he has an employment *duty* to aid the infant or there is a pre-existing doctor–patient relationship with the infant. However, if a duty to the infant does not exist prior to the delivery, then it is not suddenly created simply because an anesthesiologist works at a hospital, is in a delivery room, and has a doctor–patient relationship with the infant's *mother*.

According to the court, the question of the anesthesiologist's immunity with regard to the newborn infant turns on the issue of *duty*. Where there is a duty there can be no immunity, and vice versa.

Duty, in turn, is largely determined by the basis on which an anesthesiologist assists in neonatal resuscitation. If a jury finds that he assists by chance and on an irregular basis, then no duty will be found. On the other hand, if it finds that he assists because he is either expressly or customarily required to resuscitate, then a duty to the infant will likely be found.

The message of the appellate court to the anesthesiologist is that his duty to a particular infant is a question of fact and of individual practice, and of institutional practice rather than of law. His practice with regard to infant resuscitation *in general* will largely determine his duty to a particular infant.

Breach of Duty

Consent. Most questions about an anesthesiologist's performance are concerned with medical issues. However, the anesthesiologist's failure to obtain the patient's informed consent for an anesthetic may also be seen as actionable. The requirements of informed consent can present a confusing issue for the anesthesiologist because the standard is derived from judicial rather than medical practice. Furthermore, the stress and pain of labor have led many anesthesiologists to question whether any obstetric consent is truly "informed." Fortunately, it turns out that this issue is much easier to resolve than it first appears.

Informed Consent. In those cases addressing the adequacy of anesthetic consent during labor, the courts have not made the subjective claims of the parturient the focus of their inquiry.[7] Instead, they have noted these three common factors that *together* support a finding of informed consent: the information given to the parturient, the absence of the parturient's objection to the proposed anesthetic, and the parturient's cooperation while the procedure is performed.

This analysis favors the anesthesiologist, since two of the three factors are satisfied at the outset. It is unlikely that an anesthetic will be given over the objection of the parturient or without her cooperation.

The final factor, the information given to the parturient, also favors the anesthesiologist. This is because the courts did not base their findings exclusively on the parturient's opinion nor did they seek a specific kind of documentation. Instead, they looked mainly for assurance that reasonable information was given. Their view of reasonable information included a brief description of the anesthetic and its effects and a general acknowledgment of serious risks with the approximate chance of their occurrence. The courts also take note that an opportunity was provided for the parturient to ask questions. Once this exchange takes place, a brief notation on the chart will suffice to show that consent for an anesthetic was appropriately obtained.

Jehovah's Witnesses. People of certain religious beliefs will not consent to the administration of blood or blood products even when they are necessary to preserve life. Most physicians do not share these beliefs. Also, most physicians will, if forced to choose, prefer to preserve life rather than allow it to slip away for want of a blood transfusion.

The rights claimed here by the patient, self determination and freedom of religious expression, are among the most important in American law. On the other hand, the state also has very compelling interests in preserving life, preventing suicide, protecting the interests of innocent third parties and maintaining the ethical integrity of the medical profession.[8] The conflict between these interests can become sharp in the obstetric setting, particularly when the parties in conflict are the mother on one hand and her infant and her physician on the other.

One particular philosophy has guided the resolution of this conflict in recent decades. It is best quoted, ". . . [P]arents may be free to become martyrs themselves. But it does not follow they are free, in identical circumstances, to make martyrs of their children before they have reached the age of full and legal discretion when they can make that choice for themselves."[9] In the obstetric setting this has been interpreted to mean that a mother may not refuse the benefit of transfusion where the result would be a dependent child deprived of parental support.[10]

The case that underscores the importance of the dependent child involved a father of two children. He was allowed to refuse a transfusion, but only because his family was able to demonstrate that the children could be adequately provided for by a close extended family and with the assets of a family business.[11] It should be noted, however, that these conditions required a judicial hearing to affirm. In the emergency situation, the anesthesiologist and the obstetrician may not have the benefit of extensive fact-finding or judicial direction. In this case, the sole guidance available may be the knowledge that judicial deference has traditionally been given to the needs of dependent children.

Minors. There is no uniform guideline for obtaining a minor's consent for an anesthetic. In several states, a pregnant minor is considered completely emancipated and her consent is the same as that of an adult. There are also several states with statutes that provide a specific age at which a minor is allowed to consent to general medical treatment.

When deciding how best to handle the issue of minor consent, these considerations may be of help. First, it is most helpful to get the advice of a professional who is familiar with the issue. A local attorney who works in hospital risk management is likely to have a practical answer from his own experience. It is also important to keep in mind that while consent is an important part of patient care, it is usually not the element of negligence that controls a claim. This is another way of saying that in any clinical situation there are usually several important aspects that must all be kept in perspective. The issue of age, and its effect on consent, has its place; and so do all the other considerations that affect an obstetric patient.

Finally, the realities of society and current practice are recognized by the courts. As one attorney recently put it, "Even in the absence of statute, there have been no cases reported within the past 30 years in which a parent successfully sued a physician for nonnegligent care of an adolescent without the parent's knowledge . . . In effect, the legal principle now applied is that if a young person (aged 14 or 15 years or older) understands the nature of proposed treatment and its risks, if the physician understands the nature of proposed treatment and its risks, if the physician believes that the patient can give the same degree of informed consent as an adult patient, and if the treatment does not involve very serious risks, the young person may validly consent to receiving it."[12]

LAWS AND REGULATIONS

Not every legal issue in obstetric anesthesia is based on negligence and not everyone is resolved in a malpractice trial. Issues not involved with negligence may be decided in several contexts. The most common are case law, statutory law, and the regulatory process.

Case Law

Case law is law made by judges on the bench, one case at a time. These decisions are based on the application of legal principles to a question not answered by statute or regulation, or on the application of a statutory principle to a specific question that was not considered by the legislature. This latter is especially likely to happen when the courts are asked to adapt the existing law to a changing society.

There is one societal change that is especially familiar to obstetric anesthesiologists. As social custom has changed, the person who is expected or who may expect to be present at a delivery has also changed. This has lead to conflicts between paturients and hospitals. One of these conflicts involved a hospital whose policy allowed "immediate family" only in the delivery room. The dispute ultimately came before an appellate court for resolution.[13]

In this case the mother wanted the child's unmarried father to be present at the delivery. The hospital staff had some difficulty with this request and refused it on the grounds that hospital policy restricted the delivery room to "immediate family" only. Since the father did not technically qualify, he was refused permission to attend the delivery even though he otherwise satisfied all the hospital's requirements. The court that ultimately heard this case decided that the civil rights of the parents were at issue. The court cited a civil rights statute that forbade discrimination on the basis of marital status in places of public accommodation, and it concluded that the hospital's policy was "impermissibly discriminatory." The result was that the father could not be excluded from the delivery room solely for lack of a marriage relationship with the mother, particularly where the hospital routinely allowed other nonmedical support persons at deliveries.

Interestingly, the court decided the issue even though the delivery had already taken place at a hospital that did not contest the father's presence. The court felt a decision was needed because the civil rights issue was both publicly significant and likely to recur.

Statutory Law

State statutes can directly affect the practice of obstetric anesthesia. In California, for example, the scope of practice of nurse anesthetists is defined in the Nurse Anesthetist Act. This Act excludes nurse anesthetists from the practice of medicine or surgery. To some people, this also excluded them from performing regional anesthesia and thus, obstetric anesthesia.

This apparent exclusion, however, merely set the stage for a statutory conflict over regional anesthesia. The reason was that a second statute, the Nursing Practice Act, allowed nurses to perform "standardized procedures." Where the first statute seemed to foreclose regional anesthesia to nurses as the practice of medicine, the second statute appeared to allow nurses to perform regional procedures if the procedures were properly defined. Not surprisingly, soon after the Nurse Anesthetist Act took effect, the following question was put to California's Attorney General: May a Certified Registered Nurse Anesthetist lawfully administer regional anesthetics pursuant to a "standardized procedure?"

The Attorney General reconciled the two statutes in

an opinion that cited extensively from statutes, legislative history, court cases, and a legal nursing text. The final conclusion was that a nurse anesthetist could, indeed, "... lawfully administer a regional anesthetic when ordered by and within the scope of licensure of a physician, dentist, or podiatrist ... but not pursuant to a 'standardized procedure.'"[14]

The primary impact of this opinion was to clarify statutory intent with regard to nurse anesthetists and regional anesthesia. The opinion clearly determined that the legislature intended to allow nurse anesthetists to administer regional anesthesia in California. In fact, the scope of permissible regional procedures for the nurse appeared to encompass whatever was permitted a medical practitioner.

There is another side to this opinion, though. In considering the statutory breadth of nursing practice, the opinion also affirms the domain of medical practice. In anesthesia, the practice of medicine encompasses the decision to induce or to withhold anesthesia. This decision may not be part of a "standardized procedure," and it must be made by a medical practitioner. Only after the decision is made may the anesthetic procedure be delegated to a nurse anesthetist.

As a legal point, then, the line where anesthesia becomes the practice of medicine in California is where a medical judgment is required, rather than where a procedure occurs. As a matter of statute, the nurse anesthetist may legally perform regional anesthesia, but only based on the judgment, the initiative, and the responsibility of a medical practitioner (but not necessarily an anesthesiologist).

Regulation

The Food and Drug Administration (FDA) is one of the most influential regulatory agencies in obstetric anesthesia, primarily through its drug approval process. Unfortunately, the purpose and significance of this process is widely misunderstood, sometimes to the detriment of both anesthesiologists and their patients. For example, during the 1980s, the clinical use of epidural and subarachnoid narcotics expanded enormously, particularly in obstetric anesthesia. Despite the profession's acceptance of these techniques, many individual anesthesiologists encountered resistance to them in their own institutions. A rationale frequently cited was the lack of FDA "approval" of most narcotics for epidural or subarachnoid use. The impression given was that a lack of "approval" meant the practice was either illegal or negligent. However, neither of these implications was true, according to both the FDA and the federal courts.

FDA approval is actually *labelling* approval and not physician *usage* approval. The approval process defines what may go into a drug's labeling, and approved labelling is required before a drug may lawfully enter the marketplace.

Individual physician use is not a concern that the FDA's approval process is intended to address. The specific intent of Congress, as recorded in the legislative history of both the original Food, Drug, and Cosmetic Act and its 1962 amendments, is that the FDA *cannot* interfere in medical practice. In fact, the FDA itself has pointed out that passage of the act in 1938 was predicated on the explicit understanding that the act would not regulate the practice of medicine between physician and patient.[15]

Practically speaking, this means that once a physician has legally obtained any lawfully available medication, he does not need the approval of the FDA to vary the conditions of use from those found on the package insert. The courts have consistently upheld this right of physicians, ruling that the physician's use of legally obtained medications is the practice of medicine. As one court explained, prescribing beyond the directions in the package insert implies neither illegal nor unethical behavior. Congress did not intend the FDA to interfere with medical practice by limiting the physician's ability to prescribe according to his best judgment.[16]

With regard to obstetric anesthesia, it is clear that the careful and conscientious use of epidural and subarachnoid narcotics is not illegal, unethical, or negligent.

CONCLUSION

It is obvious that a significant number of legal issues may arise out of obstetric anesthesia practice. Taken together, they illustrate this point: Even though an anesthesiologist hardly needs to be a lawyer to practice good obstetric anesthesia, knowing certain legal principles will help a good anesthesiologist practice with that much more certainty.

REFERENCES

1. Chadwick HS, et al: A Review of Obstetric Anesthesia Malpractice Claims. p. 64. SOAP Abstracts. Seattle, 1989
2. *Fountain v. Cobb General Hospital,* 306 S.E. 2d 37 (Ga.App. 1983)
3. *Douglas v. Lombardino,* 693 P.2d 1138 (Kan. 1985)
4. Palmer SK, Gibbs CP: Risk management in obstetric anesthesia. Int Anesthesiol Clin 27(3):188, 1989
5. *Darling v. Charleston Community Memorial Hospital,* 211 N.E.2d 253 (1965)
6. *Clayton v. Kelly,* 357 S.E. 2d 865 (Ga.App. 1987)
7. Knapp RM: Legal view of informed consent for anesthesia during labor. Anesthesiology 72:211, 1990

8. *Superintendent of Belchertown v. Saikewicz,* 370 N.E.2d 417, 425 (1977)
9. *Prince v. Massachusetts,* 321 U.S. 158 (1944)
10. *Application of President & Directors of Georgetown College,* 331 F.2d 1000 (1964)
11. *In re Osborne,* 294 A.2d 372 (1972)
12. Holder AR: Minors' rights to consent to medical care. JAMA 257:3400, 1987
13. *Whitman v. Mercy-Memorial Hospital,* 339 N.W.2d 730 (Mich. App. 1983)
14. 67 Op. Atty. Gen. Cal. 122, 4–5–84
15. *Legal Status of Approved Labeling for Prescription Drugs; Prescribing for Uses Unapproved by the Food and Drug Administration,* 37 Fed Reg 16503 (1972)
16. *United States v. Evers,* 453 F. Supp. 1141, 1150 (1978)

NEUROLOGIC SEQUELAE OF CHILDBIRTH AND REGIONAL ANESTHESIA

The incidence of motor or sensory dysfunction in the lower extremity due to delivery has been reported to be as high as 1 per 2,000 in the older literature.[1–4] Most recent investigations have demonstrated an even lower rate of occurrence.[5–7] In fact, Ong et al. have found no long-term neurologic sequelae after delivery in more than 28,000 deliveries.[8] Transient neurologic dysfunction was associated with 18.9 of 10,000 deliveries. Although it is difficult to attach absolute numbers to the incidence of neurologic impairment seen with either regional anesthesia[9–12] or childbirth, some studies suggest that neurologic sequelae related to childbirth occurs more commonly than that due to regional anesthesia.[2,9,13] This discussion addresses neurologic impairment related to both regional anesthesia and delivery.

NEUROLOGIC IMPAIRMENT DUE TO CHILDBIRTH

Since childbirth itself is the more likely cause of neurologic compromise, it is discussed first. The type of delivery a parturient undergoes has a significant impact on the particular peripheral nerve involvement that can occur.

The specific neurologic impairment associated with vaginal delivery may be related to the delivery itself or to positioning for delivery. After reviewing the anatomic associations of the lumbrosacral trunk to the pelvic inlet (Fig. 10-5), one can understand why it is more commonly injured with vaginal delivery.[2,14–16] As the fetus descends through the birth canal, the fetal head exerts significant pressure on the lumosacral trunk at the level of the pelvic inlet. Lumbosacral trunk injury is a relatively common cause of neurologic impairment after delivery. Utilization of mid to high forceps delivery increases the incidence of this type of injury.[13,14] Specific neurologic compromise seen with this injury (Table 10-14) includes unilateral foot drop and weakness in hip abductors and quadriceps muscles, as well as decreased sensation over the lateral aspect of the calf and foot. Gradual resolution of symptoms is usually seen over the ensuing 2 to 4 months.

Rarely, the obturator nerve, which also traverses the pelvic inlet (Fig. 10-5), may be injured during delivery. The signs and symptoms of injury (Table 10-14) include inability to adduct the leg and decreased sensation over the medial aspect of the thigh. Complete resolution usually occurs over 2 to 4 months.

An increased incidence of neurologic problems with vaginal delivery has been associated with prolonged labor,[2,14,15] cephalopelvic disproportion,[15] and mid to high forceps delivery.[12] Aberrant maternal anatomy, such as a platypellic pelvis, is also associated with an increased incidence of neurologic dysfunction.[3,15] Pressure on the lumbosacral trunk during vaginal delivery may result from abnormal pelvic anatomy.

Positioning during vaginal delivery is associated with a variety of injuries. The common peroneal nerve is the most frequently compromised nerve in the lower limb.[15,17–19] It passes superficially over the head of the fibula (Fig. 10-5) at the lateral aspect of the knee and is most often compromised as a result of pressure at this point. Foot drop is attributed to common peroneal nerve injury when injury to the lumbrosacral trunk has not occurred.[15,17] Sensory and motor impairment seen with this injury (Table 10-14) includes foot drop and loss of sensation over the anterolateral aspect of the calf and dorsum of the foot and toes. Usually symptoms resolve completely over 2 to 4 months.[18] The saphenous nerve passes over the medial aspect of the knee (Fig. 10-5). Injury results in loss of sensation over the medial aspect of the foot and anteromedial aspect of the lower leg. Although the common peroneal nerve is injured more often, both of these nerves can be compromised, even when the patient is properly positioned in stirrups. Care must be taken to ensure stirrups are adequately padded during delivery. Bilateral peroneal palsies have been reported in patients undergoing a prolonged second stage of labor in the squatting position as a result of undue pressure exerted on the lateral aspect of both knees. Rarely, the obturator nerve may be injured in the lithotomy position.[16]

Improper positioning during delivery in stirrups may result in specific neurologic injuries. For instance, if a

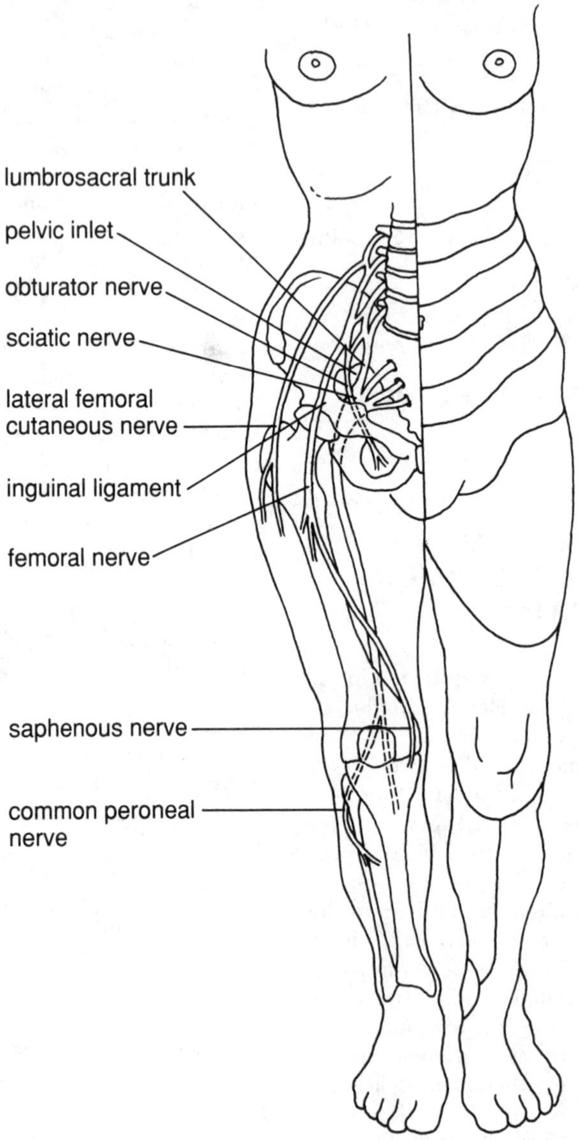

Fig. 10-5. Anatomic associations of the lumbosacral trunk to the pelvic inlet.

patient is placed in a hyperflexed lithotomy position, damage to the femoral and lateral femoral cutaneous nerves may ensue.[20,21] Both of these nerves pass superficially under the inguinal ligament and are subject to pressure at this level (Fig. 10-5). The lateral femoral cutaneous nerve contributes only sensory innervation to the leg over the anterolateral aspect of the thigh. Injury to this nerve causes numbness in the above-described distribution and is called *meralgia paresthetica.* This deficit is usually transient but may last 3 to 6 months.[21] Femoral nerve injury (Fig. 10-5) may result in quadriceps paralysis, producing an inability to extend the lower leg at the knee and decreased sensation along the anterior aspect of the thigh and medial aspect of the calf. With extension and external rotation in the lithotomy position, the sciatic nerve may be compromised.[22] Expected neurologic compromise (Table 10-14) includes sensory disturbances in the gluteal region radiating to the foot along the posterior aspect of the leg.

In patients undergoing cesarean delivery, the femoral and lateral femoral cutaneous nerves (Fig. 10-5) can be injured as a result of excessive pressure exerted by

Table 10-14. Neurologic Compromise Caused by Childbirth

Nerve	Root	Occurrence	Deficit
Lumbosacral	L4,L5	Most common in vaginal delivery; increased incidence with mid to high forceps delivery or platypellic pelvis	Hypoesthesia of lateral calf and foot; slight weakness of hip abductors; foot drop; slight weakness of quadriceps; usually unilateral involvement; resolves in 3 to 6 months
Femoral nerve	L2–L4	Injured with retractors in cesarean delivery or with prolonged lithotomy positioning; with hyperacute hip flexion in lithotomy position (kinked where it passes under inguinal ligament)	Quadriceps paralysis (no knee extension); no patellar reflex; hypoesthesia of front of thigh and medial aspect of calf
Lateral femoral cutaneous nerve	L2–L3	Injured with retractors in cesarean delivery or lithotomy positioning (pressure with passage under inguinal ligament)	Numbness over anterolateral aspect of thigh; usually transient
Sciatic nerve	L4,L5 S1–S3	Uncommonly associated with delivery; associated with incorrect lithotomy positioning with knee extension or external rotation of hips	Classic symptom: pain in posterior gluteal region radiating to foot
Obturator nerve	L2–L4	Rarely involved in vaginal deliveries; lithotomy position	Inability to adduct leg; decreased sensation over medial thigh
Common peroneal	L4,L5 S1,S2	Lithotomy positioning with pressure on nerve over fibula	Equinovarus deformity; plantar flexion with inversion; loss of sensation over anterolateral aspect of calf and dorsum of foot and toes
Saphenous		Associated with lithotomy positioning (pressure on nerve over tibia)	Loss of sensation over medial aspect of foot and anteromedial aspect of lower leg

retractors intraoperatively.[23] Signs of injury have already been described in Table 10-14.

Other causes of neurologic impairment unrelated to regional anesthesia must be entertained. Marinacci and Courville[24] demonstrated that the predominance of patients with neurologic complaints attributed to intraspinal anesthesia actually evidenced neurologic complaints due to other concurrent and unrelated conditions.[24]

In addition to the neurologic compromise occurring as a result of vaginal or cesarean delivery and positioning injuries that have already been addressed, other types of injuries may occur. They include (1) pre-existing pressure neuritis (as caused by diabetes mellitus or chronic alcoholism); (2) infectious neuritis; (3) exacerbation of multiple sclerosis; and (4) concurrent disease process such as intervertebral disc disease and spinal angioma. Differentiation between these two groups of lesions is based on the distribution of electromyographic (EMG) abnormalities and the time that these EMG abnormalities were first detected. For instance, spinal angiomas (vascular anomalies of the spinal cord) are usually associated with a history of leg weakness before onset of labor.[25] Sometimes a history of weakness is not easily elicited and the diagnosis may be difficult to establish. In this setting, EMG studies are helpful because EMG abnormalities evident immediately after delivery must be due to antecedent problems, whereas abnormal EMG studies due to intraspinal anesthesia would not become evident for at least 3 weeks.[24] The incidence of prolapsed intervertebral disc has been reported to be approximately 1 per 9,000.[26,27] This condition in the parturient is usually associated with sciatica. Most patients present with worsening back discomfort and radicular leg pain in the third trimester of pregnancy. Many patients evidence foot drop.[26] The diagnosis is confirmed by myelography.

As one might expect, certain disease processes such as diabetes and alcoholism may be associated with a higher rate of neurologic compromise in some series.[28] Underlying disease processes such as multiple sclerosis may be associated with neurologic exacerbations after the induction of regional or general anesthesia. Electrolyte abnormalities such as hypomagnesemia have also been associated with neurologic dysfunction.[29]

The pregnant patient may have a variety of complaints

irrespective of the mode of delivery or anesthetic technique utilized. The incidence of backache in the parturient is 25 to 40 percent.[30] The etiology is probably ligamentous strain from lordosis. The overall incidence of back discomfort is not increased in parturients receiving regional anesthesia for delivery. However, point tenderness in the area of needle insertion may be related to regional technique, particularly with the use of the paramedian approach. The current chloroprocaine preparation (Nescaine MPF, Astra Pharmacuticals, Inc.), has been reported to cause back discomfort after epidural anesthesia.[31]

Headache occurs commonly in the parturient after delivery regardless of whether or not regional anesthesia is utilized.[30] A detailed history, physical examination, and chart review must be performed to determine if a patient has a headache attributable to intraspinal anesthesia. The signs and symptoms of post-dural puncture headache are described in Chapter 7.

Rarely, patients may develop evidence of chemical or aseptic meningitis after intraspinal anesthesia.[32] Aseptic meningitis was reported more commonly in the older literature.[33–35] Detergents used to clean reusable spinal kits and other contaminants were often implicated. Aseptic meningitis usually presents as a severe unremitting headache accompanied by a high fever and photophobia. Other signs of meningeal irritation include nuchal rigidity, Kernig's sign, nausea, vomiting, and hypertension. Symptoms usually appear within several hours of the anesthetic and resolve within 2 to 4 days. Aseptic meningitis is characterized by high cerebrospinal fluid (CSF) pressure after dural puncture and clear to slightly cloudy CSF. Other CSF characteristics include elevated white cell count, normal glucose, increased protein, and an absence of organisms on microscopic examination or in follow-up cultures. There is usually a peripheral leukocytosis. Treatment is supportive consisting of fluids and bed rest.

Septic meningitis has been described and is exceedingly rare.[36] It may result from a breakdown in technique, faulty spinal kit preparation, direct contamination, or penetration of an infected area during needle placement. Symptoms are similar to those described above. CSF is purulent with decreased glucose content. Organisms may be seen on microscopic examination and identified with subsequent cultures. Treatment is supportive, focusing on appropriate antibiotic therapy.

A well-conducted epidural anesthetic may be associated with attendant self-limited side effects aside from the expected sympathetic blockade and sensorimotor anesthesia. The occurrence of Horner syndrome (miosis, ptosis, enopthalmos, and anhidrosis) has been described.[37,38] Explanations include reduced potential volume of the epidural space due to venous engorgement associated with labor and resulting in increased spread of local anesthetic.

NEUROLOGIC IMPAIRMENT DUE TO REGIONAL ANESTHESIA

The incidence of protracted lower extremity neurologic sequelae related to regional anesthesia is extremely low and varies depending on the series of patients studied.[8,10,12] Some occurrences are so rare that they appear only as case reports.

Prolonged anesthetic blockade secondary to high concentrations of drug administered over a long period of time has been described.[39,40] This type of blockade has been described as lasting for 48 to 72 hours after vaginal delivery with epidural anesthesia. It is often associated with use of high concentrations of local anesthetic agents and prolonged labor.[41] The resolution of the block is usually described as gradual. The cause of prolonged anesthetic blockade is unclear but may be related to local anesthetic sequestration in tissue pockets or epidural fat.

Direct trauma to nerve roots or the spinal cord by needle placement may occur after intraspinal anesthesia, however, this type of injury occurs rarely.[10,12] Nerve root injury caused by direct trauma will be limited to one nerve root and is usually associated with a sensory rather than motor deficit. Symptoms usually resolve in weeks to months.[42] Vandam has described multiple nerve root injuries that occurred in a patient who evidenced multiple paresthesias after spinal needle insertion at several different lumbar levels.[10]

Injury to the spinal cord itself has rarely been reported with spinal needle placement. Lacerating pain and loss of consciousness have been described. Neurologic injury involving multiple sensory and motor levels of the spinal cord may be involved. This injury is usually permanent. Obviously, when performing an intraspinal anesthetic, placement of the needle below the level of the termination of the spinal cord will result in a decreased likelihood of trauma. The spinal cord usually ends at the level of the first lumbar intervertebral disc but may extend to the second intervertebral disc.

Residual bladder disturbances have been reported after intraspinal anesthesia, presumably as a result of retention and overstretching of the bladder wall secondary to lack of bladder sensation. Bladder dysfunction occurs more commonly after the use of long-acting agents. However, bladder problems may also arise from trauma due to delivery.[30]

Ischemic injury to the spinal cord may occur secondary to compression of the spinal cord by space-occupying lesions such as epidural hematoma or epidural abscess.

Ischemia may also be due to compromised blood flow occurring secondary to anterior spinal artery syndrome. It must be remembered that these complications occur rarely and are not necessarily attributable to the use of regional anesthesia.

The incidence of epidural hematomas is quoted to be between 1 per 50,000 and 1 per 150,000.[9,12,43,44] Because of its infrequent appearance, it is difficult to attach an absolute incidence to this complication. More importantly, factors associated with case reports that may be responsible for increased occurrence must be identified. Spontaneous occurrence of epidural hematomas have been described.[45,46] Epidural hematoma formation has been associated with epidural catheter placement in the face of anticoagulant therapy[47] as well as occult bleeding diathesis.[48,49] Patients with pre-eclampsia with unrecognized low platelet counts and/or significantly prolonged bleeding times in whom epidural catheters are placed may be at increased risk. The clinical course usually follows the sudden onset of progressive lower extremity weakness and hypoesthesia due to cord compression. Back pain is often present. The diagnosis represents a surgical emergency that requires laminectomy, ideally within 6 hours, to prevent permanent paralysis.[50] If surgery is delayed, paralysis may be permanent.

Epidural abscess is an extremely rare complication of epidural analgesia.[12] In most series of patients reviewed, epidural abscess occurs most often as a result of seeding of the epidural space secondary to an infection elsewhere in the body, antecedent trauma, chronic debilitation, alcoholism, or diabetes mellitus, as well as some surgical procedures.[51–53] Onset may occur slowly over 1 to 3 days. Symptoms and signs of epidural abscess include severe back pain, fever, localized back tenderness, and leukocytosis, coupled with progressive flaccid paralysis and hypoesthesia of the lower extremities. Nuchal rigidity is present in over 50 percent of patients. Again, the diagnosis of epidural abscess constitutes a surgical emergency and requires urgent laminectomy. Late surgical intervention may result in permanent paralysis. The diagnosis of chorioamnionitis has raised concern about possible bacteremia and seeding of the epidural space. However, there are no reports of epidural abscess formation occurring after epidural catheter placement in parturients carrying a diagnosis of chorioamnionitis (see the discussion earlier in this chapter).

Anterior spinal artery syndrome occurs rarely and is most often observed in the older patient population with arteriosclerotic disease. It has been associated with severe atherosclerosis, profound hypotension during anesthesia, and the use of epinephrine-containing local anesthetics.[12,54,55] It has occurred as a result of aortic cross-clamping[12] as well as with prolonged hypotension without the use of regional anesthesia.[56] It involves a flaccid paralysis of the lower extremity of abrupt onset that usually persists postoperatively without improvement, however occasional partial recovery has been seen. The anterior spinal artery along with radicular artery tributaries supplies the anterior two-thirds of the spinal cord, which carries efferent motor fibers to the lower extremity. Therefore, it is not surprising that compromised blood flow to this artery would result in a flaccid paralysis occasionally accompanied by a patchy sensory deficit in the lower extremity. Unintentional subarachnoid injection of local anesthetic agents precipitating profound and prolonged hypotension have given rise to a neurologic picture consistent with anterior spinal artery syndrome.

Adhesive arachnoiditis[57,58] and cauda equina syndrome occur extremely rarely and often secondary to residual detergents or contaminants in reusable spinal or epidural kits or to occult infection.[59,60] Both syndromes were reported more commonly in the older literature.[61–63] The advent of disposable kits has decreased the reported incidence of both cauda equina syndrome and adhesive arachnoiditis. Unintentional subarachnoid administration of chloroprocaine was responsible for case reports of both syndromes in 1980.[64]

Adhesive arachnoiditis is typified by gradual progressive weakness and sensory loss of the lower extremity occurring over weeks to months after intraspinal anesthesia. This may lead to complete paraplegia and death.[59] Autopsy reveals extensive proliferation of meninges over the spinal cord. Cauda equina syndrome is characterized by urinary and fecal incontinence coupled with localized sensory loss in the perineal area with varying degrees of leg weakness. Symptoms usually occur immediately after the effects of intraspinal anesthesia wear off. These effects may be permanent or show gradual improvement over several months.

The spinal cord and nerve roots are exquisitely sensitive to the effects of detergents used to clean reusable syringes and other contaminants that have occurred with subarachnoid administration. Chloroprocaine was associated with several cases of cauda equina syndrome and adhesive arachnoiditis in 1980.[64,65] Investigations implicated the low pH of chloroprocaine coupled with sodium bisulfite, a preservative, as well as possible mechanical factors associated with high-volume injections into the epidural or subarachnoid space.[66,67] Present chloroprocaine preparations have a higher pH, are bisulfite free, and have not been associated with any case reports of these syndromes. However, the newest preparation of chloroprocaine has been associated with back pain when the block has diminished. The etiology of the back pain is unclear.

The dura appears to exert a protective effect against neurotoxic agents. Unintentional administration of potassium chloride, phenol, and thiopental in the epidural space has been tolerated with no untoward sequelae.[12] There has been a case report of severe neurologic injury occurring after epidural saline infusion.[68] The saline contained a preservative (1.5 percent benzyl alcohol). This case underlines the importance of using preservative-free drugs with both subarachnoid and epidural administration.

As has already been mentioned, postpartum neurologic deficits occur more often secondary to obstetric causes rather than to the regional anesthetic drugs or techniques. Underlying disease processes (e.g., prolapsed intervertebral disc, spinal angioma, or multiple sclerosis) may give rise to exacerbations after delivery. If a postpartum deficit is identified, a systematic form of investigation is essential to determine cause, initiate treatment, and determine prognosis. Based on the previous descriptions entailed in this section, it becomes clear that a detailed history of the patient's prior medical history, symptoms associated with pregnancy, and mode of delivery are imperative. A careful physical examination to identify specific neurologic involvement and to assess daily improvement or worsening of symptoms is necessary. Laboratory evaluations, including a glucose tolerance test, coagulation profile, complete blood count, lumbrosacral spine roentenography, computed tomographic (CT) scan, and EMG studies, when indicated are essential. A reasonable format of investigation is detailed below.

Peripartum Neurologic Complaint Following Regional Anesthesia

History. Careful history is critical

1. Antecedent medical diseases (diabetes mellitus, multiple sclerosis).
2. Neurologic complaints prior to delivery, particularly related to the lower extremity (prolapsed disc, spinal angioma, tumor, back strain from pregnancy).
3. Nature of present symptoms, distribution, onset, and *trend.*

Physical Examination.

1. Check vital signs (increased temperature, tachycardia).
2. Examine back, check for local tenderness in area of puncture sites.
3. Perform a detailed sensorimotor examination; associated bladder or bowel dysfunction.
4. Record precise distribution of symptoms in chart.

Supporting Tests.

1. Glucose tolerance test/urinalysis to rule out occult diabetes mellitus; coagulation profile to rule out bleeding diathesis (preeclampsia, HELLP syndrome).
2. Lumbar spine roentgenogram, CT scan with suspicion of disc disease.
3. Myelogram with strong suspicion of disc disease, etc.
4. Electromyogram with significant motor deficit.
5. Lumbar puncture.

Communication.

1. Discuss with obstetrician any significant neurologic impairment along with rational approach toward diagnosis with appropriate tests.
2. Consult with neurologist about significant neurologic impairment and enlist aid in determining etiology.
3. Reassure patient and institute tests and investigations to determine diagnosis; institute treatment where appropriate and determine prognosis.

REFERENCES

1. Downing JW: Bupivacaine: a clinical assessment in lumbar epidural block. Br J Anaesth 41:427, 1967
2. Hill EC: Maternal obstetric paralysis. Am J Obstet Gynecol 83:1452, 1962
3. Tillman AJB: Traumatic neuritis in the puerperium. Am J Obstet Gynecol 29:660, 1935
4. Chalmers JA: Traumatic neuritis of the puerperium. J Obstet Gynaecol Br Emp 56:205, 1945
5. Hellman K: Epidural anesthesia in obstetrics: a second look at 26,127 cases. Can Anaesth Soc J 12:398, 1965
6. Moore DC, Bridenbaugh LD, Thompson GE, et al: Bupivicaine: a review of 11,080 cases. Anesth Analg 57:42, 1978
7. Bleyaert A, Soltens M, Vaes L, et al: Bupivicaine 0.125 percent in obstetric epidural analgesia. Anesthesiology 51:435, 1979
8. Ong BY, Cohen MM, Esmail A, et al: Paresthesias and motor dysfunction after labor and delivery. Anesth Analg 66:18, 1987
9. Dawkins CJM: An analysis of the complications of extradural and caudal block. Anaesthesia 24:554, 1969
10. Dripps RD, Vandam LD: Long term follow up of patients who received 10,098 spinal anesthetics: failure to discover major neurologic sequelae. JAMA 156:1486, 1954
11. Lund PC: Peridural anesthesia: a review of 10,000 administrations. Acta Anaesthesiol Scand 6:143, 1962
12. Usubiaga JE: Neurologic complications following epidural anesthesia. Int Anesthesiol Clin 13(2):1, 1975
13. Moir DD, Davidson S: Post partum complications of forceps

delivery performed under epidural and pudendal nerve block. Br J Anaesth 44:1197, 1972
14. Donaldson JO: Neurology of pregnancy. Neuropathy 7:43, 1978
15. Murray RR: Maternal obstetric paralysis. Am J Obstet Gynecol 88:399, 1964
16. Abouleish E: Neurologic complications following epidural analgesia in obstetrics—one center's experience. Reg Anesth 7:119, 1982
17. Holdcroft A, Morgan M: Maternal complications of obstetric epidural analgesia. Anesth Intensive Care 4:108, 1976
18. Sunderland S: The relative susceptibility to injury of the medial and lateral popliteal divisions of the sciatic nerve. Br J Surg 41:300, 1953
19. Burkhart FL, Daly JW: Sciatic and peroneal nerve injury: a complication of vaginal operations. Obstet Gynecol 28:99, 1966
20. Rhodes P: Meralgia paraesthetica in pregnancy. Lancet 2:831, 1957
21. Pearson MG: Meralgia paraesthetica with reference to its occurrence in pregnancy. Br J Obstet Gynaecol 64:427, 1957
22. Nicholson MJ, Eversole UH: Nerve injuries incident to anesthesia and operation. Anesth Analg 36(4):19, 1957
23. Ruston FG, Polith VL: Femoral nerve injury from abdominal retractors. Can Anaesth Soc J 5:428, 1955
24. Marinacci AA, Courville CB: Electromyogram in evaluation of neurological complications of spinal anesthesia. JAMA 168:1337, 1958
25. Hirsch NP, Child CS, Wijetilleka SA: Paraplegia caused by spinal angioma—possible association with epidural anesthesia. Anesth Analg 64:937, 1985
26. LaBan MM, Perrin JCS, Latimer FR: Pregnancy and the herniated disc. Arch Phys Med Rehab 64:319, 1983
27. Kelsey JL, Greenberg RA, Hardy RJ, Johnson MF: Pregnancy and the syndrome of herniated lumbar intervertebral disc: an epidemiological study. Yale J Biol Med 48:361, 1975
28. Calverley JR, Mulder DW: Femoral neuropathy. Neurology 10:963, 1960
29. Ravindran RS, Carelli A: Neurologic dysfunction in postpartum patients caused by hypomagnesemia. Anesthesiology 66:391, 1987
30. Grove LH: Backache, headache and bladder dysfunction after delivery. Br J Anaesth 45:1147, 1973
31. Levy L, Randel GI, Pandit SK: Does chloroprocaine (Nesacaine^{MPF}) for epidural anesthesia increase the incidence of backache? Anesthesiology 71:476, 1989
32. Seighe TD: Aseptic meningitis following spinal analgesia. Anaesthesia 25:402, 1970
33. Goldman WW, Sanford JP: An epidemic of chemical meningitis. Anesth Analg 43:372, 1964
34. Rendell CM: Chemical meningitis due to syringes stored in Lysol. Anaesthesia 9:281, 1954
35. Livingstone H, Wellman V, Clark D, Lambrosa V: Aseptic or chemical meningitis. Surg Gynecol Obstet 77:216, 1943
36. Bonica JJ: Principles and Practice of Obstetric Analgesia and Anesthesia. FA Davis, Philadelphia, 1972
37. Skaredoff MN, Datta S: Horner's Syndrome during epidural anesthesia for elective Cesarean delivery. Can Anaesth Soc J 28:82, 1981
38. Schachner SM, Reynolds AC: Horner's syndrome during lumbar epidural analgesia for obstetrics. Obstet Gynecol 59:31, 1982
39. Bromage PR: An evaluation of bupivacaine in epidural analgesia for obstetrics. Can Anaesth Soc J 16:46, 1969
40. Cuerden C, Buley R, Downing JW: Delayed recovery after epidural block in labour. A report of four cases. Anaesthesia 32:773, 1977
41. Pathy GV, Rosen M: Prolonged block with recovery after extradural analgesia for labor. Br J Anaesth 47:520, 1975
42. Vandam LD, Dripps RD: Long term follow up of 10,098 spinal anesthetics. II. Incidence and analysis of minor sensory neurological defects. Surgery 38:463, 1953
43. Kane RE: Neurologic deficits following epidural or spinal anaesthesia. Anesth Analg 60:150, 1981
44. Skouen JS, Wainapel SF, Willock MM: Paraplegia following epidural anesthesia. A case report and a literature review. Acta Neurol Scand 72:437, 1985
45. Harik SI, Raichle ME, Reis DJ: Spontaneously remitting spinal epidural hematoma in a patient on anticoagulants. N Engl J Med 284:1355, 1971
46. Guy MJ, Zahra M, Sengupta RP: Spontaneous spinal subdural hematoma during general anesthesia. Surg Neurol 11:199, 1979
47. Mayumi T, Doki S: Spinal subarachnoid hematoma after lumbar puncture in a patient receiving antiplatelet therapy. Anesth Analg 62:777, 1983
48. Dunn D, Dhopesh V, Mobini J: Spinal subdural hematoma. A possible hazard of lumbar puncture in an alcoholic. JAMA 241:1712, 1979
49. Gustafsson H, Rutberg H, Bergtsson M: Spinal haematoma following epidural analgesia. Anaesthesia 43:220, 1988
50. Pacher NP, Cummins BH: Spontaneous epidural hematoma: a surgical emergency. Lancet 1:356, 1978
51. Danner RL, Hartman BJ: Update of spinal epidural abscess: 35 cases and review of the literature. Rev Infect Dis 9:265, 1987
52. North JB, Brophy BP: Epidural abscess: a hazard of spinal epidural anesthesia. Aust NZ J Surg 49:484, 1979
53. Baker AS, Ojemann RG, Swartz MN: Spinal epidural abscess. N Engl J Med 293:463, 1975
54. Urquhart-Hay D: Paraplegia following epidural anaesthesia. Anaesthesia 24:461, 1969
55. Harrison PD: Paraplegia following epidural anaesthesia. Anaesthesia 30:778, 1975
56. Ditzler JW, McIlver G: Paraplegia following general anaesthesia. Anesth Analg 34:501, 1956
57. Sghirlanzoni A, Marazzi R, Pareyson D, et al: Epidural anaesthesia and spinal arachnoiditis. Anaesthesia 44:377, 1989
58. Lombardi B, Girotti F: Diffuse arachnoiditis following epidural analgesia. J Neurol 230:253, 1983
59. Winkelman NW: Neurologic symptoms following accidental intraspinal detergent injection. Neurology 2:284, 1952
60. Paddison RM, Alpers BJ: Role of intrathecal detergents in

pathogenesis of adhesive arachnoiditis. Arch Neurol Psych 71:87, 1954
61. Ferguson FR, Watkins KH: Paralysis of the bladder and associated neurologic sequelae of spinal anesthesia (cauda equina syndrome). Br J Surg 25:735, 1937
62. Kennedy F, Effron A, Perry G: The grave spinal cord paralysis caused by spinal anesthesia. Surg Gynecol Obstet 91:385, 1950
63. Bergner RP, Roseman E, Johnson H, Smith WR: Severe neurological complications following spinal anesthesia: report of six cases. Anesthesiology 12:717, 1951
64. Reisner LS, Hochman BN, Plumer MH: Persistent neurologic deficit and adhesive arachnoiditis following intrathecal 2-chloroprocaine injection. Anesth Analg 59:452, 1980
65. Ravindran RS, Bond JK, Tasch MD, et al: Prolonged neural blockade following regional analgesia with 2-chloroprocaine. Anesth Analg 59:447, 1980
66. Gissen AJ, Datta S, Lambert D: The chloroprocaine controversy. I. A hypothesis to explain the neural complications of chloroprocaine epidural. Reg Anesth 9:124, 1984
67. Gissen AJ, Datta S, Lambert D: The chloroprocaine controversy. II. Is chloroprocaine neurotoxic? Reg Anesth 9:135, 1984
68. Craig DB, Habib GG: Flaccid paraparesis following obstetric epidural anesthesia: possible role of benzyl alcohol. Anesth Analg 56:219, 1977

ACUTE CARBON MONOXIDE POISONING IN PREGNANCY

Acute carbon monoxide poisoning is the leading cause of death due to poisoning, and it is estimated that between 1,500 and 3,500 deaths occur per year.[1–3] As a better understanding of this entity is realized, more accounts of true carbon monoxide poisoning during pregnancy are being reported. It is important that obstetric anesthesiologists have a thorough understanding of this clinical state, so that prompt diagnosis, appropriate monitoring, and immediate therapy may be instituted to avoid the deleterious effects of carbon monoxide poisoning on the mother and the developing fetus.

CHEMICAL ASPECTS OF CARBON MONOXIDE

Carbon monoxide poisoning and its mechanisms have been known since Claude Bernard reported in 1857 that this gas causes death by producing hypoxia.[4] Carbon monoxide is a colorless, odorless, tasteless, nonirritating gas produced by the incomplete combustion of carbonacious material. Almost any fire produces CO. Other sources of carbon monoxide include automotive exhaust, thick smoke, gas heaters (not natural gas), home and industrial heating systems, erythrocyte destruction, and cigarette smoke.[2] Automotive fumes may produce a carboxyhemoglobin (HbCO) level greater than 20 percent, erythrocyte destruction usually gives a 1 percent HbCO level, and cigarette smoke may give a HbCO level between 2 and 15 percent.[5,6]

Table 10-15. Carbon Monoxide Poisoning: Signs and Symptoms with Percentage HbCO

%HbCO	Signs and Symptoms
0–10	None
10–20	Tightness across forehead, slight headache, dilatation of cutaneous blood vessels
20–30	Throbbing headache
40–50	As above, with possibility of syncope; increased respiratory and pulse rates
50–60	Syncope, increased respiratory and pulse rates; coma with intermittent convulsions; Cheyne–Stokes respiration
60–70	Coma with intermittent convulsions; depressed cardiovascular and respiratory function, possible death
70–80	Weak pulse, slow respiratory rates; respiratory failure and death

SIGNS AND SYMPTOMS ASSOCIATED WITH CARBON MONOXIDE EXPOSURE

The signs and symptoms seen with carbon monoxide exposure relate to the percentage of carboxyhemoglobin (Table 10-15). The often-cited cherry-red appearance of the carbon monoxide poisoned patient is variable in its presentation.

DIAGNOSIS OF CARBON MONOXIDE POISONING

The diagnosis may not be immediately obvious, however, the aforementioned signs and symptoms coupled with the history usually lead to the suspicion of carbon monoxide poisoning. The definitive diagnosis is made with the HbCO level determined by multiple band spectrophotometry (vide infra).

The HbCO level is very important for diagnosis, but the presence of signs, symptoms, and history of exposure to carbon monoxide justify the institution of therapy, and any delay in administering that therapy is inappropriate.[4]

A HbCO level of greater then 20 percent is considered to be carbon monoxide poisoning. However, many victims receive supplemental oxygen therapy before blood samples are drawn, thus lowering their HbCO level upon admission. Owing to this possible reduction in HbCO level, the clinician must thoughtfully consider the diagnosis of carbon monoxide poisoning in patients with a history and presentation suggestive of this entity, even if the HbCO level is not markedly elevated. Interestingly, the $PaCO_2$ may be normal, increased, or decreased.

Included in the differential diagnosis are anemic hypoxia, circulatory hypoxia, specific organ hypoxia, and increased oxygen-requiring states (i.e., febrile states and thyrotoxicosis) and improper oxygen utilization states (i.e., cyanide poisoning). Cyanide poisoning may occur concomittantly with carbon monoxide poisoning in burn- and fume-exposed victims. These patients are unable to utilize oxygen because cyanide interferes with the electron transport of the cytochrome oxidase system.

BIOLOGIC CONSIDERATIONS OF CARBON MONOXIDE POISONING

The toxic effects of carbon monoxide are a result of tissue hypoxia. It is known that hemoglobin has an affinity for carbon monoxide that is 200 to 250 times greater than it has for oxygen. Carbon monoxide freely combines with hemoglobin (Hb) to form carboxyhemoglobin (HbCO). Carbon monoxide also interferes with the release of oxygen from hemoglobin. Carbon monoxide has this effect by shifting the hemoglobin curve to the left, thus further reducing the amount of oxygen available to the tissues and explains why tissue anoxia occurs at levels of arterial hemoglobin concentrations tolerated by anemic patients. One is better off with a 50 percent reduction in his or her hemoglobin concentration than a 50 percent level of HbCO. Carbon monoxide also interferes with cellular oxidative metabolism via the intracellular cytochrome oxidase system.[2]

Van Hoesen et al.[2] explained that the effects of carbon monoxide are dramatic for the pregnant patient and that the fetus is even more vulnerable than the mother to the hypoxic effects of carbon monoxide. Fetal HbCO concentrations depend on maternal HbCO concentration, placental diffusing capacity of carbon monoxide, endogenous fetal carbon monoxide production, and the relative affinity of maternal and fetal hemoglobin for carbon monoxide and oxygen. Normal human/maternal HbCO concentration is 1.1:1. This demonstrates that the fetal HbCO levels are 10 to 15 percent higher than maternal levels at steady state.

The fetal hemoglobin dissociation curve lies to the left of the maternal curve. Since the normal fetal arterial PO_2 is low, the fetal system normally operates on the steep part of the curve, thus a small drop in oxygen tension results in a large drop in oxygen concentration.[2]

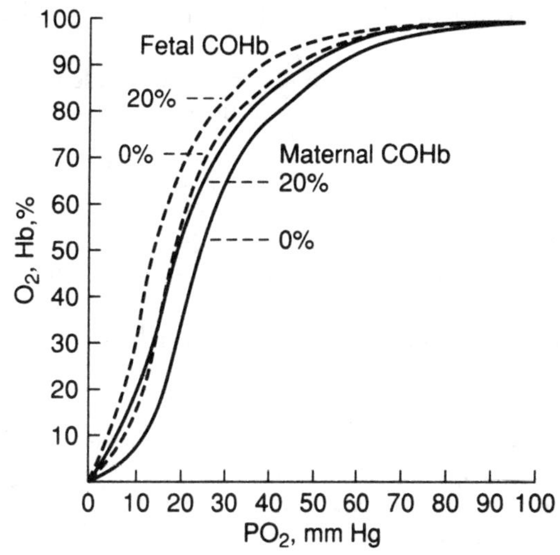

Fig. 10-6. Effect of carboxyhemoglobin on the hemoglobin dissociation curve. (From Van Hoesen et al.,[2] with permission.)

Before the fetal HbCO level has risen, there will already have been a fall in the maternal arterial oxygen content, leading to fetal hypoxia. Also, as the fetal HbCO level rises, it will further shift the hemoglobin dissociation curve to the left, making it even more difficult for the fetus to unload oxygen possibly leading to drastic hypoxia in the fetus,[2] (Fig. 10-6).

A mathematical model has been developed[7] that examines the exchange of carbon monoxide between the human fetus and the mother. Findings demonstrate that fetal HbCO levels lagged with respect to maternal HbCO levels by several hours. However, during uptake, fetal HbCO levels eventually rose above maternal HbCO levels. The elimination of carbon monoxide from the fetus considerably lagged behind the mother. With increased inspired oxygen concentration, the time for elimination of the maternal HbCO was reduced but the time for elimination of the fetal HbCO was not reduced nearly as much as that of the mother. These physiologic considerations will have important implications for the treatment of the pregnant patient exposed to carbon monoxide.

TREATMENT OF THE PREGNANT PATIENT EXPOSED TO CARBON MONOXIDE

Standard care and monitoring apply to these patients as it would to any patient with a history of smoke inhalation and possible thermal airway injury. Depending on gestational age, fetal monitoring may be appropriate. The limitations of pulse oximetry is discussed below.

The definitive treatment of carbon monoxide poisoning is to facilitate elimination of the gas via the lungs.

1. Remove the victim from the carbon monoxide source.
2. Assess ventilation and the need for intubation.
3. Increase inspired oxygen concentration to 100 percent.
4. Decrease patient activity to decrease tissue oxygen needs.

Oxygen competes with carbon monoxide for the same site on the Hb molecule so that increasing the oxygen tension will increase the competition for the sites. Removing the victim from the carbon monoxide source will decrease the alveolar partial pressure of carbon monoxide but, even with the alveolar partial pressure close to zero, there is less than a 2-mmHg gradient from blood to alveoli to remove carbon monoxide from the hemoglobin.[8] An illustration to put this elimination process in perspective: On room air the HbCO half-life is 5 hours for the nonpregnant patient; on 100 percent FiO_2, the half-life decreases to 1 hour.

Numerous studies have looked at the use of hyperbaric oxygen therapy (HBO) for the treatment of acute carbon monoxide poisoning. The first systematic studies evaluating the physiologic effects of HBO for the treatment of carbon monoxide poisoning were conducted in the 1950s.[9] HBO increases arterial and tissue oxygen tensions far in excess of that achieved with breathing 100 percent oxygen. With increasing oxygen partial pressures, the rate of release of carbon monoxide from HBO is increased, thus decreasing the HbCO half-life.[3] It has been proposed that there may be additional mechanisms by which HBO therapy functions.

Carefully conducted clinical studies have not been performed and some investigators have questioned whether HBO therapy confers a benefit over 100 percent oxygen in the treatment of acute carbon monoxide poisoning.[8,10,11] Additional concern arises with the use of HBO in the pregnant patient because of the relative lack of information on the risk of high partial pressures of oxygen on the fetus. However, there have been numerous reports that show a decrease in morbidity and mortality in patients with acute carbon monoxide poisoning who have had HBO therapy.[12–14]

It is known that carbon monoxide has toxic effects to the fetus in all stages of pregnancy.[15–17] With this in mind and the realization that carbon monoxide elimination from the fetus is much slower than in the mother, it is of considerable interest to try to hasten the carbon monoxide elimination process.

Van Hoesen et al. have reviewed numerous studies employing HBO in the pregnant patient. They remark that many of the adverse effects noted in various studies may have been secondary to the excessive hyperbaric pressures and time periods used in treatment. They also reviewed many studies that report improved fetal outcome with HBO use, without detrimental effects to the fetus. Soviet Union studies employing HBO therapy in several hundred pregnant patients during all stages of gestation report improved fetal circulation and reduced perinatal complications and mortality without any evidence of retinopathy or adverse effects secondary to HBO.[18–20] Van Hoesen et al., who have done an extensive review of the literature, believe that the benefits of HBO therapy in the pregnant patient with acute carbon monoxide poisoning far outweigh the risks and state that HBO therapy should be considered in any pregnant patient with acute carbon monoxide poisoning. They recommend the following steps (from Van Hoesen et al.,[2] with permission):

1. Administer HBO therapy if the maternal HbCO level is above 20 percent at any time during the exposure.
2. Administer HBO therapy if the patient has suffered or demonstrates signs of any neurologic injury regardless of the HbCO level.
3. Administer HBO therapy if signs of fetal distress are present (i.e., fetal tachycardia, decreased beat-to-beat variability on the fetal monitor, or late decelerations) consistent with the HbCO levels and exposure history.
4. If HBO treatment is unavailable, administer 100 percent oxygen by a tightly fitting mask for five times as long as needed to reduce maternal HbCO to normal (less than 5 percent).
5. If the patient continues to demonstrate neurologic signs or sign of fetal distress 12 hours after initial treatment, additional HBO treatments may be indicated. Multiple HBO treatments have been suggested to be beneficial in severely poisoned and nonresponsive patients exposed to carbon monoxide.

MONITORING AND CARBON MONOXIDE POISONING

Pulse oximetry has been recommended as a standard of care for every general anesthetic and is routinely used in many settings, including the obstetric operating room and recovery room.[21]

Pulse oximetry provides an instantaneous, noninvasive

means of determining the arterial oxygenation based on determining light absorption between a light-emitting diode and a nonselective photodetector. The oximeter "assumes" that there are only two species of hemoglobin present in the blood (i.e., oxyhemoglobin [HbO] and deoxyhemoglobin [Hb]). To distinguish between these two species, the oximeter emits light at two different wavelengths (i.e., one emitting red at 660 nm and the other, infrared at 940 nm). The oximeter makes use of the relative absorbance of these wavelengths of light to calculate the arterial oxygen saturation.[22] However, when another species of hemoglobin is present (i.e., HbCO, which absorbs very similarly to oxyhemoglobin at 660 nm), erroneous readings will result. Numerous studies[23–25] have demonstrated that when clinically significant quantities of HbCO are present, substantial differences may be seen between the pulse oximeter oxygen saturation reading and the actual arterial oxygen saturation. Therefore, a normal oximeter saturation reading in a patient exposed to carbon monoxide cannot be regarded as accurate, for the actual arterial saturation may be significantly lower. A "low" oximeter reading in this carbon monoxide-exposed patient may represent severe hypoxemia.

In the care of patients exposed to carbon monoxide, an arterial blood gas analysis must be immediately performed and the laboratory should be requested to report a measured HbCO level and a measured arterial oxygen saturation employing a multiple band spectrophotometer.

The accuracy of the pulse oximeter for use on the neonate has been questioned, since fetal hemoglobin differs from adult hemoglobin in its amino acid sequence and thus may differ in its absorbance characteristics. However, studies report an insignificant effect on the extinction curves employed by the pulse oximeter, with a negligible effect on the pulse oximeter reading.[22,23,26,27]

REFERENCES

1. Wharton M, Bistowish JM, Hutcheson RH, Schaffner W: Fatal carbon monoxide poisoning at a motel. JAMA 261:1177, 1989
2. Van Hoesen KB, Camporesi EM, Moon RE, et al: Should hyperbaric oxygen be used to treat the pregnant patient for acute carbon monoxide poisoning? JAMA 261:1039, 1989
3. Thom SR: Hyperbaric oxygen therapy. J Intensive Care Med 4:58, 1989
4. Winter PM, Miller JN: Carbon monoxide poisoning. JAMA 236(13):1502, 1976
5. Wald NJ, Idle M, Boreham J, Bailey A: Carbon monoxide in breath in relation to smoking and carboxyhaemoglobin levels. Thorax 36:366, 1981
6. Nordenberg D, Yip R, Binkin NJ: The effect of cigarette smoking on hemoglobin levels and anemia screening. JAMA 264(12):1556, 1990
7. Hill EP, Hill JR, Power GG, Longo LD: Carbon monoxide exchanges between the human fetus and mother: a mathematical model. Am J Physiol 232(3):H311, 1977
8. Grim PS, Gottlieb LJ, Boddie A, Batson E: Hyperbaric oxygen therapy JAMA 263(16):2216, 1990
9. Pace N, Strajman E, Walker EL: Acceleration of carbon monoxide elimination in man by high pressure oxygen. Science 111:652, 1950
10. Kumar S: Hyperbaric oxygen in the treatment of carbon monoxide poisoning [abstract]. Br Med J 289:1315, 1984
11. Raphael JC, Elkharrat D, Jars-Guincestre MC, et al: Trial of normobaric and hyperbaric oxygen for acute carbon monoxide intoxication. Lancet 2:414, 1989
12. Goulon M, Barois A, Rapin M, et al: Carbon monoxide poisoning and acute anoxia due to breathing coal gas and hydrocarbons. J Hyperbaric Med 1:23, 1986
13. Krantz T, Thisted B, Strom J, Sorenson MB: Acute carbon monoxide poisoning. Acta Anaesthesiol Scand 32:278, 1988
14. Norkool DM, Kirkpatric JN: Treatment of acute carbon monoxide poisoning with hyperbaric oxygen: a review of 115 cases. Ann Emerg Med 14:1168, 1985
15. Astrup P, Olsen HM, Trolle D, et al: Effects of moderate carbon monoxide exposure on fetal development. Lancet 2:1220, 1972
16. Ginsberg MD, Myers RE: Fetal brain injury after maternal carbon monoxide intoxication. Neurology 26:15, 1976
17. Ginsberg MD, Myers RE: Fetal brain damage following maternal carbon monoxide intoxication: an experimental study. Acta Obstet Gynecol Scand 53:309, 1974
18. Proshina IV, Kuzmina NV, Borisenko SS: Hyperbaric oxygenation in the prevention and treatment of pregnancy and placental insufficiency. Akush Ginekol 6:20, 1983
19. Aksenova A, Proshina IV, Smirnova LK, et al: Methods of prenatal diagnosis of fetal hypoxia and control of the effectiveness of its treatment with hyperbaric oxygen. Akush Binekol 11:15, 1979
20. Molzhaninov EV, Chaika VK, Domanova AI, et al: Experience and prospects of using hyperbaric oxygenation in obstetrics. p. 139. In Proceedings of the Seventh International Congress on Hyperbaric Medicine, Moscow, 1981. Moscow, Nauka 1983, vol. 1
21. Eichorn JH, Cooper JB, Cullen DJ, et al: Standards for patient monitoring during anesthesia at Harvard Medical School. JAMA 256:1017, 1986
22. Alexander CM, Teller LE, Gross JB: Principles of pulse oximetry: theoretical and practical considerations. Anesth Analg 68:368, 1989
23. Barker SJ, Tremper KK: The effects of carbon monoxide inhalation on pulse oximetry and transcutaneous PO_2. Anesthesiology 66:677, 1987
24. Tremper KK, Barker SJ: Pulse oximetry. Anesthesiology 70:98, 1989
25. Gonzalez A, Gomez-Arnau J, Pensado A: Carboxyhemoglobin and pulse oximetry (Letter). Anesthesiology 73:573, 1990

26. Pologe JA, Raley DM: Effects of fetal hemoglobin on pulse oximetry. J Perinatol 7:324, 1987
27. Anderson JV: The accuracy of pulse oximetry in neonates: effects of fetal hemoglobin and bilirubin. J Perinatol 7:323, 1987

THE OBSTETRIC PATIENT WHO IS A JEHOVAH'S WITNESS

Caring for a patient who is Jehovah's Witness can pose ethical, moral, and legal problems for the anesthesiologist. In the operating room, the anesthesiologist oversees the administration of blood and blood products. A conflict can develop as a result of the refusal of Jehovah's Witness patients to accept blood or blood products, including whole blood, packed erythrocytes, plasma, and platelets. Some, but only a small minority, will accept albumin, antihemophilic products (cryoprecipitate), or immune serum globulin.

RELIGIOUS BACKGROUND

Their refusal of blood (whole blood, packed erythrocytes, plasma, and platelets) transfusion is based on a literal interpretation of certain passages from the Bible:

> ". . . every moving thing that liveth shall be meat for you; even as the green have I given you all things. But flesh with the life thereof, which is the blood thereof, shall ye not eat." (Genesis, 9:3,4)
>
> ". . . therefore I said unto the children of Israel, ye shall eat the blood of no manner of flesh: for the life of all flesh is the blood thereof: whosoever eateth it shall be cut off." (Leviticus, 17:14)
>
> ". . . wherefore my sentence is: that they abstain from meats offered to idols, and from fornication, and from things strangled, and from blood." (Acts, 15:19,20)

ETHICAL CONSIDERATIONS

Physicians are ethically bound by the oath of Hippocrates or Maimonides to preserve life, and this may require the use of blood transfusion. Conversely, physicians have a moral obligation to respect their patients' wishes, including their religious beliefs. However, the physicians can be placed in a precarious ethical and legal position when patients endanger their lives by refusing certain medical treatments (e.g., blood transfusion).

LEGAL CONSIDERATIONS

In many situations, these decisions are made by another party, on behalf of the patient. Example include the parent deciding for a minor child, or a patient's family stating that the patient should not receive a blood transfusion. Because of these controversies, the issue of blood transfusion for these patients has been addressed by different courts of law. Unfortunately, the law has been very ambiguous, with decisions varying from case to case and from state to state. To minimize these potential problems, each hospital should develop specific protocols to guide the management of such patients who refuse blood transfusions on religious beliefs. These protocols should address both elective and emergency situations.

Pregnant Jehovah's Witnesses pose a special problem, because the mother's management also directly involves the unborn fetus. The courts seem to favor, at least at this point, the viable fetus in late gestation. The rights of the fetus early in gestation, however, have not been completely addressed, since this issue involves determining when a fetus becomes viable, as well as the rights of termination of gestation in early pregnancy.

For example, a pregnant Jehovah's Witness patient who may or may not have minor dependent children at home cannot endanger her life by refusal of blood transfusion because of religious beliefs, because she has a responsibility to the community to care for her minor, born or unborn, children. Several states have this case law. As a result, she could be forced by a court order to receive the undesired, but necessary, treatment. The interest of the unborn fetus in late pregnancy will supercede the mother's rights or wishes and the state's interests will prevail.

When admitting these pregnant patients, it should be made clear that, if the situation requires, blood will be transfused to save the life of the fetus. This issue should be addressed during the pregnancy by the obstetric care team and the position of the physician and the hospital explained to the patient. In the event that a pregnant patient refuses blood therapy, but an emergency situation ensues, a court order must be sought in order to proceed with the blood transfusion.

MEDICAL CONSIDERATIONS

The anesthesiologist should always discuss all alternatives with the patient and her family and also conduct a detailed interview to find out to what specific blood product transfusion the patient has an objection. However, it is the responsibility of the primary care physician to have already discussed the subject with the patient. For nonobstetric surgery in the pregnant patient, where the prospect of transfusion is high and the patient agrees to autotransfusion, autologous blood should be made available; if this is unacceptable to the patient, then a cell saver technique may be used during the procedure, provided there is a continuous circuit and the blood does not leave this circuit. The use of the cell saver may not be feasible at operative delivery because of contamination of the blood with amniotic fluid, fetal cells, meconium, and adipose tissue.

Plasma substitutes are another alternative that has been used to replenish blood volume; these include both crystalloid and colloid solutions. Administration of crystalloids (normal saline and lactated Ringer's) can lower the hematocrit by hemodilution, but is followed by marked intraoperative edema. Conversely, colloid administration can result in prolonged anemia and hypervolemia postoperatively, with difficulty in removing the colloid solutions by diuresis. Hetastarch (Hespan) solutions have been used successfully as plasma expanders, but they increase the risk of coagulopathy if administered in large volumes. Some of the most recent studies have concluded that a total amount of 1.5 g/kg of normal body weight of Hespan will avoid possible complications. Desmopressin (DDAVP), a synthetic vasopressin, has also been used in cases where coagulation times were prolonged, so it could have some place in the management of Jehovah's Witness patients preoperatively. Fluosol DA, a synthetic oxygen-carrying compound, has been used in certain circumstances, but it requires either general anesthesia and endotracheal intubation or a hyperbaric chamber in order to obtain PaO_2 over 300 mmHg. It has been effective in the treatment of short-term anemia, but it is not yet approved by the Food and Drug Administration for this use, because of reported anaphylactic reactions. Epsilon-aminocaproic acid (EACA), a synthetic lysine analog, is an antifibrinolytic agent that inhibits plasmin formation by binding plasminogen to fibrin. It has been used to control severe bleeding in postpartum hemorrhage, however, an increased incidence of pulmonary edema precludes its use. Recombinant human erythropoetin, immune serum globulin, danazol, conjugated estrogens, and polymerized stroma-free hemoglobin are some of the other products investigated as alternative choices for the management of nonpregnant Jehovah's Witness patients when blood transfusions are refused and emergency situations arise.

SELECTED READINGS

1. Benson KT: The Jehovah's Witness patient: considerations for the anesthesiologist. Anesth Analg 69:647, 1989
2. Samuels J: Preanesthetic assessment: the patient who is a Jehovah's Witness. Anesthesiol News 21, 1989
3. Wong DH, Jenkins LC: Surgery in Jehovah's Witnesses. Can J Anesth 36(5):578, 1989
4. Gibbs RF: Blood transfusions for Jehovah's Witnesses. p. 365. In Legal Medicine. American Society of Legal Medicine, CV Mosby, St. Louis, 1988
5. *Raleigh-Fitkin-Paul Morgan Memorial Hospital v. Anderson,* 42 N.J. 421, 201 A.2d 537 (1964)
6. *Jefferson v. Griffin Spalding County Hospital Authority,* 274 S.E. 2d. 457 (1981)
7. *Roe v. Wade,* 410 US 113, 93 S Ct 705 (1973)
8. *Application of the President and Directors of Georgetown College,* 331 F. 2d. 1000 (1964)
9. Bragg LE: Management strategies in the Jehovah's Witness patient. Contemp Surg 36:45, 1990
10. Stone DJ: DDAVP to reduce blood loss in Jehovah's Witnesses. Anesthesiology 69(6):1028, 1988
11. Howell PJ, Bamber PA: Severe acute anaemia in a Jehovah's Witness. Survival without blood transfusion. Anaesthesia 42:44, 1987
12. Sacks DA, Koppes RH: Blood transfusion and Jehovah's Witness: medical and legal issues in obstetrics and gynecology. Am J Obstet Gynecol 154(3):483, 1986
13. Brigham and Women's Hospital: Hospital Policy for Administering Blood to Jehovah's Witnesses. Brigham and Women's Hospital, Boston, 1983
14. Bonakdar MI, Ecknous AW: Major gynecologic and obstetric surgery in Jehovah's Witnesses. Obstet Gynecol 60:587, 1982
15. Tremper KK, Levine E: The preoperative treatment of severely anemic patients with a perfluorochemical blood substitute, Fluosol DA-20%. Anesthesiology 55(3):A9, 1981
16. Dixon JL: Jehovah's Witnesses. The surgical/ethical challenge. JAMA 246:2471, 1981
17. Dornette WH: Jehovah's Witnesses and blood transfusion: the horns of a dilemma. Anesth Analg 52:272, 1973
18. Jehovah's Witnesses and the Question of Blood. p. 1. Watchtower and Bible Tract Society, New York, 1977

ALTERED COAGULATION IN THE SURGICAL AND OBSTETRIC PATIENT

The most serious neurologic complication of regional anesthesia is paralysis, which, when caused by epidural or subarachnoid anesthesia, can be due to local anesthetic toxicity by direct injection into the nerve, nerve trauma caused directly by a needle or catheter, or cord compression secondary to an epidural/subarachnoid hematoma. Direct nerve injury caused by local anesthetics or by a needle or catheter has been discussed previously in this chapter. This review focuses specifically on epidural/subarachnoid hematoma.

FUNDAMENTALS OF THE CLOTTING SYSTEM

A simple but effective approach to understanding the clotting system divides the system into four components whose role is to produce a stable fibrin clot and then lyse the clot after healing has taken place.[1] The four components are vascular injury, platelet recruitment, clotting cascade, and fibrinolysis. Consideration of all components is essential in approaching any patient who may have an aberration of the clotting system.

Disruption of vascular integrity causes two separate events. First, it releases tissue thromboplastin, which serves as an activator of the extrinsic pathway of the clotting cascade. Second, it causes membrane changes in platelets that makes them adherent to the injured vascular wall and to other platelets that are brought into the area (referred to as *aggregation*). Additionally, the platelets release enzymes from granules within the platelet. Among these proteolytic enzymes is a lipoprotein released from the platelet membrane called platelet factor 3 (PF3), which is an initiator of the extrinsic pathway of the coagulation cascade. The coagulation cascade (Fig. 10-7) is a series of mainly trace proteins and calcium whose main function is to produce a fibrin clot. The intrinsic (platelet-initiated) pathway and the extrinsic (tissue thromboplastin-initiated) pathway come together in a common pathway at factor X, which when activated and along with calcium and factor V, converts prothrombin to thrombin. Thrombin leaves a peptide

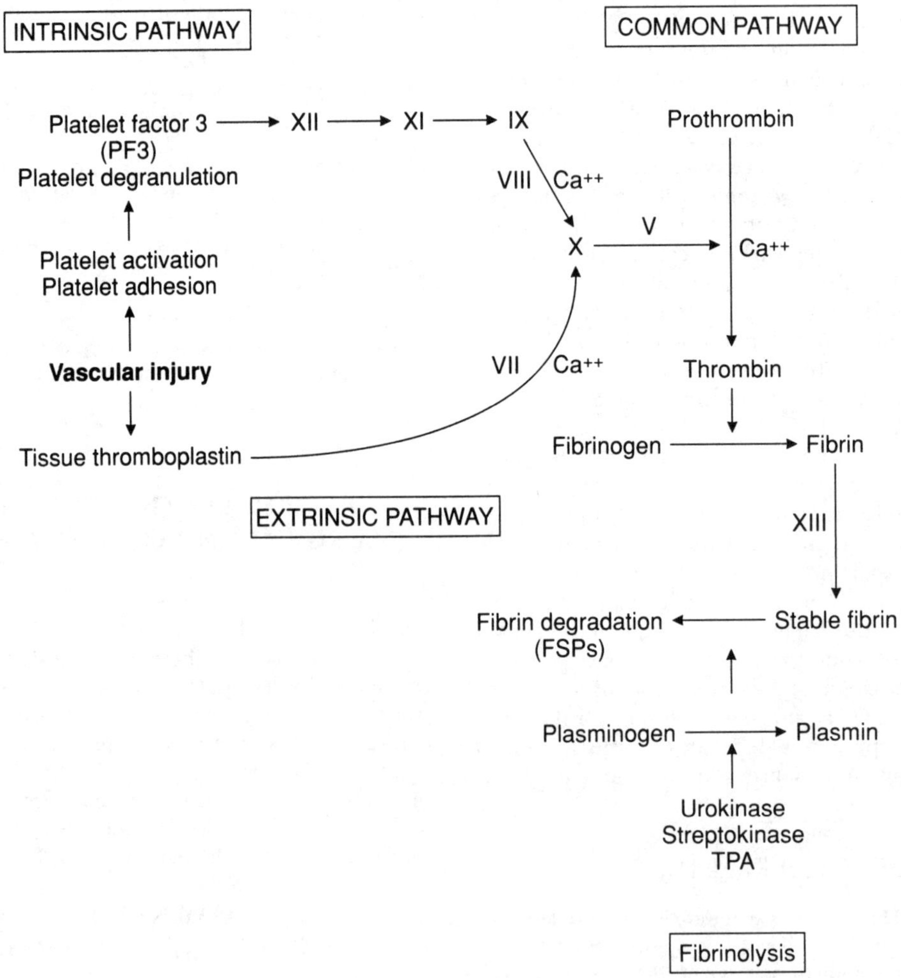

Fig. 10-7. The coagulation cascade.

off the circulating fibrinogen to form fibrin. Fibrin and stabilized fibrin are lysed by a short-lived enzyme, plasmin, which is formed from plasminogen by a rather heterogenous group of lyosomal enzymes (i.e., urokinase, streptokinase, and tissue plasminogin activator [TPA]). Although plasmin cannot be measured directly in serum, the products of fibrin degradation, fibrin split products (FSPs) and D-dimers, can. These tests of fibrinolysis are important whenever disseminated intravascular coagulation is suspected. In the parturient, this can occur with pre-eclampsia and amniotic fluid embolism.

Measurement of FSPs, partial thromboplastin time (PTT), prothrombin time (PT), platelet count, and bleeding time provide the only practical hematologic tests that can be obtained easily on the delivery floor. PT and PTT use commercially available reagents to arrive at an endpoint in the laboratory of a fibrin clot. The PTT measures activity of the intrinsic pathway and the PT measures activity of the extrinsic pathway. Platelet numbers are important in that surgical bleeding has been shown to occur with a platelet count of less than 100,000/mm^3. Bleeding times provide a crude measure of platelet function in that clinical scenarios can occur in which circulating platelet numbers are normal but the platelets are nonfunctional.

CASE REPORTS OF EPIDURAL/ SUBARACHNOID HEMATOMAS

Definition of Epidural/Subarachnoid Hematoma

For our discussion, the reported cases of epidural/ subarachnoid hematoma (Table 10-10) have been sudden catastrophes. These patients became paralyzed following subarachnoid or epidural anesthetic after an initial period of severe pain at the site of puncture. Most of these patients had myelograms, computed tomography scans, or autopsies that showed compression of the spinal cord from an extrinsic mass. All but a few of these patients underwent an emergency neurosurgical procedure for evacuation of the hematoma as, once suspected and discovered, early intervention to relieve the compression is essential (although there have been several case reports where observation rather than surgery has been done with resolution of the neurologic deficit). It is important when viewing the case report literature on epidural/subarachnoid hematoma that one adhere to the definition of epidural/subarachnoid hematoma: (a compressive mass revealed in a patient who became paralyzed after manipulation of the spinal cord area) and not mistake bleeding through needles or aspiration of blood through catheters as examples of epidural hematoma. Puncture and cannulation of epidural veins is fairly common, whereas epidural/subarachnoid hematoma is very uncommon. It has traditionally been taught that epidural/subarachnoid hematoma occurs in the following settings:

1. Difficult lumbar epidural puncture
2. Use of large-bore needles
3. Alterations in coagulation

The studies in Table 10-16 include data from six patients with no purported coagulation risk factors. As can be readily seen, with the exception of the report by Lerner et al.[2] and Rengachary et al.,[3] all patients had some severe debilitating systemic disease. Three patients had meningitis and underwent dural puncture for sub-

Table 10-16. Epidural/Subarachnoid Hematoma When No Coagulation Risk Factors Were Present

Study/Year	Disease or Procedure	Comment
Cooke[13] (1911)	TB meningitis	Hematoma at autopsy
Hammes[14] (1920)	Meningitis	Six dural punctures; no surgery
Courtin[15] (1952)	CNS syphilis	Laminectomy
Kirkpatrick[16] (1975)	Dural puncture for sciatica	CAD; Coumadin 6 months before dural puncture
Rengachary and Murphy[3] (1974)[a]	Femoral fracture	Failed dural puncture; general anesthesia; no risk factors; coagulation studies normal
Lerner et al.[2] (1973)[a]	Total knee replacement	No risk factors
King and Glass[17] (1960)[a]	Cystoscopy	Obese; HTCVD; no coagulation studies (portal cirrhosis)
Barker[5] (1988)	Total hip replacement	Prednisolone-dependent asthma; no coagulation studies

[a] Anesthetic related.

CNS, Central nervous system; CAD, coronary artery disease; HTCVD, hypertensive cardiovascular disease.

arachnoid antibiotic administration, one patient was found to have portal cirrhosis, one had a history of atrial fibrillation and exposure to warfarin 6 months prior to dural puncture, and one patient suffered from steroid-dependent asthma and had no reported coagulation profile. The major point of emphasis is that, in fact, the patients with "no risk factors' had severely debilitating diseases that may have impeded their coagulation system.

Epidural/Subarachnoid Hematoma Following Attempted Subarachnoid Puncture

As of August of 1991, there have been 36 reported cases of epidural/subarachnoid hematoma following subarachnoid puncture (Table 10-17). Thirty-four cases were reviewed by Owens et al.[4] in 1986, and since that time two more cases have been reported.[5,6] The review by Owens et al.[4] divided the cases into patients with and without coagulation associated abnormalities. Of the 36 recorded cases of epidural hematoma following subarachnoid puncture, 28 have had some recorded abnormality of their coagulation system. Nine have been inpatients with leukemia who have required dural puncture for evaluation of sepsis and whose platelet counts have all been less than 44,000/mm^3. Another 14 patients needed dural puncture for evaluation of a stroke or transient ischemic episode and received heparin, warfarin, or both temporally related to the dural puncture (only two patients received heparin before dural puncture). The remaining five patients had "miscellaneous" defects in their clotting system: one patient received aspirin after dural puncture, another was on the experimental antiplatelet drug, triclopidine, and a third was noted to have an elevated bleeding time. Two other patients had severe systemic disease: one had portal cirrhosis noted at autopsy and another had chronic renal failure requiring hemodialysis (interestingly, this patient had a normal PT and PTT).

Table 10-17 lists pertinent comments from eight reported cases of epidural hematoma associated with subarachnoid anesthesia. Of note, in all cases the dural puncture was either difficult or bloody and all (where stated) were done using a fairly large needle by 1991 standards (i.e., 23-gauge or above). The only patients without severe preexisting disease were in the report by Lerner et al.,[2] (in which the patient was reported to have had an elevated PT subsequent to developing a massive epidural hematoma, and Rengachary et al.,[3] in which no mention is made of a preoperative coagulation profile. Of note also is the conspicuous absence of any parturient who developed an epidural hematoma following subarachnoid anesthesia.

Epidural Hematomas following Epidural Anesthesia

There are 18 reported cases of epidural/subarachnoid hematoma following epidural anesthesia. The patients reported prior to 1970 (N = 8) are found in a mammoth review of over 750,000 epidural needle placements by Usubiaga[7] in several languages of the world's literature (Table 10-18). As can be seen, with one exception, all patients received heparin following epidural placement or underwent a traumatic or bloody dural puncture.

Table 10-17. Subarachnoid Hematoma after Attempted Subarachnoid Puncture (N = 8)

Study/Year	Difficult Tap	Bloody	Needle Size	Age/Sex	Procedure	Remarks
Bonica[19] (1953)	NS	Yes	NS	NS	NS	Prolonged bleeding time
King[17] (1959)	No	Yes	NS	62M	Cystoscopy	No coagulation (cirrhosis)
Lerner et al.[2] (1973)	Yes	Yes	22-g	70F	Total knee replacement	PT = 15.7 (normal = 13.5); general anesthesia
Rengachary and Murphy[3] (1974)	Yes	No	NS	64M	Femoral fracture	General anesthesia
Greensite and Katz[20] (1980)	Yes	Yes	16-g	68M	Total knee replacement	Subarachnoid catheter; ASA postdural puncture
Mayumi and Dohi[21] (1983)	Yes	No	23-g	70F	Toe amputation	Ticlopidine; general anesthesia
Barker[5] (1988)	No	No	22-g	87F	Total hip replacement	Prednisolone-dependent asthma
Carejda et al.[6] (1989)	Yes	Yes	22-g	58M	Cystoscopy	CRF; HTCVD; DM; CAD; PT WNL

NS, Not stated; PT, prothrombin time; ASA, aspirin; CRF, Chronic renal failure; HTCVD, hypertensive cardiovascular disease; DM, diabetes mellitus; CAD, coronary artery disease; PT WNL, prothrombin time within normal limits.

Table 10-18. Epidural/Subarachnoid Hematoma after Epidural Anesthesia (N = 18)

Study/Year	Age/Sex	Catheter	Blood in Catheter	Anticoagulant Postepidural	Surgery
Before 1970 (N = 18)					
All data from Usubiaga[7] (1975)	80M	No	Yes	Heparin	Exploratory laporotomy
	47F	No	No	No	Myomectomy
	28F	No	Yes	No	Nephroplexy
	72M	Yes	No	Heparin	Femoral embolectomy
	NeonateM	Yes	Yes	No	Omphalocele
	Mid-AgeF	Yes	No	Heparin	Femoral embolectomy
	73M	Yes	No	Heparin	Below-knee amputation
	48F	Yes	Yes	No	Inguinal hernia
After 1970 (N = 10)					
Dawkins[22] (1969)	NSNS	NS	NS	Yes	NS
Dawkins[22] (1969)	NSNS	NS	NS	Yes	NS
Butler and Green[23] (1970)	70M	Yes	No	Heparin	Femoral embolectomy
Helperin and Cohen[24] (1971)	76M	Yes	No	Heparin	Femoral popiteal bypass graft
Janis[25] (1972)	76M	Yes	No	Heparin	Hip reduction
Varkey and Brindle[26] (1975)	70M	Yes	No	Heparin	Pain Rx/AKA
Ballin[8] (1981)	22F	Yes(2)	Yes	No	Cesarean delivery; epidural anesthesia → general anesthesia
Wulf et al.[27] (1988)	21M	Yes	No	No (AML)	Thoracotomy
Dickman et al.[28] (1990)	67M	Yes	No	Urokinase	Catheter insertion
Dickman et al.[28] (1990)	74M	Yes	No	Heparin	Femoral embolectomy

NS, not stated; AKA, above knee amputation.

This trend holds true for the 10 reports after 1970 (Table 10-18).

One case reported by Ballin[8] deserves special consideration here because it is the only report of a parturient who ostensibly developed an epidural hematoma. This patient was a 22-year-old, small woman who underwent two attempts (L3-L4 and L4-L5) at an epidural anesthetic for relief of labor pain. After placement of the first epidural catheter "resistance to injection" was experienced upon injection of a test dose (2 ml) of 1 percent lidocaine and a clot was found in the end of the catheter when removed. The second attempt provided anesthesia until the time of cesarean delivery, whereupon pain relief was unsatisfactory and general anesthesia was required. Postoperatively, the patient had bilateral lower extremity weakness and diminished pinprick sensation, but these symptoms resolved after 2 weeks of hospitalization and was completely gone at 6 weeks. A lumbosacral series (*not* myelography) revealed a "narrow spinal canal." Because of the presence of clot in the first catheter, Ballin argued that this patient's neurologic deficit was caused by hematoma formation that spontaneously resolved. Unfortunately, this conclusion is difficult to substantiate given the fact that no myelogram was performed (the report was made prior to the CT scan era). Additionally, since no complete dosage of local anesthetic was reported for the 9-hour labor it is conceivable that the paralysis may have been due to toxic effects of local anesthetic or the volume of local anesthetic compressing the nerve roots.

IS IT SAFE TO ADMINISTER REGIONAL ANESTHESIA IN PATIENTS WHO ARE TO BE ANTICOAGULATED

In the nonobstetric literature, there are three studies that illustrate the safety with which subarachnoid or epidural anesthesia may be approached in patients who are to be anticoagulated.

Rao and El Etr[9] studied a series of patients who underwent peripheral vascular surgery requiring intraoperative heparin therapy. In this vast series of 3,164 epidural anesthetics and 847 continuous spinal anesthetics, all inserted with a 17-gauge Tuohy needle and with the catheter inserted 1 to 3 cm into the epidural or subarachnoid space, no permanent catastrophic neurologic damage occurred. This study excluded patients with leukemia, thrombocytopenia, or preoperative anticoagulation. The intraoperative heparin dosage was rigidly controlled by administering the heparin according to intraoperative anticoagulation therapy protocol. The procedure was cancelled in four patients who had a bloody dural puncture and rescheduled for the next day. The catheters were removed the following day.

Odoom and Sih[10] studied 950 patients who required 1,000 lumbar epidural anesthetics for vascular surgery. In all of these patients, who were on an unspecified dose of an unspecified oral anticoagulant (probably warfarin), the PTT and TT were 20 percent above normal. The epidural catheter was placed with a 17-gauge Tuohy needle after induction of general anesthesia. The catheter was inserted 2 to 3 cm and removed 48 hours after surgery. Patients who received aspirin or heparin preoperatively were excluded from the study as were those with thrombocytopenia or infection at the site of prospective epidural insertion. None of these patients developed an epidural/subarachnoid hematoma.

Finally, Waldman et al.[11] reported on 37 patients who required 336 caudal blocks for pain relief who had a PT or PTT 1.5 times control. In 12 of these patients, intravenous heparin therapy had been instituted and was judged to be too risky for the patient to discontinue. In 19 patients, the platelet counts were less than 50,000. By using a 25-gauge, 1.5-cm needle inserted in the caudal space, the patients were given a single-dose injection of 0.25 percent bupivacaine 20 ml with morphine 7 mg. The caudal anesthetic was administered with the patient in the prone position. The patient was then placed supine for 1 hour. In two patients hematomas were noted at the site of injection but no permanent neurologic damage was noted.

APPROACH TO THE PARTURIENT

There are several major categories of patients for whom a decision regarding epidural or subarachnoid anesthesia in the presence of a potential coagulation disorder will need to be made. First, there are a number of congenital disorders of altered plasma levels of clotting factors, the description of which is beyond the scope of this review. It is our departmental policy to make sure that all coagulation profiles (PT, PTT, platelet count, and bleeding time) are normal before initiating a regional anesthetic in patients with risk factors. We encourage our obstetricians to consult our high-risk obstetric anesthesia service prior to the onset of the patient's labor so that a plan for appropriate factor replacement may be undertaken in conjunction with the patient's hematologist.

What are the considerations for the patient who has pre-eclampsia? Kelton et al.[12] have shown in a prospective study of bleeding time of pre-eclamptic patients that these patients can have normal platelet counts but abnormally elevated bleeding times. It is our policy to measure a bleeding time in every pre-eclamptic patient before initiating a regional anesthetic if clinically indicated by history or laboratory examination.

REFERENCES

1. Fischbach D, Fogdall R: Coagulation: The Essentials. Williams and Wilkens, Baltimore, 1981
2. Lerner SM, Gutterman P, Jenkins F: Epidural hematoma and paraplegia after numerous lumbar punctures. Anesthesiology 39:550, 1973
3. Rengachary SS, Murphy D: Subarachnoid hematoma following lumbar puncture causing compression of the cauda equina: a case report. J Neurosurg 41:252, 1974
4. Owens EL, Kasten GW, Hessel EA II: Spinal subarachnoid hematoma after lumbar puncture and heparinization: a case report, review of the literature, and discussion of anesthetic complications. Anesth Analg 65:1201, 1986
5. Barker GL: Spinal subdural haematoma following spinal anaesthesia. Anaesthesia 43:663, 1988
6. Grejda S, Ellis K, Arino P: Paraplegia following spinal anesthesia in a patient with chronic renal failure. Reg Anesth 14:155, 1989
7. Usubiaga JE: Neurological complications following epidural anesthesia. Internat Anesthesiol Clin 13(2):39, 1975
8. Ballin NC: Paraplegia following epidural analgesia. Anaesthesia 36:952, 1981
9. Rao LK, El-Etr AA: Anticoagulation following placement of epidural and subarachnoid catheters. Anesthesiology 55:618, 1981
10. Odoom JA, Sih IL: Epidural anesthesia and anticoagulant therapy. Anaesthesia 38:254, 1983
11. Waldman SD, Feldstein GS, Waldman HJ, et al: Caudal administration of morphine sulfate in anticoagulated and thrombocytopenia patients. Anesth Analg 66:267, 1987
12. Kelton JG, Hunter DJS, Neame PB: A platelet function defect in preeclampsia. Obstet Gynecol 65:107, 1985
13. Cooke JV: Hemmorrhage into the cauda equina following lumbar puncture. Proc Path Soc Phila 14:104, 1911
14. Hammes EM: Hemorrhage in the cauda equina secondary to lumbar puncture. Arch Neurol 3:595, 1920
15. Courtin RF: Some practical aspects of lumbar puncture. Postgrad Med 12:157, 1952
16. Kirkpatrick D, Goodman SJ: Combined subarachnoid and subdural spinal hematoma following spinal puncture. Surg Neurol 3:109, 1975
17. King OJ, Glass WW: Spinal subarachnoid hemorrhage following lumbar puncture. Arch Surg 80:574, 1960
18. Barker 1988
19. Bonica JJ: The Management of Pain. Lea and Febiger, Philadelphia, 1953, p. 493
20. Greensite FS, Katz J: Spinal subdural hematoma associated with attempted epidural anesthesia and subsequent continuous spinal anesthesia. Anesth Analg 59:72, 1980
21. Mayumi T, Dohi S: Spinal subarachnoid hematoma after lumbar puncture in a patient receiving antiplatelet therapy. Anesth Analg 62:777, 1983

22. Dawkins CJ: An analysis of the complications of extradural and caudal block. Anaesthesia 24:554, 1969
23. Butler AB, Green CD: Haematoma following epidural anesthesia. Can Anaesth Soc J 6:635, 1970
24. Helperin SW, Cohen DD: Hematoma following epidural anesthesia: report of a case. Anesthesiology 6:641, 1971
25. Janis KM: Epidural hematoma following epidural analgesia; a case report. Anesth Analg 51:689, 1972
26. Varkey GP, Brindle GF: Peridural anesthesia and anticoagulant therapy. Can Anaesth Soc J 21:106, 1974
27. Wulf H, Maier GL, Striepling E: Epidural hematoma following epidural analgesia in a patient suffering from thrombocytopenia. Reg Anesth 11:26, 1988
28. Dickman CA, Shedd SA, Spetzler RF, et al: Spinal epidural hematoma associated with epiural anesthesia: complications of systemic heparinization in patients receiving peripheral vascular therapy. Anesthesiology 72:947, 1990

SUGGESTED READINGS

Aun C, Thomas D, St John-Jones L, et al: Intrathecal morphine in cardiac surgery. Eur J Anaesth 2:419, 1985

Baron HC, LaRaja RD, Rossi G, Atkinson D: Continuous epidural analgesia in the heparinized vascular surgical patient: a retrospective review of 912 patients. J Vasc Surg 6:144, 1987

Burrows RF, Kelton JG: Incidentally detected thrombocytopenia in healthy mothers and their infants. N Engl J Med 319:142, 1988

Casey WF, Wynands JE, Ralley FE, et al: The role of intrathecal morphine in the anesthetic management of patients undergoing coronary artery bypass surgery. J Cardiothorac Anesth 1:510, 1987

Dripps RD, Vandam LD: Long-term follow-up of patients who received 10,098 spinal anesthetics: failure to discover major neurological sequellae. JAMA 156:1486, 1954

El-Baz N, Goldin M: Continuous epidural infusion of morphine for pain relief after cardiac operations. J Thorac Cardiovasc Surg 93:878, 1987

Glass D: Management of blood and coagulation. Ch 20. In Kaplan JA (ed): Cardiac Anesthesia Vol. 2: Cardiovascular Pharmacology. Churchill Livingstone, New York, 1983

Horlocker TT, Wedel DJ, Offord KP: Does preoperative antiplatelet therapy increase the risk of hemorrhagic complication associated with regional anesthesia. Anesth Analg 70:631, 1990

Joachimsson PO, Nystrom SO, Tynden H: Early extubation after coronary artery surgery in efficiently rewarmed patients: a postoperative comparison of opioid anesthesia versus inhalational anesthesia and thoracic epidural analgesia. J Cardiothorac Anesth 3:444, 1989

Lares RK: Coagulation disorders and hemoglobinopathies in the obstetric and surgical patient. In Schnider SM, Levinson G (eds): Anesthesia for Obstetrics. Williams and Wilkins, Baltimore, 1987

Major complications in continuous epidural anesthesia. Department of Anesthesiology, First Teaching Hospital, Beijing Medical College, Chinese Med J 93:194, 1980

Mathews T, Abrams LD: Intrathecal morphine in open heart surgery. Lancet Sept. 6:543, 1980

Phillips OC, Elaner H, Nelson AT, Black MH: Neurologic complications following spinal anesthesia with lidocaine: a review of 110,440 cases. Anesthesiology 30:284, 1969

Stow PJ, Burrows FA: Anticoagulation in anaesthesia. Can J Anaesth 34:632, 1987

Turpie AGG, Robinson JG, Doyle DJ, et al: Comparison of high-dose with low-dose subcutaneous heparin to prevent left ventricular mural thrombosis in patients with acute transmural anterior myocardial infarction. N Engl J Med 320:352

Vanstrum GS, Bjornson KM, Ilko R: Postoperative effect of intrathecal morphine in coronary artery bypass surgery. Anesth Analg 67:261, 1988

11

Education, Organization, and Standards

THE ESSENCE OF CLINICAL TEACHING

In an Introductory Lecture delivered before the Medical Class of Harvard University on November 6, 1867, Oliver Wendell Holmes underscored the importance of graduate medical education. Dr. Holmes related the clinical rounds of a certain worthy Ispwich physician, Master Giles Firmin, as he rounded among his patients in 1647 with one of his "residents." Before them, a stout fellow is bellowing with colic.

> "He will die, Master, of a surety, methinks," says the timid youth in a whisper.
>
> "Nay, Luke," the Master answers, " 't is but a dry belly-ache. Didst thou not mark that he stayed his roaring when I did press hard over his lesser bowels? Note that he does not have the pulse of them with fevers. We will steep certain comforting herbs which I will shew thee, and put them in a bag and lay them on his belly. Likewise he shall have my cordial julep with a portion of this confection . . . which hath the juice of poppy in it, and it is a great stayer of anguish. This fellow said his prayers today, but I warrant thee he shall be swearing with the best of them tomorrow."[1]

Although this passage was uttered perhaps more than three hundred years ago, its message remains valid. The direct transfer of practical experience of a wise clinician into the mind of a student is the essence of clinical teaching.

Our knowledge base, particularly with regard to physiology and pharmacology; has broadened considerably over the past decade. The American Board of Anesthesiology (ABA) recognized this when it mandated a third clinical year of residency training, effective May 1986.

Enormous strides have also been made within the field of obstetric anesthesia. The approach toward educating trainees in anesthesia for the parturient must be systematic. The ABA identifies technical facility, medical judgment, and scholarship as the criteria upon which competence is based.[2]

Goals should be outlined at the outset of the training period. Instructional and technical objectives should be clearly stated (see the next section). If the trainee is undertaking either a portion or a full CA-3 or CA-4 year in obstetric anesthesia, a so-called fellowship, further administrative goals need to be addressed, as that care-provider may be called on or may be training to direct a busy obstetric anesthesia service in the future. Clinical and basic research projects are encouraged in these individuals. This may serve to elevate the appreciation for the application and acquisition of new knowledge.

REFERENCES

1. Holmes OW: Medical Essays, 1842–1882. Houghton, Mifflin, Boston, 1889
2. American Board of Anesthesiology: Quality anesthesia care: a model of future practice of anesthesiology. Anesthesiology 47:488, 1977

ORGANIZATION OF AN OBSTETRIC ANESTHESIA TEACHING SERVICE

INSTRUCTIONAL OBJECTIVES

The foundation upon which education in obstetric anesthesia rests is a core of knowledge essential to the field. The full scope of maternal physiologic alterations attendant to pregnancy and principles of perinatal pharmacology need to be understood. Management of parturition, techniques of inducing regional and general anesthesia in the parturient, and the management of their complications are basic to the practice of safe obstetric anesthesia. The fundamentals of operative delivery, management and considerations of the high-risk obstetric patient, and the anesthetic nuances for nonobstetric surgery during pregnancy and postpartum surgery need to be accentuated.

In addition to maternal, fetal, and neonatal physiologic considerations, the dynamics of the change from intra- to extrauterine life must be taught in the education program. Pre- and intrapartum assessment, effects of maternally administered drugs on the fetus and neonate, and the principles of neonatal resuscitation are particular areas for emphasis.

An understanding of the pharmacokinetics and pharmacodynamics of local anesthetics, as well as the use of epidural and subarachnoid opioids, should be incorporated into the teaching curriculum. Drug interactions to commonly used oxytocics and tocolytics deserve review.

Although drug administration is fundamental to the practice of obstetric anesthesia, a knowledge base in nonpharmacologic analgesia is as essential. Any busy obstetric anesthesiologist will confirm the fact that the patient educated in prepared childbirth classes is frequently more cooperative.[1]

With the exposure of a CA-3 and CA-4 resident to an active labor and delivery service, the value of the knowledge gained in understanding the logistics of such a service will pay handsome dividends. This trainee may someday be given the task of organizing anesthetic services in a new facility. Determining what considerations should go into the creation of the physical side of an obstetric anesthesia service cannot be taught from a textbook.

TECHNICAL OBJECTIVES

Regional anesthesia techniques play a major role in the management of the obstetric patient. Trainees in this field must have facility in the placement of epidural and subarachnoid blocks. Exposure to a large clinical service is advisable as these procedures are mastered with practice.

The administration of general anesthesia is much less common today than in the past. The skills necessary to induce and maintain a parturient with a general anesthetic, however, are vital for cesarean and, infrequently, vaginal deliveries.

The knowledge of invasive monitoring, specifically, intra-arterial and central venous monitoring, is a further technical objective in the indoctrination of trainees in obstetric anesthesia.

ADMINISTRATIVE OBJECTIVES

It is the philosophy of the Section of Obstetric Anesthesia at the Brigham and women's Hospital that CA-3 and CA-4 residents receive some training in the administration of the service itself. Residents acquire expertise in the roles of sound clinician, strategist, and diplomat when dealt the responsibility of "acting" director. Operating rooms for cesarean and vaginal deliveries, obstetric surgical emergencies, and in vitro fertilization all fall under the observant attention of the "fellow." Furthermore, the management of the labor suite for the coordination of consultations and epidural catheter placement, as well as supervision and teaching of less experienced residents, are other administrative tasks.

METHODS OF INSTRUCTION

An effective teaching program blends many sources of instruction: teaching in the labor and delivery suites, didactic programs by residents and staff, audiovisual materials, computer-assisted learning programs, and, of course, independent study.

To quote Osler, "The art of the practice of medicine is to be learned only by experience; 'tis not an inheritance; it cannot be revealed."[2] As imparted in the beginning of this chapter, even the "modest country doctor" may furnish the resident with a vital link in the education chain.[2] With stated instructional and technical objectives in mind, the resident and teacher may discuss their case in advance and apply what has been learned to the present situation.

The didactic program should consist of formal lectures given by both the attending and resident staff. Clinical case discussions and morbidity and mortality issues should be incorporated into the agenda. The capacity to discuss successes and errors of fellow trainees in such a forum is useful.

Independent study is the basis of self-education. The use of a departmental library with relevant journals, major reference texts, monographs, and books dealing with specific topics is vital to the acquisition of knowledge. Resources such as audiovisual aids, photocopying machines, and computer-assisted literature searches are invaluable.

METHODS OF EVALUATION

Cognitive skills may objectively be assessed by written examination. The ABA/ASA (American Society of Anesthesiologists) In-Training Examination attempts to accomplish this goal. A subset of questions, related to the practice of obstetric anesthesia, may audit the residents' knowledge base. Direct observation by the clinical staff may also gauge resident proficiency on the technical aspects of obstetric anesthesia care.

The judgment and attitude of the resident are not values easily measured. Evaluations of these characteristics are by definition subjective, and thus are open to bias. Periodic self-assessment, with peer and staff review, may lend objectivity.

CONTINUING MEDICAL EDUCATION

The foundation for scholarship in continuing medical education remains motivation for self-education and the maintenance of an active, alert interest in important advances in the field. If spurred by the ideal combination of curiosity and proper training, the candidate will mature into a clinical scholar.

REFERENCES

1. Bonica JJ: Obstetric Analgesia and Anesthesia. World Federation of Societies of Anesthesiologists, Amsterdam, 1980
2. Osler W: Johns Hopkins Hosp Bull 30:198–2, 1919

ACADEMIC AND CLINICAL GOALS IN OBSTETRIC ANESTHESIA

One of the basic goals of the Department of Anesthesia at the Brigham and Women's Hospital has been to develop a solid set of concepts and skills relating to obstetric anesthesia to serve as a knowledge base for our trainees. To aid in this endeavor, we have created a set of clinical and academic goals that, when mastered, will allow our residents to practice obstetric anesthesia with skill and expertise.

ACADEMIC GOALS

From the texts recommended at the end of this section, a resident should acquire a basic fund of knowledge in the following areas by the end of the rotation:

1. Maternal physiologic changes during pregnancy
   a) Cardiovascular system
   b) Respiratory system
   c) Acid-base balance
   d) Gastrointestinal system
   e) Hepatic system
   f) Neurologic system
   g) Renal system
   h) Hematologic system
2. Uterine blood flow
   a) Changes during pregnancy
   b) Effects of local/general anesthesia
   c) Effects of vasopressors/antihypertensives
3. Maternal uptake/distribution, placental drug transport, and perinatal effects (including neurobehavioral effects and transfer of drugs into breast milk) of:
   a) Volatile anesthetics, barbiturates, ketamine, muscle relaxants, narcotics, sedatives, tranquilizers, and scopolamine and their effects depending on the *route* of administration (i.e., intravenous, intramuscular, etc.)
   b) Local anesthetics
   c) Antihypertensives
   d) Anticoagulants
   e) Tocolytics
   f) Hypoglycemics/glucose administration
4. Physiology of labor
   a) Stages of labor
   b) Effects of analgesia and anesthesia on labor
   c) Suppression of preterm labor. Be able to describe mechanism(s) of action and the anesthetic considerations of:
      (1) β-sympathomimetics
      (2) Magnesium channel blockers
      (3) Calcium channel blockers
      (4) Prostaglandin synthetic inhibitors
      (5) Ethanol
      (6) Progestational agents
   d) Dystocia
      (1) Fetal

(2) Maternal
(3) Diagnosis/management
e) Induction/augmentation of labor
(1) Amniotomy and its anesthetic considerations
(2) Oxytocin and its anesthetic considerations
(3) Prostaglandins and their anesthetic considerations
(4) Ergot derivatives and their anesthetic considerations

5. Local anesthetics
a) Basic structure, properties, and mode of action of:
(1) Lidocaine with/without epinephrine
(2) Bupivacaine
(3) Mepivacaine
(4) Chloroprocaine
(5) Tetracaine
In addition, be able to discuss factors that affect toxic reactions to local anesthetics, the classification of reactions to local anesthetics, and reactions to vasopressor (epinephrine) in the local anesthetic.
b) Maternal absorption and placental transfer, including prevention and treatment of central nervous and cardiovascular system toxicities.

6. Inhaled anesthetics and ketamine
a) Uptake and distribution during pregnancy
b) Inhalational analgesia and its maternal and perinatal effects
c) Inhalational anesthesia and its maternal/perinatal effects
d) Ketamine maternal/perinatal effects

7. Use of paracervical, pudendal, and perineal infiltrative blocks
a) Anatomic landmarks
b) Drugs commonly used
c) Associated maternal and fetal complications

8. Basic concepts of major regional anesthesia in obstetrics
a) Vertebral column anatomy
b) Regional block
(1) Cardiovascular effects
(2) Respiratory effects
(3) Spinal dermatomes
(4) Pain pathways
c) Indications and contraindications, including:
(1) Coagulopathy
(2) Neurologic diseases
(3) Hypovolemia
(4) Drug allergy
(5) Fever
(6) Backache
(7) Scoliosis
Be able to discuss *why* the above may be considered absolute/relative contraindications.
d) Complications due to regional anesthesia. Be able to discuss the incidence(s), depending on the technique chosen (i.e., spinal versus epidural), and be able to formulate a treatment plan for each of the following:
(1) Cardiovascular
(2) Headache
(3) Backache
(4) Bladder dysfunction
(5) Neurologic sequelae
(6) Infection

9. Subarachnoid anesthesia
a) Techniques (preparations, landmarks, and procedures)
b) Local anesthetics used and their administration
c) Subarachnoid opioids: mechanism of action, drugs used, systemic effects, and associated complications

10. Lumbar epidural anesthesia
a) Techniques (preparations, landmarks, procedures)
b) Local anesthetics used and their administration
c) Epidural opioids: mechanism of action, drugs used, systemic effects, and associated complications
d) Use of continuous epidural infusions, including patient-controlled epidural anesthesia

11. Caudal anesthesia
a) Techniques (preparations, landmarks, procedures)
b) Local anesthetics used and their administration
c) Complications

12. Cesarean delivery
a) Indications for cesarean delivery, including:
(1) Failure to progress
(2) Breech presentation
(3) Cephalopelvic disproportion
(4) Previous cesarean delivery
(5) Fetal distress
b) Selection of anesthetic. Be able to discuss why certain techniques are chosen over others.
c) General anesthesia
(1) Management of induction, intraoperative anesthesia, and emergence
(2) Significance of delivery intervals and concentrations of volatile agents
(3) Pros and cons of nitrous oxide
(4) Complications of general anesthesia, including diagnosis and management of aspiration and failed intubation

d) Regional anesthesia
(1) Significance of delivery intervals
(2) Maternal/neonatal effects of anesthetic induced hypotension

13. Emergency delivery
a) Vaginal delivery
b) Cesarean delivery
Be able to discuss why certain anesthetic techniques are chosen over others.

14. The high-risk parturient
Be able to discuss (1) why the following maternal health complications pose problems for an obstetric anesthesiologist and (2) the anesthetic management of these patients during labor and delivery.
a) Cardiac disease, including:
(1) Congenital heart disease
(2) Valvular lesions
(3) Associated pulmonary hypertension
(4) Cardiomyopathy: restrictive
b) Respiratory disease
(1) Restrictive
(2) Obstructive
c) Diabetes
(1) Classifications
(2) Management
(3) Associated maternal/neonatal complications
d) Morbid obesity
e) Airway abnormality
f) Miscellaneous, including thyroid disease, malignant hyperthermia, coagulopathy, and neuromuscular disease

15. Obstetric complications
Be able to discuss the diagnosis, obstetric management, and anesthetic considerations/management for each of the following:
a) Abnormal presentations
(1) Breech, face, brow, and compound presentations
(2) Transverse lie
(3) Prolapsed cord
(4) Multiple gestation
b) Pregnancy-induced hypertension
(1) Classification
(2) Diagnosis
c) Premature rupture of membranes
d) Hemorrhage
(1) Placenta previa
(2) Abruptio placentae
(3) Uterine rupture
(4) Postpartum hemorrhage (uterine atony, retained placenta, birth trauma, uterine inversion, placenta accreta, disseminated intravascular coagulation).
e) Embolism: amniotic fluid, air, and thrombus

16. Anesthesia for nondelivery surgery during pregnancy
a) General surgery
(1) Preoperative evaluation and management
(2) Intraoperative management
(3) Use of tocolytics
(4) Perioperative fetal monitoring
(5) Anesthetic considerations including teratogenic effects and other problems
b) Cerclage placement
(1) Anesthetic management
c) Postpartum tubal ligation
(1) Anesthetic management

17. The fetus and the neonate
a) Physiology of fetus and newborn
b) Antepartum fetal assessment
(1) Electronic fetal heart rate monitoring
(2) Fetal pH monitoring
(3) Nonstress testing
(4) Oxytocin challenge testing
(5) Biophysical profile
(6) Fetal lung maturity testing
c) Diagnosis and management of peripartum fetal asphyxia
d) Evaluation of the neonate
e) Resuscitation of the neonate
f) Specific neonatal disorders and their management
(1) Meconium aspiration
(2) Diaphragmatic hernia
(3) Tracheoesophageal fistula
(4) Sepsis
(5) Respiratory distress syndromes

CLINICAL GOALS

1. Be able to set up an operating room to administer anesthesia for an obstetric case (vaginal or cesarean delivery).
2. Become proficient at the placement and management of an epidural anesthetic for delivery. Aim for *at least* 40 to 50 epidural catheter placements in a month-long rotation.
3. Become proficient in the performance and management of spinal anesthesia for vaginal and cesarean delivery.
4. Be able to safely administer general anesthesia for emergent and nonemergent vaginal and cesarean deliveries.
5. Be able to preoperatively evaluate and design a safe plan for the anesthetic management of:
a) a healthy parturient presenting for vaginal delivery with/without the use of forceps

   b) a healthy parturient presenting for elective cesarean delivery
   c) a healthy parturient presenting for emergency cesarean delivery
   d) a parturient with preeclampsia/eclampsia (pregnancy-induced hypertension)
   e) a parturient with antepartum/intrapartum/postpartum hemorrhage.
6. Become familiar with the diagnosis and management of a neonate in distress.
7. Be able to discuss at length the questions following the case histories below. Brief answers are provided to guide you.

Case 1

A 35-year-old parturient with a 38-week gestation has mild pregnancy-induced hypertension (BP 150/90). She fails to progress after 4 hours of labor at station +1 with cervical dilation 4 cm. She received butorphanol 2 mg IM × 2 with little relief. The obstetrician starts a oxytocin infusion, which improves the progress of labor, but the patient becomes very uncomfortable. There are intermittent type I decelerations on the fetal monitor strip. The obstetrician anticipates a vaginal delivery and requests your assistance for pain relief.

Questions

1. Why doesn't the obstetrician do a paracervical block (PCB)?

   Answer. *The main drawback to a PCB is the possible production of fetal bradycardia. This is thought to be due to fetal hypoxia/acidosis resulting from uterine artery vasoconstriction from local anesthetic applied in close location to the artery, which causes decreased uteroplacental perfusion. Second, the block is only effective during the first stage of labor because the perineal sensory fibers are not blocked with this technique.*

2. What are the advantages/disadvantages of a lumbar epidural block in this patient?

   Answer. *An epidural block is able to block pain pathways extending from T10 to S5, thus providing total pain relief during all stages of labor. Because of its continuous technique, it is especially useful in cases of prolonged labor. In the patient with pregnancy-induced hypertension, its vasodilating action and ability to lower catecholamine levels usually result in an improvement in uteroplacental perfusion and a lowering of maternal blood pressure.*

   In the inadequately hydrated patient, however, it may precipitate sudden maternal hypotension resulting in decreased uteroplacental perfusion and fetal distress.

3. What are the advantages/disadvantages of magnesium therapy in patients with pregnancy-induced hypertension?

   Answer. *Magnesium sulfate, by its effects on the peripheral neuromuscular junction, acts as an anticonvulsant and also reduces hyperreflexia. It also is a mild vasodilator and improves uterine blood flow by reducing uterine hyperactivity.*

   High doses can produce maternal muscle weakness, hypotension, and even cardiac/respiratory failure. Magnesium sulfate potentiates neuromuscular block.

Case 2

A 26-year-old primigravida at 38 weeks gestation presents in active labor with a fetus in the breech position. The obstetrician ask you to provide help with pain relief.

Questions

1. How would you proceed at this point?

   Answer: *The decision to deliver this baby by vaginal or cesarean delivery should be promptly made by the obstetrician. Vaginal delivery of a breech infant may result in umbilical cord compression or prolapse and/or a traumatic delivery for both mother and fetus.*

   If the obstetrician believes the infant can be delivered vaginally, perineal anesthesia can be supplied with a pudendal, spinal, or epidural block. On occasion, general anesthesia (following a rapid-sequence induction) may be required (rarely), using a volatile agent to relax the uterus and allow manipulation and delivery of the head.

   If obstetric indications mandate a cesarean delivery, anesthesia can be accomplished with regional or general anesthesia depending on the urgency of the situation.

2. The obstetrician specifically ask you to administer a caudal block for this patient. What are its drawbacks?

   Answer: *Because of their close proximity, the caudal needle may pierce the patient's rectum or the presenting fetal part. This may result in a toxic administration of local anesthetic to the fetus. Because a large volume of local anesthetic is required to produce analgesia using this technique, unintentional injection into the subarachnoid space would produce a high or total spinal block. In addition, unintentional intravascular injection would produce central nervous system excitation or convulsions. Most anesthesiologists believe that caudal block is technically more difficult to perform than a spinal or epidural block.*

3. After some length, vaginal delivery was accom-

plished but the infant is born with an initial Apgar score of 3. The mother is fine but only you and the obstetrician are in the room. What should you do?

Answer: *This score indicates severe cardiorespiratory depression. While you are calling for additional help, intermittent positive-pressure ventilation with 100 percent oxygen should be administered by bag and mask. If there is not an immediate response, intubation with closed chest cardiac massage should be instituted. Drug therapy with sodium bicarbonate, epinephrine, and dextrose should be considered if resuscitation is prolonged.*

REFERENCE TEXTS

Shnider SM, Levinson G: Anesthesia for Obstetrics. 2nd Ed. Williams & Wilkins, Baltimore, 1987

Datta S, Ostheimer GW: Common problems in Obstetric Anesthesia. Year Book Medical Publishers, Inc. Chicago, 1987

Albright GA, Ferguson JE, Joyce TH, Stevenson DK: Anesthesia in Obstetrics: Maternal, Fetal, and Neonatal Aspects. 2nd Ed. Butterworths, Boston, 1986

James FJ, Wheeler AS, Dewan DM: Obstetric Anesthesia: The Complicated Patient. 2nd Ed. F.A. Davis Co. Philadelphia, 1988

Crawford JS: Principle and Practice of Obstetric Anaesthesia. 5th Ed. Blackwell Scientific Publications. Oxford, 1984

Beard RW, Nathanielsz PW: Fetal Physiology and Medicine. The Basis of Perinatology. 2nd Ed. Marcel Dekker, Inc. New York, 1984

THE LABOR AND DELIVERY SUITE

QUALITY OF CARE

The regionalization of perinatal care has produced an increased demand on the anesthesiologist to participate actively in obstetric care. Fewer new facilities are constructed because they have to receive approval from a board granting a certificate of need; as a result, existing facilities are either closed or combined and upgraded to provide care for the uncomplicated to the most complex high-risk pregnancy. Regardless of the level of obstetric care, the quality of anesthetic practice in the delivery suite must be the same as that provided in the operating suite of the same institution. There cannot be two levels of anesthetic care in the same institution. The parturient and her fetus, soon to be a neonate, need and demand the highest quality of anesthetic care available to any patient in that particular institution.

LOCATION

The anesthesiologist responsible for the organization of the anesthetic services in a new hospital or facility should help coordinate the location of the delivery suite in an easily accessible area of the institution close to the admitting and laboratory facilities and equally accessible to the operating suite; ideally, it should be on the same floor. The availability of anesthesiologists is often dependent on the accessibility of the delivery rooms. The transitional nursery should be immediately adjacent to the obstetric suite with easy access to the neonatal intensive care unit. Depending on the construction of the hospital, it would be expedient to have the regular nursery and the postpartum unit on the same floor; however, in many institutions, this may be impossible. The prepartum fetomaternal intensive care unit should be part of or immediately adjacent to the obstetric suite. A schematic approach to the logistic problem is shown in Figure 11-1.

DETERMINING MATERNITY BED NEED

The overall number of beds in a maternity unit cannot be determined by a simple formula. The number of adult beds must include those in the fetomaternal intensive care unit, labor area, and postpartum units. The neonatal beds include those in the transitional, regular, and neonatal intensive care units. Each hospital must have its bed capacity calculated according to the size and geographic location of the institution, population served, accessibility, average length of stay, projections, economic factors, and regionalization requirements.

As one might expect, each state has its own formula for determining bed need. One of the early approaches was based on a set number of beds per thousand population, adjusted for the density of the particular population. Later improvements focused on future populations and suggested minimal utilization standards based on an 80 percent overall occupancy. This plan attempted to calculate total bed need for the future on a current demand basis and did not take into account the need by service.

Service-specific formulas have been recently developed. The Public Health Service formula[1] calculates an average daily census for a maternity unit by dividing the projected census days by 365. This average daily census is then divided by the expected occupancy rate to obtain the number of beds needed. This formula can only be applied when patient turnover is extremely regular and the patients do not require urgent treatment so that their admissions can be scheduled. Neither of these conditions can be applied to maternity services, in which patients' arrivals are unpredictable and unsched-

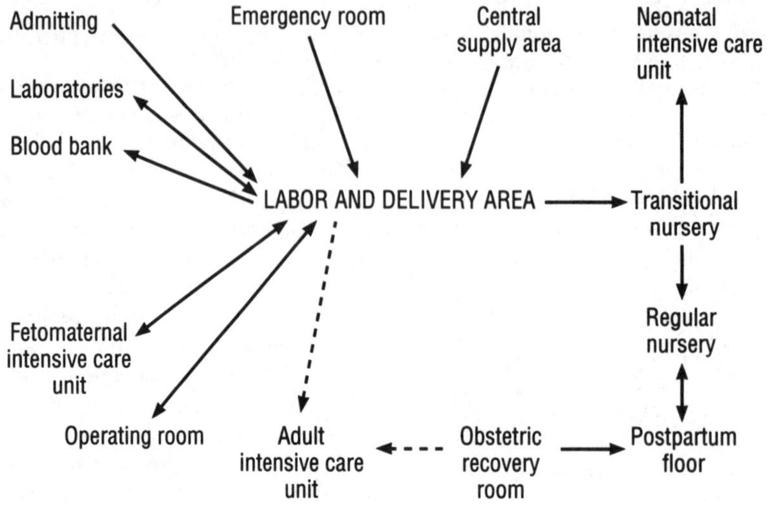

Fig. 11-1. Schematic approach to the relationship between the labor and delivery suite and the hospital.

uled. Therefore, this approach is being replaced by another formula based on the principle that patients should have equal access to beds regardless of a facility's size.

This translates into providing each unit with sufficient beds that the probability (determined by the Poisson distribution) of all beds being filled simultaneously is kept below an acceptable threshold. For larger units, the Poisson distribution can be approximated by the more convenient computer-adapted normal distribution. Thus, the number of beds required to ensure a specific probability of immediate patient access is taken from a simple formula using only the average daily census and a constant derived from the normal probability distribution. Unfortunately, maternity services do not satisfy the assumptions about length of stay that lead to a Poisson-distributed bed census and the normal distribution is not accurate for smaller services. Fortunately, mathematical models developed by statistical theorists can be used instead for maternity services analysis. The "finite-state, birth–death" queuing model has been used to plan emergency services and applies directly to maternity services. It assumes simply that patient arrivals are unpredictable and unscheduled; it imposes no restrictions on the distribution of length of stay and it assumes that the number of beds is fixed. From information on average patient arrival rates, average lengths of stay and number of beds, the queuing model will predict occupancy, or service, levels. The bed-need predictions of the complicated queuing model for specific service levels can be accurately approximated by a simple formula involving two constants, K_1 and K_2 (which depend on the service level), and the average daily census presented by the maternity unit. The higher the service level, the greater the cost and need for beds. The constants for the 99 percent and the 95 percent levels are 99 percent service level: $K_1 = 0.91$, $K_2 = 2.6$; 95 percent service level: $K_1 = 0.84$, $K_2 = 2.1$.

Sample calculations using the queuing formular for a 100-patient average daily census (ADC) are as follows:

Beds needed for a 99 percent service level:

$$= K_1 \times \text{ADC} + K_2 \times \sqrt{\text{ADC}}$$
$$= 0.91 \times 100 + 2.6 \times \sqrt{100}$$
$$= 0.91 \times 100 + 2.6 \times 10$$
$$= 91 + 26$$
$$= 117 \text{ beds}$$

Beds needed for a 95 percent service level:

$$= K_1 \times \text{ADC} + K_2 \times \sqrt{\text{ADC}}$$
$$= 0.84 \times 100 + 2.1 \times \sqrt{100}$$
$$= 0.84 \times 100 + 2.1 \times 10$$
$$= 84 + 21$$
$$= 105 \text{ beds}$$

The use of the queuing system for establishing maternity bed need will result in nearly equal service levels for all sizes of maternity units and considerable cost savings, especially with larger maternity units, because utilization will be more accurately predicted.[1]

INNOVATIONS

It is not my purpose to suggest architectural arrangements for the construction of the labor and delivery area; common sense dictates that the delivery rooms should be immediately adjacent to the labor rooms. In new facilities, some of the labor rooms should be convertible to delivery rooms with the inclusion of the appropriate beds that can function as delivery tables. This innovation will help foster the concept of family-oriented maternity care in which all the facilities of the institution such as blood banks, laboratories and intensive care units are immediately available but the parturient can deliver in a homelike environment, which may be more conducive to parent–infant bonding. Some or all of the delivery rooms should be convertible to major operating rooms for cesarean deliveries and postpartum surgical procedures. A minor operating room may be included for obstetric-related gynecologic procedures such as dilation and curettage. Regardless of the details of the arrangement of the delivery suite, one fact is clear: every full anesthetizing location must have the equipment necessary to provide complete anesthetic care from simple monitoring functions to full-scale anesthesia with the appropriate physiologic monitors for any obstetric emergency.

LABOR ROOM

What considerations should be made for anesthesia in a labor room? The amount of equipment needed depends on whether anesthesia will be inducted in a combination labor—cesarean delivery room or in a room used only for labor and vaginal delivery. In the latter situation, wall outlets must accommodate oxygen, suction, sphygmomanometer, emergency call system, and adequate lighting. Hangers for intravenous bottles can be part of the labor room or attached to the labor bed. The labor bed must be capable of being placed in a head-up or head-down position. Suction catheters and oxygen delivery systems must be in each labor room and ready for immediate use.

If the labor room is also to function as a cesarean delivery room, and therefore as a surgical location, the usual equipment found in a regular operating delivery room must be available. Compact anesthesia machines and wall-mounted cabinets can provide the essential equipment while their presence can be unobtrusive to the occupants of the labor room. Although an electrocardiograph is not mandatory for each labor–vaginal delivery room, an emergency cart must be immediately available in the labor area that will contain the standard drugs and equipment for emergency care. It should also contain a combination electrocardiographic and arterial monitor, central venous pressure equipment, a defibrillator, and a cardiac resuscitation board. Uterine displacement equipment is mandatory in each labor and delivery room. If regional blocks are initiated in the labor room, essential anesthetic and resuscitative equipment must be on a cart brought into the room before the block is performed.

In my opinion, the obstetric service should provide an electronic fetal monitor for each patient in labor. Electronic fetal heart rate monitoring provides essential information not available via auscultation, because few labor attendants—physicians, midwives, or nurses—ever listen to the entire contraction cycle. One cannot be aware of variations in fetal heart rate unless one listens from the beginning of one contraction to the beginning of the next contraction. Auscultation of the fetal heart rate between contractions will miss late decelerations and variable decelerations; it will identify only the very ominous prolonged late decelerations that demand immediate intervention, and perhaps cesarean delivery, unless vaginal delivery is imminent. Although "full-cycle" auscultation has been shown to be adequate monitoring in comparative studies, its use mandates "one-on-one" nursing, which is a luxury few hospitals can afford. Therefore, I do not see a return to auscultation in place of continuous electronic fetal heart rate monitoring.

For maternal monitoring during regional anesthesia in a labor-delivery room, I would like to see the development of a noninvasive blood pressure finger cuff to be worn on one finger accompanied by a pulse oximeter worn on another finger of the same hand. Designs attempted to date by various companies have been cumbersome and unreliable.

DELIVERY ROOM

The delivery room must be equipped to provide appropriate anesthesia for vaginal or abdominal delivery, postpartum tubal ligation, and any emergency obstetric surgery. The same quality of anesthetic equipment available in the general operating suite must be available in the delivery room.

Modern delivery rooms should have piped-in nitrous oxide and oxygen provided through an overhead unit to prevent personnel from becoming entangled in coils of tubing. Suction is most efficient if aided by gravity and led to floor bottles. There is no need to provide explosive gases in the delivery area since all procedures can be done with a variety of nonexplosive agents. The expense of conductive flooring and appropriate grounding is excessive and not justified for new or refurbished areas; most important, delivery room personnel today are unfamiliar with the precautions necessary when explosive agents are in use.

An automated noninvasive blood pressure monitor, pulse oximeter, capnograph or mass spectrometer, temperature probe, electrocardiograph, and ventilator should be mounted on the anesthetic machine, which should be equipped with fail-safe devices, an oxygen analyzer, and precision vaporizers. The availability of central venous pressure, arterial blood pressure, and pulmonary arterial blood pressure transducers would be useful. A fetal heart rate monitor must be available. The immediate availability of all necessary fluids, infusion apparatus, nerve stimulator, and other standard anesthetic equipment is essential. Scavenging devices are necessary in all anesthetizing locations to minimize the contamination of the environment by trace gases. Endotracheal intubation utilizing rapid induction and cricoid pressure is mandatory if general anesthesia is administered for vaginal or cesarean delivery. Depending on the individual needs of the institution, disposable or reusable inhalational equipment may be selected. Disposable regional anesthesia trays are recommended since aseptic meningitis appears to be related to turnover of the hospital personnel preparing the kits, because inexperienced workers may deviate from appropriate technique.

An anesthetic supply area should be easily accessible and should contain additional equipment including blood warmers and a refrigerator to keep perishable medications and cold intravenous solutions to administer during a hyperthermic crisis. This area should also have a designated shelf for specialized equipment boxes that will contain appropriate equipment and drugs to deal with difficult intubation (including fiberoptic endoscopy equipment, materials for transtracheal jet ventilation, and cricothyroidotomy/tracheotomy kits), malignant hyperthermia, and cardiac arrest. Equipment for the routine care and resuscitation of the neonate is listed in Chapter 9.

PROCEDURE ROOM

It would be to the advantage of the anesthesia team if a large room (minimum size, 400 square feet) were included in the design of the delivery suite. This area would allow the administration of multiple epidural anesthetics simultaneously, particularly in preparation for cesarean delivery. This procedure room should be fully stocked with the appropriate anesthesia equipment, including an anesthetic machine with appropriate monitoring equipment, intravenous fluids and administration sets, block trays, wall outlets for oxygen and suction and electric fetal monitors.

An efficient labor and delivery unit demands the services of the anesthetic care team coupled with skilled obstetric nursing care. Often, the labor and delivery nurses are the first to observe hypotension and fetal heart rate changes and should initiate appropriate therapy at once. This may include increasing the rate of intravenous fluid administration, giving oxygen by mask, placing the parturient in the lateral position, discontinuing the oxytocin infusion, correlating the monitoring of the uterine contractions and the fetal heart rate, and notifying the anesthetic care team about the problem.

TRANSITIONAL NURSERY

The labor and delivery suite should be on the same floor and physically connected to the neonatal intensive care unit and the regular nurseries by a transitional nursery. This area would contain bassinets to observe neonates with potential problems and incubators to facilitate transfer to the specialized acute care area. This area would provide acute intensive care from the moment the neonate arrives (minutes after delivery) until he or she has stabilized sufficiently to allow transfer to an acute care area. A small number of intensive care beds should be available at all times in the transitional nursery. Radiant heaters are essential since one of the major problems after delivery is the loss of temperature in the neonate. This factor alone can precipitate the continuation or recurrence of acidosis and hypoxia and lead to persistent fetal circulation.

RECOVERY AREA

A recovery room or area in the labor and delivery suite is essential in order to allow close observation of the mother for the first few hours after delivery. It should be immediately adjacent to the delivery and obstetric operating rooms. Ideally, there should be a separate nursing station for the recovery area, which should be as fully equipped as the postanesthetic and surgical recovery area. Accessibility to the adult intensive care areas is desirable (see Fig. 11-1). Minimal facilities include wall-mounted oxygen and suction outlets, direct and indirect lighting, sphygmomanometers, pulse oximeters, curtains to divide the room into individual private areas, routine and emergency drugs, cardiopulmonary resuscitation cart, and cardiac monitor with defibrillator. A large pleasant room is preferable to small cramped cubicles. Curtains will give the parturient, father, and neonate a chance to interact in a private area without diminishing the effectiveness of the nursing care by making observation difficult. The number of recovery room beds should equal one-third of the number of labor beds in a busy service.

Family-oriented obstetric care may allow postpartum recovery in the combination labor–delivery room or labor room if nursing coverage is sufficient. Recovery area personnel should be qualified to provide the intensive care that may be necessary in routine or emergency situations. Continuous teaching and monitoring by the obstetric anesthesia service is necessary to maintain a high quality standard of care.

ADMINISTRATION

The obstetric anesthesia section should have office facilities adjacent to the labor and delivery area. A conference room with teaching facilities and audiovisual equipment should be available and can be shared with the departments of obstetrics and neonatology. On-call rooms must be adjacent to the obstetric suite so that there can be an immediate response to an emergency call.

PERSONNEL

Determining Need

The requirements for anesthetic personnel in the labor and delivery area are difficult to ascertain. Coverage may range from the "on-call" situation, in which the anesthesiologist responds to the needs of the service from the surgical suite, to anesthetic personnel who are in attendance in the labor and delivery suite 24 hours a day. It would be very difficult to contrast our situation at the Brigham and Women's Hospital with any other hospital. At present, we are approaching 11,000 deliveries a year. We are an academic department of anesthesia that trains fellows and residents in obstetric anesthesia.

Anesthesia Care Team

Although the number of available anesthesiologists is increasing throughout the United States, I do not believe there are adequate numbers at this time to provide 24-hour-a-day coverage in the labor and delivery areas throughout the Level III hospitals in the United States, let alone the Level II or I hospitals. (A Level III hospital is able to handle any obstetric or neonatal problem and has the appropriate personnel available 24 hours a day; level II hospitals can offer advanced but not all encompassing perinatal care and level I hospitals offer routine obstetric and neonatal care.) Therefore, our initial premise in providing obstetric anesthesia care is the appropriate utilization of the anesthesia care team. Depending on the institution, the anesthesia care team may involve anesthesiologists only up to and including anesthesiologists and residents and/or nurse anesthetists. At the Brigham and Women's Hospital, the anesthesia care teams include staff anesthesiologists, fellows in obstetric anesthesia, residents on their obstetric anesthesia rotation, and, on occasion, certified nurse anesthetists. All types of obstetric pain relief are available, with the exception of inhalational analgesia, which has not been used in our institution in more than 25 years. We do not see any need to utilize an archaic form of pain relief while jeopardizing the mother's health if she has had parenteral sedatives and narcotics that in combination with inhaled analgesics may lead to a general anesthetic state, with the possibility of regurgitation and aspiration into the unprotected airway. Paracervical block is an excellent technique that is utilized as previously presented in Chapter 7 for gynecologic procedures; however, it has not been used on our obstetric service for pain relief in more than 15 years.

Coverage in the labor and delivery area is provided by a minimum of one staff anesthesiologist 24 hours a day, supplemented with a combination of fellows, residents, and nurse-anesthetists. Obviously, this is reasonable both for patient care and on a financial basis since we are administering anesthesia to approximately 70 percent of our total number of deliveries. (See the tables in Ch. 7 for our statistics on obstetric anesthesia for 1989–1990.)

Is it possible to provide adequate anesthesia care in the smaller units throughout the country? I believe adequate obstetric anesthesia care can be provided on an "on-call" basis in which the anesthesiologist is in reasonable proximity to the labor and delivery suite. The level of care provided should include major regional anesthesia and general endotracheal anesthesia for vaginal and cesarean delivery. Depending on the particular circumstances in each institution, this may not provide for the provision of continuous epidural anesthesia on a 24-hour-a-day basis.

A member of the anesthesia care team often must assist in the resuscitation of the neonate if a pediatrician or pediatric nurse trained in neonatal resuscitation is not available. Such expertise may not be available in many of the 5,000 hospitals in the United States that provide obstetric care. It must be kept in mind that "qualified personnel, *other* than the anesthesiologist attending the mother, should be immediately available to assume responsibility for resuscitation of the depressed neonate" (Standard VI of "Standards/Guidelines for Conduction Anesthesia in Obstetrics). It is the responsibility of the hospital overall to make sure that qualified personnel are available. The attending anesthesiologist acts as a "Good Samaritan" if he or she assists in the resuscitation since the primary responsibility is to the parturient.

When is it possible to provide continuous obstetric coverage other than in an academic institution? I believe that approximately 2,000 deliveries a year could be considered borderline for full-time coverage of an obstetric service by a designated anesthesiologist given:

1. A cesarean delivery rate of 20 percent (2,000 × 20 percent = 400 cesarean deliveries).
2. Fifty percent of the vaginal deliveries would require only parenteral medication: narcotics and/or tranquilizers and local infiltration or pudendal block (1,600 × 50 percent - 800 vaginal deliveries).
3. 2,000 − 400 = 1600 vaginal deliveries −800 requiring no major anesthetic = 800 deliveries that would require a major anesthetic (spinal or epidural).

We are discussing the administration of anesthesia to 1,200 parturients a year. An average of three to four deliveries a day requiring anesthesia provides enough work for the anesthesia care team.

Reimbursement

The one problem with the above calculation is that it does not take into account the reimbursement where these deliveries are taking place. Inherent to the above calculation is the factor that at least 50 percent of the population being served by obstetric anesthesia will completely pay their bill. This is presumptuous in many states.

Collections for obstetric anesthesia rarely exceed 60 percent of the total bill. Therefore, without a reasonable number of deliveries and reasonable compensation for anesthetic services, it is not difficult to understand why anesthesiologists are not that interested in providing obstetric anesthesia care. When the third-party payers and the government decide to provide appropriate reimbursement for services rendered, anesthesiologists will be more interested in providing their services for labor and delivery area.

However, let us assume that the anesthesia department in the particular hospital has decided to provide obstetric anesthesia care using an anesthesia care team. Using the figure of 2,000 as the minimal number of deliveries to make it financially feasible, we assume that at least 60 percent of the total number of women delivering must receive a major anesthetic in some form to even come close to providing satisfactory reimbursement. If the level of reimbursement is inadequate or the services are not adequately utilized and the hospital demands 24-hour-a-day coverage by the anesthesia care team, I believe it is the responsibility of the hospital to make up the difference so that the anesthesia department can break even financially given the compensation received for services provided. Only by putting the appropriate financial squeeze on the administration of the hospital will the administrators and physicians realize that perhaps regionalization of certain aspects of medical care may be more financially feasible in the long run. Obviously, hospitals in rural areas must provide Level I or routine obstetric services to their population. However, Level II or III units should have adequate populations to provide more sophisticated perinatal services. It is absurd for 8 out of 10 hospitals in a metropolitan area to provide obstetric anesthesia services and not perform more than 1,500 deliveries each.

Regionalization into Level II or III hospitals would provide an extremely high level of maternal–fetal–neonatal care and meet all the needs of the metropolitan area. State Departments of Public Health should help (force?) hospitals to consolidate their services and provide open staffing for more efficient delivery of perinatal health care. Hospital administrations must realize that they cannot provide all the services from "birth to death"; they must provide those services that they can most efficient. Therefore, while one hospital is the cardiac regional center, another hospital could be the perinatal center and have a sufficient number of deliveries to provide continuous obstetric, anesthetic, and neonatal intensive care services.

It took personnel interested in perinatal medicine many years to convince obstetricians that the uterus is the best transport incubator for the fetus. How many years will it take us to convince state and hospital administrators that the amount of money available for medical care is finite and that hard-nosed decisions must be made in order to provide the best possible medical care for the citizens of a particular area?

In summary, approximately 2,000 deliveries are required to make 24-hour-a-day obstetric anesthesia "in-house" relatively feasible, assuming that 60 percent of these patients receive a major anesthetic. Otherwise, obstetric anesthesia services should be on a consultative or per-case basis, which takes into account what other demands are being made on the anesthetic services of the hospital. If the hospital administration sees 24-hour-a-day obstetric anesthesia coverage as a selling point for their hospital over other hospitals with maternity services in the area and the number of deliveries do not come up to the rate mentioned, hospitals must supplement the income of the anesthesia department to come close to a "break even" basis. The anesthesia department cannot be in a deficit position for providing services. Obviously, 24 hour-a-day coverage of obstetric anesthesia services must be made economically feasible by direct or third-party payments.

One does not like to forecast the future, but it would appear that we are adequately training enough physicians in obstetric anesthesia to be comfortable with providing that service. However, with the exception of the Level III perinatal centers, anesthesia care for obstetrics remains the function of the anesthesiologist who is a "generalist"—trained to provide obstetric anesthesia on a "case-by-case" or consultative basis, primarily due to manpower and financial constraints.

REFERENCES

1. Department of Public Health, Commonwealth of Massachusetts: Regionalization of maternity and newborn care in Massachusetts, Final Report, August 1, 1974–September 30, 1976, Boston, 1977

STANDARDS FOR OBSTETRIC ANESTHESIA

JOINT STATEMENT ON THE OPTIMAL GOALS FOR ANESTHESIA CARE IN OBSTETRICS

After several attempts at creating standards or guidelines for the conduct of obstetric anesthesia by various groups and committees, this "Joint Statement on the Optimal Goals for Anesthesia Care in Obstetrics" was approved by the American Society of Anesthesiologists (ASA) House of Delegates on October 21, 1986, and by the American College of Obstetricians and Gynecologists (ACOG) Board of Directors on March 5, 1988. They are printed here in their entirety.

This joint statement from the ASA and the ACOG has been designed to address issues of concern to both specialties. Good obstetric care requires the availability of qualified personnel and equipment to administer general or regional anesthesia on either an elective or emergent basis. The extent and degree to which anesthesia services are available varies widely among hospitals. However, for any hospital providing obstetric care, certain optimal anesthesia goals should be sought. These include:

I. Availability of a person qualified to administer an appropriate anesthetic whenever necessary. For many women, regional anesthesia (spinal or epidural) will be the most appropriate anesthetic.

II. Availability of a person qualified to maintain support of vital functions in any obstetric emergency.

III. Availability of anesthesia and surgical personnel such that emergency cesarean deliveries can be started within 30 minutes of recognition of the need.

IV. Appointment of a qualified anesthesiologist to be responsible for all anesthetics administered. In many obstetric units, obstetricians or obstetrician-supervised nurse anesthetists administer the anesthetics. The administration of general or regional anesthesia requires numerous medical judgments and technical skills. Nurse anesthetists are not trained as physicians and cannot be expected to make medical decisions. Obstetricians seldom have sufficient training or experience in anesthesia to allow them to properly supervise nurse anesthetists.

Persons administering or supervising obstetric anesthesia should be qualified to manage the infrequent but occasionally life-threatening complications of major regional anesthesia such as respiratory and cardiovascular failure, toxic local anesthetic convulsions, or vomiting and aspiration. Mastering and retaining the skills and knowledge necessary to manage these complications require adequate training and frequent application.

To ensure the safest and most effective anesthesia for obstetric patients, the director of anesthesia services with the approval of the medical staff must develop and enforce written policies regarding provision of obstetric anesthesia. It is the responsibility of the director of anesthesia services and the medical staff to review each individual's qualifications and competence and to determine which agents and techniques may be used.

V. Availability of a qualified obstetrician during administration of anesthesia. Major conduction anesthesia (epidural, caudal, or spinal) and/or general anesthesia should not be administered until the patient has been examined, and the fetal status and progress of labor evaluated by a qualified physician who is readily available to supervise the labor and to deal with any obstetric complications that may arise.

VI. Availability of equipment, facilities, and support personnel equal to that provided in the surgical suite. This should include the availability of a properly equipped and staffed recovery room capable of receiving and caring for all patients recovering from major regional or general anesthesia. Birthing facilities, when used for anesthesia, must be appropriately equipped to provide safe anesthetic care during labor and delivery, or postanesthesia recovery care.

VII. Personnel other than the surgical team should be immediately available to assume responsibility for resuscitation of the depressed neonate. The surgeon and anesthesiologist are responsible for the mother and may not be able to leave her to care for the neonate even when a regional anesthetic is functioning adequately. Individuals qualified to perform neonatal resuscitation should demonstrate:
   A. Skills in rapid and accurate evaluation of the neonatal condition, including Apgar scoring.
   B. Knowledge of the pathogenesis and causes of a low Apgar score (asphyxia, drugs, hypovolemia, trauma, anomalies, and infection), as well as specific indications for resuscitation.
   C. Skills in airway management, laryngoscopy, endotracheal intubations, suctioning of airways, artificial ventilation cardiac massage, and maintenance of thermal stability.

In larger maternity units and those functioning as high-risk centers, 24-hour in-house anesthesia, obstetric, and neonatal specialists are usually necessary. Preferably, the obstetric anesthesia services should be directed by an anesthesiologist with special training or experience in obstetric anesthesia. These units will also frequently require the availability of more sophisticated monitoring equipment and specially trained nursing personnel.

A recent survey jointly sponsored by the ASA and ACOG found that many hospitals in the United States have not yet achieved the above goals. Deficiencies were most evident in smaller delivery units. Some small delivery units are necessary because of geographic considerations. Currently, 54 percent of hospitals providing obstetric care have less than 500 deliveries per year. Providing comprehensive care for obstetric patients in these small units is extremely inefficient, not cost-effective, and frequently impossible. Thus, the following recommendations would seem appropriate:

1. Whenever possible, small units should consolidate.*
2. When geographic factors require the existence of smaller units, these units should be part of a well-established perinatal regionalization system.

* Committee on Perinatal Health: Toward improving the Outcome of Pregnancy—Recommendations for the Regional Development of Maternal and Perinatal Health Services, The National Foundation-March of Dimes, New York, 1977.

The availability of the appropriate personnel to assist in the management of a variety of obstetric problems is a necessary feature of good obstetric care. The presence of a pediatrician at a high-risk cesarean delivery or an anesthesiologist at a breech delivery are examples. Frequently, these professionals spend a considerable amount of time but may eventually not be required to perform the tasks for which they are present. Reasonable compensation for these standby services is justifiable and necessary.

A variety of other mechanisms have been suggested to increase the availability and quality of anesthesia services in obstetrics. Improved hospital design to place labor and delivery suites closer to the operating room would allow for more efficient supervision of nurse anesthetists. Anesthesia equipment in the labor and delivery area must be comparable to that in the operating room.

Finally, interpersonal relations between obstetricians and anesthesiologists could be improved. Joint meetings between the two departments should be encouraged. Anesthesiologists should recognize the special needs and concerns of the obstetrician and obstetricians should recognize the anesthesiologist as a consultant in the management of pain and life-support measures. Both should recognize the need to provide high quality care for all patients.

STANDARDS FOR CONDUCTION ANESTHESIA IN OBSTETRICS

"Standards for Conduction Anesthesia in Obstetrics" (printed here in its entirety) were approved by the ASA House of Delegates on October 12, 1988.

These Standards apply to the use of major conduction anesthesia administered to the parturient during labor and delivery. These Standards may be exceeded based on the judgment of the responsible anesthesiologist. They are intended to encourage high-quality patient care, but cannot guarantee any specific patient outcome. They are subject to revision from time to time as warranted by the evolution of technology and practice.

Standard I

Major conduction anesthesia, (lumbar or caudal epidural, subarachnoid or bilateral lumbar sympathetic block) shall be initiated and maintained only in locations in which appropriate resuscitation equipment and drugs are immediately available to manage procedurally related problems (e.g., hypotension, respiratory depression, convulsions, and myocardial depression).

Resuscitation equipment shall include sources of oxygen and suction, equipment to maintain an airway and perform endotracheal intubation, and a means to provide positive-pressure ventilation. Drugs and equipment for cardiopulmonary resuscitation shall be immediately available.

Standard II

Major conduction blocks in obstetrics shall be initiated and maintained by or under the direction of a physician with appropriate privileges.

Physicians must be approved through the institutional credentialing process to administer or supervise the administration of obstetric anesthesia and must be qualified to manage procedurally related complications.

Standard III

Major conduction anesthesia should not be administered until the patient has been examined, and the fetal status and progress of labor evaluated by a qualified physician who is readily available to supervise the labor and to deal with any obstetric complications that may arise.

Standard IV

An intravenous infusion shall be established before initiation and maintained throughout the duration of major conduction block.

Standard V

A qualified individual shall monitor continually* the parturient's oxygenation, ventilation, and circulation.

Anesthetic techniques, drugs, and maternal vital signs shall be documented in the medical record.

Standard VI

Qualified personnel, other than the anesthesiologist attending the mother, should be immediately available to assume responsibility for resuscitation of the depressed neonate.

The primary responsibility of the anesthesiologist is to provide care to the mother. If the anesthesiologist is also requested to provide brief assistance in the care of the neonate, the benefit to the child must be compared to the risk of temporarily leaving the mother.

Standard VII

All patients recovering from major conduction anesthesia shall receive appropriate postanesthesia care.

1. A Postanesthesia Care Unit (PACU) shall be available to receive patients. The design, equipment, and staffing shall meet requirements of the facility's accrediting and licensing bodies.
2. When the PACU is not available, equivalent postanesthesia care shall be provided in a suitable location.

Standard VIII

A physician with appropriate privileges shall remain in the facility to manage anesthetic complications until the patient is accepted by the PACU or equivalent area.

Standard IX

There shall be a policy to assure the availability in the facility of a physician capable of managing anesthetic complications and providing cardiopulmonary resuscitation for patients in the PACU.

Subsequently, at the 1989 Annual Meeting of ASA, the House of Delegates directed the Committees on Standards and Obstetrical Anesthesia to re-examine the wording and meaning of Standard III. Several drafts of a new Standard III and, in fact of the entire document were compiled by both committees without reaching a consensus.

The House of Delegates at the 1990 ASA Annual Meeting approved a Reference Committee recommendation that the document entitled "Standards for Conduction Anesthesia in Obstetrics" be retitled "Guidelines for Conduction Anesthesia in Obstetrics," thus downgrading its force from "rules" to "guides for practice."

The Committee on Standards and Obstetrical Anesthesia will continue to develop a substitute document, "Guidelines for Regional Anesthesia in Obstetrics," and reach a consensus that will be presented to the 1991 ASA House of Delegates.

In addition, the 1990 House of Delegates voted not to require the use of pulse oximetry during the recovery of the obstetric patient in whom regional anesthesia was used for labor and vaginal delivery.

Further developments in this area will undoubtedly occur in the future. For clarification of any issue, please refer to the ASA Home Office for the latest information.

* Note that "continual" is defined as "repeated regularly and frequently in steady rapid succession," whereas "continuous" means "prolonged without any interruption at any time."

Index

Page numbers followed by f *indicate figures; page numbers followed by* t *indicate tables.*

F

I

p. 234
macrosomia

p.241 cactus